Neurobehavioral Toxicology

The Johns Hopkins Series in Environmental Toxicology

Zoltan Annau, Series Editor

Neurobehavioral Toxicology

edited by Zoltan Annau
Professor of Environmental Health Sciences
The Johns Hopkins University
School of Hygiene and Public Health

The Johns Hopkins University Press
BALTIMORE

The Johns Hopkins University Press, 701 West 40th Street, Baltimore, Maryland 21211

The paper used in this publication meets the minimum requirements of American National Standard for Information Sciences—Permanence of Paper for Printed Library Materials, ANSI Z39.48-1984.

Library of Congress Cataloging-in-Publication Data

Neurobehavioral toxicology.

(The Johns Hopkins series in environmental toxicology)
   Includes bibliographies and index.
   1. Behavioral toxicology.   2. Neurotoxic agents.   I. Annau, Zoltan, 1936–   .   II. Series.
RA1224.N49   1986   616.89′071   86-45452
ISBN 0-8018-3297-7 (alk. paper)

Contents

List of Figures   vii

List of Tables   xi

Introduction   xiii

1. Emerging Challenges to Behavioral Toxicology   1
   Bernard Weiss

Part I. Research Strategies

2. Reflexive Measures   23
   Laurence D. Fechter and John S. Young

3. Observational Methods   43
   Stata Norton

4. Assessment of Locomotor Activity   54
   Lee S. Rafales

5. Schedule-Controlled Behavior in Behavioral Toxicology   69
   Victor G. Laties and Ronald W. Wood

6. Learning and Memory Measures   94
   Diane B. Miller and David A. Eckerman

Part II. Exposure at Critical Periods of Development

7. Prenatal Exposure   153
   Zoltan Annau and Christine U. Eccles

8. Postnatal Exposure   170
   Patricia H. Ruppert

Part III. The Determination of Mechanisms of Toxicity

9. The Interactions of Behavior and Neurophysiology   193
   Robert S. Dyer

10. The Interactions of Behavior and Neurochemistry   214
Diane L. DeHaven and Richard B. Mailman

11. The Use of Pharmacological Challenges   244
Thomas J. Walsh and Hugh A. Tilson

12. Lesion Analysis   268
Gary L. Wenk and David S. Olton

Part IV. The Exposure of Humans to Neurotoxic Chemicals

13. Epidemiological Studies   279
Herbert L. Needleman

14. Field Testing   288
Christina M. Gullion and David A. Eckerman

15. Workplace Exposures   331
W. Kent Anger

16. Human Experimental Studies   348
Robert B. Dick and Barry L. Johnson

Part V. Regulatory and Statistical Considerations

17. Behavior as a Regulatory Endpoint   391
William F. Sette and Tina E. Levine

18. Design and Analytical Methods   404
Keith E. Muller

19. Some General Problems of Neurobehavioral Toxicology   424
Peter B. Dews

List of Contributors   435

Index   437

Figures

1.1. Schematic drawing of a system designed to present vibratory stimuli   5

1.2. The response to acrylamide treatment of a trained monkey   6

1.3. Diagram of a statistical model used to analyze response to acrylamide   7

1.4. Response rates of six rats each from one control and three different treatment groups on a fixed-interval 1-minute schedule of food reinforcement   9

1.5. Plots of linear versus quadratic coefficients for cubic fits to growth curves representing each of the six rats in each treatment group   10

1.6. The response of one subject to food-color challenge in the form of two cookies daily   13

1.7. Statistical problems of samples containing susceptible subgroups   14

1.8. Plot of the relationships between the number of additives consumed, the total burden as a percentage of ADI, and commonality of effect   15

1.9. Monte Carlo simulation based on drawing 15 randomly selected subjects from the population shown in fig. 1.7, before and after challenge   15

1.10. Plot of the multiplicative relationships among 100 additives, each consumed at 10 percent of the individual ADI   18

2.1. Stimulus conditions and the analogue response of one subject on a baseline trial and a prestimulus trial   26

2.2. Baseline startle reflex amplitudes before, during, and after exposure to TET or paired water treatment   36

2.3. Startle reflex inhibition to pure tones before treatment and during the first week of exposure to TET or paired water treatment   37

2.4. Startle reflex inhibition to pure tones before treatment and during the third week of exposure to TET or paired water treatment   37

5.1. Cumulative records of four rats working on a fixed-ratio 1 schedule of reinforcement   71

5.2. Cumulative records of one control and one rat exposed to 50 ppm lead acetate on a fixed-interval 30-second schedule of reinforcement   72

5.3. Cumulative records of one rat's performance on a fixed-interval 5-minute schedule of reinforcement during exposure to various levels of ozone   73

5.4. The 200 response runs in sequence from each of three experimental sessions for a single pigeon   74

5.5. Run-length histograms from selected 200-run sessions of two pigeons   75

5.6. Changes induced in run-length distributions by the addition of a discriminative stimulus   76

5.7. Sample cumulative records of a pigeon's performance on the multiple fixed-interval 15-minute, fixed-ratio 60 schedule of reinforcement   78

5.8. Fixed-ratio performance before, during, and after exposure to mercury vapor   79

5.9. Fixed-interval performance before, during, and after exposure to mercury vapor   80

5.10. Cumulative records of performance on the multiple fixed-interval 10-minute, fixed-ratio 50 schedule of reinforcement   81

5.11. Cumulative records of performance on the multiple FCN 8, FCN-S^D 8 schedule of reinforcement   83

5.12. Schematic drawing of the exposure chamber used to study irritant substances   85

5.13. The percentage of ammonia deliveries terminated by mice as a function of concentration   86

5.14. The effects of d-amphetamine on both heat- and food-reinforced behaviors of a single rat   87

5.15. Cumulative records showing the effects of d-amphetamine on both heat- and food-reinforced behaviors of a single rat   88

6.1. Long-lasting and temporary habituation of the whole-body acoustic startle response to a loud tone in the rat   99

6.2. The ability of phencyclidine to interfere with the habituation of the whole-body startle response   100

6.3. The effect of increasing doses of systemic aluminum lactate on classical conditioning of the nictitating membrane extension of the rabbit   102

6.4. The effect of lesions of the hippocampus on discrimination and discrimination-reversal conditioning of the nictitating membrane extension of the rabbit   103

6.5. The development of suppression of bar pressing in the presence of a tone associated with unavoidable shock, a conditioned emotional response   107

6.6. The effect of neurotoxicant-induced lesions of the ventromedial area of the globus pallidus or of the nucleus basalis magnocellularis on passive avoidance in the male rat   108

6.7. The use of a two-way conditioned avoidance paradigm to assess learning after exposure to chloramphenicol during development   110

6.8. The use of a two-way conditioned avoidance paradigm to assess learning and memory after prenatal exposure to carbon monoxide   110

6.9. The use of a multisensory conditioned pole-climb avoidance task to detect a hearing impairment induced by exposure to toluene in male weanling rats   111

6.10. The use of schedule-controlled behavior to illustrate that the degree to which a learned behavior is controlled by environmental stimuli can determine the effect of a toxicant on that behavior   112

6.11. The nearly equivalent functions obtained by the rat, the rhesus monkey, and the human in memory-scanning tasks based on the Sternberg paradigm   119

6.12. The effect of increasing the delay intervals of a delayed response on accuracy as a function of age   120

6.13. The effects of neonatal lead treatment on memory, as assessed by a delayed spatial-alternation procedure   121

6.14. The effect of age and delays between choices on performance in the radial arm maze   125

6.15. The use of a radial-arm-maze task to assess reference memory and working memory after damage to the septal area of the brain   127

6.16. The effect of damage to the hippocampus on serial-position curves in the human and the rat   128

6.17. Partial dissociation of the effect of trimethyltin on motor activity from its effect on accuracy in a radial-arm-maze memory task   130

6.18. The use of an open-field water maze to determine the effect of exposure to a steroid during development on learning spatial discrimination   131

6.19. The use of the Hamilton Search task to determine the effect of postnatal lead exposure on spatial memory in the rhesus monkey   132

6.20. The use of delayed nonmatch to sample to evaluate memory in monkeys with defined brain damage induced by thiamine deficiency   133

7.1. Rates of cell proliferation in various regions of the mouse brain during gestation and during early neonatal life   154

7.2. Time course of plasma corticosterone levels in pregnant rats on the 19th day of gestation as a function of diet   163

8.1. The brain growth spurts of seven mammalian species, expressed as first-order velocity curves of the increase in weight with age   171

8.2. Figure-eight maze activity for control and TET-exposed rats   181

8.3. Extinction scores for monomethyltin- and trimethyltin-exposed groups   183

9.1. A prototype flash-evoked potential recorded from a rat   195

9.2. Some possible patterns of evoked potential amplitude and latency changes   198

9.3. The relationship between treatment and magnitude of latency change in successive flash-evoked potential peaks   199

10.1. Model of a synapse, demonstrating many of the biochemical loci where effects of neurotoxicants have been studied   215

11.1. The effect of repeated exposure to PBBs on the responsiveness of rats to d-amphetamine and phenobarbital   249

11.2. The effect of neonatal benzene exposure on the motor-stimulant effect of d-amphetamine assessed in adulthood   251

11.3. The effect of apomorphine alone or in combination with acrylamide on VI 15-second responding   254

11.4. The effect of apomorphine on spontaneous motor activity of rats exposed to chlordecone during gestation and for the first 12 days of lactation   255

11.5. The effect of trihexyphenidyl or BC-105 on chlordecone-induced tremor   256

11.6. The effect of naloxone and chlordiazepoxide on triethyl lead–induced antinociception   261

13.1. The proportion of negative teachers' ratings on an 11-item forced-choice scale in relation to the dentine lead level   284

17.1. The decision making involved in promulgating a test rule under TSCA   395

18.1. The typical leapfrog study sequence   413

Tables

1.1. Response of monkey 948 to acrylamide treatment   7

1.2. Number of subjects required to demonstrate statistically reliable differences for various combinations of response amplitude and percentage of responders in the sample   13

6.1. Single-trial conditioning and retention of taste aversion to almond nuts in wild Japanese monkeys   105

6.2. Learned taste aversions in children receiving cancer chemotherapy   106

6.3. The use of the eight-arm radial maze and its placement in novel environments to investigate the role of opiate systems in memory   126

7.1. Mean number of pups of mice treated with methylmercury hydroxide on day 8 of gestation surviving per litter 24 hours after birth   156

7.2. Postnatal behavior measurements of exposure to 5-azacytedene during gestation in mice   159

7.3. Experimental design of fostering experiments to control for maternal treatments and postnatal conditions   164

8.1. The effect of perinatal administration of androgens to females on the development of sexually dimorphic traits   176

8.2. A comparison of the effects of hippocampal dysfunction and postnatal lead exposure in several testing situations   179

10.1. Some neurochemical strategies used to assess neuronal function in the central nervous system   216

10.2. Some neurotransmitter receptors and ligands proposed for their study.   219

11.1. Pharmacological agents that selectively interact with specific neurotransmitter systems   247

13.1. Covariates that differed between high and low lead samples at $p \leq 0.1$ and that were controlled in preanalysis   283

13.2. Outcomes that differed between high- and low-lead groups at p ≤ 0.05   283

13.3. Logistic models predicting malformations   285

13.4. The covariate-adjusted relative risk of malformation at selected blood lead levels   286

14.1. Batteries of neurobehavioral tests used in representative studies in Europe and Australia   292

14.2. Batteries of neurobehavioral tests used in representative studies in the United States   295

14.3. Some developing batteries for field testing for toxicity   299

14.4. Carroll's elementary cognitive tasks and cognitive factors   300

14.5. Test batteries used in example drug evaluations   302

14.6. Batteries for testing unusual work environments   304

15.1. Neurotoxic chemicals with estimated exposure populations over 1 million   332

15.2. Chemical groupings in which 10 or more neurotoxic chemicals are found   333

15.3. SIC classifications and industries in which neurotoxic chemicals are found   334

15.4. Neurobehavioral effects reported following chemical exposures for 25 or more chemicals   335

16.1. Criteria for human exposure studies   352

17.1. Illustrative definitions of hazards of concern and legal language for regulating exposure   393

18.1. Decision outcomes in hypothesis testing   406

18.2. Study performance ratings   411

Introduction

In 1975 the first conference devoted to behavioral toxicology was held at the University of Rochester. The proceedings of this conference were published as a book, entitled *Behavioral Toxicology,* and marked the recognition of a new branch of toxicology. Like most other developing scientific fields, behavioral toxicology was a hybrid; it rested on the behavioral sciences as well as on toxicology for its foundations, and it broadened as it moved into areas of neurochemistry, neuropathology, and other neuroscience-related disciplines. This growing association between the behavioral and neural sciences eventually led to the acknowledgment that the term *neurobehavioral toxicology* described this field more appropriately.

It is not unusual for an emerging discipline to start from a narrow view and then diverge; this has certainly happened to neurobehavioral toxicology. This is a healthy development, for one of the most obvious conclusions to emerge from the environmental crisis of the 1970s is that toxic chemicals can have extraordinarily complex effects on biological systems. Because of the complexities of the biological, ecological, and economic issues, our attempts to protect human populations from toxic chemicals have resulted in the most intricate political-scientific processes of our times.

These complexities can be seen here in the chapters devoted to the study of neurotoxic chemicals in human populations, both in the laboratory and in the field. While it has always been apparent that one end product of neurobehavioral toxicology must be the protection of humans from neurotoxic chemicals, human studies have lagged behind studies addressing animal toxicology, since the field developed from research based on animal models. This lag has occurred not only because of ethical limitations on exposing human subjects to poisonous materials but also because of the lack of proper tools for evaluating the behavior of people exposed to toxic chemicals. Most of the available techniques, such as neurological examinations or psychological testing, have not proven to be particularly useful in detecting low-level exposures. A great deal of the creative research going on in this field, especially in attempts to develop relatively portable testing devices that can measure a broad spectrum of chemical effects, is described in this book. The development of these objective measuring devices will someday bring the measurements made on animals into closer correspondence with those made on humans.

This book is divided into four major areas of neurobehavioral toxicology. Parts

I, II, and III are devoted primarily to animal studies. Part I addresses research strategies derived from the behavioral sciences and deals with the methodologies that have been employed most successfully in evaluating the behavioral effects of neurotoxic chemicals. Part II examines the effect of exposure to neurotoxic chemicals during critical periods in the development of the nervous system. Some of these chemicals, such as methylmercury, pose a far greater health hazard to the fetus than to the adult, while other chemicals, such as lead, seem to pose the greatest hazard during the neonatal period. Part III treats the mechanisms of toxicity at the neurobehavioral level and the use of noninvasive pharmacological probes to determine the underlying neurobiological alterations.

Part IV deals with epidemiological and experimental approaches to human neurobehavioral toxicity. The need for developing devices that can be used in the field and the concomitant problems of validity and reliability are also described. The final part, part V, discusses the statistical needs of this area of research as well as the impact of this new field on governmental regulations.

The first and last chapters of the book are by two of the pioneers in this field, Bernard Weiss and Peter Dews. They recognized the need for using behavioral methods to identify and describe the effects of neurotoxic chemicals before the environmental threat of these chemicals was widely accepted. Much of what is in this book can be viewed as the fruit of their labors.

It is the hope of every science to reach the stage where it becomes predictive. Many of the disciplines that are emerging as major scientific fields have not yet reached this stage; nevertheless, they have made substantial contributions to human health. This book represents the first attempt to gather a large portion of the existing knowledge base in neurobehavioral toxicology and thereby to permit a critical evaluation of this new field. It is intended, not as an exhaustive survey of the literature, but as an evaluation of the most important issues and highlights of the past few decades and a vision of the future. It is hoped that this book will be helpful not only to the present generation of neurobehavioral toxicologists but also to the students on whose shoulders the burdens of future environmental challenges rest.

Neurobehavioral Toxicology

Bernard Weiss

Emerging Challenges to Behavioral Toxicology

Behavior won its status in contemporary toxicology with two features that captured significant public concerns. One stemmed from the recognition that behavioral abnormalities express overtly a toxic state of the nervous system and, moreover, are disabling in themselves. The second stemmed from the recognition that a vast body of techniques already had been created by behavioral scientists and could be applied to measure and predict behavioral toxicity. The public issues that stimulated the acceptance of behavioral toxicology are exemplified by the debate over how to define a safe body burden of lead in children when the criterion of safety is based on psychological tests and observations; by the anxieties aroused by chemical wastes and fears about their impact on nervous-system function; by clinical entities such as the organic solvent syndrome; by the evidence implicating certain food additives in behavioral difficulties such as attention-deficit disorder.

Behavioral toxicology burgeoned so quickly that we found ourselves moving on several different fronts simultaneously. Regulatory pressures spurred efforts to develop tests for hazard prediction. Community groups promoted investigations of presumed environmental contaminants. Some neurotoxicants were adopted as models of disease or as tools for neuroscience research. Despite the distractions, all of this ferment yielded an impressive degree of progress. In this chapter, I propose to offer one view of where such progress has taken us and to speculate about the directions in which we may soon be pressed.

The accomplishments of behavioral toxicology fill this book: a technology, a mass of empirical data, a durably entrenched discipline. The next steps offer an equal, if not greater challenge. Whether or not we believe ourselves equipped to answer it, the inevitable question will arise: What are the implications for health and for governance of the environment? A substantial literature testifies to our ability to identify hazardous chemicals, that is, to confirm the actions of agents already demonstrated or suspected to be neurotoxic. Of course, we have extended these findings; in some instances we have even revealed unexpected facets of toxicity and clues to mechanisms.

Were behavioral toxicity perceived as a health threat on the scale of cancer, we would have been showered with congratulations, even if, to demonstrate effects, we had to amplify exposure levels to values hundreds of times those endured by human populations. There is no such congruence with cancer, however. Behavioral toxicity and even neurotoxicity are viewed as dangers of a different sort and will be regulated as graduated expressions of toxicity rather than as catastrophes. This dichotomy in perception evokes a dichotomy in demand. Risk-analysis models for cancer typically assume that if a substance is carcinogenic at high doses, it poses a cancer threat at much lower doses. Although the models vary as to how they extrapolate to risks, say, of 1 in 100,000, they are more similar than different in their approach.

Behavioral toxicologists will be asked to render a different kind of judgment, one that embodies risk assessment to another context. We may be asked, for example, to assign probabilities to the decline of intelligence test performance in children carrying lead body burdens equal to the current Center for Disease Control (CDC) standard of 25 µg/dl. Or what is more likely, we may be asked to assign and defend specified safety factors. We also may be asked to help identify hypersusceptible populations, to evaluate claims of incipient toxicity, to deal with problems of multiple exposures, to recommend and gauge possible therapies, to appraise the role of environmental poisons in degenerative neurological diseases. Such issues force us more visibly into the public arena, where, if we decline an immediate answer, we should be prepared both to defend our timidity and to yield the power of decision to stewards lacking our own intimacy with the science.

The Issues

Defining Safety

Dose-response (or dose-effect) functions are the beginnings of mechanistic analysis in pharmacology and toxicology and the basis of regulatory standards. Some standards embody safety margins designed to protect most members of a target population. The process by which these standards and margins are calculated usually includes estimates of the following values:

- NOEL: no observed effect level. The highest exposure level at which no detectable effects appear.
- NOAEL: no observed adverse effect level. The exposure level at which biological effects are detectable but are deemed not to be harmful; equivalent to a LOEL.
- LOEL: lowest observed effect level.
- LOAEL: lowest observed adverse effect level. The lowest exposure level producing significant toxicity.
- FEL: frank effect level. The lowest level producing clearly damaging consequences.

These values are defined with some ambiguity, because the dose or exposure levels to which they refer depend wholly on the precision with which effects are determined. These, in turn, depend on the technical details of the appropriate measures and, with conventional statistical assessment, on the size of the exposed and control samples.

How prepared is behavioral toxicology to blend its methods and findings with these criteria? A survey of papers published in one of the major publication outlets for behavioral toxicology research (*Neurobehavioral Toxicology and Teratology* 5 [1983]) indicates that it is quite unprepared. Most of the papers were still at the stage of hazard identification, and many were aimed at offering or refining variations of specific methods. Almost none would be useful for helping to estimate, say, NOAELs. This lack of adaptable data obstructs the integration of neurobehavioral observations into safety evaluation.

The process by which toxicological data evolve into standards may be ordered into three stages. The first is hazard identification, during which we might show that the agent being tested evinces behavioral toxicity. Many of the techniques described in the literature and in common use may be used to do so. The second is hazard evaluation, during which more specific information is gathered about the locus of toxicity. For behavioral toxicity, it might mean a profile of results from a screening battery of the type described by Tilson, Mitchell, and Cabe (1979). The final step is risk estimation, which depends inherently upon the dose-response or dose-effect function, especially that portion of it extending into the low dose range.

If behavioral toxicology is to earn a place in the process of standard derivation, it needs to demonstrate its ability to contribute to all three stages. Consider how neurobehavioral observations are likely to be incorporated into hazard evaluation. Given the expense and irrationality of conducting separate studies for cancer, renal toxicity, behavioral toxicity, and other specified endpoints, behavioral data are likely to emerge as part of a comprehensive toxicity assessment. Behavior might be one element in a two-year feeding study with rodents. Histopathology, reproductive efficiency, and body weight gain would be some of the other criteria. What amplification of such information is afforded by behavioral data? If a two-year feeding study of a proposed food additive showed retardation of body weight gain as the effect corresponding to the NOAEL, the typical safety factor of 100 would be applied to that dose level. From that standpoint, the other measures could be considered superfluous (except for cancer, because of its special regulatory status). By this criterion, a discouraging proportion of the neurobehavioral toxicology literature would be considered superfluous. Michaelson (1980) criticized the lead literature on this basis, pointing out that experimental regimens inducing marked absolute or relative weight loss exert profound effects on both neurochemistry and behavior.

Much of the behavioral toxicity literature lies beyond these issues because of how it uses statistics. A typical statistical approach would be, say, analyses of variance. Its aim would be to show that at an arbitrary time after the administration of an agent a behavioral endpoint reflects a significant change. Such an approach is valid if the experimenter's goal is simply to demonstrate an effect given arbitrary choices of dose, behavioral parameters, and time after treatment. It is a less useful source of data for proceeding to the later stages of toxicologic risk assessment, during which questions of progression, reversibility, exposure duration, and toxicokinetics are likely to arise.

The predominant issues facing behavioral toxicology in future years stem from the twin challenges of predictability and interpretation. As with other aspects of toxicology, the challenges will be framed in terms of human health. Whether we like it or not, our efforts will be viewed from the perspective of rubrics such as NOAELs. The implications of these views deserve discussion.

Detection of Incipient Toxicity

Some of our supporters in the toxicological and environmental health sciences welcomed our participation because they saw our techniques as keys to the early detection of toxicity. The practical contribution of such an ability in the workplace is obvious. The consequences of excessive exposure of chlordecone (Kepone) in workers examined during the investigation of the Hopewell, Virginia, episode were found to be: nervousness, tremor, ataxia, loss of weight, skin rash, sterility, abnormal liver function, hepatomegaly, opsoclonus, joint pain, and pleuritic pain (Cannon et al. 1978). The earliest indicator of toxicity was the complaint of nervousness. Psychological manifestations are also prominent during the incipient stages of lead, mercury, and manganese poisoning (Weiss 1983).

During the past decade, organic solvents have been investigated extensively for such nonspecific psychological effects. This research stimulated the formulation of organic solvent syndrome (OSS), which now is recognized in Scandinavia as a consequence of exposure and which provides eligibility for compensation benefits. The pattern of complaints associated with the syndrome is hardly distinguishable from that associated with exposure to heavy metals. It includes excessive fatigue, lack of initiative, inability to concentrate, headache, emotional instability, dizziness, and sexual dysfunction (Gregersen et al. 1984). Quantitative psychological testing, on the whole, tends to confirm these complaints—that is, it reveals depressed functioning—but there are discrepancies among studies, some arising from sharp differences in how a particular function is assessed.

The definition and boundaries of the OSS are certain to shift in the future as more data accumulate and as earlier claims are scrutinized with greater care. It probably will remain as an entity, however, and in the United States, it probably will reach the courts more and more frequently in lawsuits. An illuminating exercise is to imagine how well our discipline could fill the role of an expert witness in such a proceeding. How effectively could we respond to the question, What criteria would you use to identify a person with OSS, and how unique to solvents are these criteria? These aspects of behavioral toxicology are quite vulnerable to such questions, of course, because the assessment of human behavior is so complicated and variable. But consider a somewhat more benign setting, such as a hearing to decide whether a new solvent should be marketed with no data beyond the conventional assays of serious health effects in rodents. Should acute behavioral assessments be performed? Since volatile solvents are effective anesthetics, what else would be learned besides, perhaps, some index of relative potency? The more serious questions emerge from extended exposures: Is any special protection necessary? Are there subtle cumulative effects? Does tolerance develop? Are toxic effects reversible? Which measure or measures should be adopted for monitoring toxicity in the workplace? Do chronic toxic effects develop without accompanying histopathology at lower levels of exposure? Such questions press beyond the conventional modes of current research in behavioral toxicology, not so much in technology, but in the broader issue of methodology. Is what we have been seeking to learn, and the approaches we have chosen for this purpose, adequate for these issues?

One way in which we have limited ourselves has been our emphasis on traditional group designs and their accompanying statistical methods. Such designs typically are incompatible with the aim of tracing the progression of toxicity, because a progression is visible only in an individual organism. A special kind of information can be extracted from investigations in which single subjects, rather than groups, become the experimental unit. Maurissen, Weiss, and Davis (1983) adopted such a strategy in an experiment designed to trace the somatosensory

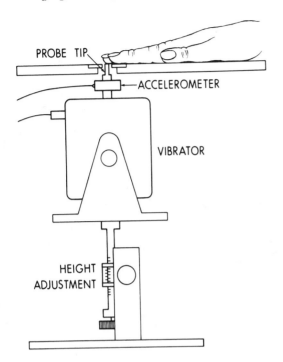

PROBE TIP

ACCELEROMETER

VIBRATOR

HEIGHT
ADJUSTMENT

Fig. 1.1 Schematic drawing of a system designed to present vibratory stimuli. The accelerometer provides a signal for monitoring frequency and amplitude. (*Source:* Maurissen, Weiss, and Davis 1983. Reprinted by permission of the publisher.)

impairment induced by acrylamide. Although exposure to this chemical, which serves as a prototype for agents inducing distal axonopathies, elicits complaints of paresthesias and hypesthesias, most of the experimental work has centered on motor deficits in rodents. Maurissen, Weiss, and Davis turned to primates (*Macaca nemestrina*) as experimental subjects because of the close correspondence between humans and macaques in somatosensory function and its nervous-system substrate. The monkeys were trained to discriminate vibratory stimuli applied to a finger. To ensure proper contact with the vibrating rod, the monkey's paw was restrained in a closely fitting plastic mold. The amplitude and frequency of vibration were controlled by the computer that governed the progress of the experimental session. (A diagram of the system appears in fig. 1.1.) Since the aim of the study was to trace the development of impairment, each experimental session was designed to provide a threshold estimate by adjusting vibration amplitude in accordance with discriminative performance. Correct detections lowered the amplitude of the next stimulus; incorrect responses raised the succeeding amplitude.

An extensive series of earlier observations devoted to the basic psychophysics of vibration in the monkey (Maurissen and Weiss 1980) had confirmed the marked differences in sensitivity to vibratory stimuli of different frequencies. On this basis, two frequencies were chosen for the acrylamide investigation: one low frequency (40 Hz) and one high frequency (150 Hz). To confirm that deficits in vibratory sensitivity would be specific to that somatosensory modality, the same monkeys were trained to discriminate electrical stimuli applied to the same finger in an equivalent system. Figure 1.2 traces the progression of impairment in one of the four treated monkeys. In addition to vibratory and electrical sensitivity data, the figure shows body weight, clinical observations, and the results of a simple visuo-

Bernard Weiss

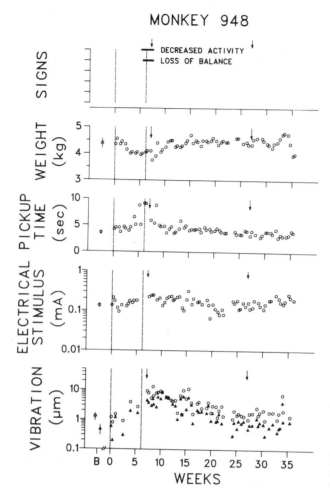

MONKEY 948

Fig. 1.2 The response to acrylamide treatment (10 mg/kg five times weekly) of a trained monkey. B = baseline (predosing). Data enclosed by vertical lines represent the period of dosing. Vibration amplitude thresholds, given in micrometers, were measured at 40 Hz (open circles) and 150 Hz (closed triangles). (*Source:* From Maurissen, Weiss, and Davis 1983. Reprinted by permission of the publisher.)

motor test in which the time taken to retrieve marshmallows from a grid was recorded. Acrylamide dosing occurred during the period defined by the vertical lines. The dose was 10 mg/kg, administered in apple juice every weekday. Dosing ceased when clinical signs became apparent. Vibration thresholds rose gradually during the course of dosing and fell slowly once dosing ended. Note that the ordinate is a logarithmic scale. Electrical sensitivity remained stable, which, along with the lack of other changes in performance (such as reaction time), indicated that loss of vibratory sensitivity was a specific effect of acrylamide treatment. Pickup test performance and body weight loss were visible toward the end of the dosing period and recovered quickly with the end of dosing.

To quantify such data requires an approach that extracts the time course information from the observations. A nonlinear regression model, charted in figure 1.3, provided this information. The model is described by six parameters: predosing baseline, latency to effect, rate of rise in threshold, latency to fall, rate of fall, and final baseline. The values computed on the basis of this model appear in table 1.1. Together with figure 1.3, table 1.1 tells us most of what we would need to know to judge whether vibration testing could serve as a noninvasive method for assessing

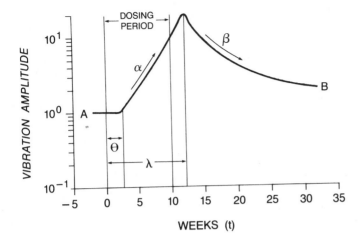

Fig. 1.3 Diagram of a statistical model (nonlinear regression) used to analyze response to acrylamide. A = predosing baseline; Θ = latency to beginning of response; α = constant representing rate (exponential) of rise of response; λ = latency, from t = 0, to peak effect; β = constant representing rate of decay of response; B = postdosing baseline.
_____Table 1.1 contains the calculated values of these six parameters, the coefficient of variation, R^2, and the results of testing the hypotheses that Θ = O and A = B. Indexes of variability are standard deviation.
(*Source:* Maurissen, Weiss, and Davis 1983. Reprinted by permission of the publisher.)

Table 1.1 Response of monkey 948 to acrylamide treatment

Parameter	Vibration (40 Hz)	Vibration (150 Hz)	Pickup	Weight
α	0.053 ± 0.013	0.053 ± 0.008	0.191 ± 0.034	−0.017 ± 0.003
β	0.125 ± 0.045	0.122 ± 0.049	0.377 ± 0.078	0.450 ± 0.230
λ	8.72 ± 1.58	10.31 ± 0.164	6.33 ± 0.72	7.43 ± 0.72
A	1.23 ± 0.04	0.45 ± 0.06	3.81 ± 0.22	4.39 ± 0.04
B	1.48 ± 0.09	0.59 ± 0.13	3.77 ± 0.13	4.46 ± 0.03
Θ	1.90 ± 1.34	0.06[a]	2.00 ± 0.43	0.43[a]
R^2 (%)	69.11	72.61	68.92	49.45
Hypothesis: Θ = 0[b]				
F test	1.33	0.0	3.97	1.27
p value	NS	NS	0.05	NS
Hypothesis: A = B[c]				
F test	0.38	0.63	0.02	1.73
p test	NS	NS	NS	NS
df	70	69	70	73

Source: Maurissen, Weiss, and Davis 1983. Reprinted by permission of the publisher.
[a]The value could not be estimated reliably because the parameter values were too close to the boundary (t = 0).
[b]Tests the hypothesis that the latency to the acrylamide effect was zero.
[c]Tests the hypothesis that the predosing baseline equaled the postdosing baseline.

incipient toxicity in exposed workers. The experiment also points to the possible morphological correlates—probably damage to the Pacinian corpuscles, the skin's acceleration receptors—because electrical sensitivity remained intact. Although the technical and procedural demands of such an experiment far exceed those of the typical investigation of neurotoxicity in rodents, only six monkeys were required to validate the technique as an index of toxicity in humans.

The issue of reversibility permeates toxicology's relationships with regulation because hazard is defined partly by permanence. Perhaps the main reason that carcinogenesis dominates risk evaluation, apart from the public's dread of cancer, is the prevailing view that the process is inexorable. As demonstrated by the experiment above, reversibility is most clearly gauged by tracking the course of performance in the individual subject. The counterpart, irreversibility, may also be difficult to judge without precisely appraising the history of individuals. Another revealing example comes from the acrylamide literature. Merigan, Barkdoll, and Maurissen (1982) trained monkeys (*Macaca nemestrina*) to perform a complex series of visual discriminations, from which they derived measures of both temporal and spatial contrast sensitivity. The animals faced a display of two oscilloscopes. To determine temporal contrast sensitivity, one of the oscilloscopes was flickered at a frequency determined by the computer program that controlled the experiment; the animal's task was to respond on a key that corresponded to the oscilloscope (randomly selected) on which the flicker appeared. Spatial contrast sensitivity was determined by programming a grating pattern of alternate light and dark strips of varying widths (i.e., varying spatial frequencies) on one of the oscilloscopes and requiring the monkey to make the corresponding key selection. Averaged visual evoked potentials also were recorded and processed, and visuomotor performance was monitored by the marshmallow-pickup test described earlier.

Acrylamide dosing led to toxic manifestations in all measures. After dosing ceased, all but one monkey recovered. Visual acuity (high contrast, high spatial frequency) remained impaired. The degree of impairment, however, was so slight that it surely would have gone undetected without the precisely determined pre-treatment baseline. It also would have gone undetected by an exposed worker and even by a thorough ophthalmological examination. It is not the kind of effect that the typical experimental design, relying on group contrasts, is equipped to distinguish. And yet, it is exactly the kind of effect that is more significant for human exposures than the motor deficits reported in the bulk of the acrylamide literature based on rodents.

Rodents are not inherently unsuitable as subjects for guides to human effects. It is simply that their relatively low cost and ease of maintenance make it tempting to substitute large samples for experimental depth or precision. But large samples only make it statistically legitimate to generalize to rat populations—hardly the reason for undertaking most of our research. Extrapolating to humans requires logical congruence at least as much as superficial statistical confidence. Consider a series of studies on the susceptibility of young rats to lead toxicity.

The prevailing view of the relation between developmental stage and sensitivity to lead is that the neonatal period, at least in rats, is the period of maximum susceptibility and that, once they are beyond weaning, their sensitivity falls sharply. This tenet was challenged by Cory-Slechta and Thompson (1979). In an experiment that initiated exposure only after weaning, they found that rates of schedule-

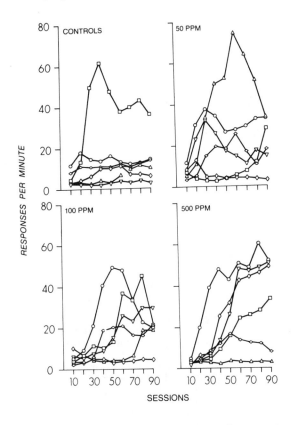

Fig. 1.4 Response rates of six rats each from one control and three different treatment groups (0, 50, 100, and 500 ppm lead acetate in drinking water) on a fixed-interval 1-minute schedule of food reinforcement.
(*Source:* Cory-Slechta, Weiss, and Cox 1983. Reprinted by permission of the publisher.)

controlled responding increased progressively during dosing with low to moderate lead concentrations in drinking water. Subsequent experiments, which incorporated additional dietary controls, assays of blood lead levels, and more precise data recording, supported and amplified the original findings (Cory-Slechta, Weiss, and Cox 1983). At 21 days of age the rats began to consume drinking-water concentrations of 0, 50, 100, or 1,000 ppm lead acetate. They were fed the American Institute of Nutrition rodent diet to avoid the problems generated by the typical commercial diet, which is grossly enhanced in mineral content (Michaelson 1980). At 55 days of age they began operant training in experimental chambers equipped with levers and pellet feeders, and they were shortly shifted to a fixed-interval, 1-minute (FI 1) schedule of food presentation.

Figure 1.4 traces the progress of this experiment over the first 90 1-hour sessions (150 days). The controls, except for one deviant animal, responded throughout at relatively low overall response rates. The group of rats exposed to 50 ppm lead acetate generally exhibited a rise in rates early in the study followed by a gradual decline. At 100 ppm and especially at 500 ppm, the rise was delayed but greater in magnitude. Capturing these features of the experiment in a quantitative analysis required something more than the usual analysis of variance, because the essence of the effect is the progression through time and the proportion of rats in each dose group displaying such a pattern. For this reason, we turned to growth curves, in the form of polynomials, to quantify the performance history. Each rat's data were fit by a three-term polynomial, providing linear, quadratic, and cubic

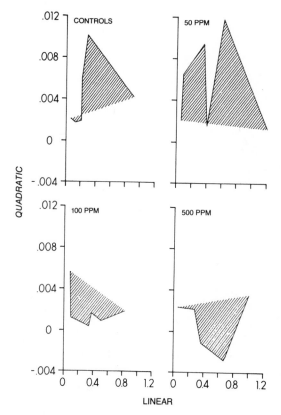

Fig. 1.5 Plots of linear versus quadratic coefficients for cubic fits to growth curves representing each of the six rats in each treatment group (cf. fig. 1.4). The quadratic coefficients significantly differentiated the two higher-dose groups from the controls.
(*Source:* Maurissen, Weiss, and Davis 1983. Reprinted by permission of the publisher.)

coefficients. A plot of the linear against the cubic coefficients is shown in figure 1.5 and indicates the difference between the two higher-dose groups and the control and 50 ppm groups. A randomization test (Edgington 1980) confirmed that the linear-coefficient values significantly separated the groups. One important outcome of this study was the finding that these performance differences occurred at blood concentrations considered to represent only a moderate elevation in humans. A subsequent experiment, by the same authors and relying on the same analytical approach, has now demonstrated effects at exposure levels of 25 ppm and accompanying blood levels of 15–20 µg/dl. Surveys of U.S. children find that half exhibit levels in that range. Given that the steepest rise in children's lead body burden occurs beyond infancy and given the presumed insensitivity of the rat to lead toxicity, these findings, in a model much more analogous to human conditions than the neonatal rodent, entail far wider implications, again, than the typical high-dose rodent study. This is especially so if the bases for prescribing safety margins are taken seriously.

These three examples illustrate behavior's most distinctive virtue as a toxicologic endpoint—its ability to track the course of a toxic process rather than to define just a single or narrow slice of time. This ability enhances behavior's contribution to toxicology because it more directly reflects those values, such as NOAELs, that link toxicology to risk estimation. The alternative—group designs and analyses—almost invariably engenders the kinds of debates that swirl about cancer risk assessment, namely, how legitimate it is to construct risk models for low-dose exposures on the basis of extremely high-dose levels. Dosing regimens common in the neurotoxicity literature could easily produce the kinds of artifacts that some investigators believe distort such extrapolation. For example, high doses of halogenated hydrocarbons in rodents could disrupt the usual metabolic pathways leading to detoxification and, instead, induce the production of toxic metabolites and misleading extrapolations. High doses can also be deceptive because damage occurs at so many sites that any specificity is buried. Much of the literature on metal toxicity suffers from this problem; a haste to achieve results may seriously deform toxicokinetic processes. Methylmercury research illustrates what may occur. Finocchio et al. (1980) administered methylmercury to monkeys at various dose levels. At the lower doses, blood levels reached a stable, asymptotic value reflecting the magnitude of the daily dose. At the highest dose level, however, the kinetics changed: blood concentration continued to rise, and death quickly ensued. The blood concentration rose beyond the level predicted by first-order kinetics; it seemed as if the dispositional and metabolic processes governing steady-state values had simply been overwhelmed. The behavioral counterpart of such an effect is quite important for standard setting, because the early signs of toxicity are apparent only when the toxic process unfolds gradually. With high doses, the spectrum of toxicity collapses into an undistinguishable mass that can be characterized only as representing a sick monkey.

Carefully calibrated dosing aimed at achieving blood levels commensurate with those measured in human victims (e.g., Bakir et al. 1973) allowed Merigan et al. (1983) to demonstrate two aspects of visual-system toxicity that had not been recognized before. First, the earliest indications of damage to the visual system consist of eccentric, not concentric, constriction of the peripheral visual field. Second, if dosing is halted at the appearance of this effect, full function can be recovered; that is, the poisoning is reversible. Moreover, such reversibility is apparent in the visual cortex, where histopathology after recovery reveals no active pathological processes or signs of previous damage. Contrast the implications of such findings for methylmercury exposure standards with the typical findings from short-term, high-dose studies.

Hypersusceptibility

Legislation such as the Clean Air Act officially recognizes the immense range of sensitivity to air pollutants by mandating protection for groups at special risk. The very young and the very old may constitute extremely sensitive groups. Persons suffering from angina are now under study because of earlier reports claiming that even modest elevations in carboxyhemoglobin could shorten the latency to anginal pains during exercise. Asthmatics have been viewed as especially susceptible to airborne oxidants such as ozone. Few chemicals have been free of speculation as to which special groups might be especially sensitive to their toxic effects.

Hardly any issue confronts toxicology with such difficult logical and experimental problems. Consider bronchial asthma and the possible hypersusceptibility of asthmatics to oxidants. The incidence in the population at large is 33 per 1,000. Randomly chosen samples of Los Angeles residents studied for effects covarying with ambient oxidant level are guaranteed to show no correlation. The alternative, of course, is a case-control study in which a group of asthmatics would be compared with controls with clinically normal pulmonary function. Most of the time, however, we do not have the luxury of identification of susceptibility beforehand. Most of the time, in fact, we would not know how to identify such individuals.

Choosing presumably homogeneous groups of experimental subjects may not be the ostensibly clear solution that it appears to be. Amdur (1980) observed that "almost all of the studies of human subjects mention some individual who was more sensitive than the rest of the subjects. Upon occasion, exposures to 5 to 10 ppm [sulfur dioxide] have been reported to cause severe bronchospasm. These individuals who were more sensitive have been 'normal, healthy subjects,' not individuals with respiratory disease" (p. 615). Figure 1.5, which plots the performance of individual rats exposed to various doses of lead, makes the same point even more graphically, perhaps, because all the rats came from the same supplier in the same shipment, belonged to the same strain, ate the same diet, and were housed in the same room; and yet, the differences among animals in the same treatment group were enormous.

There is no simple experimental strategy to overcome the intrinsic variation among organisms, and experimenters should not be lulled into smugness by submerging individual responses in group designs and analyses. The tendency to do so is responsible for a still active controversy that should have been resolved several years ago. The controversy stemmed from the claims that some of the children labeled as hyperactive or hyperkinetic actually were the victims of unusual sensitivity to certain classes of foods and food additives (Feingold 1975). I have reviewed the literature prompted by the Feingold hypothesis (e.g., Weiss 1982, n.d.) on several occasions and have concluded that in principle Feingold was right; that is, he uncovered a valid phenomenon, although his estimates of prevalence were confounded with variables typical of those intruding into uncontrolled clinical observations.

The study in which I took part (Weiss et al. 1980) sought to estimate the behavioral toxicity of synthetic food colors. It was designed, not to determine the therapeutic implications of Feingold's claims, but to explore an important toxicological issue, namely, the validity of food additive toxicity testing without the inclusion of behavioral measures. For this reason, children without clinical psychiatric or medical problems, including hyperkinesis, were enrolled as subjects. Each child was followed for an 11-week period, during which the parents made a variety of daily observations and ratings, and each child was maintained on a diet free of synthetic flavors and colors. During the middle 8 weeks of the study, on 8 randomly selected occasions, each child consumed a specially formulated and bottled soft drink containing a blend of 7 food colors. On all other days, the child consumed a control drink identical in color and taste to the experimental drink. Such a design was chosen to assess the reproducibility of effects alleged to derive from food colorings.

Out of the 22 children enrolled in the study, 2 showed significant adverse reactions. One three-year-old boy was a mild responder. One, a 34-month-old girl, was a striking responder. A careful review of the literature reveals responders in other studies as well. For example, an experiment by Williams et al. (1978) yielded an incidence of responders to food colors of about 25 percent and one subject almost as striking in his consistency as the girl in Weiss et al. (1980). Williams et al., however, apparently never examined the response patterns of the individual sub-

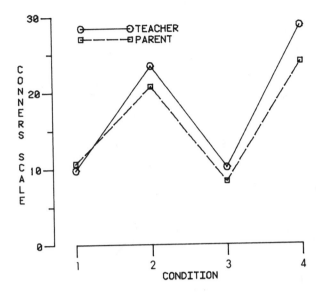

Fig. 1.6 The response of one subject to food-color challenge in the form of two cookies daily (total of 26 mg color). Conditions represent the following treatments: (1) stimulant medication plus control cookies; (2) stimulant medication plus active cookies; (3) placebo medication plus control cookies; (4) placebo medication plus active cookies.
(*Source:* the diagram, based on unpublished data from Williams et al. 1978, appeared in Weiss 1982. Reprinted by permission of the publisher.)

jects, relying instead on an analysis of variance and missing the most intriguing results of their experiment (see fig. 1.6).

Figure 1.7 reveals how little of scientific value is yielded simply by expanding the size of subject groups. It assumes a population comprising 70 percent nonresponders and 30 percent responders (top chart), a choice based on some of Feingold's assertions about the prevalence of hyperactive children sensitive to food additives. The abscissa is an arbitrary score on some measure. Assume that the responders cannot be identified beforehand and that some chemical exposure affects the responders, so that as a group they are displaced to the left by one standard deviation (middle chart). Since all the scores are combined in the statistical analysis, the total effect of the exposure is hardly distinguishable (bottom chart). The entries in table 1.2 show how large a sample would be needed to attain a 0.01 significance level 90 percent of the time given certain magnitudes of effect. For the assumptions of figure 1.8, the sample size would have to be at least 265. Of the studies relied on to reject the Feingold hypothesis, the largest examined 36 boys by

Table 1.2 Number of subjects required to demonstrate statistically reliable differences (p = 0.01) for various combinations of response amplitude and percentage of responders in the sample

Percentage of responders	Response Amplitude $\left(\dfrac{d}{\sigma}\right)$		
	1.0	2.0	3.0
10	2102	~550	265
20	~550	~150	65
30	265	65	30
40	~150	~37	16
50	90	23	12
100	23	7	4

Note: d = mean difference; σ = standard deviation.

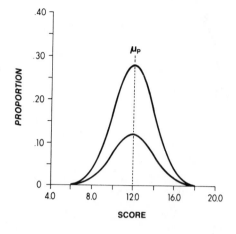

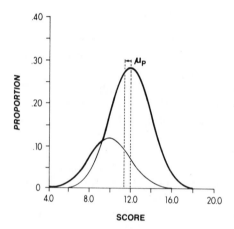

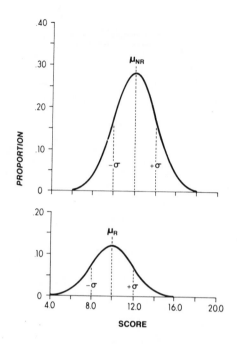

Fig. 1.7 Statistical problems of samples containing susceptible subgroups. *Top left,* hypothetical sample containing 70 percent responders and 30 percent responders (not identified to experimenter); *top right,* response to toxic (or therapeutic) challenge of hypothesized responders and nonresponders, presuming that responders, as a group, shift from baseline conditions by one standard deviation; *bottom,* distribution following challenge to total sample (heavy line). Displacement of total mean (μp) is shown by arrow.

traditional group statistics. If an experimenter had elected to study 15 subjects from a population such as that in figure 1.7, the outcome probably would resemble that plotted in figure 1.9, which represents a Monte Carlo drawing from that population.

As these models demonstrate, questions aroused by the Feingold hypothesis, by the suspected hypersusceptibility of asthmatics to air pollutants such as ozone, and by similar phenomena may require experimental designs that are unconventional for toxicology. Our approach to the Feingold hypothesis was a single-subject design, that is, a design treating each subject as an individual experiment. It was compelled by the question, Can repeated treatment with food dyes elicit a reproducible response? Another kind of single-subject design has been used by investigators studying the relations between ambient-oxidant concentrations and symptoms in patients with bronchial asthma. Their statistical approach consisted of time series analysis, that is, cross-correlations over time in the two measures. As I noted in earlier sections of this chapter, corresponding designs in animal experiments may reveal connections that also would be obscured by conventional group

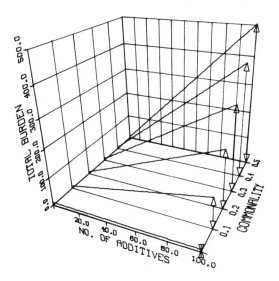

Fig. 1.8 Plot of the relationships between the number of additives consumed, the total burden as a percentage of ADI (Allowable Daily Intake), and commonality of effect (proportion of shared actions on a particular organ or system). Each additive is consumed at 10 percent of its individual ADI.

designs. Since no current investigator can be unaware of the campaigns for animal conservation, design strategies that extract the maximum information from each subject may have to be adopted simply to accommodate such pressures.

Issues Arising

Neurobehavioral toxicology is positioned to contribute to several other issues certain to pose major challenges to contemporary toxicology. One stems from our expanding aging population and the impact of that demographic shift on almost

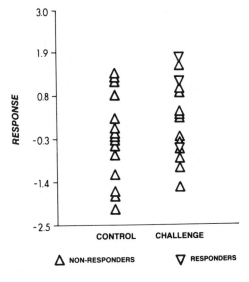

Fig. 1.9 Monte Carlo simulation based on drawing 15 randomly selected subjects from the population shown in fig. 1.7, before and after challenge.

every facet of society, including the economic and social consequences of the degenerative diseases associated with aging. It would be natural to speculate about the possible contribution of toxic processes to these diseases, many of which, such as senile dementia, reflect brain dysfunction. Calne and Langston (1983), in fact, posed the intriguing possibility that MPTP, a contaminant produced during the illicit manufacture of meperidine, may be an analogue of endogenous or exogenous substances responsible for idiopathic Parkinsonism. They noted that genetic predispositions, infectious disease, and other proposed etiologies are not tenable. At the same time, we already possess a copious literature indicating our ability to mimic at least some aspects of degenerative neurological disease. Manganese and basal ganglia dysfunction, aluminum and dementia, β,β-iminodipropionitrile and lower motor neuron disease, and other connections are intriguing, possibly fruitful guides to the sources of these diseases of the twenty-first century. And almost all of the clinical entities not only possess a major behavioral component but are manifested earliest by subtle behavioral aberrations. In this context, too, the typical group designs and short-term observations so dominant in current behavioral toxicology are less likely to yield cogent advances in understanding than careful, precise, and patient longitudinal observations aimed at tracing the disease process.

A second new issue widening in importance is how to evaluate multiple exposures. The laboratory frees us to study one toxic substance at a time under conditions as carefully controlled as we can manage. In contrast, the natural environment not only introduces disorder into the circumstances of exposure but perplexes us with multiple agents and their interactions. Drinking water in many parts of the country and chemical waste dumps contain a rich broth of toxic substances whose combined actions confront environmental health science with novel and vexing problems of evaluation.

Interactions among chemicals are hardly new to toxicology and pharmacology. Medical scientists and practitioners are sensitized to drug interactions, and toxicologists have generated a substantial literature on joint effects. It is the sheer scope of the possibilities that is so staggering. Pharmacological and toxicological studies of chemical interactions typically involve two agents. In the natural environment we face a vast array of possible interactions—drinking water from the Potomac River contains hundreds of suspected and confirmed toxic substances. I have adopted the term *conjunctive toxicology* to describe what seems to be emerging as a new toxicologic specialty. One convenient vantage point is the Allowable Daily Intake (ADI), a value typically associated with food additives. The ADI often is calculated from two-year feeding studies in rodents. The highest dose producing no detectable effects (the NOEL) is divided, typically by a factor of 100, to yield a quantity presumably safe for human consumption. It embodies a 10-fold safety margin plus a 10-fold factor to adjust for possible species differences. No safety factor is introduced to compensate for possible joint effects of additives, but closely related substances are considered as one source (e.g., BHA and BHT). Each additive ordinarily is evaluated singly, however, in the standard toxicity protocols specified by regulatory agencies. Humans, of course, consume many different additives, as packaging labels will testify; over 3,000 are approved in the United States.

Graphical displays make it easier to convey the scope and implications of conjunctive toxicity. They are meant not as mathematical models but as a context for the issues. With the ADI as its model, figure 1.8 addresses some of the implications of conjunctive toxicology. Assume that a person may consume up to 100 different additives, as on the axis labeled "No. of Additives." Assume that these additives may exert mutual actions on some biological system or process, with the degree of overlap depicted on the axis labeled "Commonality." This concept derives from the following argument. If each additive contributed 10 percent of its dose to the toxic burden of biological system S, and each were consumed at the ADI, then the "Total Burden" on that system would be $10 \times 100 = 1,000$ percent. More realistically, if each were consumed on the average at 10 percent of its ADI and each contributed one-tenth of that quantity on the average to system S (the commonality), then the total functional burden would come to 100 percent of the common ADI. If less than 100 additives were consumed or contributed to system S, then a lower total burden would be attained. If the commonality reached as high as 0.5, a functional total burden from 100 additives would come to 500 percent with the parameters chosen.

These calculations are based on the assumption that only additive interactions occur. Many interactions, however, are multiplicative. Suppose that additive A is consumed at 10 percent of its ADI and that, singly, one-tenth of that quantity is active against biological system S. Suppose that additive B is equivalent in its actions. Suppose, however, that A and B jointly are not additive but multiplicative. Instead of $A + B = 2$ percent on system S, their combination yields an effect greater than 2 percent. We can formulate the relationship as $(A + B)M = k(\text{ADI})$, where M is the multiplicative factor and k is some proportion of the functional ADI, or what I have called the total burden. If $M = 1$, we have simple summation; if $M > 1$, the relation is multiplicative; if $M < 1$, we have antagonism. Assume (fig. 1.10) exposure to 100 agents, a conservative estimate. Examining only pairs of agents, there are $(N^2 - N)/2$ possible interactions, or 4,950 pairs. If the probability of an interaction is only 0.01, that still yields 49 pairs. Suppose that the joint actions of these pairs yield an averaged multiplier across pairs of 10.0, that is, an enhancement of the burden on system S 10 times the expected contribution of their individual values. If the expected contribution were 1 percent each and the multiplicative factor were 10, we could have an equivalent functional burden of 490 percent of the presumed safe level. A factor of 10 is not startling. For example, the hepatotoxicity of chloroform in the rat is multiplied by factors of 40, 10, 100, and 60, by acetone, n-hexane, methyl-n-butyl ketone, and 2,5-hexanedione, respectively. Figure 1.10 charts these combined effects for M values of 1 to 100 and interaction probabilities ranging from 0.0001 to 0.1000, assuming a commonality of 0.1. These values are not unrealistic. The waste products from the Love Canal area clearly are not wholly independent in their effects. For example, the substances chosen there as index compounds are almost all neurotoxic, and many of them, as well as others in that area, are considered to be carcinogenic as well. The implications of these plots should be weighed carefully in decisions about risk usually derived solely from individual substances, especially since multiplicative interactions are likely to be more insidious because they are more unexpected. A recent report on Love Canal (Tarlton and Cassidy 1981) touches on such possibilities only obliquely. With thousands of wayward substances discharged into our environment from human

RISK MULTIPLE

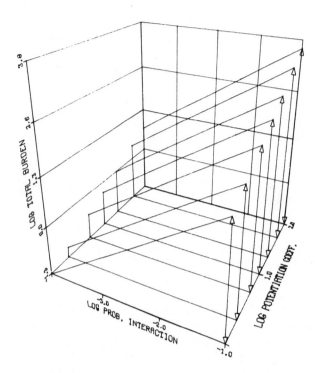

Fig. 1.10 Plot of the multiplicative relationships among 100 additives, each consumed at 10 percent of the individual ADI.

activities, and the natural poisons that already abound, even timid estimates of the likelihood of significant interactions yield a huge number of possibilities. New design strategies for such experiments (e.g., Simon 1980) need to be evolved.

New design strategies are not the total answer, however, when confronted with the collection of agents that may be found in some environmental situations, such as drinking-water supplies. Those kinds of toxicity evaluations must be made on the basis of existing sources. Toxicity estimates based on conventional rodent assays may not be feasible because of dose. How is concentration, for example, to be manipulated? One technique is to increase concentration by physical and chemical methods, but such a tactic may make the taste aversive or may modify some chemical property of the contaminants. Another tactic is to turn to behavioral techniques. Rats, at least, can be made to consume huge volumes of fluid by various experimental manipulations. They can be trained, for instance, to lick at a drinking tube to avoid unpleasant electric shocks to the feet. If the drinking tube contains a liquid diet, caloric consumption can be raised to a level that produces gross obesity. Such an avoidance paradigm could also promote the consumption of large amounts of drinking water, even, given the denser concentrations attained by chemical maneuvers, to levels perhaps hundreds of times higher than the starting concentration.

Another technique of even greater promise is adjunctive drinking. Rats consume fluid in vast amounts when it is available in conjunction with food delivery programmed under various operant reinforcement schedules, such as the fixed interval (Sanger and Blackman 1978). Such consumption is maintained by a pattern of prandial drinking synchronized with food pellet deliveries. Operant control of food delivery is not even necessary. Simply delivering a food pellet (usually 45 mg) on a periodic schedule, such as once per minute, seems sufficient to promote the adjunctive behavior of drinking, often in volumes exceeding the rat's body weight.

Such examples emphasize the potential breadth of behavioral techniques in toxicology, which need not be restricted to agents assumed to act directly on the nervous system. Some of the questions arising about the adverse consequences of ozone, for instance, are targets for behavioral methods. Tepper, Weiss, and Wood (1983) showed that some of the speculations about the source of reduced athletic performance during oxidant exposure had counterparts in rat behavior. Rats reduced spontaneous activity in a running wheel, pressed less often to release a brake on the wheel that allowed them to run, and ran less often on a fixed-interval schedule of food delivery when running was specified as the operant. Other experimenters have turned to behavioral measures to test the hypothesis that TCDD-induced body wasting is partly a loss of food-intake regulation acting through the hypothesized body weight set-point mechanism. The opportunities for translating important questions into a form accessible to behavioral technology span much of toxicology. They should not be obscured by the traditional coupling of the central nervous system and behavior.

Acknowledgments

Preparation of this chapter was supported in part by NIH grants ES-01247, ES-01248, and ES-03054 and under contract No. DE-AC02-76EV03490 with the U.S. Department of Energy at the University of Rochester Department of Radiation Biology and Biophysics and has been assigned report no. DOE/EV/03490-2413.

References

Amdur, M. O. 1980. Air pollutants. In *Toxicology: The basic science of poisons*, edited by J. Doull, C. D. Klaassen, and M. O. Amdur, 608–31. New York: Macmillan.

Bakir, F.; Damluji, S. F.; Amin-Zaki, L.; Murtadha, M.; Khalidi, A.; Al-Rawi, N. J.; Tikriti, S.; Dahir, H. I.; Clarkson, T. W.; Smith, J. C.; and Doherty, R. A. 1973. Methylmercury poisoning in Iraq. *Science* 181:230–41.

Calne, D. B., and Langston, J. W. 1983. Aetiology of Parkinson's disease. *Lancet* 2:1457–59.

Cannon, S. B.; Veazey, T. M.; Jackson, R. S.; Burse, V. W.; Hayes, C.; Straub, W. E.; Landrigan, P. J.; and Liddle, J. A. 1978. Epidemic ketone poisoning in chemical workers. *Amer. J. Epidemiol.* 107:529–37.

Cory-Slechta, D. A., and Thompson, T. 1979. Behavioral toxicity of chronic postweaning lead exposure in the rat. *Toxicol. Appl. Pharmacol.* 47:151–59.

Cory-Slechta, D. A., and Weiss, B. 1985. Alterations in schedule-controlled performance correlated with prolonged lead exposure. In *Behavioral pharmacology: The current status*, edited by L. Seiden and R. Balster, 487–501. New York: Alan Liss.

Cory-Slechta, D. A.; Weiss, B.; and Cox, C. 1983. Delayed behavioral toxicity of lead with increasing exposure concentrations. *Toxicol. Appl. Pharmacol.* 71:342–52.

Edgington, E. S. 1980. *Randomization tests*. New York: Dekker.

Feingold, B. F. 1975. *Why your child is hyperactive*. New York: Random House.

Finocchio, D. V.; Luschei, E. S.; Mottet, N. K.; and Body, R. 1980. Effects of methylmercury on the visual system of rhesus macaque (*Macaca mulatta*). I. Pharmacokinetics of chronic methylmercury related to changes in vision and behavior. In *Neurotoxicity of the visual system*, edited by W. H. Merigan and B. Weiss, 113–22. New York: Raven Press.

Gregersen, P.; Angelso, B.; Nielsen, T. E.; Norgaard, B.; and Uldal, C. 1984. Neurotoxic effects of organic solvents in exposed workers: An occupational, neuropsychological, and neurological investigation. *Am. J. Ind. Med.* 5:201–25.

Maurissen, J. P. J., and Weiss, B. 1980. Vibration sensitivity as an index of somatosensory function in monkeys and humans. In *Experimental and clinical neurotoxicology*, edited by P. S. Spencer and H. H. Schaumburg, 767–74. Baltimore: Williams & Wilkins.

Maurissen, J. P. J.; Weiss, B.; and Davis, H. T. 1983. Somatosensory thresholds in monkeys exposed to acrylamide. *Toxicol. Appl. Pharmacol.* 71:266–79.

Merigan, W. H.; Barkdoll, E.; and Maurissen, J. P. J. 1982. Acrylamide-induced visual impairment in primates. *Toxicol. Appl. Pharmacol.* 62:342–45.

Merigan, W. H.; Maurissen, J. P. J.; Weiss, B.; Eskin, T.; and Lapham, L. W. 1983. Neurotoxic actions of methylmercury on the primate visual system. *Neurobehav. Toxicol. Teratol.* 5:649–58.

Michaelson, I. A. 1980. An appraisal of rodent studies on the behavioral toxicity of lead: The role of nutritional status. In *Lead toxicity*, edited by R. L. Singhal and J. A. Thomas, 301–65. Baltimore and Munich: Urban & Schwarzenberg.

Sanger, D. J., and Blackman, D. E. 1978. The effects of drugs on adjunctive behavior. In *Contemporary research in behavioral pharmacology*, edited by D. E. Blackman and D. J. Sanger, 239–87. New York: Plenum.

Simon, W. 1980. Avoiding megamouse experiments. *J. Toxicol. Environ. Health* 6:907–10.

Tarlton, F., and Cassidy, J. J., eds. 1981. *Love Canal. Special report to the governor and legislature.* Albany: New York State Department of Health.

Tepper, J. L.; Weiss, B.; and Wood, R. W. 1983. Behavioral indices of ozone exposure. In *International symposium on the biomedical effects of ozone and related photochemical oxidants*, edited by S. D. Lee, M. G. Mustafa, and M. A. Mehlman, 515–26. Princeton, N.J.: Princeton Scientific Publishers.

Tilson, H. A.; Mitchell, C. L.; and Cabe, P. A. 1979. Screening for neurobehavioral toxicity: The need for and examples of validation of testing procedures. *Neurobehav. Toxicol.* 1, suppl. 1:137–48.

Weiss, B. 1982. Food additives and environmental chemicals as sources of childhood behavior disorders. *J. Am. Acad. Child Psychiatry* 21:144–52.

———. 1983. Behavioral toxicology and environmental health science: Opportunity and challenge for psychology. *Am. Psychol.* 38:1174–87.

———. N.d. Food additive safety evaluation: The link to behavioral disorders in children. In *Advances in clinical child psychology*, edited by A. L. Kazdin. New York: Plenum. In press.

Weiss, B.; Williams, J. H.; Margen, S.; Abrams, B.; Caan, B.; Citron, L. J.; Cox, C.; McKibbin, J.; Ogar, D.; and Schultz, S. 1980. Behavioral responses to artificial food colors. *Science* 207:1487–88.

Williams, J. I.; Cram, D. M.; Tausig, F. T.; and Webster, E. 1978. Relative effects of drug and diet on hyperactive behaviors: An experimental study. *Pediatrics* 61:811–17.

I

Research Strategies

Laurence D. Fechter and
John S. Young

2

Reflexive Measures

Reflex behaviors are receiving increasing attention from toxicologists both as screening tools for assessing neurotoxicity and as indicators of function in specific neural systems. Reflex behaviors offer certain distinct advantages that make them attractive in neurotoxicological investigations, but as with all measuring systems, the organismic and experimental factors that influence these behaviors must be understood in order to interpret the data properly. This chapter reviews the use of reflex behaviors and discusses some of the experimental variables that may also affect such behaviors. Rather than provide a survey of neurotoxicological studies employing reflex measures, the chapter seeks to identify the conditions necessary for the productive application of reflex methods to neurotoxicological investigations and to emphasize potential problems that might be considered in experimental design.

The historic definition of a *reflex behavior* given by English and English (1958) is "a very simple act in which there is no element of choice or premeditation and no variability save in intensity or time. . . . Unless qualified (as in acquired reflex) a species-specific or innate behavior is usually meant." This definition is sufficient to identify several fundamental strengths and weaknesses of reflex behaviors in elucidating neurotoxicity. In their favor, reflexes are simple acts for which underlying neuronal pathways are comparatively easy to identify. They therefore potentially can be used to identify injury in restricted areas of the nervous system and may offer unusual possibilities for distinguishing sensory and motor-system toxicity. Reflexes are readily amenable to objective quantification, with occurrence, latency, and amplitude commonly used as dependent measures. Reflex behaviors are present in all members of a species and do not require prior training. Thus, reflex assessment is typically possible in short time periods and may be accomplished using a limited sample size. Further, since these behaviors are innate, it is possible to exclude deficits in certain "higher functions," such as in learning and retention, as explanations for impaired performance by subjects receiving toxicants. As will be noted below, however, reflexes are sensitive to motivational and emotional factors and to trial effects.

The study of reflex behavior as a measure of neural function may raise fundamental questions of interpretation as well as issues of experimental design. A particularly important issue is whether a particular reflex behavior is an appropriate model for studying neurotoxicity when the reflex is found in a limited range of species. While cross-species generalizability is a recurring issue in the life sciences, the issue may become particularly acute in studying certain reflex behaviors. One might be willing to assert common mechanisms underlying cognitive functions such as learning and retention and to generalize the results of impairments in these functions (rightly or wrongly) across species, but some reflexes are so restricted phylogenetically as to impede ready generalizability. Such reflexes might include the relatively well studied Preyer's reflex (ear flick) elicited in several mammals (though not man) by sudden, loud sound stimuli; the female lordosis reflex elicited during copulation in several mammals by complex stimuli, including male mounting; and fighting behavior between male stickleback fish (*Gasterosteus aculeatus*) elicited by the red coloring of the male during the mating season (Tinbergen 1951, 1952). If one were to observe a change in one of these reflexes following a presumed toxic exposure, how should it be interpreted when one is ultimately interested in a species that does not show the particular reflex? Arguments can be made that alteration in reflex behavior is an expression of damage to the nervous system or neuromuscular unit and that as such it is a valid marker for injury. Whether injury does occur across species would depend more upon basic toxicologic and toxicokinetic determinants than upon the normal occurrence of the response in a species. Presumably, homologous behaviors, those depending upon the corresponding neuronal structure, will be altered if the toxicant produces damage in another species. An allied question concerns the functional significance of a shift in some aspect of a reflex behavior. While reflexes are thought to be indices of normal physiological function, their latency and amplitude cannot be readily characterized as good or bad. In this sense reflexes may be distinguishable from certain more complex behavioral responses such as learning, memory, motor coordination, and sensory acuity. Should any shift in a reflex resulting from exposure to some agent be taken as evidence of toxicity? One might presume that shifts in reflex behavior after exposure reflect some alteration (temporary or permanent) in nervous-system function and thereby pose a potential threat to the organism's survival. If one can identify the neurological basis for disruption of the reflex in a given species, the significance of such an effect may become more apparent.

Specification of Stimuli

While we shall discuss a number of specific factors affecting reflex behaviors, some general considerations concerning elicitation and measurement of a reflex are worth noting. First, a reflex is "a stimulus-response correlation" (English and English 1958), and the occurrence and vigor of the reflex is dependent upon the intensity of the eliciting stimulus and the stability of the organism's sensory environment. This factor, of course, has relevance for the use of reflexive tasks in assessing sensory function. It should, however, call attention to the importance of specifying and controlling the organism's sensory environment such that the intensity of the eliciting stimulus does not vary across presentations and extraneous stimuli are eliminated or controlled. The practice of good experimental control is as essential for studying "simple" reflex behaviors as it is in all scientific work. Tolman (1932) discussed the importance of *behavioral supports*, the factors in the environment necessary for a behavioral act to occur appropriately. He noted that "behavior cannot go off *in vacuo*" but, instead, is dependent upon sensory features in the environment that release the behavior, as well as other physical features that support and make possible the behavioral response. The dependence of even simple reflex behaviors on such supports has been carefully documented in certain instances and can logically be assumed to apply in certain (perhaps all) other cases.

Copulatory behavior and, specifically, male mounting and female lordosis reflexes have been very useful both for understanding neurochemical-hormonal interaction and in screening drugs for neuropharmacologic action (see Meyerson and Eliasson 1977). For such testing to be reliable, however, it must be carried out in the male rat's home cage using vigorous male subjects. In this case, while the behavioral supports are somewhat difficult to specify, test procedures can be identified that permit reliable studies to be conducted.

The behavioral supports necessary for elicitation of reliable auditory startle reflex behavior have been most carefully studied, and it is possible to identify features of the eliciting stimulus that affect the behavior in predictable ways and to pinpoint the modulating influences of extraneous environmental stimuli. The problems of startle reflex elicitation are relatively simple. All other factors being equal, the probability of reflex elicitation and reflex amplitude tend to increase with eliciting stimulus amplitude within a fairly narrow range (Hoffman and Ison 1980). The reflex begins to occur with some reliability in the rat at a stimulus intensity of 90 dBA for white noise bursts or 90 dB SPL for pure tones within the most sensitive region of the audiogram. Reflex probability is very close to 100 percent at a sound level of 110–20 dB, and reflex amplitudes are quite robust at such a stimulus intensity. Reflex amplitude is very sensitive to other environmental stimuli. Hoffman and Wible (1970) and Ison and Hammond (1971) showed that the amplitude of the acoustic startle reflex could be inhibited, and the latency reduced, by low-intensity auditory and visual stimuli presented shortly (<500 msec) before reflex elicitation. This phenomenon of reflex modulation has been studied extensively, and recent reviews are available (e.g., Ison and Hoffman 1983). The phenomenon is demonstrated in figure 2.1, in which a 60 dB SPL 10 kHz tone of 20 msec duration (top trace, right panel) presented 100 msec before a 120 dBA white noise burst (middle trace, right panel) greatly diminishes reflex amplitude (bottom trace, right panel) relative to a control condition (left panel) in which the reflex is elicited by the 120 dBA white noise burst with no prestimulus delivered. It must be appreciated that uncontrolled auditory, visual, and tactile stimuli or changes in stimulus environment have equivalent effects upon the reflex based upon their temporal relationship to the reflex eliciting stimulus. Ison (1982) and Ison and Pinckney (1983) have shown that brief gaps (4 msec) in a continuous background noise can also inhibit subsequently elicited reflex responses. To the extent that reflex modulation both within and between modalities is a general characteristic of reflex behavior, scrupulous control over the subject's stimulus environment would appear to be a critical requirement in studies of reflex behavior. Reflex modulation has been best studied using the whole-body startle reflex and the eyeblink reflex and has been reported to occur across many species, including humans (Krauter, Leonard, and Ison 1973; Graham 1975; Ison, Reiter, and Warren 1979), rabbits (Ison and Leonard 1971), guinea pigs (Young and Fechter 1983), rats (Hoffman and Searle

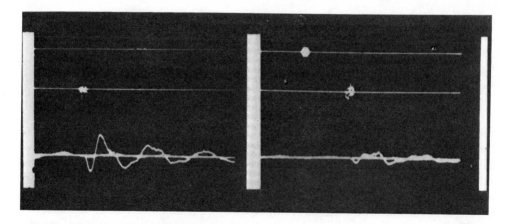

Fig. 2.1. Stimulus conditions and the analogue response of one subject on a baseline trial (*left*) and a prestimulus trial (*right*). The startle stimulus, a 20 msec 115 dBA white noise burst, was identical on both trials (*middle traces*). The prestimulus presented in the top trace of the right-hand panel was a 60 dB SPL 10 kHz tone of 20 msec duration with 5 msec onset and offset ramps. Voltage output of the response transducer is presented in the bottom traces.
(*Source:* Fechter and Young 1983. Reprinted by permission of the publisher.)

1965; Ison and Hammond 1971), mice (*Mus musculus* [Storm, Hulebak, and Fechter 1981]), and pigeons (Stitt et al. 1976), and to develop very early ontogenically (Parisi and Ison 1981).

The evidence to date does not suggest that the *general polysensory process* of reflex modulation by such prestimuli is particularly sensitive to manipulation by neurotoxicants or psychopharmacological action, although disruption of sensory function by neurotoxicants may render certain stimuli ineffective in modulating a reflex. Specifically, while a variety of drugs that affect catecholaminergic and serotonergic function markedly alter reflex amplitude, these agents are generally ineffective in altering the extent of reflex modulation (see Fechter 1974*a*). An exception to this was the finding that extreme increases in serotonin levels (100–300 percent increase in 5HT levels, depending upon brain region) following prior depletion of catecholamines and serotonin by reserpine did block prepulse inhibition (Fechter 1974*b*); however, these subjects were tested under extreme conditions.

Quantification of Reflex Behavior

As described above, the most commonly used dependent measures of reflex behavior are occurrence/nonoccurrence on one trial, probability of reflex behavior as reflected by the percentage of trials in which the reflex is elicited, reflex intensity, and reflex latency. Selection of an appropriate measure is partially dependent upon the nature of the reflex task used and the extent of experimental control exercised.

Assessment of the occurrence of a reflex response on one or more trials as the principal dependent measure requires little instrumentation and is particularly useful in more naturalistic, observational tasks. In addition to the experimental manipulation of interest, such measures may be greatly influenced by the adequacy of the eliciting stimuli and the sensitivity of the measuring system used (or subjective judgment of an observer). These need not be overwhelming problems; however, control over the stability of the eliciting stimulus is a critical concern in the evaluation of reflex behavior. Reduction of variability between subjects and within subjects in a repeated-trials design can be achieved by consistent presentation of the eliciting stimulus. Moreover, the reproduction of stimulus conditions that may be essential to the replication of experimental results requires a full description of eliciting stimulus conditions. This may be obtained easily when extremely close control can be exerted over the subjects' test environment, but substantially greater problems may arise when more naturalistic or at least less automated methods are employed for stimulus delivery and reflex assessment. Meyerson and Eliasson (1977), for example, have discussed the problems of assessing the lordosis reflex, a flexion of the spine and raising of the head and perineum elicited by male mounting in an estrous female. Their studies have been conducted for the most part in spayed female rats that have received hormone replacement to induce an intermediate probability of lordosis on mounting and a pharmacological agent to determine the consequences of neurotransmitter effects on sexual behavior. Since the complex eliciting stimuli provided by a male subject cannot be readily quantified nor assumed to be constant over repeated trials, the occurrence or nonoccurrence of the reflex on a given trial may reflect the adequacy of the eliciting stimuli as well as receptivity of the female, who is the actual test subject. Meyerson has approached this issue by assessing the occurrence of the reflex over a series of trials and using a within-subject analysis to assess increases or decreases in percentage response as an estimate of the effects of the pharmacological agent upon the reflex.

Alternative qualitative assessments of reflex strength have also been used, but it would appear that those methods may be more affected by adequacy of the eliciting stimulus and the interval between successive trials (see Meyerson and Eliasson 1977). This situation may also occur in reflex tests aimed at studying ontogeny of behavior (see below), where reflex function is observed in neonatal pups following manual placement of the subject in the test position. Occurrence versus nonoccurrence within a limited time period has frequently been used in the assessment of the ontogeny of simple reflexes in young subjects (e.g., Fechter and Annau 1980). Further, if an organism is to receive repeated testing, it is critical to assess the effects of repeated stimulus presentation upon reflex strength. While reflex behaviors are not learned, their amplitudes are well known to be altered by processes of habituation and sensitization.

Reflex Behavior as a Measure of Reactivity

Reactivity might be described most simply as the tendency to respond to sensory stimuli. It is frequently spoken of as a function of the central nervous system that can be distinguished from a purely sensory or neuromuscular process. Implicit in the use of the term is the assumption that a change in reactivity will be reflected by a generalized and consistent change in response intensity to all sensory stimuli. Unfortunately, *hyporeactivity* and *hyperreactivity* seem to be used both in a descriptive sense to note a very specific outcome on a particular task (increased or decreased response) and as a presumed descriptor of some change in the state of the nervous system. Rarely is a presumed change in the generalized reactivity level assessed using a range of sensory stimuli and motor outputs that might address the issue of locus of toxic effect. When used to screen for toxicity, the demonstration of such an altered reflex response amplitude may be quite useful, but determination of the underlying pathology and prediction of other toxic effects may be quite problematical. For example, the initial demonstrations that triethyltin (TET) reduced auditory startle reflex amplitude (Squibb, Carmichael, and Tilson 1980; Reiter et al. 1980) were extremely important in identifying neurobehavioral consequences of exposure but of themselves do not elucidate the locus of injury. A subsequent study of both startle reflex amplitude and reflex modulation audiometry (Fechter and Young 1983), discussed at greater length below, showed that the TET effects could not be explained by positing damage to the auditory periphery or ascending sensory limb of the reflex but probably reflected damage to peripheral neuromuscular elements, to motor efferents, or, less likely, to noradrenergic neurons which modulate reflex amplitude.

While the *neuronal substrate* of reactivity has not been strictly defined, the term is evocative both of the "hyperreactive syndrome" (in the rat), resulting from septal nucleus lesions, and of "state changes," reflecting some central arousal level mediated, presumably, by the reticular activating system. The so-called septal rage syndrome consists of an acute period during which the subject displays exaggerated responses to a wide range of sensory stimuli. While such animals have been described as "hyperreactive," the behavioral syndrome is marked by the presence of directed attack behavior or "rage" rather than by a generalized increase in all behaviors as a response to stimulation. Reactivity to sensory stimuli must also be seen as reflecting the arousal level of the subject. For example, active inhibition may depress responsivity to sensory stimuli more during the REM sleep period than during slow-wave or light sleep periods. Unfortunately, the imprecision in defining reactivity impedes the establishment of a firm relationship between a treatment that enhances or depresses this central state and a behavioral outcome amenable to study using reflexive or any other methods. Nevertheless, there are a number of reports in which the acoustic startle reflex has been used to assess reactivity. To the extent that the septal rage syndrome in rats is considered a model for hyperreactivity, it is clear that startle amplitude is an inappropriate measure. A series of experiments in which startle amplitudes were assessed following brain lesions showed no changes in rats following lesions in septal nucleus, amygdala, or hippocampus (Kemble and Ison 1971), despite the fact that these subjects showed classical signs of septal, amygdaloid, and hippocampal damage. Further, exposure to startle stimuli failed to reinstate the temporary septal rage syndrome observed in rats once it had subsided (Hammond and Thomas 1971). Hammond (1973) did demonstrate that the startle reaction could be enhanced by lesions in the medial frontal cortex and reduced by lesions in nucleus reticularis pontis caudalis. More recent evidence supports Hammond's findings for significant involvement of the brainstem in determining startle reflex behavior, but it is not currently possible to assume any relationship between "reactivity" and startle amplitude.

If limbic lesions do not alter startle reflex amplitude, what factors might be responsible for alteration of this measure? In addition to disruption of sensory and motor function, factors dealt with specifically below, a variety of conditions may alter startle reflex amplitude. For example, Horlington (1970) reported, and Davis and Sollberger (1971) subsequently confirmed, that startle reflex amplitudes are elevated during the dark phase of circadian rhythms in rats. Fechter and Ison (1972) demonstrated that even mild food and water deprivation (as little as 8 hr deprivation) depressed the startle reflex. Because exposure to neurotoxicants could disrupt sleep and feeding patterns, appropriate control groups must be utilized in determining the basis for alteration in startle reflex amplitude. It is interesting that another subject variable, the estrous cycle, does not alter startle reflex amplitude (Fechter, unpublished observation). This may be particularly useful, since estrous does have significant effects on many other behavioral measures, including locomotor activity.

Because unidentified subject variables can have profound effects upon reflex amplitude, it is particularly useful either to employ subjects as their own controls by means of within-subject designs or to match subjects on the basis of a pretest before assigning them to different treatment groups. Both procedures have been employed in pharmacological and toxicological investigations of the acoustic startle reflex. Fechter (1974a), for example, was able to determine that the acoustic startle could be enhanced by a monoamine depleting dosage of reserpine and that this effect was reversed by administration of the alpha adrenergic agonist, clonidine. The subjects used were four rats, which received both drug treatments after an initial test conducted prior to any drug administration. Similarly, Storm, Millington, and Fechter (1984) were able to demonstrate that diethyldithiocarbamate could depress startle amplitude using a within-subject comparison to a preliminary test conducted following saline injection. Davis (in Davis and Sheard 1974) has demonstrated the value of matching subjects in terms of acoustic startle reflex amplitude on pretests prior to assigning them to different treatment groups. He has successfully observed between-group differences following administration of a large number of pharmacological agents (see below) both by matching subjects and by employing within-subject statistical analysis.

Reflex Assessments as a Measure of Central Neurochemical Status

Perturbation of central neurotransmitter systems using a variety of pharmacological and toxicological agents has proved to yield rather predictable effects upon several reflex behaviors, including the acoustic startle reflex, which suggests the utility of this method in screening for potential effects of toxicants on these neuronal systems. While there remain some isolated results that do not readily fit the model, there is strong evidence that agents that enhance dopamine release or post-synaptic receptor activity increase startle (see Davis 1980). Thus, both apomorphine and amphetamine elevate startle, while haloperidol, a D2 receptor blocker, depresses the response. However, apomorphine enhancement of startle has a rather short time course (see Fechter 1974b; and Davis and Aghajanian 1976), and the effects of d-amphetamine are typically observed at extremely high dosage levels (3–32 mg/kg) (Kokkinidis and Anisman 1978; Davis, Svensson, and Aghajanian 1975) as compared with levels used in other experimental paradigms. Moreover, this amphetamine inducement of elevated startle behavior is not readily observed in juvenile rats (Fechter, unpublished observations). These data might suggest an indirect or at least weak effect of dopamine neurons on the reflex. That dopaminergic neurons are in fact involved in elaboration of this reflex is indicated by the ability of dopamine receptor antagonists such as pimozide (Kehne and Sorenson 1978) and haloperidol (Davis and Aghajanian 1976) to block the facilitatory effects of dopamine agonists on the reflex.

Evidence for noradrenergic involvement in the startle reflex suggests a general facilitatory role of this neurotransmitter on startle amplitude, although some contrary findings have been reported. Noradrenergic involvement in the facilitatory effects of amphetamine on startle has been suggested by experiments in which $\alpha 1$ antagonists such as phenoxybenzamine (Kehne and Sorenson 1978) and synthesis inhibitors such as FLA 63 (Kokkinidis and Anisman 1978) and α-methyl-p-tyrosine (Davis, Svensson, and Aghajanian 1975) blocked or attenuated the amphetamine effect. However, FLA 63, a DA-hydroxylase inhibitor, does not itself alter startle amplitude (Kokkinidis and Anisman 1978), nor does locus coeruleus lesioning produce significant effects on startle (a trend toward reduced startle amplitude has been reported by Davis et al. 1977).

Davis has recently published some interesting experiments in which he has evaluated the role of ascending and descending NE and 5HT fibers in mediating the startle reflex. This work has involved injection of monoamine agonists into the spinal cord (intrathecally) in comparison with intraventricular and systemic injection. Davis and Astrachan (1981) have reported that the intrathecal administration of the $\alpha 1$ agonist phenylephrine as well as d-amphetamine elevated the startle reflex and that this effect could be blocked by an $\alpha 1$ antagonist. They also showed that the depressant effects of clonidine on startle could be blocked by yohimbine, an $\alpha 2$ antagonist. Davis, Astrachan, and Kass (1980) showed that intrathecal 5HT administration enhanced startle response amplitude, while lateral ventricular placement depressed the reflex. That report helps to explain Fechter's (1974b) data showing that elevation of 5HT by enhancement of precursor levels greatly increases startle behavior, as well as the finding of a depression in startle behavior reported to result from 5HT stimulation (Davis and Sheard 1976). What is troublesome, of course, is the difficulty in predicting where the predominant effects of a serotonergic agonist, antagonist, or toxicant will occur in the central nervous system and what the behavioral result will be. For this reason, it seems particularly useful to obtain both behavioral and appropriate neurochemical data in subjects treated with a particular toxicant.

For example, Storm, Millington, and Fechter (1984) reported that diethyldithiocarbamate (DDC), a metabolite of both carbon disulfide and disulfiram, depresses acoustic startle amplitude 120, but not 30 minutes after administration. This finding is consistent both with the known inhibitory effects of this agent on dopamine-β-hydroxylase (and the subsequent decrease in norepinephrine levels in the brain) and with startle data showing that decreased NE activity at postsynaptic receptors is related to decreased startle. Storm, Millington, and Fechter (1984) were able to correlate startle levels with a decrease in NE levels in cortex and spinal cord.

In addition to data indicating catecholaminergic control of startle behavior, data have been reported suggesting serotonergic and, potentially, cholinergic and peptidergic influences on this behavior. The latter relationships are somewhat less clear than those established for the catecholamines.

Reflex Methods for Assessing Behavioral Teratology

A significant literature demonstrates the utility of reflexive tasks in studying developmental delays and disability owing to early, generally in utero, toxic exposures. Such methods are particularly important because they can be used to assess neonatal development, when the behavioral repertoire of most mammals is extremely limited. Such tests tend to be descriptive in nature and cannot be used to readily pinpoint the nature of the disability. Failure to perform well may reflect multiple sites of injury. It is not currently clear how such tests relate to subsequent neurological function. In this regard these tests appear to have much in common with clinically used indices such as the Apgar and Brazelton tests. Despite their limitations, early screening tests may be of particular value in studying transient toxic effects and in obtaining an early indication of neurological status.

As a class, the behaviors to be described are assayed by observation, with determination of occurrence versus nonoccurrence of latency used as the level of measurement. They tend, therefore, to be extremely labor-intensive. Because they are observational tests, it is essential that the observer not be aware of an individual subject's group assignment; that is, such experiments should be run "blind" to avoid experimenter bias. At times this may be a difficult condition to fulfill—if treated pups are different in size or gross appearance from controls, for example. However, since these tasks are most relevant to screening for toxicity, their value would be greatest in detecting subtle teratogenic effects of exposure in subjects whose general appearance is normal. Statistical treatment of the data also must be carefully considered. In particular, the experimenter must decide whether to test all subjects in a litter or only one. In the former case it is probably most appropriate to pool scores from individual pups into a single litter score and then use that score in statistical analysis. This method eliminates the inflation in degrees of freedom that results from inclusion of all members of a litter, where scores within the litter may well be correlated. Attention must also be paid to the rating scale used to assess behavior, since the assumptions underlying the use of parametric statistics may not be fulfilled. This is most clearly the case where occurrence-nonoccurrence measures are used, but it may also apply to latency-based measures, where many individuals fail to perform the task within a restricted time period and are subsequently assigned a score corresponding to the upper time period allowed.

Several test batteries have been described for assessing behavioral teratogenesis using reflex-based tasks (e.g., Altman and Sudarshan 1975; and Butcher and Vorhees 1979). These batteries generally include a series of tasks that sample behaviors that mature in predictable order and at different ages neonatally. It is thus possible to test subjects over a significant period of preweaning life. Often these tasks appear to rely to differing degrees upon motor and sensory function. It is rather common for a single subject or for littermates to be run on each of the tasks, although repeated testing or environmental stimulation may enhance development and tend to obscure group differences caused by prenatal treatment. Frequently used tasks include surface righting, aerial righting, negative geotaxis, placing, acoustic startle, and homing. Because these tests have been well described and their application to toxicology has been reviewed previously (Adams and Buelke-Sam 1981; Altman and Sudarshan 1975; Butcher and Vorhees 1979), additional specific review of this approach seems unwarranted here. In evaluating published studies and the above reviews, however, it is important to bear in mind experimental design, level of measurement, and subject independence.

Reflex Procedures for Evaluating Sensory Function

Attempts to make functional assessments of toxic damage to sensory systems have tended to depend heavily upon the measurement of reflexes. This reflects the fact that the more sophisticated and sensitive assays of sensory function, such as those based upon operant discrimination training, require a larger investment of time and effort than most toxicity testing laboratories are able or willing to make. A wide variety of reflexes exist for which the eliciting conditions are well specified, and several of these have a long history of clinical use for sensory evaluation. Also, various experimental animals possess specialized reflexes that provide a convenient index of sensory function. To date, most reflex procedures used in toxicity testing consist simply of a determination of the stimulus intensity required to elicit a reflex or a measurement of the amplitude of a reflexive response elicited by a fixed stimulus.

Reflex Elicitation Procedures

While the elicitation of a reflex is unambiguous evidence of the detection of the eliciting stimulus, a failure to elicit a reflex is difficult to interpret. It may in fact reflect sensory system toxicity, but it could equally well be owing to motor system damage or toxic impairment of the central nervous system pathways mediating the reflex. The investigator must also be concerned about the nature of the relationship between stimulus detection and reflex elicitation; many stimuli of intensity sufficient to be detected will not regularly elicit a reflex response.

We do not propose to catalog all the reflexes that have been used to evaluate sensory system toxicity. Rather, we concentrate on an examination of the most widely used reflex tests, with a view toward evaluating their adequacy as indicators of sensory system function. In general, one can consider three classes of reflexes. The first comprises those cases in which reflex elicitation is logically equivalent to stimulus detection; that is, if the stimulus is detected in the appropriate modality, the reflex will necessarily (barring central or motor dysfunction) be elicited. For the second class of reflexes, a clear distinction can be made between the processes of stimulus detection and reflex elicitation, yet reflex elicitation provides a reasonable index of sensory system function. Finally, there is the class of reflexes that are clearly inadequate as assays of sensory function.

Although the status of pain as a specialized sensory system is problematic, the adequacy of reflex elicitation analgesimetry, at least in animal subjects, has been generally accepted (e.g., Tilson et al. 1982; and Zagon and McLaughlin 1982). On an empirical level, the most commonly studied reflexes (tail flick, flinch jump, paw lick) correlate well with human reports of pain reduction in response to analgesics and narcotics (Beecher 1957). While animals obviously detect stimuli in the same physical continua used to elicit these reflexes at levels well below those required to produce a reflex response, it is reasonable to argue that under normal conditions such stimuli are not painful until they become sufficiently intense to elicit a reflex response. Some have argued that other procedures are more sensitive (e.g., Weiss and Laties 1970), and these operant-based psychophysical procedures do produce lower threshold values, but it is not clear that they yield as direct a measure of pain.

The utility of reflex measures for assessing nociception and analgesia depends, as in the case of the reflexes discussed earlier, on their careful implementation and interpretation. These assays are susceptible to confounding influences. For example, response in a hot-plate test may reflect an animal's reaction to a novel environment rather than a specific effect on nociception. Neither can stimulus parameters be treated cavalierly. It has recently been shown (Yoburn et al. 1984) that the effects of opiates on the tail-flick response depend critically upon the site of thermal stimulation on the tail. A given dose of morphine, for example, may induce analgesia for stimuli delivered to the most distal part of a rat's tail without apparent analgesia for stimuli applied one inch more proximally. Similarly, the development of tolerance appears to occur more slowly when stimuli are delivered to the tip of the tail than when they are delivered closer to the base of the tail.

A second case where reflex elicitation can be said to define a sensory threshold is that of upper airways irritation, as studied by Alarie and colleagues. In a number of studies (e.g., Alarie 1966, 1973; and Alarie and Anderson 1979), they demonstrated a unique pattern of reflexive respiratory changes elicited in rodents by exposure to irritants, most prominently a prolongation of the expiratory phase of respiration. These changes are clearly distinguishable from those induced by asphyxiation, which produces a pause between inspiration and expiration. There are alternative procedures that provide a sensitive measure of olfactory detection, but there is no functional measure providing a more sensitive assay of airways irritation. Such irritation is both logically and physiologically separable from olfactory detection.

A strong case can be made that both nociception and airways irritation are independent sensory systems, clearly separable from other sensory modalities. Neither, however, is a typical sensory system. In each case, the physical continuum of effective stimuli overlaps that of another sensory modality, and nociception, at least, involves a sensitivity to stimuli in several different physical continua. Both systems also have relatively high detection thresholds. Thus, the utility of reflex measures for assessing function in these systems provides little indication of their applicability to other sensory systems.

The second category of reflex assays, where one can clearly distinguish between stimulus detection and reflex elicitation but where reflex elicitation provides an adequate index of sensory function, is exemplified by the procedures used to investigate vestibular function (e.g., Naunton 1975; and McCabe 1976). While the main function of the vestibular system is its contribution to various reflexes, the most commonly studied reflex, ocular nystagmus (Jongkees 1975; Schuknecht 1975), is not elicited by stimuli in the range of intensities to which animals are normally exposed.

A variety of physiological (acceleration) and nonphysiological (thermal) stimuli are applied to the vestibular system to elicit these reflexive eye movements (Proctor 1975), which can be readily measured electrically. One can also measure a spontaneous nystagmus which is produced by certain pathological conditions (McCabe, Sekitani, and Ryu 1973; Aschan et al. 1977; Larsby et al. 1978; Aursnes 1981). In studies of nystagmus, using a constant stimulus and measuring reflex amplitude has proven more useful than attempting to determine thresholds of reflex elicitation. Finally, since a similar nystagmus can be elicited by appropriate visual stimulation, there is a straightforward control for central and motor system effects (e.g., Baarsma and Rijntjes 1979).

Nystagmography has been used successfully to investigate the basic pharmacology of the vestibular system (McCabe, Sekitani, and Ryu 1973; Blair and Gavin 1979; Gavin and Blair 1981; and for a brief review, Brown and Wood 1980), as well as the effects of ototoxic drugs in experimental animals (Mathog and Capps 1977; Wersäl 1980; Aursnes 1981) and in human patients (Lerner, Seligsohn, and Matz 1977; Winkel et al. 1978; Baarsma and Rijntjes 1979; Nordstrom et al. 1979). Reviews by Hawkins and Preston (1975) and Prazma (1981) consider drug vestibulotoxicity. Nystagmographic studies have also provided the earliest laboratory data on the ototoxicity of industrial solvents (Aschan et al. 1977; Larsby et al. 1978; Arlien-Soberg et al. 1981; Biscaldi et al. 1981; Tham et al. 1982). The procedure is commonly used clinically as well as experimentally, although it has been criticized as a human toxicity screening procedure, owing to the high degree of intersubject variability (Davey et al. 1982).

The vestibular system, in contrast to nociception and airways irritation systems, more closely resembles other sensory systems in stimulus specificity and sensitivity. It is, nevertheless, intimately involved in reflex systems, and as mentioned earlier, these reflex involvements are central to its normal function.

Probably the best example of the final class of direct reflex measures, those that are inappropriate as tests of sensory function, is Preyer's reflex, the pinna flick elicited in many rodents by sudden, intense sounds. One might also cite the use of the pupillary light reflex as an equally inappropriate index of visual toxicity (see Conquet, Tardieu, and Durand 1979; and Levett and Jerger 1980), but presumably, owing to the availability of the eye for direct in vivo anatomical evaluation by ophthalmoscopy, there does not seem to have been equal pressure to develop a rapid assay of visual function.

A search by the present authors of recent papers on ototoxicity revealed that more than half of those reporting a functional measure of hearing relied upon Preyer's reflex. The wide use of the test ignores strong evidence, some published nearly twenty years ago, that it is insensitive as a measure of hearing and ototoxicity. Thresholds of Preyer's reflex elicitation are far (60–80 dB) above detection thresholds measured using other procedures (Bobbin, Gonzalez, and Guth 1969; Baird and Carter 1979). Since most ototoxicants differentially impair hearing of low-intensity sounds, this finding suggests that only the most severe hearing impairments will influence the elicitation of Preyer's reflex. Indeed, there is direct evidence of normal Preyer's reflex elicitation in the presence of marked functional hearing impairment and severe structural damage in the cochlea (Anderson and Wedenberg 1965; Astbury and Read 1982). Other direct auditory reflexes, such as acoustic startle (Harpur 1974) and the middle-ear reflex (Jerger, Mauldin, and Igarashi 1978; Hayes and Jerger 1981; Borg and Engstrom 1982), have also been used to assess ototoxicity, without any apparent increase in sensitivity.

Reflex Modification Procedures

It is clear that direct reflex elicitation assays, while useful in a variety of areas of investigation, are not adequate tests for many types of sensory system toxicity. The difficulties involved in using the more sensitive operant psychophysical methods, as mentioned above, have motivated a search for alternatives to these two types of sensory system assays. The phenomenon of reflex modification, as described earlier in this paper, provides the basis for one such alternative.

Reflex modification was described in the scientific literature at least as early as 1862, although it has only been investigated sporadically until recently (see Ison and Hoffman 1983). Hoffman and Ison (1980) reviewed much of the recent literature on reflex modification, concentrating on the most heavily studied reflex in this area, the acoustic startle reflex of the rat. The potential of reflex modification procedures as a technique for investigating sensory function was recognized early in the century. Yerkes (1905) reported audibility data for the frog derived by reflex modification methods. Interest in the procedure lapsed for a considerable period, however (Ison and Hoffman 1983), and only recently have investigators begun again to develop psychophysical procedures based on reflex modification.

Reflex modification has several advantages as a tool for studying sensory dysfunction. One that is obvious is their efficiency. Young and Fechter (1983) were able to obtain a reasonably complete audiometric determination for four rats in two weeks, obtaining a considerable amount of data on suprathreshold hearing as well. A comparable operant study (Kelly and Masterton 1977) required 150 days of training. Similarly, Russo (1980), using a different reflex modification procedure and a more limited range of stimuli (band-limited noise of varying center frequency), was able to make audiometric determinations in four daily sessions. He was also able to determine detection thresholds for electrocutaneous stimuli with comparable efficiency. Because reflex modification is an innate feature of the vertebrate nervous system, no training of subjects is needed prior to making a psychophysical determination. Elimination of training, in addition to reducing the time required for a study, also provides a degree of independence from confounding factors that toxicant administration may introduce, such as changes in subjects' motivational level or ability to perform the trained response.

Not only are reflex modification procedures for assessing sensory function almost as efficient as direct reflex elicitation procedures but they are nearly as sensitive as procedures based upon conditioning. Both Russo (1980) and Young and Fechter (1983) report threshold values very similar to those of comparable operant studies. The slightly diminished sensitivity (10–15 dB) of Young and Fechter's procedure presumably reflects temporal integration phenomena, a by-product of employing extremely brief (20 msec) inhibitory prestimuli.

A further advantage of reflex inhibition procedures for assessing sensory function is cross-species comparability. Reflex inhibition phenomena are as evident in humans as in experimental animals and have been successfully employed in psychophysical procedures. Reiter and Ison (1977) and Reiter et al. (1980) report audiometric data, and Uhlrich (1984), in an elegant study, has determined visual spatial frequency contrast sensitivity functions that rival those obtained using classical psychophysical methods. As Uhlrich's data demonstrate, the utility of reflex modification as a psychophysical procedure is not limited to the determination of simple detection thresholds. More complex questions regarding sensory function, such as spatial acuity, can also be addressed. This is also true for studies using animal subjects. Ison (1982), for example, has investigated the temporal resolution properties of the rat auditory system.

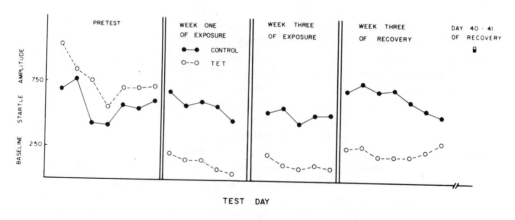

Fig. 2.2 Baseline startle reflex amplitudes before, during, and after exposure to TET (30 mg/l) (*open circles, dotted lines*) or paired water treatment (*closed circles, solid lines*).

There are also data indicating that the procedure successfully detects sensory dysfunction produced by toxic and other insults. Russo (1980) found that exposure to noise produced the expected shifts in auditory reflex inhibition thresholds and that lidocaine decreased sensitivity to electrocutaneous stimuli, as measured by their ability to inhibit startle. Young and Fechter (1983) administered neomycin to their rats and produced the expected decrease in sensitivity to low-intensity, high-frequency stimuli. Nor is the sensitivity to toxic insult limited to peripheral sensory organ damage. Kellogg, Ison, and Miller (1983) reported changes in auditory temporal processing following prenatal diazepam administration.

While reflex modification procedures detect sensory system toxicity with sensitivity, they are robust in the face of more general toxic effects, such as neuromuscular impairment. Fechter and Young (1983) investigated the effects of triethyltin (TET), a known neuromuscular toxicant, in Long-Evans hooded rats. TET administration in the subjects' drinking water (30 mg/l) over three weeks led to profound decreases in startle amplitudes followed by clinically observable hindlimb weakness (see fig. 2.2). Despite this massive damage to motor systems underlying the basic startle reflex, reflex inhibition remained normal, permitting accurate assessment of the subjects' (unimpaired) auditory sensitivity (figs. 2.3 and 2.4). This indicates that reflex modification procedures will prove especially useful in studying agents with multiple possible sites of toxic attack. The presence of control trials employing simple reflex elicitation means that the reflex modification procedure contains an inherent assay of the general sensorimotor condition of the subject.

The advantages of reflex modification methods for examining sensory function suggest that they may come to replace the commonly used reflex elicitation tests in toxicology laboratories. Several laboratories have already incorporated these tests as part of their regular procedures. While not suitable as a replacement for some more complex psychophysical procedures used to assess sensory toxicity, these methods offer an opportunity to increase considerably the effectiveness with which we monitor compounds for sensory toxicity.

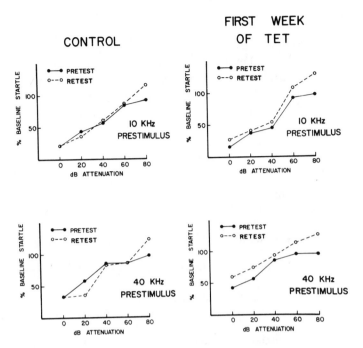

Fig. 2.3 Startle reflex inhibition to pure tones before treatment (*solid lines*) and during the first week of exposure to TET or paired water treatment (*dotted lines*). Data from TET-exposed rats are shown in the right panels, and data from paired-watered control subjects are shown in the left panels. In all cases reflex amplitude is decreased by increasing the intensity of the prestimulus (i.e., decreasing tone attenuation).

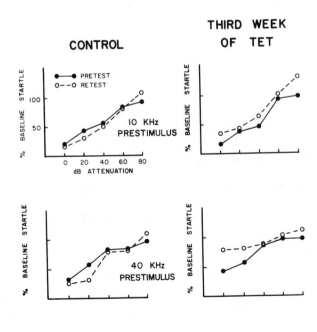

Fig. 2.4 Startle reflex inhibition to pure tones before treatment (*solid lines*) and during the third week of exposure to TET or paired water treatment (*dotted lines*). Data from TET-exposed rats are shown in the right panels, and data from paired-watered control subjects are shown in the left panels. In all cases reflex amplitude is decreased by increasing the intensity of the prestimulus (i.e., decreasing tone attenuation).

Acknowledgments

The authors wish to express their thanks to Angela James for her patience in preparing this manuscript and to their laboratory coworkers. In particular, Blair Miller, A. Gail Lee, and Tony Martin have provided invaluable help in collecting data and tracking down references. Dr. Fechter's work was supported by Research Career Development Award ES00125; Dr. Young's, by RO1-ES02852.

References

Adams, J., and Buelke-Sam, J. 1981. Behavioral assessment of the postnatal animal: Testing and methods development. In *Developmental toxicology,* edited by C. A. Kimmel and J. Buelke-Sam, 233–58. New York: Raven Press.

Alarie, Y. C. 1966. Irritating properties of airborne materials to the upper respiratory tract. *Arch. Environ. Health* 13:433–49.

———. 1973. Sensory irritation of the upper airways by airborne chemicals. *Toxicol. Appl. Pharmacol.* 24:279–97.

Alarie, Y. C., and Anderson, R. C. 1979. Toxicologic and acute lethal hazard evaluation of thermal decomposition products of synthetic and natural polymers. *Toxicol. Appl. Pharmacol.* 51:341–62.

Altman, J., and Sudarshan, K. 1975. Postnatal development of locomotion in the laboratory rat. *Anim. Behav.* 23:896–920.

Anderson, H., and Wedenberg, E. 1965. A new method for hearing tests in the guinea pigs. *Acta Otolaryngol.* 60:375–93.

Arlien-Soborg, P.; Zilstorff, K.; Grandjean, B.; and Pedersen, L. M. 1981. Vestibular dysfunction in occupational chronic solvent intoxication. *Clin. Otolaryngol.* 6:285–290.

Aschan, G.; Bunnfors, I.; Hyden, D.; Larsby, B.; Odkvist, L. M.; and Tham, R. 1977. Xylene exposure. *Acta Otolaryngol.* 84:370–76.

Astbury, P. J., and Read, N. G. 1982. Kanamycin induced ototoxicity in the laboratory rat. *Arch. Toxicol.* 50:267–78.

Aursnes, J. 1981. Vestibular damage from chlorhexidine in guinea pigs. *Acta Otolaryngol.* 92:89–100.

Baarsma, E. A., and Rijntjes, E. 1979. Vestibulo-toxicity of tobramycin. *J. Laryngol. Otol.* 93:725–27.

Baird, J. R. C., and Carter, A. J. 1979. Tests for effects of drugs on hearing and balance—A screen for assessing the ototoxic potential of aminoglycoside antibiotics. *Pharmacol. Ther.* 5:579–83.

Beecher, H. K. 1957. The measurement of pain. *Pharmacol. Rev.* 9:59–207.

Biscaldi, G. P.; Mingardi, M.; Pollini, G.; Moglia, A.; and Bossi, M. C. 1981. Acute toluene poisoning. Electrophysiological and vestibular investigations. *Toxicol. Eur. Res.* 3:271–73.

Blair, S. M., and Gavin, M. 1979. Modifications of vestibulo-ocular reflex induced by diazepam. *Arch. Otolaryngol.* 105:698–701.

Bobbin, R. P.; Gonzalez, G.; and Guth, P. S. 1969. Effects of aminooxyacetic acid on cochlear potentials and the Preyer reflex. *Nature* 223:70–71.

Borg, E., and Engstrom, B. 1982. Acoustic reflex after experimental lesions to inner and outer hair cells. *Hear. Res.* 6:25–34.

Brown, R. D., and Wood, C. C. 1980. Vestibular pharmacology. *Trends Pharmacol. Sci.,* 150–53.

Butcher, R. E., and Vorhees, C. V. 1979. A preliminary test battery for the investigation of the behavioral teratology of selected psychotropic drugs. *Neurobehav. Toxicol.* 1, suppl. 1:207–12.

Conquet, P.; Tardieu, M.; and Durand, G. 1979. Evaluation of ocular reflexes during toxicity studies. *Pharmacol. Ther.* 5:585–91.

Davey, P. G.; Harpur, E. S.; Jabeen, F.; Shannon, D.; and Shenoi, P. M. 1982. Variability and habituation of nystagmic responses to hot caloric stimulation of normal subjects. *J. Laryngol. Otol.* 96:599–612.

Davis, M. 1980. Neurochemical modulation of sensory-motor reactivity: Acoustic and tactile startle reflexes. *Neurosci. Biobehav. Rev.* 4:241–63.

Davis, M., and Aghajanian, G. K. 1976. Effects of apomorphine and haloperidol on the acoustic startle response in rats. *Psychopharmacology* 47:27–233.

Davis, M., and Astrachan, D. I. 1981. Spinal modulation of acoustic startle: Opposite effects of clonidine and d-amphetamine. *Psychopharmacology* 75:219–25.

Davis, M.; Astrachan, D. I.; and Kass, E. 1980. Excitatory and inhibitory effects of serotonin on sensory motor reactivity measured with acoustic startle. *Science* 209:521–23.

Davis, M., Cedarbaum, J. M.; Aghajanian, G. K.; and Gendelman, D. S. 1977. Effects of clonidine on habituation and sensitization of acoustic startle in normal decerebrate and locus coeruleus-lesioned rats. *Psychopharmacology* 51:243–53.

Davis, M., and Sheard, M. H. 1974. Habituation and sensitization of the rat startle response: Effects of raphe lesions. *Physiol. Behav.* 5:425–31.

———. 1976. p-chloroamphetamine (PCA): Acute and chronic effects of habituation and sensitization of the acoustic startle response. *Eur. J. Pharmacol.* 35:261–73.

Davis, M., and Sollberger, A. 1971. Twenty-four hour periodicity of the startle response in rats. *Psychon. Sci.* 25:37–39.

Davis, M.; Svensson, T. H.; and Aghajanian, G. K. 1975. Effects of d- and l-amphetamine in rats. *Psychopharmacologia* 43:1–11.

English, H. B., and English, A. C. 1958. *A comprehensive dictionary of psychological and psycho-analytic terms.* New York: Longmans.

Fechter, L. D. 1974a. The effects of l-dopa, clonidine and apormorphine on the acoustic startle reaction in rats. *Psychopharmacologia* 39:331–34.

———. 1974b. Central serotonin involvement in the elaboration of the startle reaction in rats. *Pharmacol. Biochem. Behav.* 2:161–71.

Fechter, L. D., and Annau, Z. 1980. Prenatal carbon monoxide exposure alters behavioral development. *Neurobehav. Toxicol.* 2:7–11.

Fechter, L. D., and Ison, J. R. 1972. The inhibition of the acoustic startle reaction in rats by food and water deprivation. *Learn. Motiv.* 3:109–24.

Fechter, L. D., and Young, J. S. 1983. Discrimination of auditory from nonauditory toxicity by reflex modulation audiometry: Effects of triethyltin. *Toxicol. Appl. Pharmacol.* 70:216–27.

Gavin, M., and Blair, S. 1981. Modification of the macaque's vestibulo-ocular reflex by picrotoxin. *Arch. Otolaryngol.* 107:372–76.

Graham, F. 1975. The more or less startling effects of weak prestimuli. *Psychophysiology* 12:238–48.

Hammond, G. 1973. Lesions of pontine and medullary reticular formation and prestimulus inhibition of the acoustic startle reaction in rats. *Physiol. Behav.* 10:239–43.

Hammond, G. R., and Thomas, G. J. 1971. Failure to reactivate the septal syndrome in rats. *Physiol. Behav.* 6:599–601.

Harpur, E. S. 1974. The effect of ototoxic drugs on the acoustic startle reaction of the rat. *Brit. J. Pharmacol.* 52:137.

Hawkins, J. E., Jr., and Preston, R. E. 1975. Vestibular ototoxicity. In Naunton, *The vestibular system,* 321–49.

Hayes, D., and Jerger, J. 1981. Patterns of acoustic reflex and auditory brainstem abnormality. *Acta Otolaryngol.* 92:199–209.

Hoffman, H. S., and Ison, J. R. 1980. Reflex modification in the domain of startle: I. Some empirical findings and their implications for how the nervous system processes sensory input. *Psychol. Rev.* 87:175–89.

Hoffman, H. S., and Searle, J. L. 1965. Acoustic variables in the modification of startle reaction in the rat. *J. Comp. Physiol. Psychol.* 60:53–58.

Hoffman, H. S., and Wible, B. L. 1970. Role of weak signals in acoustic startle. *J. Acoust. Soc. Am.* 47:489–97.

Horlington, M. 1970. Startle response circadian rhythm in rats: Lack of correlation with motor activity. *Physiol. Behav.* 5:49–53.

Ison, J. R. 1982. Temporal acuity in auditory function in the rat: Reflex inhibition by brief gaps in noise. *J. Comp. Physiol. Psychol.* 96:945–54.

Ison, J. R., and Hammond, G. R. 1971. Modification of the startle reflex in the rat by changes in the auditory and visual environments. *J. Comp. Physiol. Psychol.* 75:435–52.

Ison, J. R., and Hoffman, H. S. 1983. Reflex modification in the domain of startle: II. The anomalous history of a robust and ubiquitous phenomenon. *Psychol. Bull.* 94:3–17.

Ison, J. R., and Leonard, D. W. 1971. Effects of auditory stimuli on the amplitude of the nictitating membrane reflex of the rabbit (*Oryctolagus cuniculus*). *J. Comp. Physiol. Psychol.* 75:157–64.

Ison, J. R., and Pinckney, L. A. 1983. Reflex inhibition in humans: Sensitivity to brief silent periods in white noise. *Percept. Psychophysics* 34:84–88.

Ison, J. R.; Reiter, L. A.; and Warren, M. 1979. Modulation of the acoustic startle reflex in humans in the absence of anticipatory changes in the middle ear reflex. *J. Exp. Psychol.: Human Perception and Performance* 5 (1):639–42.

Jerger, J.; Mauldin, L.; and Igarashi, M. 1978. Impedance audiometry in the squirrel monkey. *Arch. Otolaryngol.* 104:559–63.

Jongkees, L. B. W. 1975. On the physiology and the examination of the vestibular labyrinths. In Naunton, *The vestibular system*, 227–47.

Kehne, J. H., and Sorenson, C. A. 1978. The effects of pimozide and phenoxybenzamine pretreatments of amphetamine and apomorphine potentiation of the acoustic startle response in rats. *Psychopharmacology* 58:137–44.

Kellogg, C.; Ison, J. R.; and Miller, R. K. 1983. Prenatal diazepam exposure: Effects of auditory temporal resolution in rats. *Psychopharmacology* 79:332–37.

Kelly, J. B., and Masterton, B. 1977. Auditory sensitivity of the albino rat. *J. Comp. Physiol. Psychol.* 91:930–36.

Kemble, E. D., and Ison, J. R. 1971. Limbic lesions and the inhibition of startle reactions in the rat by conditions of preliminary stimulation. *Physiol. Behav.* 7:925–28.

Kokkinidis, L., and Anisman, H. 1978. Involvement of norepinephrine in startle arousal after acute and chronic d-amphetamine administration. *Psychopharmacology* 59:285–92.

Krauter, E. E. 1973. Inhibition of the human eyeblink by a brief acoustic stimulus. *J. Comp. Physiol. Psychol.* 84:246–51.

Krauter, E. E.; Leonard, D. W.; and Ison, J. R. 1973. Inhibition of the human eyeblink by a brief acoustic stimulus. *J. Comp. Physiol. Psychol.* 84:246–51.

Larsby, B.; Tham, R.; Odkvist, L. M.; Hyden, D.; Bunnfors, I.; and Aschan, G. 1978. Exposure of rabbits to styrene. *Scand. J. Work Environ. Health* 4:60–65.

Lerner, S. A.; Seligsohn, R.; and Matz, G. J. 1977. Comparative clinical studies of ototoxicity and nephrotoxicity of amikacin and gentamicin. *Am. J. Med.* 62:919–23.

Levett, J., and Jerger, R. 1980. Effects of alcohol on retinal potentials, eye movements, accommodation, and the pupillary light reflex. In *Neurotoxicity of the visual system*, edited by W. H. Merigan and B. Weiss, 87–100. New York: Raven Press.

McCabe, B. F. 1976. Experimental methods in vestibular research. In *Handbook of auditory and vestibular research methods*, edited by C. A. Smith and J. A. Vernon, 551–82. Springfield, Ill.: Charles C Thomas.

McCabe, B. F.; Sekitani, T.; and Ryu, J. H. 1973. Drug effects on postlabyrinthectomy nystagmus. *Arch. Otolaryngol.* 98:310–13.

Mathog, R. H., and Capps, M. J. 1977. Ototoxic interactions of ethacrynic acid and streptomycin. *Ann. Otol.* 86:158–63.

Meyerson, B. S., and Eliasson, M. 1977. The effects of lysergic acid diethylamide on copulatory behavior in the female rat. *Neuropharmacology* 16:37.

Naunton, R. F., ed. 1975. *The vestibular system.* New York: Academic Press.

Nordstrom, L.; Christensson, P.; Haeger, K.; Juhlin, I.; Tjerristrom, O.; and Waalmar, E. 1979. Netilmicin: Clinical evaluation of efficacy and toxicity of a new aminoglycoside. *J. Int. Med. Res.* 7:117–26.

Parisi, T., and Ison, J. R. 1981. Ontogeny of control over the acoustic startle reflex by visual stimulation in the rat. *Dev. Psychobiol.* 14:311–16.

Prazma, J. 1981. Ototoxicity of aminoglycoside antibiotics. In *Pharmacology of hearing,* edited by R. D. Brown, 153–95. New York: Wiley.

Proctor, L. R. 1975. Testing the vestibular system: Value of the caloric test. In Naunton, *The vestibular system,* 249–60.

Reiter, L. A.; Goetzinger, C. P.; and Press, S. E. 1980. Reflex modulation: A hearing test for the difficult-to-test. *J. Speech Hear. Disord.* 24:262–66.

Reiter, L. A., and Ison, J. R. 1977. Inhibition of the human eyeblink reflex: An evaluation of the sensitivity of the Wendt-Yerkes method for threshold detection. *J. Exp. Psychol.: Human Perception and Performance* 3:325–36.

Reiter, L. A.; Kidd, K.; Heavner, G.; and Ruppert, P. 1980. Behavioral toxicity of acute and subacute exposure to triethyltin in the rat. *Neurotoxicology* 2:97–112.

Russo, J. M. 1980. *Sensation in the rat and mouse: Evaluation by reflex modification.* Ph.D. diss. University of Rochester. Dissertation Abstracts International, 41/01-B,392.

Schuknecht, H. F. 1975. Electronystagmography: A round table discussion. In Naunton, *The vestibular system,* 261–95.

Squibb, R. E.; Carmichael, G.; and Tilson, H. A. 1980. Behavioral and neuromorphological effects of triethyl tin bromide. *Toxicol. Appl. Pharmacol.* 55:88–197.

Stitt, C. L.; Hoffman, H. S.; Marsh, R. R.; and Schwartz, G. M. 1976. Modification of the pigeon's visual startle reaction by the sensory environment. *J. Comp. Physiol. Psychol.* 90(7):601–19.

Storm, J. E.; Hulebak, K. L.; and Fechter, L. D. 1981. Modification of acoustic startle reflex amplitude by background level and prestimuli in two strains for mice. *Soc. Neurosci. Abs.* 7:658.

Storm, J. E.; Millington, W. R.; and Fechter, L. D. 1984. Diethyldithiocarbamate depresses the acoustic startle response in rats. *Psychopharmacology* 82:68–72.

Tham, R.; Larsby, B.; Ericksson, B.; Bunnfors, I.; Odkvist, L.; and Liedgren, C. 1982. Electronystagmographic findings in rats exposed to styrene or toluene. *Acta Otolaryngol.* 93:107–12.

Tilson, H. A.; Mactutus, C. F.; McLamb, R. L.; and Burne, T. A. 1982. Characterization of triethyl lead chloride neurotoxicity in adult rats. *Neurobehav. Toxicol. Teratol.* 4:671–81.

Tinbergen, N. 1951. *The study of instincts.* Oxford: Clarendon Press.

———. 1952. The curious behavior of stickle back. *Scientific American* 187:22–26.

Tolman, E. C. 1932. *Purposive behavior in animals and man.* New York: Appleton.

Uhlrich, D. 1984. Spatial vision in humans assessed by inhibition of the blink reflex. *Eastern Psychol. Assoc.* 55:99.

Weiss, B., and Laties, G. 1970. The psychophysics of pain and analgesia in animals. In *Animal Psychophysics,* edited by W. Stebbins, 185–210. New York: Appleton-Century-Crofts.

Wersäl, J. 1980. The ototoxic potentials of netilmicin compared with amikacin. *Scand. J. Infect. Dis.,* suppl. 23:104–13.

Winkel, O.; Hansen, M. M.; Kaaber, K.; and Rozarth, K. 1978. A prospective study of gentamicin ototoxicity. *Acta Otolaryngol.* 86:212–16.

Yerkes, R. M. 1905. The sense of hearing in frogs. *J. Comp. Neurol. Psychol.* 15:279–304.

Yoburn, B. C.; Morales, R.; Kelley, D. D.; and Inturrisi, C. E. 1984. Constraints on the tailflick assay: Morphine analgesia and tolerance are dependent upon locus of tail stimulation. *Life Sci.* 34:1755–62.

Young, J. S., and Fechter, L. D. 1983. Reflex inhibition procedures for animals audiometry: A technique for assessing ototoxicity. *J. Acoust. Soc. Am.* 73:1686–93.

Zagon, I. S., and McLaughlin, P. J. 1982. Analgesia in young and adult rats perinatally exposed to methadone. *Neurobehav. Toxicol. Teratol.* 4:455–57.

Stata Norton

3

Observational Methods

Observational methods in behavioral toxicology, like those in pharmacology, have been used for several reasons. The methods often are easy to perform and do not require elaborate equipment. The degree of training or manipulation of the test animal is usually minimal. Some observational methods can be performed under circumstances where other types of tests are impossible. The most important reason is that observational tests measure unique or important aspects of the behavioral repertoire of a species.

Observational methods have assumed a greater role in toxicology than in behavioral pharmacology for some of the reasons listed above. In a chronic toxicity study, for example, there is an obvious advantage in using an observational method if the animals can be tested without being disturbed and if the method is reliable and sensitive. The latter two issues—reliability and sensitivity—are important in the evaluation of any test; unfortunately, data on these aspects are often lacking. Because there is concern for developing noninvasive methods for evaluation of toxicity from environmental or industrial exposure to chemicals, behavioral methods are being analyzed for sensitivity and reliability.

The value of observational tests in behavioral toxicology depends on the quantitative nature of the results. If behavior is observed, some permanent record must be obtained in order to evaluate the results. If the variability in repeated tests is low, the test is reproducible. If the test detects small differences in dose or duration of exposure to a toxic substance, the test is sensitive. Reliability in terms of false positives or negatives can be determined for known compounds. The meaning of the results in terms of central nervous system (CNS) actions and extrapolation to other species remains to be determined. Although considerable effort has been devoted to establishing the morphological, physiological, or biochemical bases of specific behaviors, it is safe to say that no definitive connection has been established between any complex behavior and the other parameters. Thus, in terms of CNS action of a toxic agent the meaning of all behavioral tests is in doubt.

Observational tests may be performed using animals of any age, but observational methods are particularly valuable in the study of neonates and young in the early postnatal period. In many species, such as the rat, conditioned behavioral tests are rarely attempted before weaning. The effective tests in neonates depend on observations of various behaviors, generally with behavior structured by simple environmental modifications. In studies involving animals in the juvenile or adult stage, many observational methods are based on structuring activity by control of spatial characteristics of the test environment. Other types of observational tests are designed to evaluate sensorimotor performance. A third group involves social behavior.

Juvenile and Adult Tests

Spatially Oriented Locomotion

Several of the oldest observational tests involve an environment in which the activity of an animal is recorded as it moves from place to place. The spatial arrangement may be intended to either stimulate or inhibit locomotion. Therefore, although locomotion may be a similar phenomenon in animals, the basis for locomotor behaviors in different environments and the effect of toxic agents may be different in the different tests. For example, diminished locomotor ability in response to a toxic agent would be expected to be more apparent under conditions when an animal is most active. In this case changes in activity might be more revealing than gait analysis. Changes in gait may be due to damage to the peripheral neuromuscular apparatus or to central effects on the cerebellum, the striatonigral pathway, or ascending sensory or descending motor tracts. Changes in locomotion in the open field or radial arm maze may be due to peripheral weakness or to actions on complex behaviors involving interpretation of the environment.

Gait analysis. Some years ago cerebellar ataxia was measured in young children by recording gait from inked feet. Rushton, Steinberg, and Tinson (1963) adapted this method to rats, using petroleum jelly and carbon black to record footprints. The method, this time with inked footprints, has been used to analyze the hopping gait of prenatally irradiated rats (Mullenix, Norton, and Culver 1975), the halting gait of rats treated perinatally with a goitrogen (Comer and Norton 1985), and the wide-based gait of another biped, the chicken, exposed in ovo to neurotoxic substances (Newby-Schmidt and Norton 1981; Norton and Sheets 1983).

Variability in results with the test is reduced if the foot-placement patterns are obtained as the animal walks along a corridor, which reduces lateral movement, if the home cage is placed at the far end of the corridor, if the animal is given three trials to traverse the corridor before the feet are inked for recording gait, and if data for at least six consecutive steps are obtained. For quadrupeds, only the hind feet are recorded. The method detects both acute effects on gait from pharmacological agents and chronic damage to gait from exposure to toxic agents. Various points in the neuromuscular system may be the site of action, from the peripheral neuromuscular junction to CNS damage, possibly as high as the anterior commissure (Mullenix, Norton, and Culver 1975). Although different patterns of gait abnormality have been found following the use of different agents, as noted above, anatomical correlations need to be worked out.

Open field. Probably the most widely used observational test is the open field. Its popularity derives more from the simplicity of the apparatus and method than from the sensitivity or reproducibility of the test. The test has been automated, and devices are available that record locomotion, rearing, and even grooming as separate acts. The animal, usually a rat, is placed in the center of the field, and the number of squares crossed in a limited time is recorded. The environment tends to inhibit behavior, since rats prefer to move in closed corridors and in dim lighting. A careful review of the type of data obtained using the open-field test has been published (Walsh and Cummins 1976). Examples of the use of the test in toxicology can be found in reports by Reiter et al. (1975), Butcher and Vorhees (1979), and Comer and Norton (1982). One modification in recording open-field data has been proposed. The amount of time an animal spends touching or close to the wall around the open field has been termed *barrier-directed behavior*. In addition to increasing locomotor activity, amphetamine has been shown to increase this behavior (Heimstra 1962). The generality of increases in barrier-directed behavior in response to increases in other behaviors has not been reported.

Hole-board exploration. In 1975 File and Wardill reported that head dipping into holes in a board was a measure of "exploratory behavior." This spatial modification of the open field into an open area with uniformly spaced holes increased the complexity of the open-field environment. Barrier-directed behavior decreased in this environment, and exploration of the entire field increased. The usual measure in this test was observation of the number of attempts at exploring by dipping the nose or head in the holes. Hyperactivity from amphetamine can be detected (Kokkinidis and Zacharko 1980; Daughtrey and Norton 1983), but the method has not been widely used with toxic agents.

Olton maze. An environment that encourages exploration has been proposed by Olton, Walker, and Gage (1978). The spatial arrangement of corridors in the device resembles spokes of a wheel, and the sequence of entering or exploring these corridors is recorded. Hippocampal lesions (Olton, Walker, and Gage 1978) and exposure to trimethyl tin (Walsh, Miller, and Dyer 1982) have been shown to affect exploration of the Olton maze by rodents. It has been suggested that the sequence of a complex space may be a measure of perseveration in that rats with some types of brain damage are less hesitant than control rats. Perseveration from early undernutrition (Jordan, Howells, and Cane 1980) and hypothyroidism (Comer and Norton 1985) has been discussed in recent publications. The relation to similar activity in other environments, for example, to the type of perseveration developed in the Hebb-Williams maze as reported for rats exposed to trimethyl tin (Swartzwelder et al. 1982), needs to be considered. Parallel results from different tests using the same chemical, as shown by Walsh, Miller, and Dyer (1982) and Swartzwelder et al. (1982) for trimethyl tin, are important for developing generalizations regarding the reliability of the behavioral tests, as well as for detecting toxic effects of chemicals.

Home cage activity. The diurnal cycle of activity displayed by rodents, consisting of a marked increase during the nocturnal period and relative inactivity during the diurnal period, in the home cage has been measured by various sensing devices: photocells, infrared sensors, and radio-frequency recorders. A simple, observational method of analysis of home cage activity based on time sampling can be carried out (Bindra and Baron 1959). At repeated uniform intervals the location of the animal is recorded. An estimate of amount of movement and frequency of certain behaviors can be obtained. This time-sampling observational method, while possessing the merit of identifying certain frequent behaviors as well as activity, has been supplanted by automated devices for recording diurnal-cycle activity. Depending on the toxic agent and the experimental design, residential activity of animals may be greater or less (Reiter 1977; Reiter and MacPhail 1979) than activity in a novel environment.

Behavior sequences. When an animal is placed in a new environment, several different behavioral acts are displayed. The behavior of the rat, for example, consists of various locomotor acts (e.g., walking, turning, rearing, or hopping), grooming behaviors (e.g., sitting and rubbing forepaws on face or grooming body with mouth and paws), and exploratory head movements while standing (e.g., sniffing, looking, or turning head from side to side). The sequence of production of these behaviors is not random but highly structured (Norton 1977). With repeated exposures or habituation to the environment, the degree of structure increases as activity decreases (Norton 1976). Chemicals and brain lesions, which result in hyperactivity by various methods of measurement, increase the degree of randomness in the sequences of behavioral acts. Increased activity is also associated with shortened duration of most behavioral acts (Norton, Mullenix, and Culver 1976). Although increased randomness of behavior and decreased duration of acts constitute the most uniform effects associated with behavioral "hyperactivity," the phenomenon takes its name from the shift from a predominance of static acts (sitting, standing, etc.) to an increase in movement (walking, rearing, etc.). The shift in amount of these acts is easier to observe (and easier to record) than the more complicated effects on sequence and duration of acts. Significant changes in sequences of behavior have been demonstrated from film or video records of rats following prenatal exposure to X-rays (Schneider and Norton 1979) or prenatal phenytoin (Mullenix, Tassinari, and Keith 1983). Postnatal exposure to thallium (Brown et al. 1984) or lead (Callahan et al. 1985) has also been reported to alter behavior patterns.

Tests of Sensorimotor Performance

Observational methods are particularly effective in measuring some types of sensorimotor performance. The tests can detect damage to the sensory and motor pathways involved in balancing. One condition common to these tests is that there is a marked degree of *learning*, or improvement of performance, with repeated tests. This may increase design complexity for tests of acute toxic effects and is easier to control in conditions of chronic damage.

Rotarod performance. One of the early uses of the rotarod was in evaluation of CNS depressant drugs (Kinnard and Carr 1957). The animals, usually rats, maintain balance on a rotating rod. Length of time on the rod may be measured during a period of standard rotation speed. Another endpoint, the speed of rotation at which balance is lost, may be recorded. Acrylamide is a classic example of a chemical that produces measurable effects in this test. The delayed neuropathy resulting from acrylamide includes muscle weakness, and rotarod performance is altered increasingly with increased doses (Kaplan and Murphy 1972). The classic rotarod method has been modified to measure the maximum speed at which a mouse can maintain balance (Christensen 1973). Performance of rats on an accelerating rod has been compared with performance on the standard rotarod (Bogo, Hill, and Young 1981). In the latter study, Bogo, Hill, and Young concluded that the accelerating-rod test detected lower doses of acrylamide (chronic) and ethanol (acute) than tests using the standard rotarod.

Balancing rods. Rats can be trained to negotiate a path consisting of narrow rods in order to reach food or a home cage. The ability to balance on a narrow rod—for example, a rod about 15 mm wide—develops gradually in the postnatal period (Altman and Sudarshan 1975). The method has not been widely used since its publication, probably because more common tests of visual-motor performance provide similar results. Sterman and Sheppard (1972) have used this test to detect 2,5-hexanedione neuropathy.

Tests Involving Social Behaviors

A number of observational methods are available that monitor selected social behaviors. A recent review on pharmacological tests is available (McGuire, Raleigh, and Brammer 1982). Social interactions are not necessarily more complex than behavioral acts of isolated animals, but since the social behaviors of pairs or groups involve the actions of more than one animal, the sources of variability may be increased. Whether the purpose of study of a behavior is to relate function (behavior) to the mechanism of action of a toxic agent or to establish the relative potency of two substances, variability is an important consideration. Some of the environmental conditions affecting the reproducibility of social interactions in rats, such as isolation prior to testing, light intensity during observation, and familiarity with the environment, have been considered (Niesink and van Ree 1983). Other factors affecting variability are related to the spatial environment itself. Residential mazes, with corridors resembling natural burrows, result in reliable activity levels, probably because the spatial arrangement structures behavior strongly. An example of social interaction in this environment is the dramatic increase in the activity of a naive rat when a second rat is placed in a residential maze (Reiter 1978).

Social interaction and isolation. As noted above, acute isolation in a novel environment decreases activity over the activity when a conspecific is present. Isolation prior to testing for different times has an additional effect on activity. Short-term isolation, for several days, increases social interaction with conspecifics (Niesink and van Ree 1982) and long-term isolation, for weeks or months, has effects on many social behaviors, including gregariousness (Latane et al. 1970), aggressive behavior (Valzelli 1969), and mating behavior (Hansen 1978).

Gregariousness, aggressive behaviors, and mating behaviors. Studies of social behaviors of the three types—gregariousness or conspecific investigation, aggressive behaviors, and mating behaviors—can be carried out by direct observation and a manual recording device. The behaviors are identified as separate acts. Descriptions of acts have been published for some species (Barnett 1958; Grant 1963; Richardson, Karczmar, and Scudder 1972; Norton 1976; Ciaccio, Lisk, and Reuter 1979; Lanier, Estep, and Dewsbury 1979). Sometimes a time-sampling method is used, particularly when direct observation is chosen (see, for example, Ellison 1976). The preferred method is to identify behaviors from film (Norton 1976) or videotape (Niesink and van Ree 1982). Behaviors are recorded for 5 to 15 min. Although frequency or number of behavioral acts is the usual measure, duration and sequences of acts can be determined (Norton 1977).

Some use has been made of social behaviors triggered by acute isolation from a group. These are particularly evident in young animals (Elliott and Scott 1961). One of the most reliable behaviors for study of isolated animals is isolation-induced vocalizations by chicks within 24 to 48 hrs of hatching (Panksepp et al. 1980; Newby-Schmidt and Norton 1983).

Few data address directly the relative sensitivity of social behaviors to toxic agents compared with other behavioral tests. Philosophically, there is reason to study social behaviors in conditions of acute or chronic exposure to toxic agents. As has been suggested by others (McGuire, Raleigh, and Brammer 1982), human exposure and subsequent adaptation to damage occur in a social context, and we do not know enough about potential interactions of the in vivo system with toxic substances and the environment.

Tests of Neonatal Behaviors

There is increasing interest in the consequences to the developing nervous system of exposure to toxic agents during the fetal period. These tests are of particular interest in toxicology because of concern for effects on fetal development in the presence of maternal exposure to toxic substances. There are two aspects to be considered. One is the sensitivity of the immature nervous system relative to the adult. It is possible, even probable, that the immature system is less well protected than the adult from those agents that readily cross living membranes, such as the placenta. The other consideration is the ability of the developing system to repair or compensate for damage. Depending on the developmental stage at which exposure occurs, the immature system may be less or more vulnerable than the adult. Although the neonate may seem to be a poor subject for behavioral analysis, particularly in species like the rat, which is born at an immature stage, several tests have been devised. All the tests are observational and depend on the ability of the very young mammal to respond to certain environmental stimuli.

Motor Behaviors Requiring Sensorimotor Coordination

In the early postnatal period the number of behaviors that an animal must perform is limited. The behaviors appear to be reflexive in nature; that is, they habituate slowly, if at all, occur on the first presentation of the stimulus, and, within the limits of motor ability, are performed as a complete act.

Surface righting. When neonatal rats are removed from the nest and turned on their backs, they attempt to right themselves. Control rats require an average of about 20 sec to assume a quadrupedal position within 24 hrs after birth. There is progressively more rapid righting with age, and by the tenth postnatal day the time stabilizes at about 1 sec. This test is sensitive to various toxic agents, administered to the mother (Brunner et al. 1978). A dramatic delay in development of the reflex is produced by exposing the mother to a goitrogen, methimazole, during the perinatal period (Comer and Norton 1982).

Reflex suspension. From about the seventh postnatal day, rat pups will attempt to suspend themselves by their forepaws when they are placed where they can grasp a small rod using no other support. The suspension time rises from about 5 sec to 30 sec by the end of the second postnatal week. Like surface righting, this test has been used to demonstrate developmental delay from perinatal exposure to toxic substances (Vorhees et al. 1979; Comer and Norton 1982; Daughtrey and Norton 1983).

Both surface righting and reflex suspension measure motor ability as well as a sensory component that orients the rat pup to the test environment and triggers the response. These seem to be among the simplest tests for atricial neonates. Some other, more complex behaviors have been studied, and tests have been devised for them.

Complex Behaviors Developed in the Early Postnatal Period

Some behaviors that require that the animal be able to walk have been used to monitor damage from exposure to toxic substances in the early postnatal period.

Negative geotaxis. Placing a rat pup in the early postnatal period head downward on a screen set at a 25–30° angle from the horizontal acts as a powerful stimulus that causes the animal to climb in a half-circle on the screen in order to orient with its head up. This response to gravity requires good motor control as well as integration with several sensory modalities. Some rat pups are able to complete this maneuver by the fifth postnatal day. The speed of performance improves rapidly over the next few days, as does the number of pups able to complete the turn in 120 seconds (Altman and Sudarshan 1975). Gestational exposure to some toxic agents can modify this ability (Butcher and Vorhees 1979).

Nursing behavior. Litters of nursing rats or other mammals can be observed using a time-sampling method for recording nursing (based on location of young on the mother) and arousal (eyes open or closed). It is likely that the frequency of nursing behaviors and arousal recorded in the early postnatal period for rat pups correlates with activity observed in the open field (Culver and Norton 1976).

Open field. Young animals can be tested in a miniaturized open field as soon as they can crawl. For the rat this is about the end of the first postnatal week (Culver and Norton 1976).

Conclusions

Observational behavioral methods are of particular interest in toxicology because they generally require the least manipulation of the animal in behavioral tests. Many tests begun as observational tests have proved so useful that they have been automated, and the test animals no longer need to be directly observed. Examples are numerous in tests measuring locomotor activity, such as open fields and residential mazes. There are both gains and losses with automation. The main gain is that the behavior can be recorded for long periods, and circadian rhythms can be obtained. A minor gain is in accuracy of recording with automation. The main loss is the isolation of the animal from the skilled observer, so that unique effects of an experiment cannot be detected. A machine does not generate ideas that can be proposed for subsequent exploration but only records the behavior that it was designed to record.

The issue of subjectivity in observation of animal behavior has sometimes been raised. The issue is really reliability and reproducibility, important considerations in any method or experiment. Data from observational tests are most reproducible when a permanent record is examined by one or more observers who are not aware of the treatment of the animals. Reproducibility is evaluated by repeated experiments. It is best if similar experiments are carried out by different laboratories.

Some behavioral tests have been used enough that the scientific literature offers information on reproducibility. A recent paper offers a detailed analysis of one behavioral test (Reiter 1983). Reliability of most observational methods needs additional attention. For example, the variability of the open-field test under different experimental conditions is well known (see Reiter and MacPhail 1979). This variability may sometimes preclude satisfactory evaluation of data. One recent use of the open field for behavioral evaluation in toxicology gives an example (Del Vecchio and Rahwan 1984).

One issue in many observational tests that often is not recognized is that there is a testable assumption underlying many of the methods. The assumption is that behavior consists of separate acts or units that can be identified in the continuous production of behavior. This issue is important and needs to be understood in order to eliminate subjective interpretation in observation of behavior. The basic unit of observed motor acts in animals is a brief sequence of motor acts that occur together with a probability approaching one. Such acts are kicking, biting, rearing, walking, grooming, and so on. An extension of the basic unit to groups of acts given labels, such as *aggression, investigation, dominance behavior,* and so on, may result in inaccurate definition. As long as the acts are accurately defined, the larger grouping can also be accurately defined. If, however, alteration of frequency or duration of one unit act of the group is used as a measure of increase in the group as a whole, this may lead to considerable increase in uncertainty of meaning. For example, if *aggression* is defined under condition A as a combination of kicking and biting, and kicking increases under condition B but biting does not, has aggression increased? An even more questionable interpretation of observed behavior may result from equating a word defined by one group of acts with the same word applied to another group of acts. Again, let us use *aggression* as an example, this time of a word that may be applied to groups of different acts in different species (see Scott 1966 for a review of the many phenomena included in the term *aggression*). Obviously, the use of the same word based on different unit behaviors leads to uncertain interpretation. The complexity of many behavioral phenomena must be understood before attempting seriously to translate toxicological results in one animal species to another, including man.

One reason for emphasizing the need for precise definition in recording observed behavior is that a major step in toxicology would be achieved if changes in specific behavioral acts were equated with damage to specific brain parameters following exposure to toxic agents. In this, toxicology differs from pharmacology. Most drugs cause reversible changes, by design, in behavior and leave no residual damage. On the other hand, toxic agents are of particular concern because irreversible damage may accompany serious exposure. Accumulation of precise toxicological data may lead to improved understanding of CNS function.

Observational behavior methods, as defined and described here, range from technically simple to difficult. The qualities of sensitivity for detection of behavioral effects of toxic substances, reliability and reproducibility, vary with the different tests. A common quality is that less manipulation of the test animal is required than in many tests using conditioned behavior. Finally, observation of animals exposed to toxic substances should not be forgotten as a potential tool for developing new concepts or detecting unexpected changes that may lead to new scientific concepts.

References

Altman, J., and Sudarshan, K. 1975. Postnatal development of locomotion in the laboratory rat. *Anim. Behav.* 23:896–920.

Barnett, S. A. 1958. An analysis of social behaviour in wild rats. *Proc. Zool. Soc. Lond.* 130:107–52.

Bindra, D., and Baron, D. 1959. Effects of methylphenidylacetate and chlorpromazine on certain components of general activity. *J. Exp. Anal. Behav.* 2:343–50.

Bogo, V.; Hill, T. A.; and Young, R. W. 1981. Comparison of accelerod and rotarod sensitivity in detecting ethanol- and acrylamide-induced performance in rats: Review of experimental considerations of rotating rod systems. *Neurotoxicology* 2:765–87.

Brown, D. R.; Cleaves, M.; Schatz, R.; and Callahan, B. 1984. Comparison of metal neurotoxicity: Biochemical changes in brain regions and analysis of patterns of behavior. *Toxicologist* 4:120.

Brunner, R. L.; McLean, M.; Vorhees, C. V.; and Butcher, R. E. 1978. A comparison of behavioral and anatomical measures of hydroxyurea induced abnormalities. *Teratology* 18:379–84.

Butcher, R. E., and Vorhees, C. V. 1979. A preliminary test battery for the investigation of the behavioral teratology of selected psychotropic drugs. *Neurobehav. Toxicol.* 1, suppl. 1:207–12.

Callahan, B.; Brown, D.; Schatz, R.; and Cleaves, M. 1985. Regional and temporal selectivity of lead induced neurochemical changes in neonates: Correlation with behavioral abnormalities. *Toxicologist* 5:193.

Christensen, J. D. 1973. The rotacone: A new apparatus for measuring motor coordination in mice. *Acta Pharmacol. Toxicol.* 33:255–61.

Ciaccio, L. A.; Lisk, R. D.; and Reuter, L. A. 1979. Prelordotic behavior in the hamster: A hormonally modulated transition from aggression to sexual receptivity. *J. Comp. Physiol. Psychol.* 93:771–80.

Comer, C. P., and Norton, S. 1982. Effects of perinatal methimazole exposure on a developmental test battery for neurobehavioral toxicity in rats. *Toxicol. Appl. Pharmacol.* 63:133–41.

———. 1985. Behavioral consequences of perinatal hypothyroidism in postnatal and adult rats. *Pharmacol. Biochem. Behav.* 22:605–11.

Culver, B., and Norton, S. 1976. Juvenile hyperactivity in rats after acute exposure to carbon monoxide. *Exp. Neurol.* 50:80–98.

Daughtrey, W. C., and Norton, S. 1983. Caudate morphology and behavior of rats exposed to carbon monoxide *in utero. Exp. Neurol.* 80:265–68.

Del Vecchio, F. R., and Rahwan, R. G. 1984. Teratological evaluation of a novel antibortifacient, dibenzyloxyindanpropionic acid. II. Postnatal morphological and behavioral development. *Drug Chem. Toxicol.* 7:357–81.

Elliott, O., and Scott, J. P. 1961. The development of emotional distress reactions to separations in puppies. *J. Genet. Psychol.* 99:3–22.

Ellison, G. 1976. Monoamine neurotoxins: Selective and delayed effects on behavior in colonies of laboratory rats. *Brain Res.* 103:81–92.

File, S. E., and Wardill, A. G. 1975. Validity of head-dipping as a measure of exploration in a modified hole board. *Psychopharmacologia* 44:53–59.

Grant, A. C. 1963. An analysis of the social behaviour of the male laboratory rat. *Behaviour* 21:260–83.

Hansen, S. 1978. Mounting behavior and receptive behavior in developing female rats and the effect of social isolation. *Physiol. Behav.* 19:749–52.

Heimstra, N. W. 1962. Social influence on the response to drugs: I. Amphetamine sulfate. *J. Psychol.* 53:233–44.

Jordan, T. C.; Howells, K. F.; and Cane, S. E. 1980. Hippocampal and spatial memory deficits resulting from early undernutrition. In *Multidisciplinary approach to brain development*, edited by DiBenedetta, R. Balazs, G. Gombos, and G. Parcellati, 347–48. New York: Elsevier.

Kaplan, M., and Murphy, S. D. 1972. Effects of acrylamide on rotarod performance and sciatic nerve β-glucuronidase of rats. *Toxicol. Appl. Pharmacol.* 22:259–68.

Kinnard, W. J., Jr., and Carr, C. J. 1957. Preliminary procedure for the evaluation of central nervous system depressants. *J. Pharmacol. Exp. Ther.* 121:354–61.

Kokkinidis, L., and Zacharko, R. M. 1980. Intracranial self-stimulation in mice using a modified hole-board task: Effects of d-amphetamine. *Psychopharmacology* 68:169–71.

Lanier, D. L.; Estep, D. Q.; and Dewsbury, D. A. 1979. Role of prolonged copulatory behavior in facilitating reproductive success in a competitive mating situation in laboratory rats. *J. Comp. Physiol. Psychol.* 93:781–92.

Latane, B.; Cappell, H.; and Joy, V. 1970. Social deprivation, housing density and gregariousness in rats. *J. Comp. Physiol. Psychol.* 70:221–27.

McGuire, M. T.; Raleigh, M. J.; and Brammer, G. L. 1982. Sociopharmacology. *Annu. Rev. Pharmacol. Toxicol.* 22:643–61.

Mullenix, P.; Norton, S.; and Culver, B. 1975. Locomotor damage in rats after X-irradiation *in utero*. *Exp. Neurol.* 48:310–24.

Mullenix, P.; Tassinari, M. S.; and Keith, D. A. 1983. Behavioral outcome after prenatal exposure to phenytoin in rats. *Teratology* 27:149–57.

Newby-Schmidt, M. B., and Norton, S. 1981. Detection of subtle effects on the locomotor ability of the chicken. *Neurobehav. Toxicol. Teratol.* 3:45–48.

———. 1983. Drug withdrawal prior to hatch in the morphine tolerant chick embryo. *Pharmacol. Biochem. Behav.* 18:817–20.

Niesink, R. J. M., and van Ree, J. M. 1982. Short-term isolation increases social interactions of male rats: A parametric analysis. *Physiol. Behav.* 29:819–25.

———. 1983. Normalizing effect of an adrenocorticotropic hormone (4-9) analog ORG 2766 on disturbed social behavior in rats. *Science* 221:960–62.

Norton, S. 1976. Hyperactive behavior of rats after lesions of the globus pallidus. *Brain Res. Bull.* 1:193–202.

———. 1977. The study of sequences of motor behavior. In *Handbook of psychopharmacology*, vol. 7, edited by L. L. Iverson, S. D. Iverson, and S. H. Snyder, 83–105. London: Plenum Press.

Norton, S.; Mullenix, P.; and Culver, B. 1976. Comparison of the structure of hyperactive behavior in rats after brain damage from X-irradiation, carbon monoxide and pallidal lesions. *Brain Res.* 116:49–67.

Norton, S., and Sheets, L. 1983. Neuropathy in the chick from embryonic exposure to organophosphorus compounds. *NeuroToxicology* 4:137–42.

Olton, D. S.; Walker, J. A.; and Gage, F. H. 1978. Hippocampal connections and spatial discrimination. *Brain Res.* 139:295–308.

Panksepp, J.; Bean, N. G.; Bishop, P.; Vilberg, T.; and Sahley, T. L. 1980. Opioid blockage and social comfort in chicks. *Pharmacol. Biochem. Behav.* 13:673–83.

Reiter, L. W. 1977. Behavioral toxicology: Effects of early postnatal exposure to neurotoxins on development of locomotor activity in the rat. *J. Occup. Med.* 19:201–4.

———. 1978. Use of activity measurements in behavioral toxicology. *Environ. Health Perspect.* 26:9–20.

———. 1983. Chemical exposures and animal activity: Utility of the figure-eight maze. In *Developments in the science and practice of toxicology*, edited by A. W. Hayes, R. C. Schnell, and T. S. Miya, 76–84. Amsterdam: Elsevier.

Reiter, L. W.; Andersen, G. E.; Laskey, J. W.; and Cahill, D. F. 1975. Developmental and behavioral changes in the rat during chronic exposure to lead. *Environ. Health Perspect.* 12:119–23.

Reiter, L. W., and MacPhail, R. C. 1979. Motor activity: A survey of methods with potential use in toxicity testing. *Neurobehav. Toxicol.* 1, suppl. 1: 53–66.

Richardson, D.; Karczmar, A. G.; and Scudder, C. L. 1972. Intergeneric behavioral differences among methamphetamine treated mice. *Psychopharmacologia* 25:347–75.

Rushton, R.; Steinberg, H.; and Tinson, C. 1963. Effects of a single experience on subsequent reactions to drugs. *Br. J. Pharmacol.* 20:99–105.

Schneider, B. F., and Norton, S. 1979. Postnatal behavioral changes in prenatally irradiated rats. *Neurobehav. Toxicol.* 1:193–97.

Scott, J. P. 1966. Agonistic behavior of mice and rats: A review. *Amer. Zool.* 6:683–701.

Sterman, A. B., and Sheppard, R. C. 1972. A neurobehavioral model of 2,5-hexanedione-induced neuropathy. *Neurobehav. Toxicol. Teratol.* 4:567–72.

Swartzwelder, H. S.; Hepler, J.; Holahan, W.; King, S. E.; Leverenz, H. A.; Muller, P. A.; and Myers, R. D. 1982. Impaired maze performance in the rat caused by trimethyltin treatment: Problem-solving deficits and perseveration. *Neurobehav. Toxicol. Teratol.* 4:169–76.

Valzelli, L. 1969. Aggressive behaviour induced by isolation. In *Aggressive behaviour*, edited by S. Garattini and E. B. Sigg, 70–76. Amsterdam: Exerpta Medica.

Vorhees, C. V.; Butcher, R. E.; Brunner, R. L.; and Sobotka, T. J. 1979. A developmental test battery for neurobehavioral toxicity in rats: A preliminary analysis using monosodium glutamate, calcium carrageenan and hydroxyurea. *Toxicol. Appl. Pharmacol.* 50:267–82.

Walsh, R. N., and Cummins, R. H. 1976. The open-field test: A critical review. *Psychol. Bull.* 83:482–504.

Walsh, T. J.; Miller, D. B.; and Dyer, R. S. 1982. Trimethyltin, a selective limbic system neurotoxicant, impairs radial-arm maze performance. *Neurobehav. Toxicol. Teratol.* 4:177–83.

Lee S. Rafales

4

Assessment of Locomotor Activity

The measurement of locomotor activity (LA) is perhaps the most frequently used behavioral method in toxicological studies. As with other neurobehavioral methods and procedures, LA's value can be measured in terms of its contribution toward (1) establishing the neurotoxic potential of compounds, (2) determining the locus of a neurotoxic lesion, or (3) providing indications as to the mechanism(s) of action of neurotoxicants (Tilson, Cabe, and Burne 1980; Tilson and Mitchell 1980; Tilson and Harry 1982; Pryor et al. 1983). LA's effectiveness in providing meaningful information in these areas has been a source of controversy. Concern over this method had greatly focused on the proper use and control of environmental and organismic factors that influence LA (Reiter and MacPhail 1982). Concern over these factors has been well founded, and the discussion of their use in toxicology has undoubtedly contributed toward more robust experimental designs and less equivocal interpretations as to the significance of changes in LA resulting from a toxicant.

Every method has certain limitations, and use of a method without regard for these limitations constitutes a waste of valuable effort and resources. Even well-controlled and well-designed studies may generate equivocal or misleading information when they rely on inappropriate methodologies for the questions asked. Given the prevalent use of LA in toxicological research, it is perhaps time to consider some of its limitations and to delineate those areas of investigation for which it is best suited.

A method's limits are determined by both theoretical and practical concerns of measurement. Theoretical issues revolve around (1) the sensitivity of the method, (2) its ability to resolve certain classes of information, (3) its stability and reliability, and (4) its validity in providing data that correspond in an absolute or proportional way to known quantities. Practical issues are concerned with the amount of time and/or resources needed to reach a theoretically limiting condition, as well as whether an improvement in the methodology will bear upon the resolution of an important question for which other approaches are less feasible.

It is important to distinguish two different ways in which theoretical concerns of measurement relate to LA. In one context it is the adequacy of a device to measure some form of animal movement that is of interest. In another context the adequacy of changes in movement to accurately reflect neurotoxicity is of concern.

Measuring Animal Movement

Narrowly defined, locomotor activity represents horizontally directed movement using the limbs. Operational definitions usually rely on some measure of the frequency of movement, that is, spatial displacement per unit of time. Spatial displacement of an animal has been measured visually—for example using open-field devices—by scoring the number of discrete locations in which an animal moves. Automated devices such as tilt cages record the number of crossings between two discrete areas of a rectangular box that pivots according to the distributed weight of an animal. Other devices rely on various "proximity detectors," such as photosensitive diodes or fluctuations in weak magnetic fields (based on the Hall effect), to document an animal's spatial displacement. In running wheels an animal does not actually change its spatial position, and wheel displacement itself (recorded as revolutions per unit time) serves as the operational measure of activity.

It has been emphasized that the kinds of movement transduced by these various devices are not equivalent (Reiter and MacPhail 1979, 1982). In some cases, rearing or grooming movements may be scored as a component of LA. Tremor may also contribute to some measures of activity. An investigator's failure to recognize which components of behavior are being measured can lead to the selection of a device that does not provide sufficient or optimal sensitivity for the movement under study. The sensitivity and reliability of the measurement can also be degraded, since procedural controls instituted to equate influences on one movement may be ineffective in controlling other body movements transduced by the measuring device.

Measuring Neurotoxicity

The suitability of a device to accurately and reliably provide quantitative correlates of LA is an important concern. However, even a perfect measuring device would only provide data about overt patterns of movement. The interpretation of LA, in conjunction with other sources of data, constitutes one basis for evaluating substances with regard to their neurotoxicity. The following discussion addresses this latter issue as it relates to the effectiveness of LA (1) in identifying neurotoxic substances, (2) in identifying discrete neural lesions, and (3) in determining the mechanisms by which substances impair neurological function.

Screening for Neurotoxicants

Procedures for screening for neurotoxicants have been and continue to be devised in an effort to identify neurotoxic compounds (Tilson, Mitchell, and Cabe 1979; Mitchell, Tilson, and Cabe 1982; Pryor et al. 1983; Voorhees et al. 1979). It is reasonable to expect that these procedures should, at a very minimum, be capable of identifying potent neurotoxicants while minimizing the false categorization of compounds as neurotoxic when they are not (false positive results). As one component of a screening procedure, LA should also meet these minimal requirements. Failure to detect a disruption in neural function that is apparent using other methods would demonstrate a lack of sensitivity, while frequent alterations in LA by compounds believed to be nonneurotoxic would constitute a lack of validity for this method.

It would be fairly easy to assess these issues of measurement, and ultimately the utility of LA in screening for neurotoxic substances, if this behavioral procedure were uniformly applied to test many compounds known to be neurotoxic, as well as an equivalent number of negative control substances. Problems regarding dosage, species, and sex differences and a host of procedural and instrument controls would obviously need to be considered. However, some probabilistic determination could be made as to the empirical occurrence of correct detections, instances in which known neurotoxicants were not detected (false negative results), and instances in which neurotoxicity was attributed to compounds without neurotoxic properties (false positive results). The absence of such information poses a substantial impediment to an intelligent discussion of LA's utility for screening neurotoxicants. Remaining are anecdotal instances of its success or failure under idiosyncratic experimental conditions for compounds that often have unknown or marginal neurotoxic actions. Arbitrary selection of examples from this literature can serve to support a reviewer's personal bias but cannot justifiably be used to establish LA's real value. Failure to show significant detection can always be countered with claims that the experimental manipulations and/or the instruments used had minimal sensitivity, were prone to high levels of background noise, or failed to control some contributory influence on LA. Alternatively, citing isolated instances of the successful detection of a neurotoxicant using LA requires consideration of the relative doses required to produce the effect and the possibility that nonneural effects may underlie the observed changes in this behavior.

The outlook on LA that follows should be considered an interim, or perhaps speculative, evaluation that of necessity relies on a very limited amount of "hard" data. Two approaches have been used in this evaluation. One approach reviews some of the ways in which LA is affected by manipulations of nonneural systems. These data are meant to highlight the fact that observations of altered LA need not be directly related to the neurotoxic action of a compound. Such data suggest that in a more systematic study of LA's value for screening neurotoxicants many false positive results would likely be obtained. A second approach considers some comparative data on the sensitivity of LA and other behavioral methods in detecting known neurotoxicants. Studies that allow such comparisons represent a first step in acquiring the kind of quantitative information needed to estimate the true validity and sensitivity of LA.

Influences of Nonneural Origin upon Locomotor Activity

LA, like any other behavior, represents some interactive outcome of information processing. Since the nervous system is involved in such processing, it is reasonable to assume that at least certain disruptions of this system would alter LA. It is perhaps less obvious that relevant changes in the information used by the nervous system can alter the processing outcome even though the nervous system remains intact. Hormonal and nutritional influences are two prominent sources of information used to initiate and direct an animal's behavior. The nervous system acquires such information through the use of specialized receptors which are collectively used to establish aspects of an animal's *internal milieu.*

Ovarian and testicular secretions are one subset of hormonal influences that affect LA. For example, the LA of female rats measured in revolving drums displays a cyclicity that corresponds to the estrous cycle (Richter 1932). The activity cycle does not appear until puberty and disappears during pregnancy and lactation and after cessation of ovulation. The peak phase of activity corresponds to the cornification period of estrus (Wang 1923). These and other observations (Munn 1950) suggest that ovarian secretions, particularly estrogen, can regulate the activity cycle. Adult male rats are also subject to modification of LA by hormonal influences. Injections of estrone increase LA (Hoskins and Bevan 1941), and castration decreases activity in proportion to the amount of testicular tissue removed (Hoskins 1925; Gans 1927; Richter 1933). Testicular grafts can reinstate normal levels of activity (Richter and Wislocki 1928), although testosterone injections alone do not (Heller 1932). LA can also be affected by removal or manipulation of the thyroid, adrenal cortex, or anterior pituitary; a reduction in secretions from these glands results in attenuated activity levels (Munn 1950). Many of these effects, it should be noted, are device-dependent, and some measures of activity are minimally affected by these or similar manipulations (Reiter and MacPhail 1982). It may eventually be concluded that all of these effects are the results of pituitary influences. It is apparent, however, that the direct or indirect effects of a substance on endocrine glands or gonads, or presumably on hormone kinetics, may affect the frequency of ambulation.

Dietary and nutritional factors that are directly or indirectly modified by toxicant exposure may also affect measurement of LA. The particular direction of change, whether it be an increase or decrease in activity, is highly dependent upon the measuring device used. For example, decreases in food or water availability result in increased measures of activity using running wheels or stabilimeter cages (Tapp 1969). However, decreases are evident using some photocell cages or a circular open field, and no differences have been detected using a Williamson tiltcage (ibid). Although the brain uptake of dietary constituents such as tryptophan involve complex interactions with other plasma amino acids (Fernstrom and Wurtman 1972), modification of dietary constituents such as phenylalanine (Thurmond et al. 1979, 1980) or tryptophan injections (Jacobs et al. 1974; Marsden and Curzon 1976) have been shown to affect some measures of locomotion. Early nutritional deficiencies also cause long-term alterations in the pattern (Barnett, Smartz, and Widdowson 1971) and frequency (Dobbing and Smart 1973; Schenck, Slob and Busch 1978) of LA.

Several critical reviews (Bornschein et al. 1977; Mahaffey and Michaelson 1980; Michaelson 1980) have emphasized the need to consider a toxicant's influence on nutritional and dietary factors, since these can confound interpretations of both behavioral changes and associated neurochemical measures. Perhaps these reviews have not gone far enough in extrapolating the ramifications of these factors on the use of LA in evaluating neurotoxicants. Changes in vascular permeability, flow rate, or gastrointestinal absorption could readily affect the delivery of essential precursors such as phenylalanine or tryptophan and thereby affect LA. Alternatively, a variety of vascular and nonneural metabolic effects could alter the distribution of one or more endogenous hormones to affect LA. It is possible to conceive of several other manipulations of nonneural systems that could be shown to affect this behavior as well.

The point of this discussion is to emphasize that a change in any aspect of the internal milieu of an animal represents a change in what may be relevant information used and operated upon by the nervous system in establishing an organism's needs and directing appropriate behavior. As such, behavioral changes in general—and modifications of LA in particular—do not necessarily represent the *neurotoxic action* of a chemical substance on the nervous system.

Comparative Data on the Sensitivity of Locomotor Activity for Screening Neurotoxic Compounds

Given the nervous system's reliance upon varied sources of information and the sensitivity of LA to many of these, it might seem paradoxical that a direct insult to the nervous system would *not* be detected by LA. However, alterations in neurocellular organization can occur with little impact on some behaviors. For example, it has been observed that comparable neural destruction (e.g., using electrolytic or radio-frequency lesions), when it occurs over a more extended period of time with many smaller (multistage) lesions, can produce less extensive functional deficits (Finger, Walbran, and Stein 1973; Corwin et al. 1982). Two processes that have been suggested to account for preserving or reinstating lost functions are denervation supersensitivity and axonal regeneration (Schoenfeld and Hamilton 1977). Exposure over extended periods of time to low doses of neurotoxicants represents a condition that may approximate that of multistage lesions. Over time, neural damage produced in this way could be extensive, and yet functional deficits would not be apparent.

At least one comparative study also suggests that LA may be relatively insensitive to some potent neurotoxicants (Pryor et al. 1983). This study warrants particular attention because it evaluated substances that differed in their neurotoxic effects using several behavioral measures, including LA. As a result, it is one of the few studies to provide comparative data regarding the ability of several neurobehavioral methods to detect, or fail to detect, known neurotoxicants and to establish the occurrence of false positive results for nonneurotoxic substances, data previously suggested to be most relevant in evaluating the utility of LA for screening purposes.

In this study nine behavioral measures were used to rate the relative neurotoxicity of eight compounds. The compounds included acrylamide, methylmercury, chlordecone, tetraethyltin, triethyl lead chloride, inorganic lead acetate, arsenic trioxide, and monosodium salicylate. The test battery included behavioral measures of grip strength (fore- and hindlimb), thermal sensitivity (tail flick response), negative geotaxis, startle (acoustic and airpuff), conditioned avoidance responding, escape activity and LA. *LA activity was not generally responsive to any compound examined, and changes in this measure did not correspond to the final relative toxicities of the eight compounds.* It is worth noting that LA was not affected by the three compounds that were shown to significantly reduce hindlimb grip strength in the same animals. The apparatus used to measure activity in this study was a field-measuring device not specific for ambulation. It transduced both vertical and horizontal movements and probably could detect higher-frequency grooming movements as well. Since drugs and toxicants may increase some components of movement (e.g., tremor, grooming) while concurrently decreasing others (e.g., ambulation), this particular device may not have been well suited for the compounds examined. However, the compound rated most neurotoxic in this study, acrylamide, has also been used in other studies employing LA. In these studies as well, LA has been shown to be relatively insensitive to neurological damage. For example, dosages of acrylamide that caused hindlimb splay (Rafales, Bornschein, and Caruso 1982) or were reported to cause as much as a 10 percent incidence of peripheral nerve degeneration (Rafales et al. 1983) were not effective in changing the normative pattern of locomotion as recorded by photocells. Furthermore, activity in running wheels was only transiently affected after several weeks of exposure to acrylamide. With continued exposure to this neurotoxicant there were quantifiable changes in hindlimb posture, although activity measures for acrylamide-exposed and control rats were not significantly different (Rafales, Bornschein, and Caruso 1982). In Pryor et al. 1983 there were indications that LA was more responsive to one compound, arsenic, which is not believed to be neurotoxic in the rat.

At least three different measures of LA, therefore, have shown a limited sensitivity for detecting the neurotoxic effects of a highly potent neurotoxicant, while other dependent measures were effective in demonstrating a functional motor impairment or an observable histopathological alteration for nervous-system tissue. In addition, LA was responsive to at least one compound that ostensibly was not neurotoxic, thus leading to false positive results.

Increasing the Sensitivity of LA

Subtle changes in neural function that are not manifest under conditons of spontaneous LA can become evident with the addition of an interactive stress on the central nervous system. Pharmacological agents, in particular, offer a means of selectively perturbing the central nervous system and eliciting differences in LA between control and toxicant-exposed animals. For example, lead-exposed animals who have spontaneous levels of LA equivalent to that of controls display an altered responsiveness to psychomotor stimulants such as d-amphetamine (Cahill et al. 1976; Kostas, McFarland, and Drew 1978; Rafales et al. 1979; Rafales et al. 1981). Similarly, the spontaneous LA of animals exposed to acrylamide is not distinguishable from that of negative controls when tested in photocell activity chambers; but differences in LA are demonstrable when animals are challenged with d-amphetamine or apomorphine (Rafales, Bornschein, and Caruso 1982; Rafales et al. 1983).

Toxicant-related alterations in LA that are evident only after pharmacological manipulations must be interpreted with caution. Altered drug responsiveness may reflect compromised neural function; however, it is also possible that drug distribution and/or metabolism are substitutively different for control and toxicant-exposed cohorts as a consequence of some nonneural influence of the compound under study. Making more specific conclusions regarding a compound's *neurotoxic* potential requires additional information. For example, neurochemical data can be collected under pharmacological conditions equivalent to those that produce alterations in LA. This allows for certain inferences to be made regarding the neurological basis for observed changes in LA. (This topic is discussed in more detail below.)

Determining the Locus of a Neurotoxic Lesion

It has been suggested that in addition to their use in screening for neurotoxicants, neurobehavioral procedures can contribute toward identifying the locus or loci of a neurotoxic lesion. How effective can LA be in this regard? To answer this question it is first necessary to consider what is known about the neurological control of this behavior.

Primary Control over Locomotion

LA and other simple components of motor behavior are organized in the lower brainstem (Bernston and Micco 1976). Cats with only spinal cord and hindbrain structures (cerebellum, pons, medulla) intact can be stimulated to right themselves and perform unsteady ambulatory movements (Bazett and Penfield 1922; Bard and Macht 1958). These animals cannot, however, perform goal-oriented movements, since a number of sensory inputs needed for *guidance control* are absent. When more anterior lesions are made that spare the superior and inferior colliculi, these partially decerebrate animals retain the ability to perceive distant stimulus events and have functional locomotor abilities (Bard and Macht 1958; Woods 1964; Grill and Norgren 1978). Transections of the spinal cord below the hindbrain restrict the input of sensory information and obviate even the most rudimentary voluntary movements (Kuhn 1950). Simple stereotyped movements that rely upon stretch reflexes and reciprocal inhibitory connections of opposing muscle groups remain intact. However, elicitation of these movements requires direct sensory stimulation and rarely lasts beyond the duration of stimulation. The coordinated movement necessary for locomotion is not possible in spinally transected animals.

Deficits in Ambulatory Control

In a technical sense, then, direct control over ambulation and other simple motor acts probably resides at the level of the hindbrain. LA impaired as a result of damage to this region or relevant areas within this region may be considered to represent a *pure* or specific, deficit to the locomotor control apparatus. Infectious agents and chemical substances have been known to concentrate in discrete brain areas (Norton 1980), and it is perhaps feasible that a few neurotoxic agents would selectively affect the unique centers responsible for primary control over ambulation. However, compounds that have been shown to affect ambulation have diverse chemical properties, kinetics, and metabolic fates. Given this diversity, it seems highly improbable that aberrant patterns of locomotion will typically represent a deficit in the neural assemblies directly involved in the explicit coordination of this behavior. More probable areas of dysfunction would be in (1) subordinate neural assemblies and musculature relied upon by hindbrain coordinating centers and necessary for affecting limb movement, (2) sensory systems needed for proper guidance control in three-dimensional space, or (3) superordinate or higher-level organizing functions in the di- and tel-encephalon that initiate, maintain, and otherwise affect purposeful movement.

A considerable body of information is available to suggest that LA is affected by (1) manipulations of several forebrain areas, including the hippocampus (Kimble 1963; Teitelbaum and Milner 1963), caudate nucleus (Ungerstedt and Arbuthnott 1970), and nucleus accumbens (Pijnenburg et al. 1976); (2) manipulations of visual and acoustic systems (Grossman 1967); and (3) impairments to lower-order systems such as stretch receptors and peripheral sensory afferent nerves (Moruzzi 1950a, 1950b).

Given the diversity of neural influences affecting LA, it is difficult to conceptualize how this behavior can be effectively used to determine the locus of a neurotoxic lesion. A pattern of histopathology or unequal regional concentrations of a suspected neurotoxicant in the brain might be of value in identifying a neural locus. Correlative changes in LA could provide an indication that such measures were related to a disruption of normal brain function, but LA would not add additional information regarding the locus at which such a disruption occurred. This does not mean that functional indications serve no purpose in assessing neurotoxicants, only that functional alterations of LA do not readily contribute the information needed to identify the *locus* of a neurotoxic lesion.

Mechanisms of Neurotoxicity

The focus of a neurotoxic lesion may be chemical as well as anatomical. The extent to which a neurotoxicant affects one chemical locus, or group of neurons charac- terized by their utilization of a class of related chemical substances, can suggest several things about the compound being evaluated. It can provide indications about a neurotoxicant's distribution or metabolism in neural tissue. It can also relate to the ability of a substance to interfere with biochemical processes necessary for the viability of nerve cells or required to support effective, chemically mediated neurotransmission.

A prodigious body of research has been directed at establishing the influences of several neurotransmitter systems of LA (see Cole 1978). This research has relied most heavily on experiments using centrally acting pharmacological agents and neurotoxicants that are selectively accumulated by certain populations of neurons. The volume of information accrued in this area is by no means definitive. However, it is generally believed that manipulations of monoamine systems have predomi- nant influence over LA, while cholinergic, serotonergic, and amino acid–based transmitter systems have more modest, modulatory roles (ibid).

One research strategy that neurotoxicologists have used relies on the assump- tion that changes in LA produced by a compound can be explained by establishing associated changes in neurochemical systems that influence this behavior. How useful are the relationships between LA and chemical indications of altered neural function in establishing causal models for the neurotoxicity of a compound?

Neurochemical and behavioral measures may be related in three basic ways: (1) behavioral measures may follow the occurrence of changes in neurochemical sys- tems; (2) behavioral measures may precede neurochemical events and act to initiate changes in neurochemical systems; and (3) behavioral and neurochemical mea- sures may be correlated because they are consequences of some event common to them both (Russell 1969). The research strategies typically used to establish associa- tions between LA and neurochemical measures provide no basis for distinguishing among these three possibilities, yet it is widely believed that neurochemical-behav- ioral associations constitute general support for the *neurotoxicity* of a compound as well as provide specific information with regard to the chemical locus by which a compound affects changes in LA (Sauerhoff and Michaelson 1973; Golter and Michaelson 1975; Silbergeld and Goldberg 1975; Jason and Kellogg 1977; Dubas and Hrdina 1978; Hrdina, Hanin, and Dubas 1980).

The problems that neurotoxicologists face in attempting to make causal in- ferences from these correlative associations are perhaps best illustrated by consid- ering two studies in which it was possible to approach *concurrent* assessment for both measurement of neurochemical and behavioral variables (Yamamoto and Freed 1982; Yamamoto, Lane, and Freed 1982). These studies were devised to demonstrate changes in brain dopamine metabolism associated with asymmetric body movement. Animals were trained to circle in one of two directions by selectively reinforcing them using a sucrose-water reward. Animals retained their turning responses without regular training sessions for one month or longer. Trained animals were subsequently sacrificed at different times during a test for circling behavior, and their caudate nuclei were dissected and assayed for dopamine (DA) and dihydroxyphenylacetic acid (DOPAC) concentrations (Yamamoto and Freed 1982). In animals sacrificed prior to turning, caudate DA and DOPAC levels were the same bilaterally. However, animals sacrificed after 20 minutes of circling showed a 67 percent increase in DA and a 46 percent increase in DOPAC concentrations for the caudate contralateral to the direction of movement. Ipsilateral caudate concentrations did not reflect any differences from preturning values. The assessment of DA and DOPAC in this study was not really concurrent with the behavioral assessment, since some time elapsed between the last behavioral observation and the removal of caudate tissue. However, in a subsequent study (Yamamoto, Lane, and Freed 1982) indwelling electrochemical electrodes were bilaterally implanted in the caudate and used to assess the relative concentrations of DA and DOPAC in vivo and concurrent with the assessment of circling movement. Under these conditions it was also possible to show a strong relationship between the magnitude of circling movements and the magnitude of the differential concentrations of DA and DOPAC in the caudate nuclei.

These studies are subject to certain criticisms, most notably with regard to the adequacy of concentration data for determining neural activity and, in the latter study, for utilizing a methodology concerning which there is considerable controversy (Falat and Cheng 1982; Plotsky 1982). If, however, we suspend such criticism and accept the data as they are presented, then we have a concurrent neurochemical and behavioral measurement rarely, if ever, encountered in neurotoxicological studies. Even under these relatively optimal conditions of measurement, however, it cannot be determined whether increases in DA concentration reflected neural activity that subsequently initiated the movement or whether the changes in DA concentration occurred as a consequence of the movement.

Given this situation, it is difficult to attribute alterations in LA following exposure to a suspected neurotoxicant to related changes in neurochemical systems. Consider, for example, a study by Dubas and Hrdina (1978) in which the LA of developing rats was measured at various ages after exposure to lead. At 8 weeks of age, lead-exposed rats were significantly more active than control animals; regional levels of NE, DA, 5HT, and 5HIAA also differed. By 12 weeks of age, however, the activity of lead-exposed rats was equivalent to that of controls, and their levels of DA and NE were also similar. Although changes in 5HT and 5HIAA continued to be present, these changes appeared to be unrelated to the frequency of LA exhibited by the lead-exposed animals.

Were the changes in LA observed for lead-exposed rats mediated by changes in monoamine function? or were the changes in monoamine steady-state levels an indirect response to altered levels of activity? Unfortunately, the experimental design of this and similar correlative studies does not allow a test of these hypotheses.

Using Pharmacological Probes to Determine Mechanisms

A related strategy of many neurotoxicological studies uses the responsiveness of LA to drugs that affect neurochemically discrete pathways as a means of identifying altered transmitter systems (Sobotka et al. 1975; Cahill et al. 1976; Kostas, McFarland, and Drew 1978; Rafales et al. 1981). Responsiveness is typically determined by measuring LA alone or in combination with dependent neurochemical measures such as neurotransmitter and metabolite concentrations, calculated turnover rates, or the binding properties of pre- and/or postsynaptic receptors. Problems similar to those mentioned above must be considered when attempts are made to interpret the basis for changes observed in drug responsiveness as a result of the administration of a compound. In addition, this strategy requires that pharmacological agents used as probes be fairly well characterized with respect to their effects on neural function. However, there are some distinct advantages to this methodology. One advantage, mentioned earlier, is that drug challenges can unmask latent alterations produced by a neurotoxicant. Another advantage is that a drug challenge provides a reference point from which temporal relationships between behavioral and neurochemical observations can be made. For example, if toxicant-exposed animals are found to have neurochemical alterations that precede overt differences in LA, then one can be more confident that neurochemical events precede behavioral differences and are not secondary to differential muscular activity and associated changes in proprioceptive feedback. If concern over issues of differential drug distribution and metabolism can be eliminated, then one comes closer to identifying the "cause" of the altered LA as the neurotoxic action of an administered substance.

A study on acrylamide conducted by the author provides one example of the use of pharmacological probes, in conjunction with neurochemical measures, to identify mechanisms by which a toxicant affects LA (Rafales et al. 1983). In this study male rats received acrylamide in their drinking water for a six-week period. Spontaneous LA, assessed both before the onset of exposure and at weekly intervals during the exposure, was not altered. However, LA following low doses of d-amphetamine was significantly greater for exposed rats than for animals assigned as negative controls. Acrylamide facilitated the psychomotor stimulant properties of d-amphetamine during a 50-minute interval beginning 15 minutes after the administration of the drug. Neurochemical data were collected for animals under the same conditions of handling, exposure, and drug administration as those in the LA phase of the study. In this way it was possible to assess the regulatory responses of several neuronal systems as they responded to the drug probe and then returned to baseline levels. Neurochemical measures consisted of regional, steady-state concentrations for tyrosine, DA, DOPAC, HVA, NE, tryptophan, and 5HT. These were acquired at four time intervals after drug administration: 0 (saline), 15, 80, and 120 minutes.

Neurochemical differences between control and acrylamide-exposed rats were evident in the absence of drug (time = 0 minutes; saline) and at 15, 80, and 120 minutes postinjection. The earliest neurochemical differences consisted of increased levels of 5HIAA for acrylamide-exposed animals after vehicle injections only. This neurochemical observation corresponds in time to a period when differences in LA were not yet apparent. The second earliest neurochemical distinction between control and exposed rats occurred at 15 minutes after d-amphetamine injection. At this time, control animals displayed a substantial drop in their 5HIAA concentration in three of the four brain regions examined. It is not clear whether this event represented a direct effect of d-amphetamine on the serotonergic system or whether it was a secondary response following dopaminergic or some other activity. It is significant, however, that acrylamide-exposed animals did not evidence a similar drop in their 5HIAA concentration and that their increased locomotor response to the drug corresponded in time to this negative neurochemical response.

Definitive conclusions regarding the mechanism(s) by which acrylamide "caused" increased LA to occur are not possible from this study because (1) steady-state levels of neurotransmitters and their metabolites may not be adequate indicators of neuronal activity; (2) as mentioned repeatedly, consideration must be given to drug metabolism and kinetics in exposed animals; and (3) several additional experiments can be proposed to test specific hypotheses regarding acrylamide's effects on serotonergic function. However, this study should make it clear that heuristic information can be acquired that bears upon mechanistic interpretations for toxicant-induced alterations in LA.

Summary

Measures of LA are widely used in toxicology because motor activity occurs naturally and because it is ostensibly easy to obtain some measure of activity (Reiter and MacPhail 1982). There has not, however, been adequate empirical or theoretical justification for the prevalent use of this behavioral methodology in toxicological research. This chapter has considered how appropriate LA may be in providing relevant information in three areas: (1) establishing the neurotoxic potential of compounds, (2) determining the locus of a neurotoxic lesion, and (3) providing indications as to the mechanism(s) of action of neurotoxicants.

In general, the use of LA in addressing these questions has been of limited value. This is not to say that innovative experimental designs cannot be devised to take advantage of this methodology. However, the existing base of literature suggests that LA is not uniquely sensitive to, or specific for, the neurotoxic properties of compounds. In addition, the organization and interrelationships of neural control over LA are such that functional alterations in this behavior produced by a neurotoxic substance are not likely to allow for a determination as to which level or locus of the nervous system has been affected. It is equally unlikely that correlative observations of LA and neurochemical measures in themselves can provide indications as to the mechanism(s) by which LA is altered by suspected neurotoxicants.

Pharmacological probes can be used in some instances to increase the sensitivity of LA for detecting toxicant-related changes. Pharmacological probes can also be used to help identify neural systems that may be preferentially or uniquely affected by a neurotoxicant. However, it should be cautioned that such studies must be capable of distinguishing alterations in LA owing to the *neuro*toxic properties of a substance from indirect effects.

Perhaps the greater value of LA for behavioral toxicology is not in this method's use in assessing nervous system function per se but rather in assessing factors that influence toxicity. Once it can be determined that a substance alters LA, then several questions may be posed. These may be related to the exposure situation and may be used to assess threshold levels and/or durations of exposure necessary to see alterations in LA. Alternatively, they may be related to several subject-related factors such as sex, genetic status, age, species, and strain (Doull 1980). Social factors (e.g., housing) and several environmental concerns (e.g., noise, light, and ambient atmospheric conditions) can also be evaluated if there is reason to believe that they are important in providing a clear picture of the toxicity of a compound. Other questions that may be posed include How persistent is the alteration in this behavior following termination of exposure? and Are there critical periods, levels, and/or durations of exposure necessary to see alterations in LA?

Acknowledgments

The author would like to thank Drs. Kathleen Krafft, Daniel Minnema, and Arthur Michaelson for their helpful comments and suggestions.

References

Bard, P., and Macht, M. B. 1958. The behavior of chronically decerebrate cats. In *Ciba Foundation symposium on neurological basis of behavior,* edited by G. E. Woshlstenholm and C. M. O'Connor. London: J. and A. Churchill.

Barnett, S. A.; Smart, J. L.; and Widdowson, E. M. 1971. Early nutrition and the activity and feeding of rats in an artificial environment. *Dev. Psychobiol.* 4:1–15.

Bazett, H. C., and Penfield, W. G. 1922. A study of the Sherrington decerebrate animal in the chronic as well as the acute condition. *Brain* 45:185–265.

Bernston, G. G., and Micco, D. J. 1976. Organization of brainstem behavioral systems. *Brain Res. Bull.* 1:471–483.

Bornschein, R.; Michaelson, I. A.; Fox, D. A.; and Loch, R. 1977. Evaluation of animal models used to study effects of lead on neurochemistry and behavior. In *Biochemical effects of environmental pollutants,* edited by S. D. Lee. Ann Arbor: Ann Arbor Science Publishers.

Bornschein, R.; Pearson, D.; and Reiter, L. 1980. Behavioral effects of moderate lead exposure in children and animal models: Part 2, animal studies. *CRC Crit. Rev. Toxicol.* 8:101–52.

Cahill, D. F.; Reiter, L. W.; Santolucito, J. A.; Rehnberg, G. I.; Ash, M. E.; Favor, M. J.; Bursian, S. J.; Wright, J. F.; and Laskey, J. W. 1976. Biological assessment of continuous exposure to tritium and lead in the rat. In *Biological Effects of Low Level Radiation. Proc. Int. At. Energy Agcy.* 2:65–78.

Cole, S. O. 1978. Brain mechanisms of amphetamine-induced anorexia, locomotion, and stereotypy: A review. *Neurosci. Biobehav. Rev.* 2:89–100.

Corwin, J. K.; Vicedomini, J. P.; Nonneman, A. J.; and Valentino, L. 1982. Serial lesion effect in rat medial frontal cortex as a function of age. *Neurobehav. Aging* 3:69–76.

Dobbing, John, and Smart, J. L. 1973. Early undernutrition, brain development and behavior. In *Ethology and development,* edited by S. A. Barnett, 16–36. London: Spastics International Medical Publications with Heinemann Medical Books.

Doull, J. 1980. Factors influencing toxicology. In *Casarett and Doull's toxicology: The basic science of poisons,* edited by J. Doull, C. D. Klaassen, and M. O. Amdur, 70–83. New York: Macmillan.

Dubas, T. C., and Hrdina, P. D. 1978. Behavioral and neurochemical consequences of neonatal exposure to lead in rats. *J. Environ. Pathol. Toxicol.* 2:473–84.

Falat, L., and Cheng, H.-Y. 1982. Voltammetric differentiation of ascorbic acid and dopamine at an electrochemically treated graphite/epoxy electrode. *Anal. Chem.* 54:2108–11.

Fernstrom, J. D., and Wurtman, R. J. 1972. Brain serotonin content: Physiological regulation by plasma neutral amino acids. *Science* 178:414–16.

Finger, F. W. 1972. Measuring behavioral activity. In *Methods in psychobiology,* edited by R. D. Meyers. 2:1–19. New York: Academic Press.

Finger, S.; Walbran, B.; and Stein, D. G. 1973. Brain damage and behavioral recovery: Serial lesion phenomena. *Brain Res.* 63:1–18.

Gans, H. M. 1927. Studies on vigor: XIV. Effects of fractional castration on voluntary activity of male albino rats. *Endocrinology* 11:145–48.

Golter, M., and Michaelson, I. A. 1975. Growth, behavior and brain catecholamines in lead-exposed neonatal rats: A reappraisal. *Science* 187:359–61.

Grill, H. J., and Norgren, R. 1978. Neurological tests and behavioral deficits in chronic thalamic and chronic decerebrate rats. *Brain Res.* 143:299–312

Grossman, S. D. 1967. *A textbook of physiological psychology,* 241–87. New York, London, and Sydney: John Wiley & Sons.

Heller, R. E. 1932. Spontaneous activity in male rats in relation to testis hormone. *Endocrinology* 16:626–32.

Hoskins, R. G. 1925. Studies on vigor: II. The effects of castration on voluntary activity. *Am. J. Physiol.* 72:324–30.

Hoskins, R. G., and Bevan, S. 1941. The effect of fractionated chorionic gonadotropic extract on spontaneous activity and weight of elderly male rats. *Endocrinology* 27:929–31.

Hrdina, P. D.; Hanin, I.; and Dubas, T. C. 1980. Neurochemical correlates of lead toxicity. In *Lead toxicity,* edited by R. L. Singhal and J. A. Thomas, 273–300. Baltimore and Munich: Urban & Schwarzenberg.

Jacobs, B. L.; Eubanks, E. E.; and Wise, W. D. 1974. Effect of indolalkylamine manipulations on locomotor activity in rats. *Neuropharmacology* 13:575–83.

Jason, K., and Kellogg, C. 1977. Lead effects on behavioral and neurochemical development in rats. *Fed. Proc.* 36 (abstr. 388): 1008.

Kimble, D. P. 1963. The effects of bilateral hippocampal lesions in rats. *J. Comp. Physiol. Psychol.* 56:273–83.

Kostas, J.; McFarland, D. J.; and Drew, W. G. 1978. Lead-induced behavioral disorders in the rat: Effects of amphetamine. *Pharmacology* 16:226–36.

Kuhn, R. A. 1950. Functional capacity of the isolated human spinal cord. *Brain* 73:1–51.

Mahaffey, K. R., and Michaelson, I. A. 1980. The interaction between lead and nutrition. In *Low level lead exposure: The clinical implications of current research,* edited by H. L. Needleman. New York: Raven Press.

Marsden, C. A., and Curzon, G. 1976. Behavioral effects of tryptophan and parachlorophenylalanine. *Neuropharmacology* 15:165–71.

Michaelson, I. A. 1980. An appraisal of rodent studies on the behavioral toxicity of lead: The role of nutritional status. In *Lead toxicity,* 301–65. *See* Hrdina, Hanin, and Dubas 1980.

Mitchell, C. L.; Tilson, H. A.; and Cabe, P. A. 1982. Screening for neurobehavioral toxicity: Factors to consider. In *Nervous system toxicology,* edited by C. L. Mitchell, 237–45. New York: Raven Press.

Moruzzi, G. 1950a. Effects at different frequencies of cerebellar stimulation upon postural tonus and myotatic reflexes. *EEG Clin. Neurophysiol.* 2:463–69.

———. 1950b. *Problems in cerebellar physiology.* Springfield, Ill.: Thomas.

Munn, N. L. 1950. *Handbook of psychological research on the rat,* 52–83. Boston: Houghton Mifflin Co.

Norton, S. 1980. The central nervous system. In *Casarett and Doull's toxicology. See* Doull 1980.

Pijnenburg, A. J. J.; Honig, W. M. M.; Van der Heyden, J. A. M.; and Van Rossum, J. M. 1976.

Effects of chemical stimulation of the mesolimbic dopamine system upon locomotor activity. *Europ. J. Pharmacol.* 35:45–58.

Plotsky, P. M. 1982. Differential voltammetric measurement of catecholamines and ascorbic acid at surface-modified carbon filament microelectrodes. *Brain Res.* 235:179–84.

Pryor, G. T.; Uyeno, E. T.; Tilson, H. A.; and Mitchell, C. L. 1983. Assessment of chemicals using a battery of neurobehavioral tests: A comparative study. *Neurobehav. Toxicol. Teratol.* 5:91–117.

Rafales, L. S.; Bornschein, R. L.; and Caruso, V. 1982. Behavioral and pharmacological responses following acrylamide exposure in rats. *Neurobehav. Toxicol. Teratol.* 4:355–64.

Rafales, L. S.; Bornschein, R. L.; Michaelson, I. A.; Loch, R. K.; and Barker, G. F. 1979. Drug induced activity in lead-exposed mice. *Pharmacol. Biochem. Behav.* 10:95–104.

Rafales, L. S.; Greenland, R. D.; Zenick, H.; Goldsmith, M.; and Michaelson, I. A. 1981. Responsiveness to d-amphetamine in lead-exposed rats as measured by steady levels of catecholamines and locomotor activity. *Neurobehav. Toxicol. Teratol.* 3:363–67.

Rafales, L. S.; Lasley, S. M.; Greenland, R. D.; and Mandybur, T. 1983. Effects of acrylamide on locomotion and central monoamine function in the rat. *Pharmacol. Biochem. Behav.* 19:635–44.

Reiter, L. W., and MacPhail, R. C. 1979. Motor activity: A survey of methods with potential use in toxicity testing. *Neurobehav. Toxicol.* 1, suppl. 1:53–66.

———. 1982. Factors influencing motor activity measurements in neurotoxicology. In *Nervous system toxicology*, 45–65. *See* Mitchell, Tilson, and Cabe 1982.

Richter, C. P. 1932. Symposium: Contributions of psychology to the understanding of problems of personality and behavior. IV. Biological foundation of personality differences. *Am. J. Orthopsychiatry* 2:345–54.

———. 1933. The role played by the thyroid gland in the production of gross bodily activity. *Endocrinology* 17:73–87.

Richter, C. P., and Wislocki, G. B. 1928. Activity studies on castrated male and female rats with testicular grafts in correlation with histological studies of the grafts. *Am. J. Physiol.* 86:651–60.

Robbins, T. W. 1977. A critique of the methods available for the measurement of spontaneous motor activity. In *Handbook of psychopharmacology*, edited by L. L. Iversen, S. D. Iversen, and S. H. Snyder, 7:37–82. New York: Plenum Press.

Russell, Roger W. 1969. Behavioral aspects of cholinergic transmission. *Fed. Proc.* 28:121–31.

Sauerhoff, M., and Michaelson, I. A. 1973. Hyperactivity and brain catecholamines in lead-exposed developing rats. *Science* 182:1022–24.

Schenck, P. E.; Slob, A. K.; and Bosch, J. J. 1978. Locomotor activity and social behavior of old rats after preweaning undernutrition. *Dev. Psychobiol.* 11:205–12.

Schoenfeld, T. A., and Hamilton, L. W. 1977. Review: Secondary brain changes following lesions: A new paradigm for lesion experimentation. *Physiol. Behav.* 18:951–67.

Silbergeld, E. K., and Goldberg, A. M. 1975. Pharmacological and neurochemical investigations of lead-induced hyperactivity. *Neuropharmacology* 14:431–44.

Sobotka, T. J., Brodie, R. E., and Cook, M. P. 1975. Psycho-physiologic effects of early lead exposure. *Toxicology* 5:175.

Tapp, J. T. 1969. Activity, reactivity, and the behavior-directing properties of stimuli. In *Reinforcement and behavior*, edited by J. T. Tapp. New York: Academic Press.

Teitelbaum, H., and Milner, P. 1963. Activity changes following partial hippocampal lesions in rats. *J. Comp. Physiol. Psychol.* 56:284–89.

Thurmond, J. B.; Kramarcy, N. R.; Lasley, S. M.; and Brown, J. W. 1980. Dietary amino acid precursors: Effects on central monoamines, aggression and locomotor activity in the mouse. *Pharmacol. Biochem. Behav.* 12:525–32.

Thurmond, J. B.; Lasley, S. M.; Kramarcy, N. R.; and Brown, J. W. 1979. Differential tolerance to dietary amino acid induced changes in aggressive behavior and locomotor activity in mice. *Psychopharmacology* 66:301–08.

Tilson, H. A.; Cabe, P. A.; and Burne, T. A. 1980. Behavioral procedures for the assessment of neurotoxicity. In *Experimental and clinical neurotoxicology,* edited by P. S. Spencer and H. H. Schaumburg, 758–66. Baltimore: Williams & Wilkins.

Tilson, H. A., and Harry, G. J. 1982. Behavioral principles for use in behavioral toxicology and pharmacology. In *Nervous system toxicology,* 1–27. See Mitchell, Tilson, and Cabe 1982.

Tilson, H. A., and Mitchell, C. L. 1980. Models of neurotoxicity. In *Biochemical toxicology,* edited by E. Hodgson, J. R. Bend, and R. M. Philpot, 265–94. New York: Elsevier.

Tilson, H. A.; Mitchell, C. L.; and Cabe, P. A. 1979. Screening for neurobehavioral toxicity: The need for and examples of validation of testing procedures. *Neurobehav. Toxicol.* 1, suppl. 1:137–48.

Ungerstedt, U., and Arbuthnott, G. W. 1970. Quantitative recording of rotational behavior in rats after 60HDA lesions of the nigrostriatal dopamine system. *Brain Res.* 24:485–93.

Voorhees, C. V.; Butcher, R. E.; Brunner, R. L.; and Sobotka, T. J. 1979. A developmental test battery for neurobehavioral toxicity in rats: A preliminary analysis using monosodium glutamate, calcium carrageenan and hydroxyurea. *Toxicol. Appl. Pharmacol.* 50:267–82.

Wang, G. H. 1923. Relation between "spontaneous" activity and oestrus cycle in the white rat. *Comp. Psychol. Monogr. Ser.* 2:6.

Woods, J. W. 1964. Behavior of chronic decerebrate rats. *J. Neurophysiol.* 27:634–44.

Yamamoto, B. K., and Freed, C. R. 1982. The trained circling rat: A model for inducing unilateral caudate dopamine metabolism. *Nature* 298:467–68.

Yamamoto, B. K.; Lane, R. F.; and Freed, C. R. 1982. Normal rats trained to circle show asymmetric caudate dopamine release. *Life Sci.* 30:2155–62.

Victor G. Laties and
Ronald W. Wood

5

Schedule-Controlled Behavior in Behavioral Toxicology

Behavioral toxicologists study behavior in all its complexity. Here we focus on behavior that has been placed on a schedule of reinforcement: following an animal's responses with reinforcing stimuli according to an explicit schedule produces orderly patterns of behavior (Ferster and Skinner 1957; Thompson and Grabowski 1972). The history of behavioral pharmacology has demonstrated the utility of schedule-controlled behavior for evaluating the behavioral effects of chemicals. In this context, such behavior has several advantages (Morse 1975; Laties 1982). Relatively small numbers of animals can be used, with these studied intensively. Both the arrangement of environmental contingencies and the collection of data are done with automatic equipment, thereby diminishing the biases that can be introduced when reliance is placed on human interventions and observations. Animals can be used as their own controls, and this exclusion of between-subject variability enhances sensitivity. In addition, the contingencies of reinforcement themselves restrict variability within the individual animal, both within an individual session and across sessions. Excellent general introductions to the use of schedule-controlled behavior in pharmacology have been written by Kelleher and Morse (1968), Thompson and Schuster (1968), McMillan and Leander (1976), Seiden and Dykstra (1977), Thompson and Boren (1977), McKearney and Barrett (1978), Iversen and Iversen (1981), and Carlton (1983), among others. All of these are quite relevant to the needs of those interested in toxicology.

Most chemicals administered at high enough doses will have untoward behavioral effects. Many of these effects may not be of scientific interest or concern because they only predict impending death. They may serve an important alerting function, however, by indicating either that the central nervous system may be the target organ at lower doses or that some other toxic process is impairing behavior indirectly. Behavioral effects are of greater concern when they occur at low fractions of the minimal lethal dose, especially if they occur only after chronic exposure and are insidious in character. Although manipulations of dose and exposure are important, a detailed discussion of exposure protocols is beyond the scope of the present chapter (see Dews 1972; and NAS 1977).

We offer some examples of how workers in behavioral toxicology have used schedules of reinforcement. In some cases the schedule-controlled behavior is itself the immediate subject of interest; schedules can generate behavior worth studying in its own right. In others, a controlling variable is the focus, the schedule allowing its easy manipulation; here the emphasis is on discovering the relative importance of different behavioral variables in determining the substance's behavioral effects. In still other studies schedules are used to change the sensitivity of performance or to control behavior so that another variable can more easily be manipulated. Taken together, the experiments discussed below should introduce the reader to a few of the behavioral variables that engage the interest of behavioral toxicologists. Finally, we address the role of schedule-controlled behavior in the regulation of chemicals.

Following the assumption that most people reading this chapter are not active in this area, we examine only a small number of studies and do so in a somewhat didactic fashion. We make no attempt to survey all the many ways in which schedule-controlled behavior has been used in the field. Indeed, all the examples have been drawn from our own work and from that of our colleagues and predecessors at the University of Rochester. This choice has been made for our own convenience and does not mean that we think these studies superior to the numerous other exemplars that could have been used to make our points. In fact, the ubiquity of the schedules approach is such that similar articles limited to other geographical locales could easily be written.

Simple Schedules of Reinforcement

Fixed-ratio and fixed-interval schedules are conceptually the simplest schedules, and it is not surprising that they have been widely used in behavioral toxicology.

The Fixed-Ratio Schedule

The simplest reinforcement schedule of all arranges for each single response to produce a single reinforcer. This is fixed-ratio 1 (FR 1), or as it is sometimes called, continuous reinforcement (see Ferster and Skinner 1957, chap. 4, pp. 39–132, for the original analysis of the determinants of behavior on this schedule). This simple arrangement has been used to study the effects of microwaves on thermoregulatory behavior. It was appropriate for this experiment because reinforcements are directly proportional to responses and because in this experiment the major dependent variable was to be reinforcement rate. It has long been known that a rat will take advantage of the opportunity to warm itself while in a cold room by pressing a lever that operates a heat lamp (Weiss and Laties 1961). Stern et al. (1979) used this fact to assess the heat output associated with microwave radiation. They arranged alternating 15-minute periods during which 2,450 MHz continuous-wave microwaves were or were not present. By varying microwave power density, they examined how this source of heat, which did not depend upon any response on the part of the animal, altered operant behavior on the FR 1 schedule for heat reinforcement. Cumulative records for four rats are shown in figure 5.1. The steeper the slope, the higher was the rate. It is clear that response rate moved lower as the amount of heat from the microwave generator increased. An effect from as little as 5 mW/cm^2 could be distinguished. This finding allowed the authors to conclude that previously reported actions of microwaves that had been attributed to nonthermal effects may have been secondary to thermal effects similar to those detected here by the FR schedule of heat-reinforced behavior.

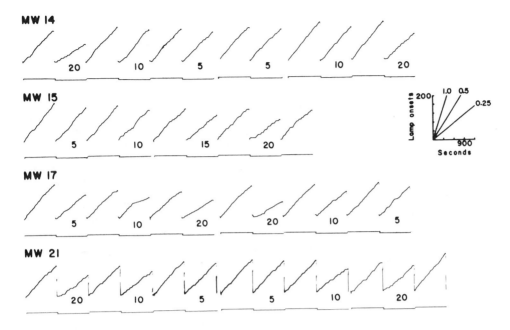

Fig. 5.1 Cumulative records of four rats working on a fixed-ratio 1 schedule of reinforcement are shown as the upper of each pair of records. Each response that turned on a heat lamp for two seconds moved the pen vertically. The recorder paper moved at a constant speed, and the inset gives some examples of the slopes produced by various reinforcement rates. The pen reset to the baseline at the end of each 15-minute period. The lower record of each pair shows when microwave exposure was occurring; it was deflected downward at those times, and the power densities (in mW/cm^2) are given below the appropriate sections of the record. When not in the down position, no microwave radiation was present.
(*Source:* adapted from Stern et al. 1979. Copyright 1979 by the American Association for the Advancement of Science. Reprinted by permission of the publisher.)

The Fixed-Interval Schedule

Much work in behavioral pharmacology and toxicology has used the fixed-interval (FI) schedule. For example, Cory-Slechta and colleagues have examined the effects of lead on the FI performance of rats (Cory-Slechta and Thompson 1979; Cory-Slechta, Weiss, and Cox 1983; Cory-Slechta 1984). One finding was that lead acetate would produce large changes in response rate—either increases or decreases, depending upon exposure level—without interfering with the response distribution within the interval. They chose to use this schedule because of its demonstrated sensitivity to many drugs and because of its wide species generality (Weiss and Laties 1967; Kelleher and Morse 1968; Dews 1976). In addition, they chose the FI schedule because any changes induced in response rate would not produce large changes in the number of reinforcers delivered, since reinforcement requires but a single response after the specified time interval has elapsed. (A ratio schedule is more appropriate when interest is focused on how frequently reinforcement occurs; cf. Stern et al. 1979, discussed above.) Only very severe rate reductions have any effect upon the animal's meeting this quite modest requirement. This feature helps experimenters interpret response rate data, since any changes are unlikely to be dependent upon a chemically induced reduction in reinforcement frequency: a

CONTROL

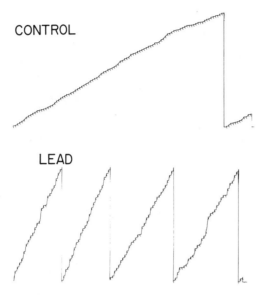

LEAD

Fig. 5.2 Cumulative records of one control (*top*) and one rat exposed to 50 ppm lead acetate (*bottom*) on a fixed-interval 30-second schedule of reinforcement. The session duration was one hour. The short oblique lines on the records indicate deliveries of food reinforcers. The response pen reset to the baseline after 550 responses. An approximately fourfold increase in response rate after a 65-day exposure to lead acetate can be seen. This response rate increase did not change the rate at which the subject earned reinforcers.
(*Source:* data from Cory-Slechta and Thompson 1979.)

minor performance alteration is not magnified by a precipitous change in the frequency of the event responsible for maintaining the behavior. This removes the confounding effects of reinforcement frequency alterations. Figure 5.2 shows how chronic exposure to 50 ppm lead acetate produced a large increase in response rate on an FI 30-second schedule with no concomitant change in reinforcement rate (Cory-Slechta and Thompson 1979).

The FI schedule was also chosen in order to maintain a relatively constant food reinforcement rate in a study of ozone's behavioral effects (Weiss et al. 1981). Figure 5.3 shows the cumulative records for a single rat exposed to various ozone concentrations for six hours. Note that the basic response pattern on the FI 5-minute schedule did not change greatly during exposure, intervals usually showing a pause followed by a rapid rate increase. The main effect was that higher concentrations produced severe response rate reductions sooner in the session. Using the FI schedule guaranteed that food delivery during sessions remained quite constant until responding practically ceased. In subsequent experiments to characterize the nature of the rate reductions produced by ozone, Tepper and colleagues observed that activity measured in a running wheel was more sensitive than schedule-controlled lever pressing maintained by food (Tepper, Weiss, and Cox 1982; Tepper, Weiss, and Wood 1983). The authors noted that the less sedentary behavior of running most likely led to inhalation of more ozone. They then made the opportunity to run in the wheel contingent upon lever pressing and demonstrated that this schedule-controlled behavior was equally sensitive to the activity measure (Tepper, Weiss, and Wood 1983).

More Complex Schedules of Reinforcement

The Fixed-Consecutive-Number Schedule

A more involved schedule, the fixed-consecutive-number (FCN) schedule, was used to examine the effects of a toxic substance, methylmercury, upon the ability of

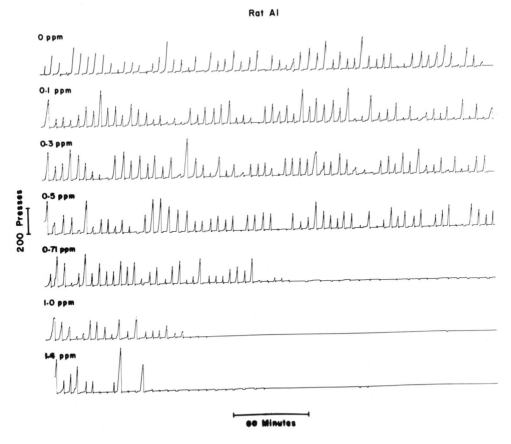

Fig. 5.3 Cumulative records of one rat's performance on a fixed-interval 5-minute schedule of reinforcement during exposure to various levels of ozone. Each lever press moved the response pen vertically a small amount while the recorder paper moved at a constant speed. The pen reset to the baseline when the first response was made following the end of each interval. Timeout periods of variable duration occurred after pellet deliveries. The height of each interval therefore gives the number of responses made during that period.
(*Source:* Weiss et al. 1981. Reprinted by permission of the publisher.)

an organism to discriminate its own behavior (Laties 1975; Laties and Evans 1980). This example also demonstrates how the addition of external discriminative stimuli can produce a profound change in methylmercury's effects. The subject, a pigeon, had to make a certain number of responses by pecking one key, followed by a peck on a second key, which gave it a few seconds' access to grain. Switching to the second key without successfully completing the requirement on the first reset the number and forced the bird to start all over again. This arrangement can also be described as a tandem schedule, since completion of the requirement on one schedule produced a second schedule, with no discriminative stimulus being correlated with the change from one to the other (Ferster and Skinner 1957, pp. 415–58). In this study, the requirement was to make at least eight but not more than nine responses on the first key before making the peck on the second. Switching after making seven or fewer, or ten or more, responses merely reset the requirement

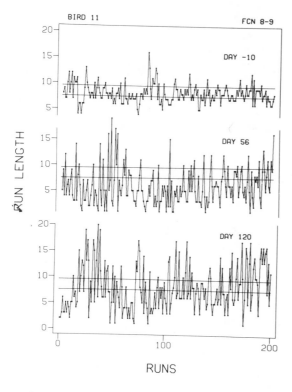

Fig. 5.4 The 200 response runs in sequence from each of three experimental sessions for a single pigeon. The horizontal bands enclose runs of eight and nine responses, the only ones reinforced. Methylmercury had been given on days 1–39. "Day -10" refers to a control session ten days before exposure began.
(*Source:* Laties and Evans 1980. Copyright by the Williams & Wilkins Co., Baltimore. Reprinted by permission of the publisher.)

without presenting the bird the opportunity to gain access to food by pecking the second key once. When exposed to such contingencies, a pigeon will readily learn to do what is required.

Figure 5.4 (top) shows how well a pigeon could perform on this schedule before being given any methylmercury. This bird started its experimental session by successively making 8, 9, 7, 7, 10, 12, and 8 responses on the first key, each of these runs being followed by a single response on the second key. Of course, only runs of 8 or 9 pecks—here enclosed by the horizontal lines—led to the presentation of grain. The next two panels show how methylmercury affected this performance. At its height, chronic exposure to the substance produced both a decrease in the length of the response runs made by the pigeon and an increase in within-session variability.

These results are presented in a different fashion in figure 5.5, where histograms of run lengths for selected sessions are shown both for the pigeon we have been discussing (11) and for a second pigeon (12), one not given methylmercury. Histograms for the three sessions in figure 5.4 are included (days 10, 56, and 120). The relatively high day-to-day reliability shows why this type of schedule-controlled behavior is so attractive as a baseline performance, especially when it is necessary to work with only a few animals, an almost inevitable limitation if one wishes to follow recovery over many months or years.

We have described this schedule partly because it gives us the opportunity to make a point about other factors that can modify the sensitivity of a schedule. Figure 5.6 shows some histograms of sessions from an experiment with a pigeon that showed approximately the same degree of performance impairment as pigeon

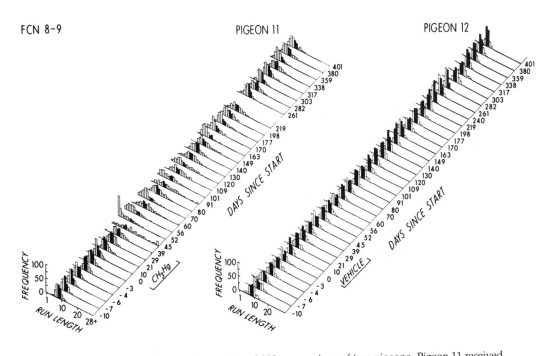

Fig. 5.5 Run-length histograms from selected 200-run sessions of two pigeons. Pigeon 11 received methylmercury during the time indicated, and pigeon 12 received the control vehicle during the same period. The filled bars represent run lengths of eight or nine responses, the only ones that were reinforced.
(*Source:* Laties and Evans 1980. Copyright by the Williams & Wilkins Co., Baltimore. Reprinted by permission of the publisher.)

11. Recall that only runs of 8 or 9 were reinforced and that the bird had only discriminative stimuli arising out of its own behavior to rely upon. Suppose that external stimuli correlated with the opportunity for reinforcement had been present. There is much evidence that behavior under the strong control of discriminative stimuli is more resistant to change by many, but not all, drugs (Laties 1972, 1975; Thompson 1978). Laties and Evans (1980) did not study whether methylmercury would have initially produced a lesser effect upon strongly controlled behavior, but they did ask whether the effect already shown by pigeons that had been given methylmercury could be modified by the addition of stimuli correlated with the opportunity for reinforcement. Figure 5.6 shows what happened when, starting with day 275, the key that the bird pecked turned red with the eighth response and back to its original white with the tenth. Key color soon took control of the switch to the second key; by day 284 (which was actually the eleventh session with the added discriminative stimulus) control was fairly strong, and by day 296 (the seventeenth session with the red key) it was excellent. When the added stimulus was removed, performance returned to its previous state, as can be seen in the final two histograms in the bottom panel. The top panel shows how a few months later, still with no discriminative stimulus signaling when reinforcement was available, the pigeon continued to show profound changes in its behavior. Once again, however, adding the discriminative stimulus led to behavior quite similar to that of unexposed birds working on such a schedule.

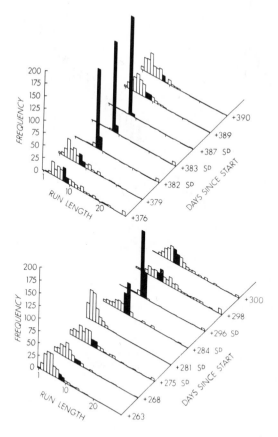

Fig. 5.6 Changes induced in run-length distributions by the addition of a discriminative stimulus (S^D). This stimulus was present after the eighth response and before the tenth on the fixed-consecutive-number schedule of reinforcement during sessions labeled "S^D." During other sessions no stimulus was correlated with any of the response runs. In all cases only runs of eight or nine responses were reinforced with a few seconds' access to mixed grain; these are indicated by the dark bars.
(*Source*: Laties 1975. Copyright by the Federation of American Societies for Experimental Biology. Reprinted by permission of the publisher.)

If behavior like that under control of the added discriminative stimulus had been chosen for examining the effects of methylmercury, very little change would have been detected. Would a general conclusion that the substance had no behavioral effect have been justified? Of course not. This points up the importance of a thorough exploration of just which variables modulate any observed behavioral effects (Ferster and Appel 1963; Sidman 1963). Without such a search, one can easily be fooled.

The work with the FCN schedule can be used to make another point about the usefulness of reinforcement schedules in toxicology. Because the toxicologist occasionally must study the effects of chronic exposure to a chemical, techniques that promise to maintain some specified behavior in a relatively constant state over prolonged time periods are of great interest. An animal that has been trained to work on a schedule of reinforcement will usually retain that training for a lifetime and will perform on call whenever required to do so. These attributes are particularly useful for the study of delayed or cumulative effects. We shall return to this point when discussing the role of schedule-controlled behavior in the regulation of chemicals.

Multiple Schedules

Starting with Ferster and Skinner (1957), reinforcement schedules have been combined in ways that bewilder the uninitiated. Here we shall limit ourselves to a few examples of combinations that have proven useful in illuminating questions in toxicology in the Rochester laboratories.

Behavioral changes have long been recognized as important consequences of human exposure to mercury vapor (Evans, Laties, and Weiss 1975). Nevertheless, it is somewhat surprising to find that a study by Armstrong et al. (1962, 1963) was, according to the authors, the very first to examine how chronic mercury poisoning affected any aspect of an intact animal's biological functioning, as well as apparently the first to use schedule-controlled behavior to study a toxic substance. Appropriately enough, given his pivotal position in the development of behavioral pharmacology, this early study of behavioral toxicology was partially designed by Peter B. Dews, who served as a consultant for the group at Rochester.* In fact, Armstrong spent some time with Dews and his colleague W. H. Morse, during which time Armstrong was introduced to the mysteries of operant conditioning. The behavior and the organism both reflected Dew's interests: key pecking in the pigeon. And so did the reinforcement schedules selected for the research: fixed-interval (FI) and fixed-ratio (FR), combined into what was already a staple in the field of behavioral pharmacology, the multiple FI-FR schedule (Dews 1956; Morse and Herrnstein 1956).

The object of the research was to discover whether the mercury vapor affected key pecking. In addition, it was meant to discover whether the effect depended upon the precise way in which the key-pecking response was maintained. Previous research, by Dews and others, had pointed to the fundamental importance of the schedule of reinforcement in determining what effect many drugs that influenced the central nervous system had upon behavior. The two ways chosen here for arranging for food delivery differed greatly. With the FR schedule the food hopper rose to a position accessible to the pigeon after each sixtieth peck. This schedule was in force whenever the key was transilluminated with red light. With the FI schedule food delivery occurred following the first key peck made after the key had been green for 15 minutes. After each food reinforcement, either the key remained the same color that it had been before reinforcement, in which case the pigeon remained on the same schedule, or it changed to the other color, meaning that the schedule had also changed. In order to ensure that the two colors were in control of the two schedules, they and their associated schedules were programmed to change together in an irregular fashion throughout the experimental session.

The two reinforcement schedules did indeed produce very different behaviors. Some cumulative records of one bird's behavior on these schedules are shown in figure 5.7. The last responses on one interval, a complete interval, six ratios, another complete interval, a single ratio, and then part of another interval are shown, with the position of these within a daily experimental session indicated at the top of the figure. Differences in the patterns of behavior determined by the schedules are immediately evident. First, the bird pecked at a very high rate on the

---

*Dew's contribution is described in a technical report in the following way: "A visit to the laboratory of P. B. Dews by one of us (HCH) led to the suggestion that operant behavior analysis might detect and characterize some of the chronic effects of mercury exposures in an animal. Following discussions with Dr. Dews a preliminary study was planned, making full use of his suggestions as to the selection of equipment and the design of behavioral testing programs" (Armstrong et al. 1962). "HCH" refers to Harold C. Hodge, then in the Department of Radiation Biology, who served as first chairman of the Department of Pharmacology at Rochester. In 1961–62 Hodge served as the first president of the Society of Toxicology.

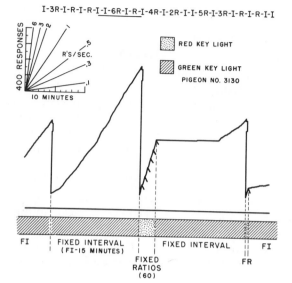

Fig. 5.7 Sample cumulative records of a pigeon's performance on the multiple fixed-interval 15-minute, fixed-ratio 60 schedule of reinforcement. The pen reset to the baseline at the end of each fixed interval. Diagonal slashes indicate reinforcements.
(*Source:* Armstrong et al. 1963. Reprinted by permission of the publisher.)

ratio schedule. Note that it made two or more responses per second while completing the six ratios in a row. (Compare the slope of the record with the slopes of the reference lines in the upper left corner of the figure.) Second, it responded at a much lower rate when on the fixed-interval schedule. Also, variability was great from interval to interval, with responding starting almost immediately within the first complete interval but in the next interval only after much of the interval had elapsed. And the rate achieved during the last parts of the intervals never exceeded about one response per second.

Note that performance on the two schedules was under very close control of key color; when the key was made red, the bird immediately started to peck the key in a manner "appropriate" for the FR schedule. When it turned green, the pigeon instantly stopped its rapid responding and changed to a low or even zero rate. This strong control of key pecking by the stimuli correlated with the two component schedules is what made it possible to examine repeatedly the two very different types of behavior within a single experimental session, merely by changing key color. The multiple schedule, consisting of a combination of two or more schedules, each under the control of its own unique stimulus, is one of the most powerful tools available to the behavioral investigator, making possible the elimination of confounding factors associated with the passage of time.

The changes produced by the mercury are shown in figure 5.8, where the ratio records for one pigeon are reproduced for the last session of each week's experimentation. Each vertical cumulative record represents key pecking during a single session, with the horizontal lines showing where fixed-interval records have been cut out (sample interval records are described below). The four control sessions shown (labeled "Chamber conditioning") display the high steady rate typically associated with the FR 60 schedule in the pigeon. Ten weeks of such control responding yielded a mean rate of 2.7 responses per second, and this rate never fell below 2.3 responses per second during several months of training on the schedule. Within three weeks of exposure to mercury vapor, the rate fell below this level, and

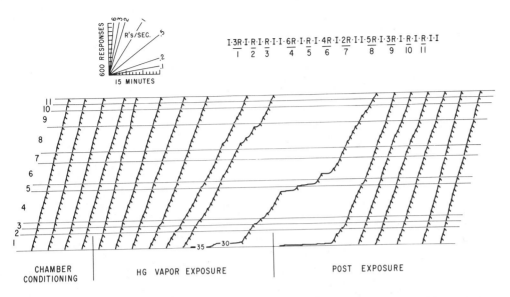

Fig. 5.8 Fixed-ratio performance before, during, and after exposure to mercury vapor, 2 hours per day, 5 days per week, at 17 mg Hg vapor/m³. The cumulative record of all the ratios from the last experimental session of each week are presented with the intervals removed. The diagonal slashes indicate reinforcements.
(*Source*: Armstrong et al. 1963. Reprinted by permission of the publisher.)

over the next several weeks it gradually fell even further, until exposure was stopped. Behavior then recovered in a few weeks.

Sample cumulative records of performance on the interval schedule are shown in figure 5.9. These are for the second interval of each session for which ratio behavior was presented in figure 5.8. The generally positively accelerated responding under control conditions was rapidly replaced by an almost complete suppression of responding. Although the particular intervals shown here indicate that intervals were more sensitive than ratios, these investigators concluded that the two schedules were affected equally by the vapor. If true, this would be somewhat surprising. The two schedules usually differ in sensitivity to both drugs (e.g., Kelleher and Morse 1968) and environmental toxicants (e.g., Levine 1976; see also below), with the interval schedule more likely to be disrupted than the ratio. However, since only the weekly overall response rate data were presented, not enough detail was provided to make any further analyses. Daily rates would have been more informative, since the effects came on rapidly. Unfortunately, the study by Armstrong et al. has never been replicated, and we are loath to conclude that the lack of specificity reported is truly a hallmark of mercury vapor. If it is, it would be an important finding. The general point we wish to make here is that using a multiple schedule allowed the investigators to compare two very different kinds of behavior during a single experimental session, switching from one to the other simply by changing the color of the response key.

The more usual differential sensitivity of the fixed-interval and fixed-ratio schedules was seen by Levine (1974, 1976) when she examined the effects of carbon disulfide on these two schedules, again using them as components of a multiple schedule. The essential findings are illustrated in figure 5.10, which shows repre-

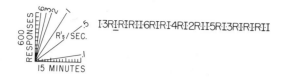

I3RIRIRII6RIRI4RI2RII5RI3RIRIRII

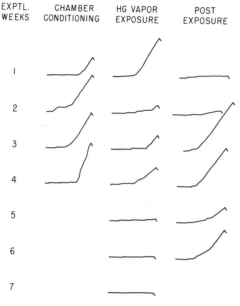

Fig. 5.9 Fixed-interval performance for four weeks before, seven weeks during, and six weeks after exposure to mercury vapor. The diagonal slash at the end of each interval's cumulative record indicates reinforcement.
(*Source:* Armstrong et al. 1962. Reprinted by permission of the publisher.)

sentative cumulative records for one pigeon under control conditions (top two records) and after either one or two days' eight-hour exposures to the carbon disulfide. The ratio performance withstood the toxicological insult much better than did the interval performance. The factors underlying this differential sensitivity are complex, involving the controlling variables associated with the two types of scheduled behavior (Kelleher and Morse 1968).

While the particular combination of schedules just discussed, multiple FI FR, has proven very popular, it is only one of a very large number of possible combinations. The particular combination used in an experiment naturally reflects the purpose of the investigation. Choice of the multiple FI FR offers the opportunity to compare results with those obtained by many other workers on many other substances. Partly for that reason, it is occasionally recommended as a general screening technique in behavioral toxicology (see NAS 1977). But other factors may outweigh the importance of this virtue and lead to the choice of a different combination.

The Role of Reinforcement Schedules in Investigating Behavioral Mechanisms of Action

Some experiments are not directed simply at screening for behavioral toxicity but are attempts to learn more about which aspects of behavior appear to be responsible for the behavioral changes that are seen. The investigator may try to learn how a

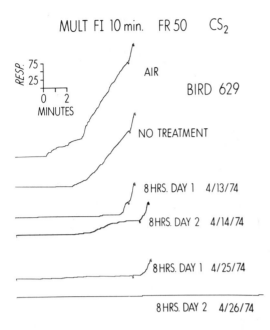

MULT FI 10 min. FR 50 CS$_2$

RESP.

AIR

BIRD 629

NO TREATMENT

8 HRS. DAY 1 4/13/74

8 HRS. DAY 2 4/14/74

8 HRS. DAY 1 4/25/74

8 HRS. DAY 2 4/26/74

Fig. 5.10 Cumulative records of performance on the multiple fixed-interval 10-minute, fixed-ratio 50 schedule of reinforcement. A single interval followed by a single ratio has been taken from the middle of each behavioral session. A diagonal slash indicates reinforcement, and the immediately following upward pen movement signals the change in schedule. (*Source:* Levine 1974. Reprinted by permission of the author.)

specific behavioral variable is affected by the toxic substance. This effort to understand the behavioral mechanisms underlying the observed effects requires knowledge of the determinants of the behavior under study. There is nothing unique about behavior in this regard; to understand the physiological or biochemical mechanisms of action of a chemical, knowledge of a system's physiology or biochemistry is required. Two quotations from the literature of behavioral pharmacology will serve to introduce this approach. The first, by Murray Sidman, puts the case well for first acquiring a thorough understanding of the behavior that is being investigated before proceeding to the study of a chemical's interactions with that behavior:

In establishing relations between drugs and behavior, it is necessary first to investigate the behavior intensively and to identify the specific variables which control it. Each drug must then be checked out against each known behavioral variable in order to determine which variable or combination of variables, changes its mode of control over the behavior. Functional relations must be determined, relating specific variables to behavior and these relations must then form the baseline from which to evaluate and classify the action of a drug. . . . One cannot simply adopt a behavioral technique as a means for evaluating drugs on the basis of some superficial characteristic of the technique. And after the behavioral spadework has been accomplished, the range of functional relations that will have to be investigated with each drug will greatly increase the complexity and amount of labor involved in drug-behavior investigations. Perhaps this is a discouraging prospect. But a subject matter cannot be simplified by ignoring its methodological problems. The only eventually effective approach will be to face these problems squarely and to devise more rapid and efficient methods for solving them. (Sidman 1963, pp. 168–69)

Travis Thompson and John Boren introduced their discussion of the role of this type of analysis in behavioral pharmacology this way:

It is important to keep in mind the principle that a drug cannot cause a biological system to respond in a qualitatively new way. That is, a drug may increase or decrease values of dependent variables but may not cause a fundamental change in the operation of the biological system. As a consequence, we must ask ourselves, "With which of the existing systems that regulate behavior is a drug interacting to produce the observed behavioral change?" This is the fundamental question to which we must address ourselves when we ask, "What is the behavioral mechanism by which this drug effect is brought about?" (Thompson and Boren 1977, p. 541)

Some pages later, they suggested the following:

Arriving at an understanding of the mechanisms by which drugs modify behavior is as complex as the permutations and combinations of variables which interact at any moment in time to engender a particular performance. . . . The rate, pattern, and form of current operant behavior are determined by certain antecedent factors, the current stimulus conditions, and the maintaining consequences of behavior. Drugs, as independent variables, interact with any or all of these classes of factors to determine the particular behavioral outcome. A better grasp of the meaning of a particular finding in behavioral pharmacology can be had if one asks, "With which of these factors that regulate behavior has the drug interacted?" Has the drug altered the deprivation state (an antecedent variable), stimulus control (a current stimulus variable), response topography (a property of the response), or the reinforcer or schedule control (a consequent variable)? (p. 553)

The multiple-schedule technique can be a powerful tool in such work. For instance, it allows one to vary one feature of a particular schedule in order to explore that feature's importance in determining the effects of a substance. The multiple schedule can thus be formed from two (or more) versions of a single schedule, the difference representing the variable under study. Any aspect of the schedule can be investigated. The number of responses required before the reinforcer is presented on a fixed-ratio schedule; the number of seconds that must pass before a response produces the reinforcer on a fixed-interval schedule; the minimum delay required between responses on an interresponse-time schedule; time-related stimuli that are available to the organism during, say, fixed-interval performance; the type of reinforcement presented at the end of each component—all such variables can be studied using the multiple schedule.

Examples abound of how a behavioral analysis contributes to the understanding of pharmacological agents (e.g., Dews 1958; Sidman 1959, 1963; Laties and Weiss 1969; Ferster and Appel 1963; and Harvey 1971; consult also the references listed in the introduction to this chapter). Rather few studies in behavioral toxicology can now be cited. In association with D. C. Rees, we recently studied whether the effects of the common solvent toluene on performance on the fixed-consecutive-number (FCN) schedule would be modified by the addition of a discriminative stimulus that indicated the completion of the minimum response requirement. The same technique had previously been used to study various drugs (Laties 1972; Laties, Wood, and Rees 1981). We varied one aspect of the stimuli being used to demarcate the component schedules within a multiple schedule (Wood, Rees, and Laties 1983). Two versions of FCN were used. In one version, FCN, a run of eight or more responses on the left of two levers followed by a response on the right lever was reinforced. No external stimulus indicated when the eight-response requirement had been satisfied. In the second version, FCN-SD, a complex stimulus consisting of a tone and a light came on with the eighth response, signaling the availability of reinforcement for making the right-lever response. (In Ferster and Skinner's terminology, these two schedules would be

R19

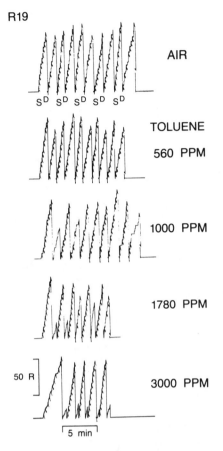

AIR

S^D S^D S^D S^D S^D

TOLUENE

560 PPM

1000 PPM

1780 PPM

50 R

3000 PPM

5 min

Fig. 5.11 Cumulative records of performance on the multiple FCN 8, FCN-S^D 8 schedule of reinforcement. The first, third, fifth, seventh, and ninth series of ten runs were on FCN-S^D 8, the others on FCN 8. The diagonal slashes indicate reinforcements for meeting the minimum response requirement. In each schedule component the pen reset to the baseline upon completion of the tenth run. Two-hour exposures to air or various concentrations of toluene preceded these performances. The FCN 8 schedule component shows much the greater sensitivity to toluene.
(*Source:* Wood, Rees, and Laties 1983. Reprinted by permission of the publisher.)

tandem FR8 FR1 and chain FR8 FR1, respectively.) Every ten runs these two slightly different schedules alternated. Under these conditions, the rats produced performances comparable to those obtained when the schedules were studied separately in earlier work, demonstrating that joining the schedules in this fashion did not compromise the experimental conclusions. Exposure to toluene produced performance impairment that was greater in the absence of the added external cues (fig. 5.11), an effect that was interpreted in terms of stimulus control, the behavioral variable that had been manipulated. This finding confirmed some results obtained when the schedules were studied independently, again verifying the choice of the multiple-schedule procedure. Moreover, combining the two schedules made it possible to gather the data in about half the time and to avoid the problems inherent in running experimental conditions serially.

Incidentally, on the more sensitive schedule used by Wood et al. (1963) some measures of toluene's effects showed changes at 560 ppm, which is close to the level reported to affect human behavior. One usually expects rodents to be substantially less sensitive to toxicants than humans; in this case, rodents and humans appear to display almost comparable sensitivity, although, of course, type of behavior as well as species is varying here.

The Use of Schedules to Increase the Sensitivity of a Behavioral Performance

Besides providing behavioral baselines for testing the effects of chemicals or other environmentally important factors, reinforcement schedules can prove useful in enhancing the sensitivity of a behavioral performance. In fact, assessment of the effects of a toxicant can sometimes depend crucially upon a seemingly insignificant characteristic of the schedule. Parametric variation such as that recommended above in the discussion of behavioral mechanisms of action and multiple schedules can be quite important. Thompson and Boren (1977) make the point that the effects of morphine on fixed-ratio behavior in the rat differ greatly depending upon the value of the ratio required; FR 40 was much more sensitive to the drug than was FR 10.

Wood (1979, 1981) found that modification of the response requirement on FR was very useful in decreasing the rate of a response, an effect that then made it possible to detect a substance's effects more easily. The study was concerned with describing a chemical's irritant properties. Wood was interested in developing a sensitive measure of irritation in the mouse. He adopted an escape procedure according to which the irritant would remain present until the animal performed a simple response. The irritant thus served as a negative reinforcer whose removal (for a one-minute period) served as the reinforcer. He used the apparatus shown in figure 5.12 to demonstrate that a mouse would readily learn to shut off the flow of a substance such as ammonia by interrupting a light beam with its nose.

A troublesome feature of the first experimental work was the high rate of response shown by the mouse even in the absence of the irritating substance. In this work, a single nose poke sufficed to shut off the substance; the schedule was therefore simply fixed-ratio 1, or FR 1. As can be seen in figure 5.13, about 50 percent of the occasions on which air alone was blown into the chamber were terminated with a nose poke. This left uncomfortably little room for maneuver for the determination of a concentration-effect curve, which would, of course, top out at close to 100 percent. The solution was to increase the response requirement to five light beam interruptions in a row (FR 5), a change that reduced terminations under control conditions to about 5 percent and made possible the very satisfactory curve shown in the figure.

There are many other ways in which schedules can be used to change sensitivity. Permitting performance on two schedules concurrently can, under some circumstances, uncover an effect that would not appear under simpler conditions. We have not yet used concurrent schedules with toxic substances, so an example will be drawn from some work on the effects of d-amphetamine on behavioral thermoregulation (Laties 1971). The question was whether the drug's effect upon lever pressing for heat reinforcement would be changed by the opportunity to work for food. Therefore, two reinforcement schedules were arranged to operate concurrently. On one, FR 1, a rat could warm itself by turning on two heat lamps (one below and one above the open chamber) for a brief period (2 seconds) by pressing a lever once. On the other, FR 75, the rat could earn a food pellet by pressing a different lever 75 times. Behavior in this situation was compared with that shown when only the heat lever was present. Since these two conditions were alternated every 15 minutes, with a retractable lever being introduced whenever the food reinforcement schedule was to be available, the whole experimental pro-

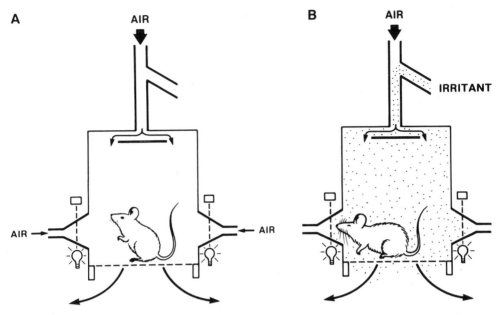

Fig. 5.12 Schematic drawing of the exposure chamber used to study irritant substances. Part A shows the situation before irritant delivery, and part B, the situation during irritant delivery. The chamber atmosphere was introduced at the top and struck a baffle, which ensured even mixing. The mouse stood on a perforated stainless-steel platform through which the atmosphere exhausted. The irritant was added to the dilution air immediately above the chamber. Delivery of the irritant could be terminated by the mouse's interrupting a light beam located in a conical recess in the wall. Only one of these sensors was active; the other served to measure the specificity of any behavioral changes. When the irritant was shut off, either by a nose poke or at the end of 60 seconds, a one-liter-per-minute stream of clean, humidified air was delivered through each cone in order to minimize the delay of irritant termination after a response had occurred.
(*Source:* Wood 1979. Reprinted by permission of the publisher.)

cedure may be considered to be a multiple schedule, one component being the concurrent FR 1 (heat), FR 75 (food) and the other being FR 1 (heat).

The drug experiments were done after the well-trained rats had been working on these schedules for about four hours and were making very few responses on the food lever but were responding on the heat lever about five times per minute. Figure 5.14 shows how various doses of the drug affected behavior. When only the heat lever was available (top graph), all but the lowest doses reduced response rate initially. The other two graphs summarize the results on the concurrent schedule, heat data in the center and food data at the bottom. The initial decrease in heat-reinforced responding seen when only the heat lever was available was now prolonged, and no large increases were seen. The bottom graph shows that the rat was working on the food lever when it was available. It was this behavior, brought on by the drug, that was competing with responding on the heat lever.

The effect was most dramatic at 1.5 mg/kg, and cumulative records for a single session at this dose are given in figure 5.15. The rat worked hardly at all for food during the predrug period (right column, top). Under drug, during the alternate 15-minute periods when the food lever was made available, the rat responded for food rapidly and rarely moved over to the heat lever. Thus the drug-induced decrease in heat-reinforced behavior was enhanced by the presence of the oppor-

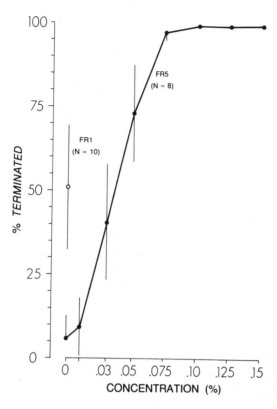

Fig. 5.13 The percentage of ammonia deliveries terminated by mice as a function of concentration when either one (FR 1) or five (FR 5) nose-poke responses were required to terminate the ammonia delivery. Mean +/− 2 SE. (*Source:* Wood 1981. Reprinted by permission of the publisher.)

tunity to work for food. (That increased sensitivity of a schedule-controlled performance is not the inevitable consequence of requiring performance on a second schedule was shown in some work with ethanol in humans by Laties and Weiss 1962: interresponse time distributions on the differential-reinforcement-of-low-rate schedule were not changed by the addition of a concurrently programmed fixed-interval schedule.)

The Role of Schedule-Controlled Behavior in the Regulation of Chemicals

A wide variety of chemicals in commerce, food additives, cosmetic ingredients, and pesticides remain to be evaluated for their neurobehavioral toxicity and constitute a high-priority testing need (NAS 1984). The authority to regulate these forms of toxicity resides in a variety of regulatory agencies, the principal ones being the Food and Drug Administration, the Consumer Product Safety Commission, and the Environmental Protection Agency (EPA). In an attempt to prevent hazardous chemicals from escaping regulation, Congress gave EPA overall authority for the prevention of the adverse effects of chemicals under the Toxic Substance Control Act of 1976. When it was adopted, behavioral toxicity was explicitly recognized as an adverse health effect, the incidence of which was to be minimized under the general provisions of the act. In one of the first proposed test rules issued under this act (Environmental Protection Agency 1980), EPA reaffirmed congressional concern about behavioral disorders and neurotoxicity when it asserted that

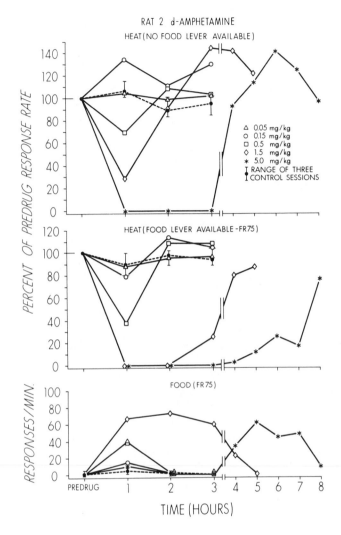

RAT 2 d-AMPHETAMINE
HEAT(NO FOOD LEVER AVAILABLE)

Δ 0.05 mg/kg
○ 0.15 mg/kg
□ 0.5 mg/kg
◇ 1.5 mg/kg
* 5.0 mg/kg
Ⅰ RANGE OF THREE
Ⅰ CONTROL SESSIONS

HEAT(FOOD LEVER AVAILABLE -FR75)

FOOD (FR75)

PERCENT OF PREDRUG RESPONSE RATE

RESPONSES/MIN.

PREDRUG   1   2   3   4   5   6   7   8

TIME (HOURS)

Fig. 5.14 The effects of d-amphetamine on both heat- and food-reinforced behaviors of a single rat. The curves for 0.05 and 1.5 mg/kg represent means of two sessions. The other drug curves represent single sessions. Mean heat-response pre-drug rates were 5.0 resp/min (range: 3.6–6.2) when no food lever was available and 5.1 resp/min (range: 4.1–6.3) when the food lever was available.
(*Source:* Laties 1971. Reprinted by permission of the publisher.)

the size of the exposed population was of less concern when deciding to test an existing chemical suspected of inducing such disorders.

[This] seems well founded since, if the testing reveals a serious hazard, some restrictions undoubtedly would be considered appropriate to reduce the risk when weighed against the alternative of doing nothing. Of course, economic, technological, and other considerations would influence the degree to which the risk could be reduced or eliminated. Even if there were an extraordinary case where no control options existed at present, the knowledge that people were exposed to a very hazardous chemical may create a substantial incentive to develop substitute products and processes. (Ibid., p. 48529)

Elsewhere in this book (chap. 17), Sette and Levine address the general question of how behavior is used in governmental regulation of chemicals. Here we consider the role that schedule-controlled behavior has been recognized to play in the regulatory process.

By 1977, three expert committees had recognized the contribution that schedule-controlled behavior could make to toxicity evaluation (NAS 1975, 1977; U.S.

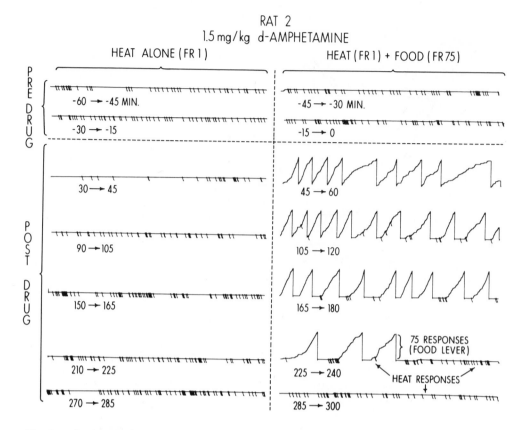

Fig. 5.15 Cumulative records showing the effects of 1.5 mg/kg d-amphetamine on both heat- and food-reinforced behaviors of a single rat. Alternate half-hour sections of the post-drug record have been omitted so as to avoid inordinate reduction in size. The rat had worked for three hours before the first records shown here. Each time it satisfied the 75-response requirement, the rat received a pellet and the pen returned to the baseline. The pen also returned to the baseline at the end of each 15-minute period.
(*Source:* Laties 1971. Reprinted by permission of the publisher.)

Department of Health, Education, and Welfare 1977). For instance, the *Report of the Second Task Force for Research Planning in Environmental Health Science* had asserted that "schedule-controlled behavioral baselines have been one of the principal research tools of behavioral pharmacology. With the methodology of operant behavioral pharmacology as a starting point, such tools should be adapted to serve as a sensitive general screen for safety evaluation and as a means for studying mechanisms of toxicity" (U.S. Department of Health, Education, and Welfare 1977, recommendation 13-5, p. 337).

The expert committees formed under the auspices of the Committee on Toxicology of the National Academy of Sciences prepared a document to assist the Consumer Product Safety Commission in implementing the Federal Hazardous Substances Act (NAS 1977). This committee agreed that the study of some type of operant behavior was necessary and recommended the use of a multiple schedule consisting, perhaps, of fixed-interval and fixed-ratio components. The argument was made there that a multiple schedule would yield a relatively broad sample of behavior, one likely to turn up many of a chemical's behavioral effects on complex operant behavior at the exposure level tested.

Although much concern has been expressed that the adoption of strictly prescribed testing procedures might not protect the public health and might retard the continuing growth of an interesting toxicological literature, and although we ourselves originally had grave doubts about arbitrary rules issuing from a central source (e.g., Weiss and Laties 1979), this concern seems to have been quite misplaced. EPA has resisted rigidification by adopting general guidelines rather than promulgating rigid test standards. Furthermore, the amount of toxicity evaluation actually required has been negligible. Given the great amount of information now needed, requiring more testing would be extremely desirable, since virtually any reliable information would aid in identifying the toxicity of whole classes of chemicals, as well as the toxicity of specific chemicals in need of more detailed examination.

The extent of this need for testing has recently been emphasized by a group that assessed the toxicity-testing needs for substances to which there is known or anticipated human exposure (NAS 1984). They identified a select universe of chemicals consisting of a wide variety of those used in commerce, food additives, cosmetic ingredients, and pesticides and inert ingredients. Reference protocol guidelines were established against which to determine the adequacy of existing neurobehavioral toxicity evaluation. These guidelines included neuropathological evaluation and functional evaluation of samples of both unconditioned and conditioned behavior. Neurobehavioral toxicity evaluation was the area of greatest testing need in two categories: pesticides and inert ingredients in pesticide formulations and cosmetic ingredients. For food additives and for three separate categories of chemicals in commerce, neurobehaviroal toxicity evaluation ranked in the top five areas of greatest testing need. Only for drugs and excipients used in drug formulations did the need for neurobehavioral toxicity information approach the median rank of the set of approximately 30 types of toxicity evaluation.

Having established that there is a need for such testing and that techniques are readily available for implementation, we turn now to how the regulator can interpret chemically induced changes in schedule-controlled behavior as findings that are predictive of unreasonable risk of injury to health. Although the health relevance of results generated using these testing procedures is frequently self-evident, some regulatory problems offer complex interpretive challenges.

It is self-evident that schedule-controlled behavior is useful in evaluating acute behavioral effects of chemicals. This has been demonstrated repeatedly throughout the 30-year history of modern behavioral pharmacology. The rates and patterns of behavior generated using schedules of reinforcement are repeatable both within an individual session and across a series of sessions. This makes possible the description of time-effect relationships both within a single session and across sessions. And since many acute effects are reversible, it may permit redeterminations within the individual subject. Stability is particularly important in studying the acute effects of agents given by inhalation. Duration of exposure is then an important determinant of the effect's concentration dependency during and following exposure. It is much easier to study these effects on endpoints that do not display marked trends across control exposures, since such trends confound the estimation of the magnitude of the effect with the initial value of the endpoint.

We have previously noted that schedule-controlled behavior in rodents can be affected by solvent exposure at concentrations relatively close to those demonstrated to alter human behavior (Wood, Rees, and Laties 1983). Information of this sort would be particularly useful in providing data for the establishment of short-term-exposure-limit (STEL) values. These are established by the American Conference of Governmental Industrial Hygienists (ACGIH) to prevent "narcosis of sufficient degree to increase accident proneness, impair self-rescue, or materially reduce work efficiency" (ACGIH 1983). In this case, the interpretation of changes in the temporal structure of behavior can be unambiguously interpreted as toxicity; no one exposed to chemicals involuntarily should expect to experience an alteration in reaction time or pattern of behavior that might interfere with the operation of heavy machinery on the factory floor, highway, or elsewhere where the consequences of impaired performance could have disastrous consequences. Nor should workers be expected to tolerate involuntary exposure to chemicals that could alter intellectual function or emotional behavior.

Schedule-controlled behavior can be used to characterize behavioral changes produced by pharmaceuticals, food additives, and cosmetics, just as it can be used to evaluate the adverse effects of environmental chemicals. However, the interpretation of changes in schedule-controlled behavior after exposure to chemicals intended for human use or consumption offers a more complex series of regulatory decisions. Few would consider acceptable any changes in behavior caused by appropriately chosen levels of a food additive whose sole function is to change color or flavor or to extend shelf life. Similarly, although the sole purpose of cosmetics is to change the behavior of others, no untoward behavioral effects on the wearer would be acceptable. On the other hand, a great deal of behavioral toxicity would not cause the removal of a drug from medical practice if the toxic pharmaceutical was the only alternative for patients with life-threatening or irreversibly debilitating disease.

Difficult decisions must also be made during the development of drugs intended to exert behavioral effects and in the evaluation of other therapeutic agents with undesirable side effects. One might be willing to accept moderate behavioral effects from over-the-counter medications marketed as hypnotics, analgesics, or cold remedies. However, few would consider a given formulation acceptable if it produced cumulative toxicity at moderate doses or, worse, irreversible changes or if it had abuse potential.

Summary

Schedules of reinforcement can be useful in evaluating the behavioral effects of chemicals. We have illustrated this usefulness with examples drawn from the experience of a single laboratory. The schedules approach has several advantages: relatively small numbers of animals are usually studied intensively with automatic data-collection equipment, so that the bias and unreliability associated with human observational data are eliminated. Animals can be used as their own controls, and this exclusion of between-subject variability enhances sensitivity. In addition, the contingencies of reinforcement themselves restrict variability within the individual animal, both within an individual session and across sessions. These procedures can be used to bring phenomena of interest under control in a laboratory setting, where the effects of toxicants can be thoroughly examined. Perhaps the greatest strength of these procedures lies not in their demonstrated ability to detect toxicity but in their ability to characterize its functional significance and to do this in terms derived from a coherent, systematic approach.

References

American Conference of Governmental Industrial Hygienists (ACGIH). 1983. *TLV's. Threshold limit values for chemical substances and physical agents in the work environment with intended changes for 1983–84.* Cincinnati, Ohio.

Armstrong, R. D.; Leach, L. J.; Belluscio, P. R.; Maynard, E. A.; Hodge, H. C.; and Scott, J. K. 1962. *Behavioral changes in the pigeon following inhalation of mercury vapor.* AEC Research and Development Report UR-578. Rochester, N.Y.: University of Rochester Atomic Energy Project.

Armstrong, R. D.; Leach, L. J.; Belluscio, P. R.; Maynard, E. A.; and Hodge, H. C. 1963. Behavioral changes in the pigeon following inhalation of mercury vapor. *Am. Indus. Hyg. Assoc. J.* 24:366–75.

Carlton, P. E. 1983. *Behavioral pharmacology.* New York: W. H. Freeman.

Cory-Slechta, D. A. 1984. The behavioral toxicity of lead: Problems and perspectives. In *Advances in behavioral pharmacology,* vol. 4, edited by T. Thompson, P. B. Dews, and J. E. Barrett, 211–55. Orlando, Fla.: Academic Press.

Cory-Slechta, D. A., and Thompson, T. 1979. Behavioral toxicity of chronic postweaning lead exposure in the rat. *Toxicol. Appl. Pharmacol.* 47:151–59.

Cory-Slechta, D. A.; Weiss, B., and Cox, C. 1983. Delayed behavioral toxicity of lead with increasing exposure concentration. *Toxicol. Appl. Pharmacol.* 71:342–52.

Dews, P. B. 1956. Modification by drugs of performance on simple schedules of positive reinforcement. *Ann. N.Y. Acad. Sci.* 65:268–81.

———. 1958. Analysis of effects of psychopharmacological agents in behavioral terms. *Fed. Proc.* 17:1024–30.

———. 1972. Assessing the effects of drugs. In *Methods in psychobiology,* edited by R. D. Myers, 2:83–124. New York: Academic Press.

———. 1976. Interspecies differences in drug effects: Behavioral. In *Psychotherapeutic drugs,* edited by E. Usdin and I. Forrest, 175–224. New York: Dekker.

Environmental Protection Agency. 1980. Chloromethane and chlorinated benzene: Proposed test rule. *Federal Register* 45:48524–66.

Evans, H. L.; Laties, V. G.; and Weiss, B. 1975. Behavioral effects of mercury and methyl mercury. *Fed. Proc. Am. Soc. Exp. Biol.* 34:1858–67.

Ferster, C. B., and Appel, J. B. 1963. Interpreting drug-behavior effects with a functional analysis of behavior. In *Psychopharmacologic methods,* edited by Z. Votava, M. Horvath, and O. Vinar, 170–81. New York: Macmillan.

Ferster, C. B., and Skinner, B. F. 1957. *Schedules of reinforcement.* New York: Appleton-Century-Crofts.

Harvey, J. A., ed. 1971. *Behavioral analysis of drug action: Research and commentary.* Glennview, Ill.: Scott, Foresman.

Iversen, S. D., and Iversen, L. L. 1981. *Behavioral pharmacology.* 2d ed. New York: Oxford University Press.

Kelleher, R. T., and Morse, W. H. 1968. Determinants of the specificity of behavioral effects of drugs. *Ergebn. Physiol.* 60:1–56.

Laties, V. G. 1971. Effects of *d*-amphetamine on concurrent schedules of heat and food reinforcement. *J. Physiol.* (Paris) 63:315–18.

———. 1972. The modification of drug effects on behavior by external discriminative stimuli. *J. Pharmacol. Exp. Ther.* 183:1–13.

———. 1975. The role of discriminative stimuli in modulating drug action. *Fed. Proc.* 34:1880–88.

———. 1982. Contributions of operant conditioning to behavioral toxicology. In *Nervous system toxicology,* edited by C. L. Mitchell, 67–79. New York: Raven Press.

Laties, V. G., and Evans, H. L. 1980. Methylmercury-induced changes in operant discrimination by the pigeon. *J. Pharmacol. Exp. Ther.* 214:620–28.

Laties, V. G., and Weiss, B. 1962. Effects of alcohol on timing behavior. *J. Comp. Physiol. Psychol.* 55:85–91.

———. 1969. Behavioral mechanisms of drug action. In *Drugs and the brain,* edited by P. Black, 115–33. Baltimore: Johns Hopkins Press.

Laties, V. G.; Wood, R. W.; and Rees, D. C. 1981. Stimulus control and the effects of *d*-amphetamine in the rat. *Psychopharmacology* 75:277–82.

Levine, T. E. 1974. Effects of carbon disulfide on operant behavior in pigeons. Ph.D. diss., University of Rochester, Rochester, N.Y.

———. 1976. Effects of carbon disulfide and FLA-63 on operant behavior in pigeons. *J. Pharmacol. Exp. Ther.* 199:669–78.

McKearney, J. W., and Barrett, J. E. 1978. Schedule-controlled behavior and the effects of drugs. In *Contemporary research in behavioral pharmacology,* edited by D. E. Blackman and D. J. Sanger, 1–68. New York: Plenum.

McMillan, D. E., and Leander, J. D. 1976. Effects of drugs on schedule-controlled behavior. In *Behavioral pharmacology,* edited by S. D. Glick and J. Goldfarb, 85–139. St. Louis: C. V. Mosby.

Morse, W. H. 1975. Schedule-controlled behaviors as determinants of drug response. *Fed. Proc.* 34:1868–69.

Morse, W. H., and Herrnstein, R. J. 1956. Effects of drugs on characteristics of behavior maintained by complex schedules of intermittent positive reinforcement. *Ann. N.Y. Acad. Sci.* 65:303–17.

National Academy of Sciences (NAS). 1975. Effects on behavior. In *Principles for evaluating chemicals in the environment,* 198–216. Washington, D.C.

———. 1977. Behavioral toxicity tests. In *Principles and procedures for evaluating the toxicity of household substances,* 111–18. Washington, D.C.

———. 1984. *Toxicity testing: Strategies to determine needs and priorities.* Washington, D.C.

Seiden, L. S., and Dykstra, L. A. 1977. *Psychopharmacology: A biochemical and behavioral approach.* New York: Van Nostrand Reinhold.

Sidman, M. 1959. Behavioral pharmacology. *Psychopharmacologia* 1:1–19.

———. 1963. Some technical problems in evaluating the behavioral effect of drugs. In *Psychopharmacological methods,* 162–69. *See* Ferster and Appel 1963.

Stern, S.; Margolin, L.; Weiss, B.; Lu, S. T.; and Michaelson, S. M. 1979. Microwaves: Effect on thermoregulatory behavior in rats. *Science* 206:1198–1201.

Tepper, J. L.; Weiss, B.; and Cox, C. 1982. Microanalysis of ozone depression of motor activity. *Toxicol. Appl. Pharmacol.* 64:317–26.

Tepper, J. L.; Weiss, B.; and Wood, R. W. 1983. Behavioral indices of ozone exposure. In *International symposium on the biomedical effects of ozone and related photochemical oxidants,* edited by S. D. Lee, M. G. Mostafa, and M. A. Mehlman, 515–26. Princeton, N.J.: Princeton Scientific Publishers.

Thompson, D. M. 1978. Stimulus control and drug effects. In *Contemporary research in behavioral pharmacology,* 159–207. *See* McKearney and Barrett 1978.

Thompson, T., and Boren, J. J. 1977. Operant behavioral pharmacology. In *Handbook of operant behavior,* edited by W. K. Honig and J. E. R. Staddon, 540–69. Englewood Cliffs, N.J.: Prentice-Hall.

Thompson, T., and Grabowski, J. G. 1972. *Reinforcement schedules and multioperant analysis.* New York: Appleton-Century-Crofts.

Thompson, T., and Schuster, C. R. 1968. *Behavioral pharmacology.* Englewood Cliffs, N.J.: Prentice-Hall.

U.S. Department of Health, Education, and Welfare. 1977. *Human health and the environment—some research needs. Report of the Second Task Force for Research Planning in Environmental Health Science.* DHEW Pub. No. NIH 77-1277. Washington, D.C.: Government Printing Office.

Weiss, B.; Ferin, J.; Merigan, W.; Stern, S.; and Cox, C. 1981. Modification of rat operant behavior by ozone exposure. *Toxicol. Appl. Pharmacol.* 58:244–51.

Weiss, B., and Laties, V. G. 1961. Behavioral thermoregulation. *Science* 133:1338–44.

————. 1967. Comparative pharmacology of drugs affecting behavior. *Fed. Proc.* 26:1146–56.

————. 1976. *Behavioral pharmacology: The current status.* New York: Plenum. Originally published in *Fed. Proc.* 34 (9) (August 1975).

————. 1979. Assays for behavioral toxicology: A strategy for the Environmental Protection Agency. In *Neurobehav.* 1, Toxicol. suppl. 1, *Test methods for definition of effects of toxic substances on behavior and neuromotor function,* edited by I. Geller, W. C. Stebbins, and M. J. Wayner, 213–15.

Wood, R. W. 1979. Behavioral evaluation of sensory irritation evoked by ammonia. *Toxicol. Appl. Pharmacol.* 50:157–62.

————. 1981. Determinants of irritant termination behavior. *Toxicol. Appl. Pharmacol.* 61:260–68.

Wood, R. W.; Rees, D. C.; and Laties, V. G. 1983. Behavioral effects of toluene are modulated by stimulus control. *Toxicol. Appl. Pharmacol.* 68:462–72.

*Diane B. Miller and
David A. Eckerman*

6

Learning and Memory Measures

Impaired cognitive function often numbers among the adverse effects associated with exposure to toxicants. The predominance of symptoms associated with impaired cognitive function requires that measures designed to identify deficits in learning and memory be included in the determination of an agent's neurotoxic potential (Cabe and Eckerman 1982; Dewar 1983; Anger 1984; Anger and Johnson 1985). Such impairments have ranged from the frank mental retardation and diminished intellectual capacity found in the offspring of victims of methylmercury exposures that occurred in Canada, Minimata Bay, Iraq, Pakistan, and Guatemala (Takeuchi 1972, 1977; Harada 1977; Amin-Zaki et al. 1979; McKeown-Eyssen and Ruedy 1983; Marsh 1985) or in children exposed to high levels of lead (Pentschew 1965; Perlstein and Attala 1966; Center for Disease Control 1978) to the mental confusion accompanied by problems in concentrating, remembering, and thinking expressed after exposure to organic solvents (Hane et al. 1977; Arlien-Søborg et al. 1979; Mikkelsen 1980), organophosphates (Holmes and Gaon 1956; Gershon and Shaw 1961; Dille and Smith 1964; Metcalf and Holmes 1969; Levin and Rodnitzky 1976; Duffy et al. 1979; Sterman and Varma 1983), polybrominated biphenyls (PBBs) (Valciukas et al. 1978; Brown and Nixon 1979), chlordecone (Kepone®) (Taylor et al. 1978) inorganic lead, and mercury (Hanninen et al. 1979; Smith and Langolf 1981; Hogstedt et al. 1983; Smith, Langolf, and Goldberg 1983).

With human exposures, an anecdotal report or complaint of memory loss (e.g., Valciukas et al. 1978) is frequently the first step in an evaluative sequence. Epidemiological assessment follows, and finally assessment culminates in actual laboratory testing for memory impairment. The Michigan PBB episode (see Brown and Nixon 1979; and Brown et al. 1981) is of particular interest not only because it illustrates this sequence but also because it illustrates one of the major problems in this specialized area: the problem of unequivocally demonstrating a *direct effect* of a toxic agent *on learning or memory*. In some cases the sequence from anecdote to actual laboratory testing affirms and documents the initial reports of impaired cognition (e.g., mercury [see Smith and Langolf 1981]). In the Michigan episode, on the other hand, further testing revealed that the initial complaints could be accounted for as reactions to the stress of the situation rather than a direct result of exposure to PBB (Brown et al. 1981). While some of the measured changes in behavior at first appeared to involve deficits in learning and memory, these changes eventually proved to be secondary to a shift in attention or motivation. Thus it was finally concluded that for the individuals exposed in the Michigan PBB incident, rather than a direct memory impairment, other "factors affecting psychological functioning may [have been] more important causes of memory complaints and low scores on objective tests of memory than [was] the level of PBB contamination" (ibid.).

The PBB episode in Michigan highlights the pivotal issue in the use of measures of learning and memory in neurotoxicity—unequivocal demonstration that a toxic insult has changed these attributes. To adequately test an effect on the ability to learn and remember requires a series of tests for the direct as well as the indirect effects of an agent. It is our hope that this review will aid in improving future evaluations of toxic impairment of learning and memory. To meet this goal, the dual purposes of this chapter are (1) to consolidate and integrate the available literature, both human and infrahuman, on learning and memory measures in the detection and characterization of neurotoxicant exposure effects and (2) to make suggestions for the future use of learning and memory measures in neurotoxicology.

This review also has several limits. First, we do not attempt to review the effects of specific agents; rather, we draw examples from the toxicology literature to illustrate issues relevant to the measurement of learning and memory effects in neurotoxicology. We also draw examples from the considerable literature evaluating effects of pharmacological agents, aging, and relatively specific disease states such as Alzheimer's disease or Korsakoff's syndrome. Many issues and problems in detecting and characterizing cognitive deficits explored in these literatures are the same as those faced in neurotoxicology. Further, the effects of a toxic agent may mimic those of a pharmacological agent, aging, or disease states. Second, we attempt to build on, rather than duplicate, the recent reviews of neurotoxic effects provided by Feldman, Ricks, and Baker 1980; Cabe and Eckerman 1982; Weiss 1983a, 1983b; and Anger and Johnson 1985.

Neurotoxicity can be defined as any unwanted change in the functional status of the nervous system. As such, changes in learning and memory after toxic insult are neurotoxic effects. Such changes may be either relatively permanent or quite reversible in nature and still be considered as evidence of neurotoxicity (Dewar 1983), although irreversible effects are of greater concern. The long-term effect of exposure is not always immediately apparent. An agent may have insidious, slowly accumulating effects that are irreversible, as well as readily observed reversible effects. For example, solvents (including the aromatic hydrocarbons, aliphatic hydrocarbons, and alcohols) can produce acute or reversible central nervous system (CNS) effects that include headache, dizziness, nausea, drunken feeling, and absent-mindedness. Continued exposure to these same agents, however, results in apparently irreversible symptoms, including difficulty in sleeping, chronic tiredness, difficulty in concentration, and impaired memory, as well as possible structural damage to the nervous system (see Arlien-Søborg et al. 1979; Husman 1980; and Seppäläinen 1981). In the present paper, any unwanted change in learning and memory, whether reversible or irreversible, is considered a neurotoxic effect. Also, somewhat more emphasis is placed on memory measures than on learning measures, since these deficits are frequently the focus of interest after toxicant exposure in humans.

Definition of Learning and Memory

An attempt to integrate the existing literature on the use of learning and memory measures in the assessment of neurotoxicity must begin by specifying the meaning of these commonly used terms. Since the terms are appropriate for many behavioral changes, however, no exact and exhaustive definition of either is uniformly agreed upon. We shall therefore start with a general specification: *learning* is a relatively long-lasting change in behavior resulting from a change in the environment, while *memory* is the retention of that change (McGaugh 1973; Cabe and Eckerman 1982). It should be clear from a logical standpoint that memory is impossible without learning, and learning cannot occur if there is no long-term impact of prior events (i.e., memory). While these statements specify an area of interest, the exact definition of either *learning* or *memory* is difficult because these effects cannot be directly measured. Rather, they indicate complex changes in behavior over time. Behavior is influenced by myriad environmental changes, with only some of these influences being long-lasting changes classified as learning or memory. Changes affecting behavior not classified as learning include changes in motivation, arousal, attention, and sensory capacity. These factors are described as nonassociative effects (note that these effects are different from those described below under the topic of nonassociative learning: habituation and sensitization). A toxic agent may, for example, reduce the palatability of food reinforcers, alter locomotor ability, or decrease control exerted by particular stimuli—all effects that can alter performance. Such nonassociative effects of toxicants are of interest in themselves. Yet, to draw conclusions regarding effects of toxicants on learning and memory, nonassociative effects must be dissociated. Stated broadly, if a learning or memory task requires locomotion and the agent in question prevents completion of the task by paralysis, it would be erroneous to conclude that it has a direct effect on learning or memory (see Rodier 1978 for a discussion of these issues in behavioral teratology). It should be noted, then, that in practice, since measurement of learning and memory depends on adequate functioning in other categories, attribution of a change as a learning and memory effect will be completely clear only when these other functions are relatively unimpaired (see Izquierdo et al. 1983).

The Role of Human versus Nonhuman Subjects in Assessing Toxic Effects on Learning and Memory

Human exposure is frequently the impetus for the study of a particular toxic agent, with anecdotal reports serving to identify agents of concern to the health of human populations. Learning and memory impairments are generally described by exposed individuals using subjective terms such as impaired concentration, increased distractibility, mental confusion, difficulty in thinking, and slowed thoughts or mental functioning (Weiss 1983*a,b*; Anger and Johnson 1985). Adequate characterization of effects and dose-response relations rarely can be constructed from available field and clinical data (see Fein et al. 1983). Different durations of exposure, as well as exposure during different periods of the life span, can result in different patterns of effect from the same neurotoxicant (e.g., methylmercury [Reuhl and Chang 1979]). In addition, other determining factors, such as prexisting disease states, motivation to perform, and personality factors, contribute significantly to deterioration of function. For example, subjects may be motivated to do poorly, or they may refuse to cooperate at all. In a discussion of memory evaluation in the elderly, Crook and colleagues (e.g., Crook 1979; Crook, Ferris, and McCarthy 1979; Crook et al. 1980) note several relevant issues. To engage the subject in a task, it may be particularly important that an evaluation have face validity and that the subjects be able to relate the test to everyday activities. The elderly frequently score poorly, not because their ability to do memory tasks has deteriorated, but because they are not interested in doing well on that particular task. On the other hand, if the test is transparent, poor performance might occur if the subjects will profit from the handicap or merely if they believe that they have been exposed to toxic agents. While there are testing strategies that seek to reduce the effects of motivation (Gullion and Eckerman, chap. 14 in this volume), such complexities cloud most clinical and field studies. Determination of the effects of motivational factors is somewhat easier in studies using nonhuman subjects, although here, too, caution is needed.

It is sometimes possible to search for patterns of effects with exposed humans if the causal agent has been identified (see Schaumburg, Spencer, and Arezzo 1983). Given the complexities of assessment, however, both human and nonhuman studies are typically needed to adequately characterize a neurotoxic effect. While research with nonhumans may never totally mimic effects observed in the human population, animal studies allow the researcher more control over possible contributing factors as well as dose and duration of exposure to the putative toxicant. The ability to manipulate these dosing and testing parameters allows the researcher to evaluate patterns of effects not available in exposed human populations (see Morris 1983).

Learning Measures

Many methods are available for assessing learning. They are generally categorized as ways to evaluate either nonassociative or associative learning, with the major emphasis being on the acquisition of the behavior.

Nonassociative Learning

The nonassociative, simple forms of learning—habituation and sensitization—are rudimentary types of response change (e.g., increased heart rate, orienting, whole-body startle, limb withdrawal) that occur with repeated presentation of stimuli (e.g., light, shock, flavor, complex stimuli such as an entire test chamber) that are explicitly unpaired with an outcome such as food (Kandel 1979). Organisms at all points on the phylogenetic scale, from invertebrates (e.g., *Aplysia*) to man, are capable of nonassociative learning. Its ubiquity as well as its occurrence early in ontogeny of many species suggests that it is an evolutionarily useful way of adapting to changes in the environment. At a theoretical level (see Groves and Thompson 1970; and Thompson et al. 1973) stimulation of any sensory system affects dual processes in the CNS. The first of these is an enhanced excitability of the system to stimulation—sensitization. The second effect of the same stimulation is a decremental process—habituation—resulting in decreased responsiveness of the system to stimulation. There are still some arguments as to whether habituation and sensitization are really primitive forms of learning, because the response form does not change with repeated stimulation (see Shepard 1983). Nonassociative learning, especially in invertebrates, has been the focus of recent research owing to the belief that an understanding of the neural and biochemical substrates of learning and memory may be best approached through the use of simple model systems (e.g., Kandel and Schwartz 1982). Current work with the mollusc *Aplysia* suggests that the same molecular mechanisms are involved in sensitization, habituation, and classical conditioning and that the same unifying principles may serve both associative and nonassociative learning, that is, that there is a common mechanism that can account for all learning (see Hawkins and Kandel 1984). Habituation (a decrease in responsiveness) and its opposite, sensitization (an increase in responsiveness), are short-lived changes. Sensitization is usually the briefer of the two, frequently enduring only for minutes; the intensity and duration of the response are directly related to the strength of the eliciting stimulus. While habituation endures longer than does sensitization, there appears to be both a temporary and a long-lasting form.

Temporary and long-lasting habituation of the acoustic startle response are nicely illustrated by Leaton (1976) (see fig. 6.1). In the first phase, whole-body startle to a single presentation of a loud tone was measured. Although the tone occurred only once in each 24-hour period, habituation still occurred. The amplitude of the response, while not totally abolished, decreased with repeated presentations. Because the amplitude on a given day was lower than that of the preceding days, this decrease can be described as a long-lasting habituation of the startle response; and because the tone presentations were 24 hours apart, the decrease cannot be attributed to fatigue. However, when the tone was presented 300 times with 3 seconds between presentations, the startle response quickly habituated, and virtually no response was observed by the end of phase 2. That the habituation observed in this phase was temporary was demonstrated in the next phase, where the tone was again presented only once in 24 hours. Since the startle amplitude here and at the end of phase 1 are similar, it can be concluded that the phase 2 decrease after massed presentation was a temporary habituation and that recovery had occurred. Although recovery did occur, note that the amplitude of the whole-body startle was never as great as after the first few tone presentations. Dishabituation can also be used to demonstrate that habituation of a response is a result of nonassociative learning and not fatigue. For example, if a novel stimulus had been presented during phase 2 of the Leaton experiment, the amplitude of the startle response could have increased almost to the level observed at the beginning of tone presentations.

The startle response can be used to evaluate pharmacological and toxicological treatments and in fact has been suggested as an ideal measure of sensory stimulation for assessment in toxicology. Essentially the same procedure could be used to evaluate both adaptation and the functioning of sensory systems across species (see Adams and Buelke-Sam 1981; and Cabe and Eckerman 1982). Certain CNS-active compounds, such as LSD and phencyclidine, appear to prevent the habituation of the startle response (Geyer et al. 1978; Geyer, Segal, and Greenberg 1984). For example, phencyclidine in a dose that does not affect the initial response to an airpuff stimulus does prevent the habituation of the startle response (Geyer, Segal, and Greenberg 1984) (see fig. 6.2). The amplitude of the response is almost the same at both the beginning and the end of testing. These nonassociative forms of

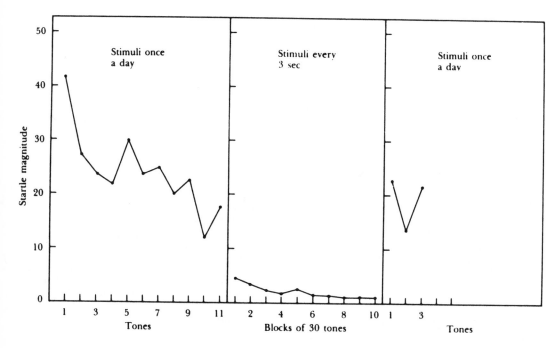

Fig. 6.1 Long-lasting and temporary habituation of the whole-body acoustic startle response to a loud tone in the rat. Amplitude of the response was measured following each tone presentation, but the period of time separating these presentations varied. In phase 1 (*left panel*) the tone was presented once every 24 hours, and over successive days the amplitude of the startle response gradually diminished to about half of its original strength. In phase 2 (*middle panel*) the tone was presented 300 times a day with a 3-second separation between presentations. This massed presentation resulted in an almost total cessation of the response. However, a return to a single presentation of the tone every 24 hours (*right panel*) caused the startle to recur, demonstrating the temporary nature of the habituation engendered by massed tone presentations (*middle panel*). The results from phase 3 also demonstrate the presence of long-lasting habituation, because the amplitude of the response was less than that seen with the initial presentation of the tone.
(*Source:* Leaton 1976. Reprinted by permission of the publisher.)

learning, because of their generalized occurrence and apparent simplicity, have provided the means, across a broad spectrum of research settings, for answering practical as well as theoretical questions concerning learning and memory in organisms ranging from the blowfly (*Calliphora vomitoria*) to the preverbal human infant. The discriminative capabilities of human infants have been detailed using these procedures, which have also provided evidence for how well a particular sensory system functions (see Cabe and Eckerman 1982). The retention capabilities of the human infant have also been addressed using nonassociative learning paradigms. For example, if infants are repeatedly shown the same visual stimulus, the gaze response habituates. If the previous stimulus is then paired with a novel one, the infant will gaze at the new one rather than the old. This suggests that there is some mechanism for a comparison between the old and the new stimulus (i.e., recognition memory). Infants with known CNS disabilities or developmental disorders, such as Down's syndrome, are delayed in the development of this type of memory capacity (Miranda and Fantz 1973, 1974; Miranda, Hack, and Fantz 1977; Harmant et al. 1983). While Bornschein, Pearson, and Reiter (1980a, 1980b), in their

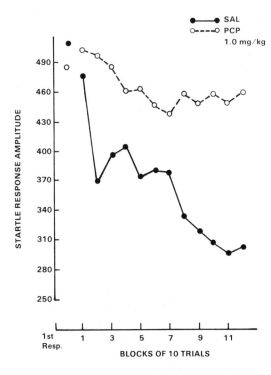

Fig. 6.2 The ability of phencyclidine (PCP) to interfere with the habituation of the whole-body startle response. When compared with saline controls, subjects injected with 1.0 mg/kg PCP s.c. 35 minutes before the first trial showed little diminution in the amplitude of their startle response with repeated presentations (12 blocks of 10 trials) of a tactile stimulus (15 p.s.i. airpuff). The amplitude of the startle response for the control and groups treated with drug was the same on the initial trial.
(*Source:* Geyer, Segal, and Greenberg 1984. Reprinted by permission of the publisher.)

review of the lead toxicity literature, conclude that objective means for assessing the impact of neurotoxic agents on learning and memory in children, especially in the preverbal stages, would be useful, there appears to have been no attempt to apply nonassociative learning paradigms to these types of neurotoxicology problems.

Associative Learning

Associative learning, usually categorized as either classical conditioning or instrumental learning, as the name implies, is a formed association between a stimulus and an outcome when they are explicitly paired. However, what is associated in the two categories differs.

Classical Conditioning. In classical conditioning, also referred to as Pavlovian or respondent conditioning, an association develops between a previously neutral stimulus and a response as a function of repeated pairing. The organism is often considered to have a passive role, because the stimulus is responded to rather than acted on. Initially, an unconditioned stimulus (UCS) such as food will elicit a reflex such as salivation. If a stimulus such as a buzzer predicts an increased likelihood of the UCS, the buzzer comes to elicit a conditioned reflex (CR), in this case also salivation. A consideration of the important parameters in classical conditioning is presented in Cabe and Eckerman (1982).

Certain classical conditioning paradigms have value in the analysis of the neuronal substrates of learning and memory, much as nonassociative habituation and sensitization paradigms have been used as model systems. In particular, the rabbit eyeblink or nictitating membrane response has utility because of some special characteristics of this preparation. Rabbits rarely blink so it is easy to distinguish the conditioned or learned response over baseline responses of the same type: in other classical conditioning situations this is not so easily accomplished. More important perhaps is the relatively small role that motor systems have in the display of this response.

While Gormezano and colleagues have made ample use of the rabbit nictitating membrane system to delineate the role of various neural systems in the classical conditioning of this response and in a characterization of the effects of numerous pharmacological agents (e.g., morphine, LSD), little use of this particular classical conditioning paradigm has been made in neurotoxicology (Gimpl, Gormezano, and Harvey 1978; Harvey, Gormezano, and Cool 1982). Of course, nonassociative learning can be studied within the context of classical conditioning. For example, habituation and sensitization to the unconditioned stimulus occur, and Harvey, Gormezano, and Cool-Hauser (1983) have made use of this in elucidating the role of cholinergic systems in this response. Specifically, scopolamine, a cholinergic antagonist, retards the acquisition of the conditioned eyelid response in rabbits but has little or no effect on the development of long-lasting habituation to the tone or aversive shock when they are presented separately. In effect, scopolamine interferes with the learning of the association between the signal and the aversive event.

In part because of historical and theoretical issues, Soviet scientists more than their Western counterparts have applied classical conditioning procedures in the field of neurotoxicology. Recent work, however, does suggest the potential for use in evaluating classical conditioning preparations in which the conditioned response has only a small motoric component, for example, the rabbit nictitating membrane extension (Yokel 1983, 1985). Adult rabbits exposed to repeated injections of aluminum, a suspected etiological factor in the mental and neurological deterioration sometimes accompanying kidney dialysis, did not condition as well as controls (i.e., the percentage of responses exhibited in response to the tone signaling shock was higher for the control group than for the high-dose aluminum group) (Yokel 1983) (see fig. 6.3). Aluminum can affect peripheral motor function, and since previous attempts to clarify its effects on learning and memory have relied on conditioned responses requiring significant motor movement, the deficits observed may be owing to the effect of aluminum on motor responses rather than learning. The Yokel (1983) study suggests that these deficits may indeed be mediated centrally.

Otto and colleagues, in a unique application of classical conditioning methodology in conjunction with human electrophysiology techniques, were able to demonstrate long-term deficits in the sensory conditioning of children exposed to nonencephalopathic lead levels. The application of classical conditioning techniques allowed the demonstration of learning deficits in an experimental setting where the subjects were required to make neither verbal nor motor responses (Otto et al. 1981; see also Cabe and Eckerman 1982).

In another application of classical conditioning methodology a discrimination variation of the standard rabbit nictitating membrane procedure was used to assess the impact of brain lesions on the formation of the conditioned blink (Berger and Orr 1983; Orr and Berger 1985) (see fig. 6.4). During conditioning two stimuli or tones were used. One of these (CS+) was always followed by the UCS; the other (CS−) was never followed by the UCS. Brain lesions made prior to discrimination

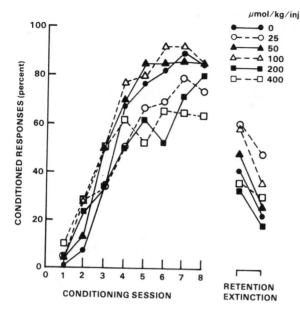

Fig. 6.3 The effect of increasing doses of systemic aluminum lactate (0.0, 25.0, 50.0, 100.0, 200.0, 400.0 μmol/kg per injection 5 times a week for four weeks) on classical conditioning of the nictitating membrane extension (NME) of the New Zealand white rabbit. The data are expressed as (*left*) the mean percentage of NMEs conditioned with 50 pairings of paraorbital shock (UCS) and tone (CS+) interspersed with 50 trials of a different tone (CS−) not paired with shock in each of 8 conditioning sessions and (*right*) the percentage of conditioned NMEs that occurred with 100 presentations of the CS+ alone. All groups receiving aluminum lactate exhibited classical conditioning of the NME, but the mean percentage conditioned responses (CR) for the 400.0 μmol/kg group were only 75 percent of those for the control group. Because no substantial motor movement is necessary for the NME and because all groups exhibited conditioning of the NME, the deficits in acquisition of the CR probably cannot be attributed to effects of aluminum on motor or sensory systems. The results suggest that systemic exposure to this compound may interfere with the learning of the association between the shock and tone. In contrast, extinction of the conditioned NME was not retarded by aluminum treatment. (*Source:* Yokel 1983. Reprinted by permission of the publisher.)

training had little obvious effect on formation of the conditioned eyeblink, but when the CS+ and CS− were reversed, the development of this new association was severely compromised in animals with lesions of the hippocampus (left panel). Additional information was provided by assessing which components of reacquisition were most affected. Although the rabbits were able to form an association between the previously neutral tone and an aversive event, they also continued to respond to the tone that formerly had signaled the airpuff (right panel). There was some individual variation in the degree to which lesions of the hippocampus affected reversal learning (right panel). Discrimination and discrimination-reversal variants of classical conditioning procedures do not appear to have been applied extensively in neurotoxicology settings.

Conditioned taste aversion is the one classical conditioning preparation that has received a fair amount of use in both the detection and the characterization of neurotoxicity. In the hallmark study demonstrating this phenomenon, a known emetic agent, lithium chloride, was paired with novel saccharin-flavored water. In later testing the decreased consumption of the saccharin-flavored water was interpreted as a classically conditioned aversion. Thus, an association is formed between the novel flavor—saccharin—the (CS), and the effect of the lithium chloride—the UCR (illness, gastrointestinal stress, etc.). Suppression of a consum-

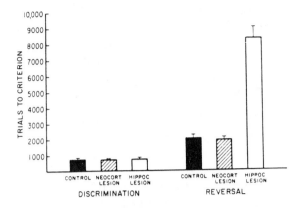

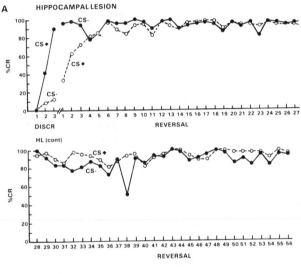

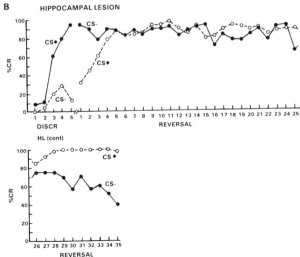

Fig. 6.4 The effect of lesions of the hippocampus on discrimination and discrimination-reversal conditioning of the nictitating membrane extension of the rabbit. New Zealand white rabbits received lesions in the neocortex or the hippocampus or served as sham controls. Post-surgical training consisted of 12 daily blocks of trials (16 trials/block) in which a 1 or 10 kHz tone served as the CS+ and was paired with an airpuff to the eye (UCS); the remaining tone served as the CS−. Discrimination training continued until a conditioned NME occurred in at least 85 percent of the CS+ trials and less than 15 percent on the CS− trials. When the criterion was reached, the CS+ and CS− stimuli were reversed. The data are expressed as trials to criterion. Lesions had no effect on acquisition of the initial discrimination; all groups required 1,000 or fewer trials to reach the criterion. All groups required more trials to learn the reversal of this discrimination, but lesions of the hippocampus substantially increased the number of trials necessary (*top*). Although these subjects (*bottom*) were able to develop a conditioned NME to the former CS−, they also continued to show a NME to the previous CS+ when it was no longer associated with the airpuff. This difficulty persisted for long periods, although in some cases training continued for as long as 56 sessions (*A of bottom illustrations*).
(*Source:* Berger and Orr 1983. Reprinted by permission of the publisher.)

matory response is, however, used as the index of conditioning because of the difficulty in objectively quantifying an internal state such as gastrointestinal distress. Note that the use of a subject-initiated response, drinking or eating, also allows conditioned taste aversion to be considered a passive-avoidance or instrumental-learning paradigm. The subject "passively" avoids by not drinking or eating (see the discussion of passive avoidance below).

That centrally active pharmacological agents such as amphetamine can also serve as the UCS for the demonstration of taste aversions suggests that internal states other than nausea and so on may be sufficient for conditioning (see Berger 1972; Wise, Yokel, and deWit 1976; Booth et al. 1977; Gamzu 1977; and Miller and Miller 1983). While high doses of amphetamine can cause nausea, this drug can induce taste aversions at doses well below those necessary to induce gastrointestinal distress, a common side effect of high doses (see Cappell and LeBlanc 1975). Lesions of the area postrema, a chemoreceptive brainstem emetic region, will abolish the effectiveness of lithium chloride in inducing taste aversion but have little effect on amphetamine-induced aversions (see Berger, Wise, and Stein 1973). As has been suggested, taste aversion is multifaceted in nature and clearly may be induced by mechanisms other than malaise or sickness (Gamzu 1977).

Conditioned taste aversion is a form of learning that can be demonstrated early in ontogeny (Rusiniak et al. 1983; Vogt and Rudy 1984) and across the phylogenetic scale including invertebrates like the terrestrial slug, amphibians, fish, reptiles, birds, and mammals including humans (Garcia, Ervin, and Koelling 1966; Capretta and Moore 1970; Burghardt, Wilcoxon, and Czaplicki 1973; Garb and Stunkard 1974; Gustavson et al. 1974; Mackay 1974; Brett, Hankins, and Garcia 1976; Gustavson et al. 1976; Bernstein 1978; Bernstein and Webster 1980; Mikulka, Vaughan, and Hughes 1981; Sahley, Gelperin, and Rudy 1981; Matsuzawa et al. 1983). What is interesting is that humans have reported taste aversions as long as 50 years after the initial pairing (see Garb and Stunkard 1974).

This particular associative learning paradigm has several unique characteristics: (1) learning can require as few as one pairing between the CS and UCS; (2) association or conditioning can still occur when there are long delays between the pairing of the CS and UCS; and (3) the association is retained over particularly long periods of time, for example, months or years. The single-trial nature and long retention of conditioned taste aversion are shown in table 6.1, which shows the effects of giving wild monkeys novel food paired with cyclophosphamide, a toxic agent known to produce gastrointestinal stress. Most monkeys receiving the single pairing of the flavor with the toxic agent were still avoiding almond nuts three months later (Matsuzawa et al. 1983).

Taste aversion has been used in two different ways in neurotoxicology. In its simplest and most frequently used application, taste aversion is used to assess the toxic properties of a treatment; the question is simply whether that manipulation can serve as the UCS in the production of a conditioned taste aversion. A wide array of treatments including solvents, organic and inorganic metals, herbicides, as well as exposure to gamma irradiation, rotation, vitamin deficiency, and tumor growth, will produce taste aversions (Garcia and Koelling 1966; Rozin 1967; Braun and Snyder 1973; Sjoden and Archer 1977; Snyder and Braun 1977; Levine 1978; Kutscher, Yamamoto, and Hamburger 1979; Sjoden, Archer, and Carter 1979; Dantzer 1980; Leander and Gau 1980; McCoy, Nallan, and Pace 1980; MacPhail and

Table 6.1 Single-trial conditioning and retention of taste aversion to almond nuts in wild Japanese monkeys

Subject	Age	Sex	Before Poisoning	After Poisoning			
				1st Day	2d Day	1 Month	3 Months
Experimental							
Ibu	5	F	0	1*	1*	1*	1*
Togakushi	6	M	0	1*	1*	1*	1*
Wagunah	5	F	0	1*	1*	1	1
Keito	5	F	0	1*	1	1	1
Kehrii	5	M	0	1*	1*	1	1
Mugi	9	F	0	1*	1*	0	0
Musubi	3	F	0	1	1	0	0
Control							
Nagaenmamushi	2	F	0	0		0	0
Momiji	4	F	0	0		0	0
Moano	1	M	0	0		0	0

Source: Matsuzawa et al. 1983. Reprinted by permission of the publisher.

Note: Conditioned taste aversions (TAs) were being studied as a means for controlling crop raiding. Monkeys were living in a natural-setting park, and members of the troop could be identified; park staff periodically provided food at specific areas. During the test period 4 novel foods were made available (peanuts, almond nuts, marshmallows, and red beans). On the basis of the preference shown for almond nuts, this item was chosen to pair with cyclophosphamide, an agent known to produce gastrointestinal distress and vomiting. Almond nuts were made available, and the monkey was then captured and moved to an injection cage, where 20 mg/kg cyclophosphamide (N = 7) or saline (N = 3) were administered. Testing for conditioned TAs took place 1 day, 2 days, 1 month, and 3 months after the pairing. Data are presented for individual monkeys and are expressed as: no aversion (0), almond nuts not eaten (1), almond nuts avoided by sight (1*), and other novel foods avoided (1). A single pairing of almond nuts and cyclophophamide was sufficient to induce a conditioned aversion in all monkeys for at least 2 days and in 5 of the monkeys for as long as 3 months. One or two pairings of the flavor and gastrointestinal distress is usually sufficient for conditioning TAs in most species.

Leander 1980; Reiter et al. 1980; Landauer et al. 1982; MacPhail 1982; Rabin, Hunt, and Lee 1982).

In a practical sense, taste aversions may be an unwanted side effect of toxic treatments whether exposure is for toxicity testing purposes (e.g., when exposure to the agent is by inclusion in food or water [see Cory-Slechta and Weiss 1981]) or therapeutic purposes, such as cancer chemo- or radiation therapy. It has been proposed that the severe anorexia often accompanying cancer therapy may in fact be a result of conditioned taste aversions. Bernstein (1978) has experimentally tested the notion that typical cancer chemotherapy regimens can alter preference for a particular food item, leading to avoidance of that food. Children tested 2–4 weeks after a treatment session that has been preceded by the eating of a novel flavor of ice cream were more likely to choose playing a game (79 percent) than eating the same flavor of ice cream. In a later retest they were offered a choice between the flavor previously paired with chemotherapy and a new flavor (see table 6.2). Although at least 4.5 months had passed between the pairing of the aversive event and the novel flavor, conditioned aversions were quite evident. Learning did not result from exposure to the cancer chemotherapy agent alone (group 2) or to the novel flavor alone (group 3); it resulted only when the two were paired (group 1). The retest provides greater support for a learned aversion because the choice was between two food items.

The second way that conditioned taste aversion can be used in neurotoxicity

Table 6.2 Learned taste aversions in children receiving cancer chemotherapy

Treatment in Session 1	Total Number of Patients	Patients Selecting Ice Cream in Session 2	
		Number	Percentage
Group 1			
Mapletoff ice cream paired with GI toxicity	14	3	21
Group 2			
GI toxicity alone	12	8	67
Group 3			
Mapletoff ice cream alone	15	11	73

Source: Bernstein 1978. Copyright 1978 by the American Association for the Advancement of Science. Reprinted by permission of the publisher.

Note: Prior to treatment with antineoplastic agents, patients in a cancer clinic were offered a novel flavor of ice cream (Mapletoff) or were allowed to play a game. Antineoplastic drugs causing gastrointestinal symptoms were thus paired with ice cream (group 1) or with game playing (group 2). Another group (group 3) had ice cream paired with a drug that had no gastrointestinal side effects. When they next returned to the clinic, patients were allowed to choose between eating Mapletoff ice cream and playing a game.

assessment is to determine whether a given agent interferes with or prevents the learning or retention of such an aversion. In essence, it is treated like any other associative paradigm. Immediate testing assesses whether learning occurred at all, while testing at set intervals after the initial pairing assesses retention capability. For example, taste aversion may be included as one of a number of memory paradigms to date. "Old" rats have been found to be similar to young rats in their ability to retain a taste aversion for as long as 12 weeks after the initial pairing, although they are severely impaired in other retention tasks (see Martinez and Rigter 1983). This particular use of the conditioned taste aversion paradigm has not found wide applicability in toxicology.

Another potentially useful classical conditioning paradigm is the conditioned emotional response or conditioned suppression. In general, shock or some other punishing event is used as the UCS, and the disruption of ongoing operant behavior is the measure of conditioning. If an animal receives food consequential to bar pressing but at some time during the session a tone or other signal is followed by an inescapable shock, bar pressing will eventually be suppressed as soon as the signal comes on. Shock is generally used as the aversive event, but food has been used as the UCS on occasion (see Miczek 1973). As in the taste aversion paradigm, where learning is evidenced by suppression of drinking, here it is evidenced by suppression of bar pressing during the tone (Thomas and Riccio 1979) (see fig. 6.5). The signal alone comes to suppress the ongoing behavior. It takes a relatively small number of pairings to CS and UCS to form a conditioned emotional response, and once established, these responses, like taste aversions, are maintained over long periods (Hoffman, Selekman, and Jensen 1966; Gleitman and Holmes 1967; Coulter, Collier, and Campbell 1976; Thomas and Riccio 1979). Although this procedure has been used extensively to evaluate the effect of pharmacological agents on learning and memory (e.g., Miczek 1973), it apparently has not received wide application in neurotoxicology (see Cabe and Eckerman 1982).

Operant Conditioning. In a classical conditioning paradigm the stimulus events occur regardless of the organism's behavior while in an operant conditioning pro-

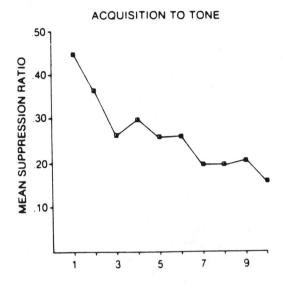

ACQUISITION TO TONE

MEAN SUPPRESSION RATIO

Fig. 6.5 The development of suppression of bar pressing in the presence of a tone associated with unavoidable shock, a conditioned emotional response (CER). Male Holtzman albino rats were trained on a VI 1-minute schedule for water reward during daily 30-minute sessions. On the seventh day a 3,160 Hz tone (the conditioned stimulus) was presented during the twelfth and twenty-fourth minutes of the session; a 0.5 mA shock (the unconditioned stimulus) was presented immediately after the tone stopped. Data are presented as suppression ratios for each stimulus presentation, that is, the rate of bar pressing during the tone divided by the rate of bar pressing during the minute immediately preceding the tone plus the rate during the tone as a function of the number of pairings. A ratio of 0.5 indicates little suppression; one of 0.0, complete suppression. Only a few pairings of tone and shock are necessary for almost complete cessation of bar pressing during the tone. CERs of this type are retained over long periods and have been used to study memory for the conditioned stimulus. (*Source:* Thomas and Riccio 1979. Reprinted by permission of the publisher.)

cedure, also called instrumental learning, the outcome of a behavior is changed by its consequences. Thus, in a classical conditioning preparation a buzzer may signal food, resulting in the response of salivation, while in an operant conditioning procedure a specific response is necessary to produce the stimulus or outcome condition. The measure taken is the frequency, rate, or probability of the response that produces the change.

Perhaps the most commonly used instrumental learning paradigm for the assessment of learning and/or memory is passive avoidance. Rodents are typically used, and on the training trial they will emerge from a lighted chamber into a dimly lit one or will step down from a small platform into a larger, open area. In the step-through passive avoidance procedure, shock is administered when the dimly lit chamber is entered; in the step-down passive avoidance procedure, the animal is shocked after stepping off the small platform (Jarvic and Kopp 1967). To determine whether learning has occurred, the animal is placed back into the lighted chamber or on the small platform (usually 24 hours later), and the time to emerge or step down is recorded. A shorter latency than that of control subjects is taken to imply a deficit in retention or memory. But decreased latency may also be the result of impaired learning. Flicker et al. (1983) made lesions in various brain areas hypothesized to have a role in memory and then used the step-through passive avoidance procedure to test for retention deficits (fig. 6.6). While the lesioned groups clearly were compromised relative to the controls, the deficit was the same whether testing occurred 1 or 24 hours after training. Thus the passive avoidance deficit could be explained as a failure to learn rather than a failure to remember (see Erickson and Scott 1977; and Bammer 1980 for a discussion of the training-testing interval and its

PASSIVE AVOIDANCE RETENTION

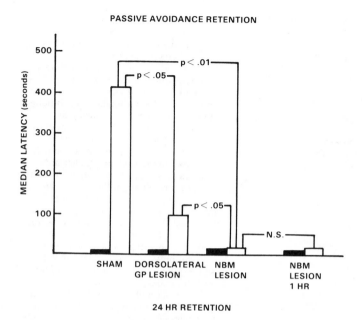

24 HR RETENTION

Fig. 6.6 The effect of neurotoxicant-induced lesions (direct infusion of 0.4 µl of a 6.0 mg/ml of ibotenic acid into the brain area) of the ventromedial area of the globus pallidus (GP) or of the nucleus basalis magnocellularis (NBM) on passive avoidance in the male Fischer-344 rat. Data are expressed as the median latency in seconds to enter the rear shock chamber of a two-compartment apparatus. On the conditioning trial (*left bar*) a 3-second 1.0 mA foot shock was received when the rear chamber was entered. Damage to the GB or NBM did not affect initial latencies, but at retest 24 hours later (*right bar*) both groups with lesions entered the rear compartment significantly faster than the control group. Because the testing occurred 24 hours after training, the increase in latency is usually referred to as a retention or memory deficit. However, an NBM group that was tested only 1 hour after training showed equally short latencies. Thus, the failure of the NBM group to passively avoid is more accurately considered as a deficit in initial learning rather than memory. A group tested shortly after training is rarely included when passive avoidance is used as a method for assessing memory. The failure to include a group tested shortly after training makes it difficult to conclude with certainty that a specific treatment or manipulation does affect memory. (*Source:* Flicker et al. 1983. Reprinted by permission of the publisher.)

relationship to the interpretation of learning and memory deficits in human and animal test situations).

Passive avoidance, because of ease of measurement and brevity of training, is used as a simple method for assessing whether a particular manipulation (pharmacological agent, toxicant, lesion) alters learning and memory. It should be noted, however, that the intersubject variability is frequently quite substantial, making the use of large groups necessary. Also, if a manipulation alters activity, response to stress or sensitivity to shock, or influences motor competence, then conclusions about effects on either learning or memory are not so easily drawn. Additional control groups and procedures (e.g., recording partial entries into the lighted chamber [see Walsh et al. 1984]) or inclusion of the passive avoidance procedure in a battery of tests (e.g., Flicker et al. 1983) allows for a clearer interpretation of effects (see Bammer 1980 for an elucidation of these issues and pharmacological agents). For example, it has been shown that even when a deficit in retention is demonstrated, the performance may be reinstated by presentation of noncontingent shock or by exposure of the animal to some other aspect of the training situation. This implies that the association was learned but not *retrieved* (see the discussion of retrieval deficits below). The amelioration of retention deficits or *reinstatement of memory* by *probe* stimuli (e.g., the *selective reminding* technique of Buschke [see Buschke 1973; or Buschke and Fuld 1974]) has been demonstrated for amnesia or retention deficits in humans and in appetitive analogues of passive avoidance (Miller and Springer 1972; Miller et al. 1974; Devietti and Bucy 1975; Spear and Parsons 1976; Gordon and Mowrer 1980; Gordon 1981; Block and Berchous 1984).

Another instrumental paradigm commonly used in evaluating learning deficits is conditioned avoidance (Bertolini and Pogglioli 1981; Nelson et al 1981; Mullin and Krivanek 1982; Mactutus and Fechter 1984; Mactutus and Tilson 1984). As with passive avoidance, an event like shock is used, but in this case the animal can avoid the shock by making a specific response (hence the term *active* avoidance). In pole or platform active avoidance, for example, the animal is placed in a chamber and then a tone is sounded, followed by shock presentation. Shock is terminated if the animal jumps onto the pole or a small elevated platform; the animal can "escape" the shock by making a specific response. Eventually the animal performs the response as soon as the tone is sounded and avoids shock altogether. Failure to acquire avoidance while adequately developing escape performance indicates learning deficits. For example, exposure to either chloramphenicol (Bertolini and Pogglioli 1981) (see fig. 6.7) or carbon monoxide (Mactutus and Fechter 1984) (see fig. 6.8) during gestation impairs acquisition of a conditioned avoidance response but does not affect escape performance. Figure 6.8 also suggests that a two-way conditioned avoidance response (the animal must return to the compartment where it was just shocked when the signal occurs) is difficult for very young rats (16–23 days of age) to learn and that additional deficits may be demonstrated if retention is included as part of the procedure.

Other applications of the conditioned avoidance paradigm are possible. By using multiple simultaneous stimuli to signal the shock and then testing for avoidance to each stimulus separately, the effect of a toxic agent on various sensory systems can be evaluated (Pryor et al. 1983) (see fig. 6.9). The failure to avoid on the trials signaled by tone alone relative to on the trials signaled by a nonaversive current or light suggests that repeated exposure to the solvent toluene may result in hearing impairment.

The control over rate and patterning of behavior by reinforcer schedules (e.g., every fifth press of a bar results in a food pellet or bar pressing will result in a food pellet when the red but not the green light is lit) is typically demonstrated through the *steady-state performance* of an organism. The *sensitivity* of the organism's behavior to environmental conditions (perhaps akin to orientation, concentration, and attention), rather than the ability to acquire such a relation, is measured. Some use has been made in neurotoxicity assessment of the acquisition of simple conditioning or patterns of behavior maintained by schedules of reinforcement (Sobotka, Brodie, and Cook 1975; Petit, Alfano, and LeBoutillier 1983), though the preponderance of the literature does not directly address matters of acquisition (see Cabe and Eckerman 1982). No clear resolution has occurred to the following puzzle: Steady-state performances offer the best opportunities to witness small changes in performance, for they are very reliable (i.e., the error variance is small). Yet, well-learned behaviors might be particularly robust and therefore difficult to disrupt

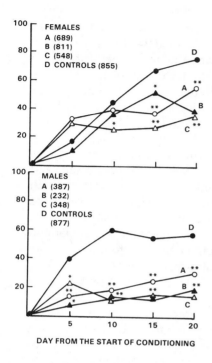

Fig. 6.7 The use of a two-way conditioned avoidance paradigm to assess learning after exposure to chloramphenicol during development. This broad-spectrum antibiotic was given to gravid Wistar rats on gestation days 7–21 and to the offspring of nontreated females on postnatal days 1–3. Two-way shuttle-box conditioned avoidance (CA) training (10 trials daily for 20 days) began at 60 days of age. A trial began when a buzzer sounded, and if the adjacent compartment was not entered in 5 seconds, the rat received a 1.8 mA shock. Data are expressed as the number of CA responses for an entire group on days 5, 10, 15, and 20 of testing. Rats given chloramphenicol in utero (A) or postnatally (B—50 mg/kg; C—100 mg/kg) were unable to learn the avoidance task as well as untreated rats (D). Numbers in parentheses indicate the total number of avoidances for a given group summed over the training period. Note that the chloramphenicol-treated male rats did not perform as well as their female counterparts. (*Source:* Bertolini and Pogglioli 1981. Copyright 1981 by the American Association for the Advancement of Science. Reprinted by permission of the publisher.)

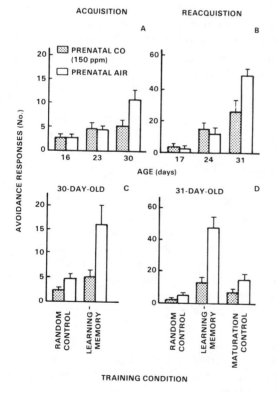

Fig. 6.8 The use of a two-way conditioned avoidance (CA) paradigm to assess learning and memory after prenatal exposure to carbon monoxide. Gravid Long-Evans hooded rats were exposed throughout gestation to 150 ppm carbon monoxide (CO), a level that produces maternal carboxyhemoglobin concentrations of approximately 16 percent but results in only minor birth weight reduction in the pups. Learning and retention of the CA was assessed at several postnatal ages. A trial began with the presentation of a compound stimulus of tone-light and was followed 5 seconds later by a 1.0 mA constant current foot shock. Shock terminated if the other of a two-compartment chamber was entered or if the animal remained in the original compartment for 30 seconds. Shock could be avoided totally by entering the other compartment during the initial 5 seconds during which the tone-light was on. Each session comprised 100 trials separated by an intertrial interval that varied from 35 to 85 seconds. Data are presented as the number of trials during which shock was avoided. CO during gestation impaired both the acquisition and the retention of the CA (*top, left and right*). Reacquisition is used as the index of retention, but differences in initial acquisition require a correction (e.g., covariance analysis) for this problem. Rats 24 days or younger show little learning of the contingencies, as evidenced by the small number of trials during which they avoid. The addition of a maturation control, a group tested only on day 31 (*bottom right*) lends further support to the idea that exposure to CO during gestation impairs both learning and memory. (*Source:* Mactutus and Fechter 1984. Copyright 1984 by the American Association for the Advancement of Science. Reprinted by permission of the publisher.)

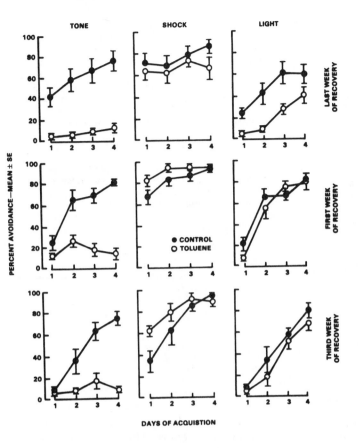

Fig.6.9 The use of a multisensory conditioned pole-climb avoidance task to detect a hearing impairment induced by exposure to toluene (1,200 ppm for 14 hours per day for 5 weeks) in male weanling Fischer-344 rats. Acquisition of the response during the last week of toluene exposure, as well as during the first and third weeks following the cessation of exposure, is presented as the mean percentage of the 60 daily trials on which a 1 mA shock is avoided by climbing a 13 cm pole suspended from the chamber ceiling. During the trials signaled by a pure tone (20 kHz) (*left*), the group exposed to toluene was unable to learn the avoidance response during or after exposure, suggesting that this solvent may have ototoxic effects. When shock was signaled by a nonaversive current (100 uA) on the chamber floor (*middle*) or an increase in the chamber lighting (*right*), the exposed group was equivalent to the control group once toxicant exposure had ceased. Thus, toluene had no long-term effects on other sensory systems. (*Source:* Pryor et al. 1983. Reprinted by permission of the publisher.)

(i.e., true variance would also be small, since the performance would be less sensitive). Thus, tests relying on recall of long-held information such as vocabulary and general information—*hold tests*—do not show change, while tests requiring learning of new associations such as symbol digit or block design—*don't-hold tests*—do (Lezak 1984).

It has been speculated that the demonstration of a deficit using well-learned tasks may require a challenge to the organism and that an increase in task complexity or a shift in the task requirements will accomplish this. Complexity or challenge can be introduced in a number of ways, for example, by requiring discrimination between fewer or less well distinguished stimuli or by changing the task requirements by requiring the subject to reverse what has already been learned, *reversal learning*, or to learn a new behavior during each test session, *repeated acquisition*. Thus, pharmacological agents are known to more easily disrupt behaviors under internal or weak stimulus control (see Thompson 1978). In one study (Wood, Rees, and Laties 1983), toluene, a lipophilic solvent known to produce nervous system dysfunction, differentially affected behavior, depending on the degree of stimulus control. Rats learned to respond on one lever after having responded on another lever at least eight times (a fixed-consecutive-number schedule). In one component a signal was provided to indicate when eight presses had been made, and a shift to the other lever would be reinforced (signaled component). In another component

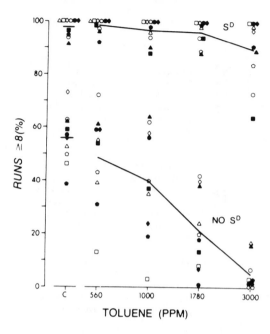

Fig. 6.10 The use of schedule-controlled behavior to illustrate that the degree to which a learned behavior is controlled by environmental stimuli can determine the effect of a toxicant on that behavior. Long-Evans rats were trained on a multiple fixed-consecutive-number (FCN8) schedule of reinforcement in which eight presses on one lever must be followed by a switch to an alternative lever to receive milk. In one component of the multiple schedule lights and tone signaled (S^D) that eight presses had been made. In the other component no cues (NO S^D) were given to signal when the switch to the other lever could be made. Training continued until no systematic changes in behavior were observed; all 10 subjects were then exposed to the solvent toluene. Each subject was exposed twice to each concentration of toluene. The individual and group data are expressed as the percentage of runs that were equal to or greater than eight as a function toluene concentration (0.0, 560, 1,000, 1,780 and 3,000 ppm). Performance was consistently better during the signaled component of the schedule (S^D); deficits in this component were observed only at the higher concentrations of toluene. In contrast, only about 60 percent of the runs were at or greater than 8 during the unsignaled component; performance was disrupted even at the low toluene concentrations.
(*Source:* Wood, Rees, and Laties 1983. Reprinted by permission of the publisher.)

during the same session there was no cue to indicate when eight lever presses had been made (unsignaled component). During the unsignaled component some internal cue comes to determine when the rat switches levers. The percentage of times the animal was able to make runs of eight or more and appropriately switch to the alternate lever was affected by toluene in both components (see fig. 6.10), but the behavior in the unsignaled component was disrupted at much lower doses than that in the signaled component. What is important is that since the subjects were responding under both conditions, this differential effect of toluene was demonstrated within individual subjects.

Like reversal learning, repeated acquisition paradigms require the adaption of performance to new requirements. In such procedures a new sequence or chain of responses is acquired within a session (within-session acquisition). For example, three response levers are made available, and after the animal has learned to respond on all levers, it receives a reward only if it responds with the sequence 3–2–1; the next day a new sequence, 1–3–2, is correct. Every time this sequence occurs, a reward is available; thus, within a given session the acquisition of the new response sequence can be gauged by the decrease in the number of errors as the session continues. If an additional response is required that remains invariant from session to session, then the effect of compounds on both acquisition and steady-state performance can be accomplished. The additional response could be merely responding on an additional set of three levers for which the correct sequence is always 1–2–3. Repeated acquisition learning has been demonstrated in pigeons, monkeys, rats, and humans and is affected by pharmacological and toxicological treatments as well as environmental manipulations (for further discussion see

Cabe and Eckerman 1982. See also Thompson 1973, 1974; Dietz, McMillan, and Mushak 1979; Moerschbaecher et al. 1979; Thompson and Moerschbaecher 1979, 1984; Schrot, Thomas, and Banvard 1980a, 1980b; Pollard et al. 1981; Desjardins, Moerschbaecher, and Thompson 1982; and Schrot and Thomas 1983).

Memory Measures

Approaches to the Evaluation of Memory

Toxic exposures can create severe memory losses, sometimes quite insidiously, without the individual or his associates having a clear idea as to the source of the disorder. High levels of mercury vapor, for example, can produce significant memory deficits. Vroom and Greer (1972) report that in a plant where workers were exposed to extremely high levels of mercury vapor, young mothers would forget to retrieve children from baby-sitters on the way home from work, and many workers became much more dependent on lists for shopping, became lost in familiar surroundings, and misplaced commonly used objects. Neuropsychological testing confirmed that there were problems with recent memory for both verbal and nonverbal material, while intellectual function was otherwise well preserved.

We are likely to attribute declining memory to other sources such as age, perhaps in part because memory is always variable and loss is frequently gradual and almost always only partial. As has been noted by Hirst in his review of amnesia (1982) and by Squire in his review of the neuropsychology of human memory (1982a, 1982b), even severe amnesia and memory disorders rarely result in a total loss of memory; various aspects of memory are preserved. Substances affect only some of the many types of learning and memory. It may, in fact, take close scrutiny to establish that there is a deficit. It is increasingly clear that memory failure may take many forms. A close inspection of deficits that at first glance appear to be similar may well reveal that they differ (Mair and McEntee 1983; Weingartner et al. 1983). Gross-performance measures and simple clinical impressions have not served well in diagnosing and rehabilitating disorders (Erickson and Scott 1977). It becomes important, then, to carefully distinguish the possible deficits and to evaluate each of these possibilities.

The following sections introduce some of the issues in the field of memory assessment. The goal is to alert individuals first considering this topic to the complexities involved and to the methods that are available. The references given to both memory and behavioral toxicology literatures should provide information to resolve these issues. We shall have succeeded if we have provided a road map to this terrain.

How Many Types of Memory Are There?

Many different abilities are subsumed under the general heading "memory." We remember how to do things, language, events, formulae, and so on. A thorough assessment of toxic impairment of memory, then, requires that we assess potential impairment for several partially separable abilities. In designating these abilities, we turn to basic research on memory. A number of viewpoints have provided direction for this research and for the application of theory to account for deficits in memory: stage models of memory suggest that deficits are owing to decreased ability to store or retrieve information (e.g., Atkinson and Shiffrin 1968); a levels-of-processing approach points to deficiencies in encoding as a source of deficits (Craik and Lockhart 1972); interference theory suggests that a retrieval deficit accounts for much memory loss (Baddeley 1976); and context theory proposes that an inability to discriminate past events on the basis of spatial and temporal contextual cues results in memory deficits (Bransford et al. 1977; for a more complete discussion of the relation of memory theories to amnesia see Hirst 1982). In this present chapter, we could list different types of memory according to these current cognitive-theoretical accounts, according to current biological knowledge, or according to more procedural variations that appear to represent different variables determining the phenomenon. The last approach may be most useful at present, since theoretical and biological accounts are currently quite controversial. The separable procedural variations are enumerated below under a general stage approach to understanding memory. First we shall review work using human subjects, and then we shall try to apply this same organization to the literature using nonhuman subjects.

Sorting out different stages of remembering. By and large, we are *directly* influenced by events for only a limited period. This period is called primary memory. The period of primary memory may be further subdivided into a phase in which sensory impressions are still available for "re-reading" (a sensory, or *iconic-store*, stage) and a phase in which we are potentially controlled by only part of the now unavailable sensory array (for a general review of issues in the study of memory see Puff 1982). During this latter phase, called *short-term* or *working memory*, the event itself is said to be replaced by images, codes, or descriptions—that reduced set of attributes that control behavior. Although this stage can be prolonged by rehearsal and sustained attention, eventually our attention shifts—we come under control of other events. Subsequent to this period of primary memory, the impact of a past event on performance is said to be a result of recall into working memory of information from a much less labile *secondary memory*.

Which attributes of sensory memory might a toxicant affect? Sperling (1960, 1963) developed a procedure that revealed some attributes of this sensory store. He demonstrated that although we can recall only a small part of a matrix of stimuli (limited span of apprehension), for a brief period following the flash of a matrix of stimuli a subject can be directed to recall from many different parts of this matrix. Thus, he concluded that there must be a clear sensory store which can later be "read." He measured the time of availability for this sensory store by determining how much information was lost as the direction to attend to a particular part of the display was delayed. A toxicant might well reduce this time of availability for the sensory store, but there appear to be no studies clearly showing this loss.

Short-term memory, the stage said to immediately follow the sensory store, is notably limited in capacity. The common *digit span* included in most measures of intellect appears to measure how much information we can hold onto in this temporary memory. In the usual version of this task, digit series of increasing length are presented, and the subject is required to repeat them immediately; the longest series repeated without error is the measure of span. Variations include backward digit span and running digit span. Many studies evaluating memory deficits have incorporated a measure of digit span, and sometimes this method has revealed a deficit (Hänninen et al. 1976; Lindström, Härkönen, and Hernberg 1976;

Hane et al. 1977). The general conclusion drawn from the literature, however, is that although frequently used, digit span is relatively insensitive in detecting memory deficits. This insensitivity is found, for example, when seeking to detect memory deficits owing to natural aging, Alzheimer's disease, or amnesias resulting from brain damage (Erickson and Scott 1977; Crook et al. 1980), though Crook et al. (1980) have some suggestions for making the test more sensitive. Because of its limited sensitivity, other measures of short-term capacity have been developed (Eckerman 1986).

That exposure to a toxicant decreases a measure of short-term memory capacity does not, it should be emphasized, prove a *memory* deficit. A toxicant might reduce span directly, or it might affect span indirectly, for example, by reducing the vigor or efficiency of coding and/or rehearsing. Since rehearsing prolongs the time of *direct* influence of events, the span is decreased, though whether memory is impaired is questionable. Similarly, if a sequence of separable events (e.g., letters) is grouped and then remembered as a unit (e.g., a word), the capacity increases. Such *chunking* appears to be an important strategy in maximizing capacity in digit span. A toxicant might decrease alertness to such groupings and thereby reduce short-term memory. Whether such a decrease should be attributed to decreased memory or to a changed response strategy is open to question.

Besides capacity, the *process* of control in short-term memory might be affected by a toxicant. Sternberg (1966, 1975) developed a procedure that offers a description of the timing characteristics of the scanning process. The procedure involves determining how long it takes to review various types and numbers of items. A list of items is presented, followed by a probe item. The subject is asked to determine whether the probe was contained in the prior list. The longer the prior list, the longer it takes the subject to make this determination—presumably because the memory set has to be scanned. The procedure does not measure capacity, since accuracy is high for all subjects. The focus is on characterizing the speed of this scanning process. Sternberg's account is plausible (though not without challengers, e.g., Townsend [1971]), and the measures from this procedure have proven to be sensitive to impairment by toxicants. Mercury exposure slows the scanning rate. The work by Langolf, Smith, and their colleagues with workers from chlor-alkali factories has consistently confirmed the effects of a body burden of elemental mercury on memory function. Although tremor occurred in workers with elevated urinary mercury levels, memory impairment occurred in workers with lower levels (Langolf et al. 1981; Smith and Langolf 1981; Smith, Langolf, and Goldberg 1983).

Although one account for the change in time measured by the Sternberg procedure is that memory scanning rate is altered, another plausible account for the data is that longer lists take longer to report on because they represent more difficult problems. By this account, mercury might be interpreted as producing confusion (making decisions more difficult) rather than impairing memory. That Smith and Langolf (1981) found scanning times to correlate with other measures of memory, however, supports Sternberg's interpretation. Subjects in speeded tasks must, however, always choose between responding quickly and responding accurately. A toxicant's change in reaction time might in fact represent a shift in the resolution of this *speed-accuracy tradeoff*. Because of this potential confounding, it is important to measure several aspects of memory before reaching a conclusion regarding memory functioning. In addition to using the simple scanning rate for sub-span lists, other interesting variations of this same procedure might be used. One can present the test probe following presentation of lists too long to remember by mere scanning (supra-span lists). Such searching appears to be different in kind (Murdock 1982). We might also test for control by other aspects of the stimuli: Can the subject report which of two items came earlier, which item followed a particular item, or which item was at position X in the list (as in the game Concentration)? We could ask for recall rather than recognition of the item (see below).

Short-term control is quite disrupted when rehearsal is prevented. In the Peterson-Brown short-term-forgetting paradigm, an item is presented to the subject and then the subject is involved in a task that prevents rehearsal. It is common to find that information is gone when the subject is tested after as short a time as 12–15 seconds (Peterson and Peterson 1959). It is important that the filler tasks typically used have *no direct interference* with the items to be remembered; the loss therefore appears to represent a simple loss of information rather than a masking. Would this curve be even steeper following impairment by a toxicant? The rate of loss does seem to be increased by some drugs (Mohs et al. 1980). Again a caution needs to be raised, however, before such a change can be interpreted. To truly measure forgetting, rehearsal during the retention interval must be prevented; that is, the subject must be completely engaged in the competing task. Were a toxicant to increase this engagement, it might affect remembering without affecting the rate of loss directly. It should be noted that there is evidence that the task is not completely free from direct-interference effects. The slope of the loss function over time steepens over the first several successive trials (Keppel and Underwood 1962), an effect interpreted as a build-up of proactive interference across trials.

Events continue to control behavior long after they have passed from primary memory. Such control is said to require retrieval from *long-term memory*, often considered metaphorically to be like retrieving an item from a warehouse. Whether an item or event continues to exercise control depends on both the item and the way it was coded and rehearsed. For example, material is more likely to continue its control when it is easily imaged, more meaningful, more elaborately "processed," more common, more slowly presented, or more tied to other items. Those aspects of the material that continues to control behavior are said to be "encoded." These codes are "stored" and then "retrieved" (a process considered to require both memory and decision making). The types of information that can be stored may include *item information* (e.g., face, word, etc.) and *associative information* (e.g., other items or events related to this item). Associations can be along chronological as well as other dimensions of the stimuli. Thus, we can remember which of several events came first, and we can remember the age at which we learned something (autobiographical memory). Such associations need not be simple associations but can be more complex networks of associations (knowledge). Coding of words, for example, is usually by semantic categories. Such a relation is witnessed by the improvement in learning of words that differ in semantic category from words learned in prior lists (release from proactive inhibition [Wickens 1970]).

Whether memory is shown depends greatly upon the characteristics of the test used. Material is more easily remembered when prompts are given (cued recall, recognition) than when prompts are minimal ("free" recall). When an item is tested through seemingly unprompted recall, we test its "availability"; when we test using a great deal of prompting, we test its "accessibility." Useful prompts can include the name of a category into which the event fits (i.e., an association), an image used at the time of processing, an associate of the event (e.g., synonym, homonym, antonym), or some aspect of the environment present at the time of intial exposure (e.g., a drug state). One procedure for assessing memory—recognition—uses the event itself as a prompt (by placing it in a "line-up" of other events with the instruction to indicate which event was previously presented). Such prompts can *reinstate* control by an item that could not previously be recalled. Perhaps reinstatement occurs because recall actually represents two steps (*searching* the alternatives and then *recognizing* the correct item or items from among them). The universality of this plausible proposal is called into question, however, by findings that recall is sometimes superior to recognition (Tulving and Thomson 1973). The relations between recall, cued recall, and recognition are thus not straightforward. Further, even if there is no recall or recognition of an item, memory for that item may be demonstrated if it is easier to learn than it would have been had there been no prior presentation, that is, if there is a "savings" in re-learning. Memory is thus demonstrable even when the individual is unconscious of prior exposure to the material. Given these complexities, it is clear that no single measure or approach will provide all the answers regarding the effect of a toxicant on secondary remembering. A multiplicity of measures will be required for a thorough account. (For further examples see Drachman 1977; Ferris et al. 1980; Weingartner et al. 1983; Williams and Rundell 1983; Block and Berchous 1984; Ghoneim, Hinrichs, and Mewaldt 1984; and Majkowski 1984.)

In detecting neurotoxicity of learning and memory in humans, much testing has used existing memory scales developed for determining potential for training (intelligence tests) or neuropsychological diagnosis. Little attempt has been made to differentiate between impairment of short-term and of long-term memory. Recall for the items to be remembered almost always occurs immediately after exposure to the items; very rarely is it hours or days later (see Erickson and Scott 1977; and Hirst 1982). Rarely have multiple tests been used. Further, a population of individuals exposed to a particular substance may well include a diversity of impairments, perhaps representing different stages in the process of impairment. Mikkelsen (1980) notes that initial minor impairments in solvent workers develop into disabling chronic brain damage. Organophosphates, after chronic exposure, appear to differ in effect from other cholinergics acutely given (Rodnitzky, Levin, and Mick 1975; Levin and Rodnitzky 1976).

Memory for skills and procedures. The conceptualizations above have, for the most part, been derived from work with "meaningful material," that is, words or pictures. We might call that *declarative memory.* How about memory for other sorts of materials? How do we remember *procedures* like riding a bike, swinging a golf club, mirror-tracing, solving a puzzle such as the Towers of Hanoi? Such procedures can be learned even by individuals without apparent long-term memory for recently experienced events, individuals who are unaware that they have performed the task before.

It is also noteworthy that the ability to learn new skills and retain these skills is preserved in amnesias resulting from brain lesions, herpes, hypoxia, Korsakoff's syndrome, and aneurysms (Brooks and Baddeley 1976; Hirst 1982) even when the patients report no knowledge of having learned the skill. For example, Weiskrantz and Warrington (1979) have reported that amnesic patients will show typical acquisition for classical eyelid conditioning even though they have no recall of ever having performed the task.

Memory Assessment in Infrahumans

The study of memory in humans is characterized by a primary emphasis on verbal and language-related aspects of memory. Consequently, the terminology, procedures, and aspects of memory studied in the human are quite different from those emphasized in memory research with nonverbal organisms. These differences make it difficult to compare research in these separate literatures, although there are some exceptions. A first area of comparability is found in the work of Squire and his colleagues. In their description of the different types of amnesias associated with various disorders, including chronic alcoholism, they noted that memory for "knowing how" (i.e., procedures) remains intact, while memory for "knowing that" (i.e., verbal knowledge) is compromised (see Cohen and Squire 1980; Squire 1982*a*, 1982*b*; and Cohen et al. 1985). For example, H.M., a subject who had received a bilateral surgical resection of the medial temporal lobe as treatment for intractable seizures, remembers very little of an event immediately after it has occurred (Scoville and Milner 1957). H.M. displays a learning curve (i.e., a decrease in time to solve the puzzle) for the manual skills necessary to trace a pattern visible only in a mirror (mirror-tracing task) but cannot remember ever having performed the task (Milner 1962). With nonhuman subjects, Mishkin and Squire have exploited this type of distinction in their exploration of the changes produced in short-term, long-term, and procedural memory by ablation of the hippocampus and other limbic structures in the primate (see Zola-Morgan and Squire 1984; and Murray and Mishkin 1985). Second, Kesner and colleagues have ingeniously devised a rodent analogue of the Sternberg paradigm (widely used to study memory scanning in humans). For humans, monkeys, and rats, the same function is obtained that relates set size and decision time (Sands and Wright 1981; Ellis, Clegg, and Kessner 1984) (see fig. 6.11). That is, the larger the set of items to be scanned, the longer time required for a decision. This type of approach is useful because it places the emphasis on a comparison of procedures and outcomes between species rather than considers the concept of memory as a concrete thing (see Branch 1977 for a discussion of reification of the concept of memory). However, it should be noted that attempting to use similar memory procedures for both humans and infrahumans adds considerably to the training time needed for the infrahuman subjects (see Ellis, Clegg, and Kesner 1984).

Delayed response. The remainder of this report offers a brief review of paradigms used to assess short-term or working memory. In this review we build on the review provided by Cabe and Eckerman (1982), emphasizing more recent work while providing a thorough outline of the approaches that have been taken. The emphasis is on working memory, since most of the literature on changes in memory addresses short delays. Memories of longer duration (e.g., reference memory)

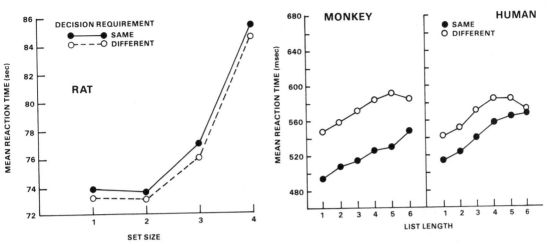

Fig. 6.11 The nearly equivalent functions obtained by the rat, the rhesus monkey, and the human in memory-scanning tasks based on the Sternberg paradigm. A series of stimuli (words, letters, digits, pictures, colors, shapes, or sounds) are shown as an array or sequentially for study. A probe stimulus is then presented which must be identified as the same or different from the study items. Decision (reaction) time increases as the number of items in the study set increases, although the error rate remains the same. Ten different foods (e.g., Kelloggs Froot Loops, General Mills Cocoa Puffs, Frito's Corn Chips, etc.) and 211 color slides (e.g., fruits, flowers, people, etc.) served as the stimulus sets for the rat and monkey or human, respectively. Set size was 1–4 for the rat and 1–6 for the monkey or human. The human and the monkey studied the set items by visually observing them; study of items for the rat consisted in eating them. The monkey and the rat were rewarded with food for correctly identifying a probe stimulus as being the same as or different from a study item. The human was simply informed about the correctness of the response.
(*Sources*: Sands and Wright 1981, copyright by the American Association for the Advancement of Science; and Ellis, Clegg, and Kesner 1984. Reprinted by permission of the publishers.)

can be assessed by noting loss of previously acquired discriminative control (for an example see the discussion on the radial arm maze below).

Delayed-response techniques are nicely illustrated in work by Bartus and colleagues (e.g., Bartus, Dean, and Beer 1980). In this study, *Cebus* monkeys were trained to locate a lighted panel in a matrix of nine panels; the response was simply the pressing of the panel, which was followed by a food reward. Variable lengths of delay were interposed between the lighting of the panel and the opportunity to respond. The monkey thus was required to remember the panel location over varying lengths of time. Aged monkeys had more difficulty in retaining the location of the lighted panel over delay periods; the longer the delay, the less accurate were their choices (Bartus, Dean, and Beer 1980) (see fig. 6.12). Complete retention curves for individual subjects could be generated in single sessions allowing for the comparison of individual dose-response functions for chemical agents (thus, comparisons could be made between "responders" and "nonresponders" [see Bartus, Dean, and Beer 1980). Such delayed-response techniques have been used mainly to determine the length of delay that can be tolerated by various species and have received little attention in toxicological settings (Maier and Schneirla 1964; Beck 1967). Since these techniques have proved useful in the study of other neurobiological problems, such as aging and therapeutic amelioration of the effects of

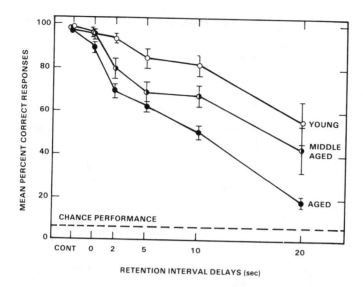

Fig. 6.12 The effect of increasing the delay intervals of a delayed response on accuracy as a function of age. Young, middle-aged, and aged Cebus monkeys were initially trained to press a lighted panel in a matrix of nine panels for a food reward. The task was arranged so that a limited motor movement and agility were required. This made the level of task effort equivalent for monkeys at the three different age levels. A varying delay interval (2–20 seconds) was then interposed between the lighting of the panel and the point at which the monkey was allowed to respond. The monkey indicated by pressing which of the panels had been lit; thus, the location had to be "remembered" over the delay interval. The data are presented as the percentage of correct responses as a function of the delay. Accuracy declined for all ages as the delay increased, but the decline occurred more rapidly for aged monkeys (i.e., the curves for the three age levels are not parallel). This suggests a memory impairment in the older monkeys.
(*Source:* Bartus, Dean, and Beer 1980. Reprinted by permission of the publisher.)

aging, their application to neurotoxicological problems may prove useful (see Bartus and Johnson 1976; Bartus 1979; and for further discussion, Cabe and Eckerman 1982).

Delayed alternation. In this paradigm the subject is required simply to alternate between response choices (e.g., 2 levers or buttons with the sequence left, right, left, right, . . .), but with varying delay intervals interposed between response choices. Because there is no explicit stimulus or cue to indicate which of the levers is currently correct, the animal must rely on "memory" of the previous correct response to serve as the cue for which of the two responses is currently the correct one. Varying the delay interval between responses within a test session allows one to determine the effect of delay interval on accuracy. As would be expected, the longer the delay between choices, the less accurate the performance (Heise et al. 1969; Heise, Conner, and Martin 1976; Milar, Krigman, and Grant 1981). The results obtained with this paradigm are interesting because they illustrate that "memory" effects are often specific to the procedure used to assess them. With this procedure, rats typically decrease to chance accuracy after delay intervals greater than around 10 seconds. Later we shall review procedures with which much longer delays can be tolerated. Perhaps the difference derives in part from the fact that in this procedure hundreds of trials are given the subject in a session, producing proactive

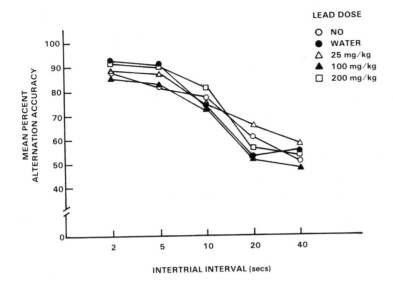

Fig. 6.13 The effects of neonatal lead treatment on memory, as assessed by a delayed spatial-alternation procedure. Long-Evans rat pups were dosed orally with lead acetate (0.0, 25.0, 100.0, and 200.0 mg/kg) from post-natal day 3 to day 30 and then trained as adults on a bar-press-alternation task. Further training required alternation between the two levers, with the interval between trials varying from 2 to 40 seconds in length. This variable intertrial interval serves as a retention interval, over which the rat must "remember" which lever was pressed on the previous trial. Individual memory curves can be obtained because each subject is tested at all retention intervals. The data are expressed as the mean percentage of alternation accuracy as a function of the intertrial interval. Typical memory curves were displayed. That is, as the retention interval increased, the percentage of accuracy with which lever alternation occurred declined; at the 40-second interval all groups were performing at chance level. However, lead acetate during development had no effect on performance in this memory task.
(*Source:* Milar, Krigman, and Grant 1981. Reprinted by permission of the publisher.)

interference. The advantage is that an entire memory-decay function may be mapped in one session.

While delayed-response alternation has been used to evaluate the role of cholinergic neurotransmitter systems in the storage and retrieval of memory, it has rarely been used to assess toxicant effects (see Ksir 1974; and Heise, Conner, and Martin 1976). In one study, daily exposure to lead acetate in the developing rodent had no effect on retention in this measure of memory; treated and control animals showed the typical within-session retention curve (Milar, Krigman, and Grant 1981) (see fig. 6.13).

Complex delayed or spatially-cued discriminations: the radial arm maze. A recent innovative method developed for the analysis of memory function in the rodent is the radial arm maze (RAM). This paradigm has been used to address questions in several areas: spatial behavior, mnemonic processes in infrahumans, the neural substrates for learning and memory, and the action of several drugs and toxic substances on memory processes. That rodent behavior comes quickly under the control of spatial location is used to advantage in this procedure developed by Olton and colleagues (Olton and Samuelson 1976; Olton, Collison, and Werz 1977; Olton 1979). Although the importance of spatial location in animal discrimination learning has been documented frequently, in many animal learning and memory paradigms an attempt is made to eliminate spatial cues. The RAM, in contrast, utilizes spatial cues as part of the paradigm (see Olton 1978 and 1979 for an extensive discussion of animal spatial learning). Generally the maze is open to the room, and there is no sound- or light-attenuating chamber surrounding it, although there are a number of variations (see Bureŝová 1980; Bureŝová and Skopková 1982; Miller et al. 1982; Winocur 1982; and Foreman, Arber, and Savage 1984). The typical RAM consists of an open, central platform from which 8 arms radiate like spokes of a wheel. Food-deprived rats are allowed to choose freely from among the 8 arms, but only 1 piece of food is available at the end of each. Increasing the number of arms increases the difficulty of the task but also increases the training time necessary to reach asymptotic performance. Versions with 4, 6, 12, 17, and as many as 24 arms have been used (Olton, Collison, and Werz 1977; Ingram, London, and Goodrick 1981; Bureŝ and Skopková 1982; Bureŝ and Bureŝová 1984). An animal is typically allowed 1 trial per day; to reach asymptotic performance of 4 out of 4 requires 10 trials, while a performance of 15 out of 17 requires 50 trials (Olton, Collison, and Werz 1977; Olton 1978).

Typically the rat is allowed to select arms continuously until all novel arms have been visited and food collected; in general, no constraints are placed on this selection other than a cutoff time or total number of visits allowed. The total number of arms visited or the number of novel arms selected in the first 8 choices then serves as the index of accuracy (Olton and Samuelson 1976). Revisiting arms before all "novel" arms have been selected can, however, be interpreted as being a result of factors other than an interference with the ability to remember which arms have already been visited. Other explanations are possible, for there are several ways in which the goal of entering each arm only once can be realized. Other than relying on memory for arms visited, efficient maze performance can be accomplished through control by discriminative stimuli (e.g., odor trails) or response patterning strategies (e.g., always turn right after exiting from an arm or select every third arm). Although normal rats will sometimes exhibit patterned response, and selection of adjacent arms will occur frequently, in general, the sequence of choices made from one daily trial to the next is unsystematic enough to suggest that reliance on response strategies is uncommon (Olton, Collison, and Werz 1977; Olton and Werz 1978; Eckerman et al. 1980). There are, however, certain physical aspects of the maze's configuration, as well as certain treatments, that seem to be determinants in eliciting response strategies or stereotypies. For example, changing the size of the central platform affects whether an adjacent arm is chosen; the larger the center, the greater the probability of an adjacent arm's being chosen. In some instances, pharmacological and other treatments, such as specific brain lesions, increase or alter the use of response strategies and stereotypies (Beatty and Carbone 1980; Eckerman et al. 1980; Walsh, Miller, and Dyer 1982; Devenport and Merriman 1983; Devenport, Merriman, and Devenport 1983; Hall and Macrides 1983; Walsh et al. 1984). Even the strain of animal employed appears to be a partial determinant of the degree of patterning exhibited; avians and fish appear to rely on response strategies more than rodents do (Bond, Cook, and Lamb 1981; Roitblat, Tham, and Golub 1982). Mice appear to adopt response patterns if the maze is enclosed, and this may result in performance levels at little better than chance (Mizumori, Rosenzweig, and Kermisch 1982; Levy, Kluge, and Elsmore 1983; Reinstein et al. 1983; see also Pico and Davis 1984). Introducing a delay between each choice aids evaluation of the role of response patterning, since confinement forces an almost exclusive dependency on environmental cues. Usually confinement is carried out by placing doors at the entrance to each arm, preventing access to the arms for a certain period. But the maze may also be configured such that the rat does not go back to the central platform by retraversing the chosen arm (see Olton, Collison, and Werz 1977; Magni, Krekule, and Bureŝ 1979; Bureŝová 1980; and Bureŝová and Bureŝ 1980, 1982).

Various reinforcers have been used, including standard and sucrose Noyes pellets (see Miller et al. 1982; and Miller 1984), chocolate chips (Staubli, Baudry, and Lynch 1984), Froot Loops (Kesner and Novak 1982), and water (Eckerman, personal communication). It is interesting that unlike in most food-motivated memory paradigms (e.g., delayed match to sample), in the typical RAM procedure rats are required to use a "win-shift" strategy, that is, *not* to go back to a place where they have previously obtained food. It should be noted that the basic demand characteristics of the task can be restructured in a "win-stay" mode (e.g., Collier et al. 1982; and see below).

Although most of the studies in the literature use food reinforcement, there has been no attempt to address the issue of quality or magnitude of reinforcement effects and their possible interactions with the demands of the task (but see Gaffan, Hansel, and Smith 1983). In point of fact, the RAM can be considered a complex alternation paradigm in which the animal visits all the novel arms before repeating entries, and in this context it has been used to study the spatial patterning of rodents not deprived of food or water in the absence of reinforcement (Golub 1982; Bruto and Anisman 1983; Bruto et al. 1984; Laughlin, Finger, and Bell 1984). In essence, nonnovel, or "old," arms are avoided. When food or other reinforcers are provided, they strengthen this initial response bias.

There are many available cues (including visual, olfactory, auditory, and distal room cues and intramaze cues such as odors of food or of odor trails left by the organism itself) that could be utilized to avoid entering old arms. Considerable research has shown, however, that accurate performance in most cases is controlled by extramaze spatial cues, that is, visual aspects of the test room. Odors and intramaze cues appear to play a very small part in controlling accurate choice behavior. In fact, forcing an exclusive reliance on intramaze cues may lead to performance accuracy that is little above chance (Zoladek and Roberts 1978; Maki, Brokofsky, and Berg 1979; Olton and Collison 1979; Winocur 1982; Maki et al. 1984).

The RAM procedure has advantages over other, more traditional methods for assessing memory function in infrahumans (e.g., delayed match to sample) in that it (1) is rapidly acquired (Olton 1978, 1979); (2) can be acquired by a variety of species, including rats, mice, and gerbils (Olton and Samuelson 1976; Olton 1977; Kjellstrand et al. 1980; Levy, Kluge, and Elsmore 1983; Wilkie and Slobin 1983; Pico and Davis 1984), as well as pigeons and ring doves (Bond, Cook, and Lamb 1981; Wilkie, Spetch, and Chew 1981) and fish (Roitblat, Tham, and Golub 1982); and (3) affords a method for the study of memory across the life span of particular species. Rats can begin training immediately prior to or at the time of weaning (see Olton and Schlosberg 1978; and Rauch and Raskin 1984).

The ability to study memory for lists of items allows manipulations to be made that are similar to those explored in the work on human memory. This comparability might be of value in cross-species comparisons (see Morris 1983; and Kesner 1985). Memory for items as well as order of items can be evaluated. Certain characteristics of human memory for lists of items, such as *recency-primacy effects* and *proactive* and *retroactive inhibition* can be studied. These have typically been considered difficult to investigate using a rodent (but see Roberts and Smythe 1979; and Roberts and Dale 1981). That rats display what appears to be a typical serial position curve and that memory for the list of places is altered by manipulations that alter human memory for lists is demonstrated rather convincingly by Kesner and Novak's (1982) application of the RAM task.

Further evaluation of the control of maze performance, including mnemonic aspects of the task, can be accomplished by the use of delays. Delays can be inserted after each choice or between certain choices (e.g., 5 and 6). The type of delay procedure used is dictated in part by the particular aspect of maze performance being addressed. Introducing delays, as well as other ways of arranging or restructuring the demands of the task, is an important part of using the RAM to study mnemonic processes, for such manipulations provide a way to unconfound other sources of control than memorial processes (see Gallagher, King, and Young 1983; and Kesner 1985). Of course the interaction of compounds with response patterning or other strategies employed in the RAM are of legitimate research interest in their own right (e.g., Devenport and Merriman 1983).

Several different ways of restructuring the RAM task have been described. Perhaps the most commonly used variation is the introduction of a delay (minutes to hours) between choices 4 and 5 (Olton and Samuelson 1976; Zoladek and Roberts 1978; Maki, Brokofsky, and Berg 1979; Beatty and Shavalia 1980; Wallace, Krauter, and Campbell 1980; Roberts and Dale 1981; Roitblat, Tham, and Golub 1982; Gallagher, King, and Young 1983; Pico and Davis 1984). In general this variation has been used to explore the length of delay that can be tolerated and how this decline in accuracy is altered by variables related to the procedure itself (e.g., drugs given during the delay interval) or the organism tested (e.g., species or age). Aged rats, for example, perform more poorly on both continuous and delay versions of the RAM tasks. However, the delay itself does not differentially affect the old rats more than the young ones (Wallace, Krauter, and Campbell 1980) (see fig. 6.14). Exposure to a wide variety of manipulations and activities during the delay (e.g., running of a smaller radial arm maze) appears to have surprisingly little effect on performance (Zoladek and Roberts 1978; Maki, Brokofsky, and Berg 1979). It appears to make little difference whether the first four choices are determined by the animal or the experimenter (Roberts and Dale 1981).

In one particularly innovative application of the RAM task the role of opiate systems in memory processes was investigated by training a delayed performance in a series of novel environments (Gallagher, King, and Young 1983). Control by the new set of cues had to be reacquired in each new environment. Training was continued in one environment until accurate performance was attained for a six-hour delay interposed between choices 4 and 5. The maze was then moved to a new room, where training continued until accurate delay performance was again acquired. The speed with which the criterion was reached depended on the drug treatment given prior to each training session. When naloxone (an opiate antagonist) was given, reacquisition was faster than when saline was administered

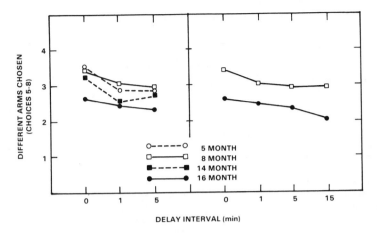

Fig. 6.14 The effect of age and delays between choices on performance in the radial arm maze. Male Fischer-344 rats of different ages (5, 8, 14, and 16 months) were given 10 daily training trials in an 8-arm maze in which continuous choices were allowed. On days 11–20 a delay of 1 minute was interposed between choices 4 and 5; the delay was increased to 5 minutes on days 21–25 and to 15 minutes for the 5- and 16-month-old animals on days 31–35. Data are expressed as the number of different arms chosen on selections 5–8, with 4 being the best possible score. The younger rats performed better on the task than did the older rats; regardless of the delay interval, they made more different choices after the delay (*left*). However, performance of all rats declined as the delay interval increased (*left and right*). It is interesting that the performance of the older rats did not worsen significantly with the longer delay intervals (*right*), suggesting that retention at these intervals is impaired selectively in older rats.
(*Source:* Wallace, Krauter, and Campbell 1980. Reprinted by permission of the publisher.)

(ibid.) (see table 6.3), confirming previous reports that endogenous opiate systems play a role in retention of information.

The RAM can also be used to sort out effects on *reference memory* versus *working memory* (see Honig 1978). If the same four arms are always baited, and the remaining four always unbaited, rats learn to always avoid the unbaited set (reference memory), as well as arms from which the bait was already obtained that day (working memory). In general, this configuration of the RAM task, as well as reversals of the baited and unbaited arms, has been used in neurobiological settings to determine the role of particular neurological systems or substrates, especially the hippocampal formation and other structures of the limbic system, in short-term, or working, memory (Olton and Papas 1979; Jarrard 1980; Harrell, Barlow, and Davis 1983; Harrell et al. 1984). Rats have no difficulty mastering this task (Harrell, Barlow, and Davis 1983) (see fig. 6.15); the frequency of entering never-baited arms or revisiting arms from which the food has been collected is low. Note also that almost no visits are made to the never-baited arms after training. Lesions or other neurobiological manipulations are almost always made after the animal has reached asymptotic performance. In part this is because of attempts to model or operationally duplicate effects observed in human amnesic syndromes, such as the episodic memory impairments described by Tulving (1972) or the "knowing how" and "knowing that" distinction reported by Cohen and Squire (1980); that is, in many human amnesic syndromes retention of new information is difficult or impossible, while experiences prior to brain damage are recalled with

Table 6.3 The use of the eight-arm radial maze and its placement in novel environments to investigate the role of opiate systems in memory

Treatment	Trials to Criterion	Errors to Criterion
Experiment 1 (N = 8)		
Saline	5.38 ± 0.71	12.0 ± 2.89
Naloxone	3.25 ± 0.63[a]	4.4 ± 2.74[a]
Experiment 2 (N = 10)		
Saline	4.90 ± 0.70	12.2 ± 3.03
Diprenorphine	3.60 ± 0.49[a]	5.8 ± 2.89[a]

Source: Gallagher, King, and Young 1983. Copyright 1983 by the American Association for the Advancement of Science. Reprinted by permission of the publisher.

Note: Values are means ± standard errors. In the usual RAM procedure the maze remains in the same room throughout the experiment, with performance being at optimum, highly accurate levels. Male Sprague-Dawley rats were trained to continuously select arms in the RAM until no more than two arm reentries were made on three consecutive days. A gradually increasing delay (1 minute, then 30 minutes, then 6 hours) was then interposed between arm choices 4 and 5; the delay period increased when the criterion was met. When the criterion at the longest delay was reached, the RAM was moved, and training continued in two totally novel rooms. Accurate performance is considered to depend on the use of spatial cues in the environment around the maze. Thus, placement of the maze in a new environment requires learning of new spatial cues, and performance after the 6-hour delay initially will be less than optimum. Because endogenous opiate systems are hypothesized to have a role in memory, the ability of opiate antagonists (naloxone, 2 mg/kg, or diprenorphine, 1 mg/kg) to optimize performance was evaluated. Either the antagonist or saline was administered after the first four choices immediately before the start of the 6-hour delay period. The same animals were trained in both of the novel environments; saline was given in one of the rooms, an opiate antagonist in the other. Data are presented as trials (days) to criterion and errors to criterion. Less trials and errors were necessary to reach optimum performance in a new environment after administration of either antagonist.

[a]Significantly different from saline treatment.

relative ease (see Kesner 1985). In the Harrell study lesions of the medial septal area of the limbic system disrupted performance in both the reference memory (unbaited arms) and working memory (baited) components, as reflected in the increase in both errors and arm selections; in essence, the lesion produced a nonspecific effect. Subsequent training facilitated recovery, and although recovery after septal lesions has been observed previously, compromised performance is generally observed in the working, not the reference, component of other spatial memory tasks after this particular brain insult (see Milner 1978; and Thomas et al. 1982).

Similarly, Wirsching et al. (1984) found that low doses of scopolamine (0.1 and 0.4 mg/kg) injected selectively disrupted the working memory component of the radial-maze task (reentries into the four baited arms) and not reference memory (entry into the four never-baited arms). This same selective effect was noted by Brito et al. (1983), using a contingently reinforced T-maze alternation procedure. They compared the effect of intrahippocampal injections of scopolamine on alternation when visual cues indicated the correct arm (reference memory) with the effect when no external cues were provided and therefore the rat's past selections were the only cue (working memory). A dose as low as 12 mg/μl produced a significant decrease in working memory but not in reference memory.

Other innovative applications have made use of the fact that in the RAM task the arms can be considered to be a list of places visited in a temporal sequence (Kesner and Novak 1982). For humans, the accuracy with which an item is recognized or recalled from a serial list of items (usually words) is determined by the

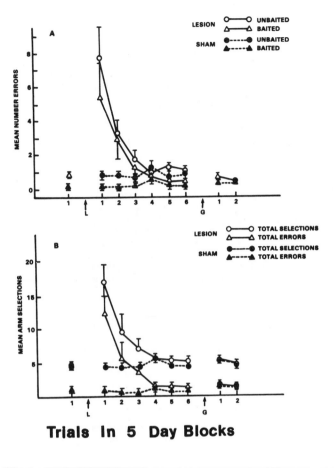

Fig. 6.15 The use of a radial-arm-maze task to assess reference memory and working memory after damage to the septal area of the brain. Male Sprague-Dawley rats were trained in an eight-arm maze in which food was always available in four of the arms and never available in the others. Entry into a never-baited arm is considered a reference memory error, because this information remains invariant throughout the study. However, a working memory error occurs when an arm from which food has been collected is revisited, because this information changes during each daily trial. Daily training in which arm choices were allowed until all baited arms were visited and the food had been consumed or 10 minutes had passed continued until a criterion of four correct choices in the first five arm visits for five consecutive days was achieved. Then sham operations or lesions in the septal area were made. Following recovery, training was continued until the preoperative criterion was again met. Data are expressed as the mean number of errors and as the total arm selections. Lesions in the septum increased both working (baited) memory and reference (unbaited) memory errors (*top*), indicating that this type of damage had a nonspecific effect. Total selections and total errors (*bottom*) showed a concomitant increase. With additional training, however, lesioned animals were able to reattain preoperative baselines (*top and bottom*). (*Source:* Harrell, Barlow, and Davis 1983. Reprinted by permission of the publisher.)

Trials In 5 Day Blocks

position the item occupies in the list. Accuracy is better for items at the beginning (*primacy effect*) and end of the list (*recency effect*); this configuration of accuracy effects for a serial list of items is known as a serial position curve (Milner 1978) (see fig. 6.16). These positional effects can be encompassed under several different theoretical frameworks, including information-processing and stimulus-control explanations. For example, items at the beginning and end of the list are more easily remembered because those positions in the list are in themselves more distinctive (see Kesner 1985 for a discussion).

Kesner and Novak (1982) studied serial-position effects in the rat by utilizing the RAM task as one in which a sequential list of items was remembered. The exact sequence of the eight arms visited was controlled by opening the doors into the alleys one at a time. Immediately after the eighth pellet was collected, rats were presented with two open doors, at positions 1 and 2, 5 and 6, or 7 and 8 in the

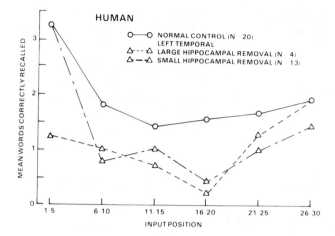

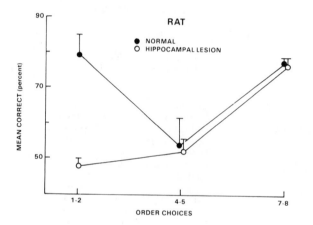

Fig. 6.16 The effect of damage to the hippocampus on serial-position curves in the human and the rat. Humans were presented with a list of words to remember. Accuracy (the mean words correctly recalled) depended on the position of the word in the original list; words at the beginning and end of the list are recalled more accurately than those in the middle (*top, normal control*). Persons who have had a large portion of the hippocampus removed do not show a primacy effect. Male Long-Evans rats trained on an analogue of the serial-position task using a radial-arm-maze task also display primacy and recency effects (*bottom, normal*). Animals were allowed to visit arms of the maze in a sequence predetermined by the experimenter (i.e., the list of items to be "remembered"). Doors to two arms (either first and second, fourth and fifth, or seventh and eighth visited in the sequence) were then opened. Choosing the arm that had been visited earliest in the sequence was rewarded. Removal of a large portion of the dorsal hippocampus eliminated the primacy effect (*bottom, normal*), as it does in humans. (*Sources:* Milner 1978; and Kesner and Novak 1982, copyright 1982 by the American Association for the Advancement of Science. Reprinted by permission of the publishers.)

previous sequence of arms visited. An additional pellet was earned if the arm presented earlier in the sequence was chosen. Thus, Novak and Kesner were able to demonstrate that (1) the accuracy with which a rat chooses arms in a radial arm maze when confronted by a choice between two previously visited arms is determined by the serial position of the arm in the original visit, that is, that rodents display a serial position curve; and (2) the primacy effect is disturbed by hippocampal lesions, which lower the accuracy with which items at the beginning, but not the end, of the list are identified (see fig. 6.16).

Although the RAM paradigm has been used in neurotoxicity assessment following the exposure of adult and developing animals to known or putative neurotoxicants, there has been no careful analysis to determine whether the neurotoxicant in question actually affects mnemonic processes (Kjellstrand et al. 1980; Alfano and Petit 1981; Golub 1982; Miller et al. 1982; Stiglick and Kalant 1982, 1983; Walsh, Miller, and Dyer 1982; Miller 1984; Miller and O'Callaghan 1984; Walsh et al. 1984). While these studies document that RAM performance can be disrupted following exposure to neurotoxic agents and thus may have utility in detecting and characterizing memory deficits induced by neurotoxicants, the lack of manipulation of any of the memory components of the task prevents any real conclusions about the effects of the compound on memory.

Does the RAM procedure provide a measure of learning, as well as a measure of memory? Learning to enter all arms and eat all available food within a short time period can occur quite rapidly in this task (although some strains of rat are notoriously slow to cease freezing and begin any exploration upon placement into a novel environment, especially if room illumination is bright). Drug treatment or CNS lesions can be made after asymptotic performance has been attained and acquisition of the task not of concern. However, in a setting where toxic agents are administered to developing animals or where exposure is made prior to training, acquisition effects can be both a focus of study and a serious concern regarding assessment of memory effects. Toxicants may interfere with the ability to habituate to certain nonessential aspects of the task or with motivational parameters. These effects are separable from those on memory. For example, exposure to the organotins triethyl- and trimethyltin during the first 30 days of life retards acquisition of RAM: however, it appears that when training is continued to asymptote, the exposure has only a small effect on the accuracy with which the task is performed (see Cabe and Eckerman 1982; and Miller et al. 1982).

That there is a large motoric component in the execution of the RAM task cannot be discounted, especially when this procedure is used in a toxicological setting. Changes or deficits in motoric competence after toxicant exposure constitute a potential confounding that should not be overlooked. Many toxicants and pharmacological agents affect activity; consequently, an effect on the accuracy of performance could be secondary to this activity effect. Rats can, however, have greatly increased or decreased activity levels without altering the accuracy of RAM performance (Eckerman et al. 1980; Miller 1984; Miller and O'Callaghan 1984). Acute early postnatal exposure to the organotins will increase activity in the juvenile and adult rat, as detected by a variety of monitoring methods, including the RAM (Reiter et al. 1981; Ruppert, Dean, and Reiter 1983; Miller 1984; Miller and O'Callaghan 1984; Ruppert, chap. 8 in this volume). Exposure to 4 or 6 mg/kg of trimethyltin on postnatal day 5 will produce increases in activity in an automated RAM, but only the higher dose compromises accuracy when a continuous selection procedure is used (Miller and O'Callaghan 1984) (see fig. 6.17). Whether the introduction of delays or other variations on the basic procedure would produce a decreased accuracy in a lower dose group has not been evaluated.

The Morris water tank maze. The Morris water tank maze, like the RAM, can be used to assess memory for spatial location. In this task, the rat must swim to a submerged platform in a large tank filled with opaque water. Since escape from the water is the reward, no food deprivation is required. The starting position in the tank varies from trial to trial, and latency to reach the platform, as well as directness of the route, can be measured. Animals are removed from the tank if they have not located the platform within a certain period of time. Because the starting position is varied from trial to trial and there are no explicit cues in the tank, it is assumed that room or spatial cues are used to navigate (Morris 1981; Morris et al. 1982; Sutherland and Lingard 1982). Performance can be affected by specific brain lesions and treatments that interfere with development of the nervous system (e.g. deKosky, Nonneman, and Scheff 1982; and Sutherland,

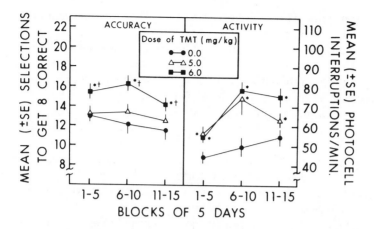

Fig. 6.17 Partial dissociation of the effect of trimethyltin (TMT) on motor activity from its effect on accuracy in a radial-arm-maze memory task. In the RAM a small amount of food is available at the end of eight equidistantly spaced arms radiating from a central platform, and efficient performance requires the animal not to reenter arms from which food has already been obtained; that is, the animal must "remember" which arms have already been visited. Photocells are located throughout the maze to monitor movement. Accuracy (mean total selections required to collect food from the eight arms) and activity (mean photocell interruptions per minute) are both expressed as a function of the dose of TMT (0.0, 5.0, and 6.0 mg/kg i.p.) given on postnatal day 5 to Long-Evans rats. Although the groups exposed to TMT were more active than the group given just vehicle (*right*), only the group given 6.0 mg/kg TMT showed accuracy deficits (*left*). This suggests that in the automated RAM apparatus the effect of TMT on activity can be separated from its effect on accuracy. (*Source:* Miller and O'Callaghan 1984. Copyright 1984 by the American Society for Pharmacology and Experimental Therapeutics. Reprinted by permission of the publisher.)

Whishaw, and Kolb 1983). Early postnatal treatment with the glucocorticoid dexamethasone increased both the initial number of days to reach performance equivalent to that of controls and the number of days to reacquire performance after the platform was moved (deKosky, Nonneman, and Scheff 1982) (see fig. 6.18). Although this procedure has not been applied to neurotoxicology, it may have some utility.

The Hamilton Search task. The delayed match-to-sample procedures are among the more frequently used procedures in the analysis of infrahuman primate memory; however, there are some procedures in which the emphasis is memory for spatial location (see Hamilton 1911; and Menzel 1973). The Hamilton Search task (Hamilton 1911; Levin and Bowman 1983) is an interesting analogue of the RAM task for primates. The monkey is required to locate food in a series of boxes, each occupying a distinct spatial location and containing only one reward. The most efficient performance, as for the RAM, is to open, or "visit," each box only once. Monkeys exposed postnatally to lead had great difficulty in performing under the most difficult of the task parameters (Levin and Bowman 1983) (see fig. 6.19). Animals exposed to high doses of lead required almost twice as many trials as controls to obtain the rewards from the six boxes with no repeat visits. Less stringent criteria did not differentiate between the groups, nor were there any differences in the ability to acquire the rudiments of the task (go to different boxes, etc.) (Levin and Bowman 1983). Although the authors report that no response patterning strategies (e.g., sequence left to right) were used and a 20-second delay

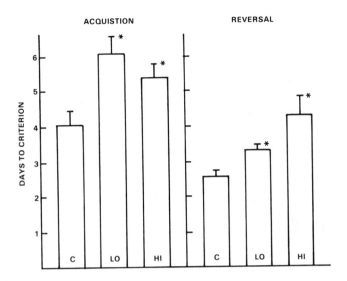

Fig. 6.18 The use of an open-field water maze to determine the effect of exposure to a steroid during development on learning spatial discrimination. Sprague-Dawley rat pups were given a single treatment of the glucocorticoid dexamethasone or vehicle on postnatal day 4. This resulted in permanent decreases in the brain, including the hippocampus and cerebellum, and body weight. At 90 days of age animals were tested for their ability to acquire and reverse a spatial discrimination. A circular tank was filled with opaque water, forcing the rat to utilize distant or spatial cues to navigate to a submerged platform. Eight acquisition trials were given daily until the platform was reached in less than five seconds on six of eight trials for two consecutive days. The platform was then moved to a different section of the tank, and testing continued until criterion was again reached. Data are expressed as the days to criterion during acquisition (*left*) and reversal (*right*) as a function of dose. Animals treated with dexamethasone, whether given a low (1.0 mg/kg) or high (100.0 mg/kg) dose, were compromised in both their ability to acquire the initial spatial discrimination and their ability to learn the reversal of the original discrimination.
(*Source:* deKosky, Nonneman, and Scheff 1982. Copyright 1982, Pergamon Press, Ltd. Reprinted by permission of the publisher.)

was interposed between choices, no formal analysis of the memory component of the task was conducted.

Match to sample and delayed match to sample. In matching to sample the subject is reinforced for selecting a stimulus that matches a sample (either a physical match or an arbitrary associate, generally visual). Rodents are rarely used for such tasks, since a lengthy training time is usually involved for these subjects. In the typical match-to-sample experiment the subject is confronted with the sample stimulus or standard (e.g., a red light). After a period of "study" the standard is withdrawn, and the subject is immediately presented with a pair, set, or matrix of stimuli that includes the standard (e.g., red, blue, and green lights). Selecting the correct light indicates that this stimulus can be discriminated from the others in the set (see Cumming and Berryman, 1965; and Carter and Werner 1978). If a delay is interjected between the time when the standard is presented and the time when it must be selected from among the set of stimuli, then short-term memory for the standard can be evaluated. The introduction of a delay makes this a memory task; thus, this procedure can be used to evaluate the effect of various manipulations on memory (McMillan 1981, 1982; Bartus, Dean, and Beer 1983; Witt and Goldman-Rakic 1983).

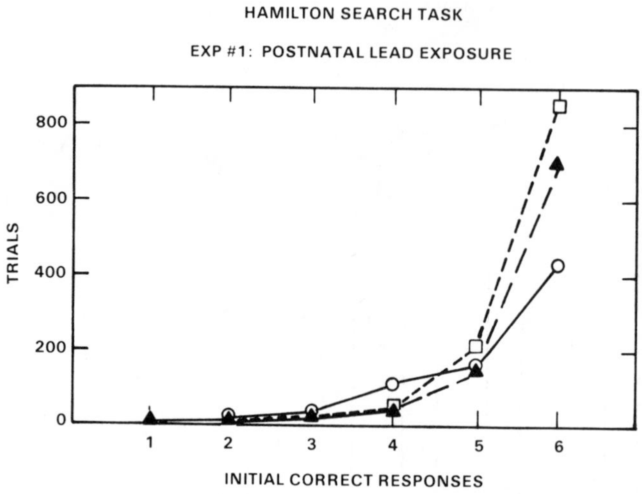

HAMILTON SEARCH TASK

EXP #1: POSTNATAL LEAD EXPOSURE

Fig. 6.19 The use of the Hamilton Search task (HST) to determine the effect of postnatal lead exposure on spatial memory in the rhesus monkey. During training the monkey is confronted with a linear arrangement of lidded boxes baited with food; on a given trial only one box can be opened, and the food retrieved if available. Once food is removed from a box, it is not replaced; for efficient performance the location of the already visited box must be "remembered" on subsequent trials. Infant monkeys were exposed to no lead (circle) or a low (triangle) or high (square) level of lead acetate in their Similac milk diet for the first year of life; blood lead levels of 40 and 85 μg/dl were attained in the low- and high-dose groups, respectively. When they were tested on the HST at 4–5 years of age, their blood lead levels were equivalent to those of controls (1–10 μl/dl). Data from the HST are expressed as the number of total trials required to reach increasingly more difficult criteria, the most difficult being no boxes revisited out of the six available. The effect of postnatal lead was apparent only when the most difficult criterion was used.
(*Source:* Levin and Bowman 1983. Reprinted by permission of the publisher.)

It should be noted, however, that some consider delayed matching to sample to be a measure of stimulus control rather than of short-term memory (see Thompson 1978).

The delayed nonmatch to sample is a variation on the same procedure, with the subject being rewarded for choosing not the matching stimulus but the nonmatching stimulus (Mishkin and Delacour 1975). Memory loss in rhesus monkeys following intermittent thiamine deficiency has been found using this procedure (Witt and Goldman-Rakic 1983). It is interesting that deficits depended on the novelty of the test stimuli used. If the monkey was required to remember which of two highly familiar objects had occurred most recently, then the thiamine-deficient monkeys had great difficulty in identifying the nonstandard member of such a set; few met criterion. No deficits were found if the pairs were composed of new, or "novel," stimuli; neither control nor thiamine-deficient monkeys had trouble identifying the nonmatch (Witt and Goldman-Rakic 1983) (see fig. 6.20). The response of non-matching highly familiar stimulus pairs seems more disruptive, perhaps because the correct choice cannot be made on the novelty or unique aspects of the stimuli, but rather on the basis of which alternative appeared more recently. Thus, the thiamine-deficient monkeys appeared to have difficulty remembering the temporal ordering of information, a type of memory deficit noted in certain human amnesic

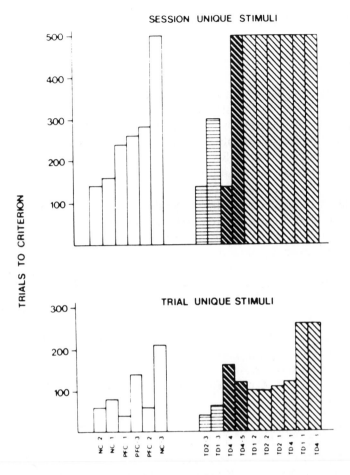

Fig. 6.20 The use of delayed nonmatch to sample to evaluate memory in monkeys with defined brain damage induced by thiamine deficiency. Juvenile male rhesus monkeys were maintained on normal (NC or PFC) or thiamine-deficient diets for one (TD1), two (TD2), three (TD3), or four (TD4) bouts. At the end of each deficiency period symptoms (e.g., collapse, ataxia, severe weight loss) were reversed with thiamine injections and normal diet. Behavioral testing was conducted after recovery from the final bout of thiamine depletion to ensure that deficits were attributable to the chronic rather than acute effects. Testing was conducted using a Wisconsin General Testing Apparatus, in which 500 small sample objects were used. On the pretrial a stimulus object was used to cover a baited well; the object was removed by the monkey to retrieve the bait. Following a delay of 10, 15, or 20 seconds, a pair of objects was then shown, one a match, the other a nonmatch. The nonmatch stimulus covered the baited food well, and choice of this stimulus resulted in reward. Training (20 trials per session) continued until a criterion of 90 trials correct in 100 or until a total of 500 training trials had occurred; correction of errors was not allowed. Training in which the pair of sample objects changed on each trial preceded training in which the sample pair remained the same throughout the session. After-autopsy groups were formed on the basis of the following defined neuroanatomical damage: control (open bars); basal ganglia, thalamus, and brainstem damage (horizontally striped bars); brainstem and cerebellum damage (light diagonally striped bars); thalamus, brainstem, and cerebellum damage (dark diagonally striped bars). The data are presented as trials to criterion and are collapsed across all delay intervals. Delayed nonmatch-to-sample with the same stimulus pair was difficult to learn if the brainstem was damaged. This suggests memory impairment. When unique pairs are used for each trial (bottom), choice of the nonmatch stimulus can be made on the basis of novelty. But when the same pair is used throughout the session, each becomes equally familiar, and "memory" for the stimulus most recently associated with reward must be used to choose (top).
(Source: Witt and Goldman-Rakic 1983. Copyright 1983 by Little, Brown & Co. Reprinted by permission of the publisher.)

disorders (see Witt and Rakic-Goldman 1983; for further discussion see Cabe and Eckerman 1982).

Conclusion and New Directions

It should be apparent that the area of learning and memory assessment is complex and that no single test or small subset of tests will serve to indicate all forms of impairment that might follow toxicant exposure. Rather, the identification and characterization of such dysfunction in neurotoxicity should be made on the basis of an evaluation using a battery of measures. Reasons for selecting a particular test include: (1) demonstrated *sensitivity* (especially important during screening for detecting an effect); (2) *reliability;* and (3) *validity* (for a discussion of these issues in a field-testing arena see Gullion and Eckerman, chap. 14 in this volume). The characterization of an effect requires considerably more research than does its detection, especially to determine if there is really a change in learning or memory as a result of exposure. Challenging the subject by difficult tasks or rearranging task requirements may aid in sorting out learning and memory effects from others. It is important to assess more than one type of learning and more than one aspect of memory.

References

Adams, J., and Buelke-Sam, J. 1981. Behavioral assessment of the postnatal animal: Testing and methods development. In *Developmental toxicology,* edited by C. A. Kimmel and J. Buelke-Sam, 233–58. New York: Raven Press.

Alexinsky, T., and Chapouthier, G. 1978. A new behavioral model for studying delayed response in rats. *Behav. Biol.* 24:442–56.

Alfano, D. P., and Petit, T. L. 1981. Behavioral effects of postnatal lead exposure: Possible relationship to hippocampal-dysfunction. *Behav. Neural Biol.* 32:319–33.

Amin-Zaki, L.; Majeed, M. A.; Elhassani, S. B.; Clarkson, T. W.; Greenwood, M.; and Doherty, R. A. 1979. Prenatal methylmercury poisoning. *Am. J. Dis. Child* 133:172–77.

Anger, W. K. 1984. Neurobehavioral testing of chemicals: Impact on recommended standards. *Neurobehav. Toxicol. Teratol.* 6:147–53.

Anger, W. K., and Johnson, B. L. 1985. Chemicals affecting behavior. In *Neurotoxicity of industrial and commercial chemicals,* edited by J. L. O'Donoghue, 421–29. Boca Raton, Fla.: CRC Press.

Arlien-Søborg, P. A. 1984. Chronic toxic encephalopathy. In *Third workshop on memory functions,* edited by Karl-Axel Melin, *Acta Neurol. Scand.* 69, suppl. 99:105–14.

Arlien-Søborg, P. A.; Bruhn, P.; Gyldensted, C.; and Melgaard, B. 1979. Chronic painters' syndrome: Chronic toxic encephalopathy in house painters. *Acta Neurol. Scand.* 60:149–56.

Atkinson, R. C., and Shiffrin, R. M. 1968. Human memory: A proposed system and its control processes. In *The psychology of learning and motivation,* edited by K. W. Spence and J. T. Spence, vol. 2. New York: Academic Press.

Baddeley, A. D. 1976. *The psychology of memory.* New York: Basic Books.

Bammer, G. 1980. Pharmacological investigations of neurotransmitter involvement in passive avoidance responding: A review and some new results. *Neurosci. Biobehav. Rev.* 6:247–96.

Bartus, R. T. 1979. Physostigmine and recent memory: Effects in young and aged non-human primates. *Science* 206:1087–89.

Bartus, R. T.; Dean, R. L.; and Beer, B. 1980. Facilitation of aged primate memory via pharmacological manipulation of central cholinergic activity. *Neurobiol. Aging* 1:145–52.

———. 1983. An evaluation of drugs for improving memory in aged monkeys: Implications for clinical trials in humans. *Psychopharmacol. Bull.* 19:168–84.

Bartus, R. T., and Johnson, H. R. 1976. Short-term memory in the rhesus monkey: Disruption from the anti-cholinergic agent scopolamine. *Pharmacol. Biochem. Behav.* 5:39–46.

Beatty, W. W., and Carbone, C. P. 1980. Septal lesions, intramaze cues and spatial behavior in rats. *Physiol. Behav.* 24:675–78.

Beatty, W. W., and Rush, J. R. 1983. Spatial working memory in rats: Effects of mono-aminergic antagonists. *Pharmacol. Biochem. Behav.* 18:7–12.

Beatty, W. W., and Shavalia, D. A. 1980. Spatial memory in rats: Time course of working memory and effect of anesthetics. *Behav. Neural Biol.* 28:454–62.

Beck, B. B. 1967. A study of problem solving in gibbons. *Behaviour* 28:95–109.

Berger, B. 1972. Conditioning of food aversions by injections of psychoactive drugs. *J. Comp. Physiol. Psychol.* 81:21–25.

Berger, B.; Wise, C. D.; and Stein, L. 1973. Area postrema damage and bait shyness. *J. Comp. Physiol. Psychol.* 82:475–79.

Berger, T. W., and Orr, W. B. 1983. Hippocampectomy selectively disrupts discrimination reversal conditioning of the rabbit nictitating membrane response. *Behav. Brain Res.* 8:49–68.

Bernstein, I. L. 1978. Learned taste aversions in children receiving chemotherapy. *Science* 200:1302–3.

Bernstein, I. L., and Webster, M. M. 1980. Learned taste aversions in humans. *Physiol. Behav.* 25:363–66.

Bertolini, S., and Pogglioli, R. 1981. Chloramphenicol administration during brain development: Impairment of avoidance learning in adulthood. *Science* 213:238–39.

Block, R. D. I., and Berchous, R. 1984. Alrazolam and loazepam effects on memory acquisition and retrieval processes. *Pharmacol. Biochem. Behav.* 20:233–41.

Bolhuis, J. J.; Bureŝová, O.; and Bureŝ, J. 1985. Persistence of working memory of rats in an aversively motivated radial maze task. *Behav. Brain Res.* 15:43–49.

Bond, A. B.; Cook, R. G.; and Lamb M. R. 1981. Spatial memory and the performance of rats and pigeons in the radial arm maze. *Anim. Learning Behav.* 9:575–80.

Booth, D. A.; Pilcher, C. W. T.; d'Mello, G. D.; and Stolerman, I. P. 1977. Comparative potencies of amphetamine, fenfluramine, and related compounds in taste aversion experiments in rats. *Br. J. Pharmacol.* 61:669–77.

Bornschein, R.; Pearson, D.; and Reiter, L. W. 1980*a*. Behavioral effects of moderate lead exposure in children and animal models: Part 1, clinical studies. *CRC Crit. Rev. Toxicol.* 8:43–99.

———. 1980*b*. Behavioral effects of moderate lead exposure in children and animal models: Part 2, animal studies. *CRC Crit. Rev. Toxicol.* 8:101–52.

Bornstein, M. H. 1981. Psychological studies of color perception in human infants: Habituation, discrimination and categorization, recognition, and conceptualization. In *Advances in infancy research*, vol. 1, edited by L. P. Lipsitt and C. K. Rovee-Collier. Norwood, N.J.: Ablex.

Brady, K.; Herrera, Y.; and Zenick, H. 1976. Influence of parental lead exposure on subsequent learning ability of offspring. *Pharmacol. Biochem. Behav.* 3:561–65.

Branch, M. N. 1977. On the role of "memory" in the analysis of behavior. *J. Exp. Anal. Behav.* 28:171–79.

Bransford, J. D.; McCarrell, W. S.; Franks, J. J.; and Nitsch, K. E. 1977. Towards unexplaining memory. In *Perceiving, acting, and knowing*, edited by R. Shaw and J. Bransford. Hillsdale, N.J.: Erlbaum.

Braun, J. J., and Synder, D. R. 1973. Taste aversions and acute methylmercury poisoning in rats. *Butl. Psychon. Soc.* 1:419–20.

Brett, L. P.; Hankins, W. G.; and Garcia, J. 1976. Prey-lithium aversions. III. Buteo hawks. *Behav. Biol.* 17:87–98.

Brito, G. N. O.; Davis, B. J.; Stopp, L. C.; and Stanton, M. E. 1983. Memory and the septo-hippocampal cholinergic system in the rat. *Psychopharmacology* 81:315–20.

Brooks, D. N., and Baddeley, A. D. 1976. What can amnesic patients learn? *Neuropsychologia* 14:111–22.

Brown, G. G., and Nixon, R. K. 1979. Exposure to polybrominated biphenyls: Some effects on personality and cognitive functioning. *JAMA* 242:423–526.

Brown, G. G.; Preisman, R. C.; Anderson, M. D.; Nixon, R. K.; Isbister, J. L.; and Price, H. A. 1981. Memory performance of chemical workers exposed to polybrominated biphenyls. *Science* 212:1413–15.

Bruto, V., and Anisman, H. 1983. Acute and chronic amphetamine treatment: Differential modification of exploratory behavior in a radial maze. *Pharmacol. Biochem. Behav.* 19:487–96.

Bruto, V.; Beauchamp, C.; Zacharko, R. M.; and Anisman, H. 1984. Amphetamine-induced perseverative behavior in a radial arm maze following DSP4 or 6-OHDA pretreatment. *Psychopharmacology* 83:62–69.

Burešová, O. 1980. Spatial memory and instrumental conditioning. *Acta Neurobiol. Exp.* 4:51–65.

Burešová, O., and Bureš, J. 1980. Capacity of working memory in rats as determined by performance on a radial maze. *Behav. Proc.* 7:63–72.

―――. 1982. Radial maze as a tool for assessing the effects of drugs on the working memory of rats. *Psychopharmacology* 77:268–71.

Burešová, O., and Skopková, J. 1982. Vasopressin analogues and spatial working memory in the 24-arm radial maze. *Peptides* (Fayetteville) 3:725–27.

Burghardt, G. M.; Wilcoxon, H. C.; and Czaplicki, J. A. 1973. Conditioning in garter snakes: Aversion to palatable prey induced by delayed illness. *Anim. Learning Behav.* 1:317–20.

Buschke, H. 1973. Selective reminding for analysis of memory and learning. *J. Verb. Learn. Verb. Behav.* 12:543–50.

Buschke, H., and Fuld, P. A. 1974. Evaluating storage, retention, and retrieval in disordered memory and learning. *J. Verb. Learn. Verb. Behav.* 24:1019–25.

Butters, N., and Cermak, L. S. 1980. *Alcoholic Korsakoff's syndrome: An information processing approach to amnesia.* New York: Academic Press.

Cabe, P. A., and Eckerman, D. A. 1982. Assessment of learning and memory dysfunction in agent-exposed animals. In *Nervous system toxicology,* edited by C. L. Mitchell, 133–98. New York: Raven Press.

Cappell, H., and LeBlanc, A. E. 1975. Conditioned aversion by amphetamine: Rates of acquisition and loss of the attenuating effects of prior exposure. *Psychopharmacology* 43:157–62.

―――. 1978. Gustatory avoidance conditioning by drugs of abuse: Relationships to general issues in research on drug dependence. In *Food aversion learning,* edited by N. W. Migram, L. Krames, and T. M. Alloway, 133–67. New York: Plenum Press.

Capretta, P. J., and Moore, M. J. 1970. Appropriateness of reinforcement to cue in the conditioning of food aversions to chickens (*Gallus gallus*). *J. Comp. Physiol. Psychol.* 72:85–89.

Carter, D. E., and Werner, T. J. 1978. Complex learning and information processing by pigeons: A critical analysis. *J. Exp. Anal. Behav.* 29:565–601.

Castellucci, V., and Kandel, E. 1976. An invertebrate system for the cellular study of habituation and sensitization. In *Habituation,* edited by T. J. Tighe and R. N. Leaton, 1–47. New York: Wiley.

Center for Disease Control. 1978. Preventing lead poisoning in young children. *J. Pediatr.* 93:709–20.

Charlebois, C. T. 1978. High mercury levels in Indians and Inuits (Eskimos) in Canada. *Ambio* 7:204–10.

Cohen, N. J.; Eichenbaum, H.; Deacedo, B. S.; and Corkin, B. 1985. Different memory systems underlying acquisition of procedural and declarative knowledge. In *Memory dysfunctions: An integration of animal and human research from preclinical and clinical perspectives*, edited by D. S. Olton, E. Gamzu, and S. Corkin, 54–71. New York: New York Academy of Sciences.

Cohen, J. J., and Squire, L. R. 1980. Preserved learning and retention of pattern-analyzing skill in amnesia: Dissociation of knowing how and knowing that. *Science* 210:207–10.

Collier, T. J.; Miller, J. S.; Travis, J.; and Routtenberg, A. 1982. Dentate gyrus granule cells and memory: Electrical stimulation disrupts memory for places rewarded. *Behav. Neural Biol.* 34:227–39.

Cory-Slechta, D. A., and Weiss, B. 1981. Aversiveness of cadmium in solution. *Neurotoxicology* 2:711–24.

Coulter, X.; Collier, A. C.; and Campbell, B. A. 1976. Long-term retention of early Pavlovian fear conditioning in infant rats. *J. Exp. Psychol.: Anim. Behav. Proc.* 2:48–56.

Craik, F. I. M., and Lockhart, R. S. 1972. Levels of processing: A framework for memory research. *J. Verb. Learn. Verb. Behav.* 1:671–84.

Crapper, D. R., and Dalton, A. J. 1973. Alterations in short-term retention, conditioned avoidance response acquisition and motivation following aluminum-induced neurofibrillary degeneration. *Physiol. Behav.* 10:925–33.

Crook, T. 1979. Psychometric assessment in the elderly. In *Psychiatric symptoms and cognitive loss in the elderly*, edited by A. Raskin and L. F. Jarvik, 207–20. Washington, D.C.: Hemisphere.

Crook, T.; Ferris, S.; and McCarthy, M. 1979. The misplaced-objects task: A brief test for memory dysfunction in the aged. *J. Am. Ceriatr. Soc.* 27:284–87.

Crook, T.; Ferris, S.; McCarthy, M.; and Rae, D. 1980. Utility of digit recall tasks for assessing memory in the aged. *J. Consult. Clin. Psychol.* 48:228–33.

Cumming, W. W., and Berryman, R. 1965. The complex discriminated operant: Studies of matching-to-sample and related problems. In *Stimulus generalization*, edited by D. Mostofsky, 284–330. Stanford: Stanford University Press.

Dantzer, R. 1980. Conditioned taste aversion as an index of lead toxicity. *Pharmacol. Biochem. Behav.* 13:133–35.

deKosky, S. T.; Nonneman, A. J.; and Scheff, S. W. 1982. Morphological and behavioral effects of perinatal glucocorticoid administration. *Physiol. Behav.* 29:895–900.

Desjardins, P. J.; Moerschbaecher, J. M.; and Thompson, D. M. 1982. Intravenous diazepam in humans: Effects on acquisition and performance of response chains. *Pharmacol. Biochem. Behav.* 17:1055–59.

Devenport, L. D., and Merriman, V. J. 1983. Alcohol and behavioral variability in the radial-arm maze. *Psychopharmacology* 79:21–24.

Devenport, L. D.; Merriman, V. J.; and Devenport, J. A. 1983. Effects of ethanol on enforced spatial variability in the 8-arm maze. *Pharmacol. Biochem. Behav.* 18:55–59.

Devietti, T. L., and Bucy, E. E. 1975. Recovery of memory after reminder: Evidence for two forms of retrieval deficit induced by ECS. *Physiol. Psychol.* 3:19–25.

Dewar, A. J. 1983. Neurotoxicity. In *Animals and alternatives in toxicity testing*, edited by M. Balls, R. J. Riddell, and A. N. Worden, 229–84. New York: Academic Press.

Deweer, B.; Sara, S. J.; and Hars, B. 1980. Contextual cues and memory retrieval in rats: Alleviation of forgetting by a pretest exposure to background stimuli. *Anim. Learning Behav.* 8:265–72.

Dietz, D. D.; McMillan, D. E.; and Mushak, P. 1979. Effects of chronic lead administration of acquisition and performance of serial position sequences by pigeons. *Toxicol. Appl. Pharmacol.* 47:377–84.

Dille, J. R., and Smith, P. W. 1964. Central nervous system effects of chronic exposure to organophosphate insecticides. *Aerospace Med.* 35:475–78.

Dimattia, B. V., and Kesner, R. P. 1984. Serial position curves in rats: Automatic versus effortful information processing. *J. Exp. Psychol.: Anim. Behav. Proc.* 10:557–63.

Drachman, D. A. 1977. Memory and cognitive function in man: Does the cholinergic system have a specific role? *Neurology* 27:783–90.

Drachman, D. A., and Leavitt, J. 1972. Memory impairment in the aged: Storage versus retrieval deficit. *J. Exp. Psychol.* 93:302–8.

Dubowitz, L. M. S.; Mushin, J.; Morante, A.; and Placzek, M. 1983. The maturation of visual acuity in neurologically normal and abnormal newborn infants. *Behav. Brain Res.* 10:39–45.

Duffy, F. H.; Burchfiel, J. L.; Bartels, P. H.; Gaon, M.; and Sim, V. M. 1979. Long-term effects of an organophosphate upon the human electroencephalogram. *Toxicol. Appl. Pharmacol.* 47:161–76.

Eckerman, D. A. 1980. Monte Carlo estimation of chance performance for the radial arm maze. *Bull. Psychon. Soc.* 15:93–95.

———. 1986. Cognitive effects of neurotoxic agents. Proceedings of a workshop on cognitive testing methodology—Committee on Military Nutrition Research, National Academy of Science, 11–12 June 1984. Washington, D.C., National Academy Press, 129–61.

Eckerman, D. A.; Gordon, W. A.; Edwards, J. D.; MacPhail, R. C.; and Gage, M. I. 1980. Effects of scopolamine, pentobarbital and amphetamine on radial arm maze performance in the rat. *Pharmacol. Biochem. Behav.* 12:595–602.

Ellis, M.; Clegg, D.; and Kesner, R. 1984. Exhaustive memory scanning in *Rattus norvegicus:* Recognition for food items. *J. Comp. Psychol.* 98:194–200.

Erickson, R. C., and Scott, M. L. 1977. Clinical memory testing: A review. *Psychol. Bull.* 84:1130–49.

Fein, G. G.; Schwartz, P. M.; Jacobson, S. W.; and Jacobson, J. L. 1983. Environmental toxins and behavioral development. *Am. Psychol.* 38:1188–97.

Feldman, R. G.; Ricks, N. L.; and Baker, E. L. 1980. Neuropsychological effects of industrial toxins: A review. *Amer. J. Ind. Med.* 1:211.

Ferris, S. H.; Crook, T.; Clark, E.; McCarthy, M.; and Rae, D. 1980. Facial recognition memory deficits in normal aging and senile dementia. *J. Gerontol.* 35:707–14.

Flicker, C.; Dean, R. L.; Watkins, D. L.; Fisher, S. K.; and Bartus, R. T. 1983. Behavioral and neurochemical effects following neurotoxic lesions of a major cholinergic input to the cerebral cortex in the rat. *Pharmacol. Biochem. Behav.* 18:973–81.

Foreman, N.; Arber, M.; and Savage, J. 1984. Spatial memory in preschool infants. *Dev. Psychobiol.* 17:129–37.

Gaffan, E. A.; Hansel, M. C.; and Smith, L. E. 1983. *Learn. Motiv.* 14:58–74.

Gallagher, M.; King, R. A.; and Young, N. B. 1983. Opiate antagonists improve spatial memory. *Science* 221:975–76.

Gamberale, F., and Hultengren, M. 1972. Toluene exposure II. Psychophysiological functions. *Work Environ. Health* 9:131–39.

Gamzu, E. 1977. The multifaceted nature of taste-aversion-inducing agents: Is there a single common factor? In *Learning mechanisms in food selection,* edited by L. M. Barker, M. R. Bert, and M. Domjan, 477–509. Waco, Tex.: Baylor University Press.

Garb, J. L., and Stunkard, A. J. 1974. Taste aversions in man. *Am. J. Psychiatry* 131:1204–7.

Garcia, J.; Ervin, R. R.; and Koelling, R. A. 1966. Learning with prolonged delay of reinforcement. *Psychon. Sci.* 5:121–22.

Garcia, J., and Koelling, R. A. 1966. Relation of cue to consequence in avoidance learning. *Psychon. Sci.* 4:123–24.

Gershon, S., and Shaw, R. H. 1961. Psychiatric sequelae of chronic exposure to organophosphorus insecticides. *Lancet* 1:1371–74.

Geyer, M. A.; Petersen, L. R.; Rose, G. J.; Horwitt, D. D.; Light, R. K.; Adams, L. M.; Zook, J. A.; Hawkins, R. L.; and Mandell, A. J. 1978. The effects of lysergic acid diethylamide and mescaline-derived hallucinogens on sensory-integrative function: Tactile startle. *J. Pharmacol. Exp. Ther.* 207:837–47.

Geyer, M. A.; Segal, D. S.; and Greenberg, B. D. 1984. Increased startle responding in rats treated with phencyclidine. *Neurobehav. Toxicol. Teratol.* 6:161–64.

Ghoneim, M. M.; Hinrichs, J. V.; and Mewaldt, S. P. 1984. Dose-response analysis of the behavioral effects of diazepam: I. Learning and memory. *Psychopharmacology* 82:291–95.

Gimpl, M. P.; Gormezano, I.; and Harvey, J. A. 1978. Effects of LSD on learning as measured by classical conditioning of the rabbit nictitating membrane response. *J. Pharmacol. Exp. Ther.* 208:33–334.

Gleitman, H. 1971. Forgetting of long-term memories in animals. In *Animal memory*, edited by W. K. Honig and P. H. R. James, 1–44. New York: Academic Press.

Gleitman, H., and Holmes, P. 1967. Retention of incompletely learned CER in rats. *Psychon. Sci.* 7:19–20.

Glosser, G.; Butters, N.; and Samuels, I. 1976. Failures in information processing in patients with Korsakoff's syndrome. *Neuropsychologia* 14:327–34.

Godding, P. R.; Rush, J. R.; and Beatty, W. W. 1982. Scopolamine does not disrupt spatial working memory in rats. *Pharmacol. Biochem. Behav.* 16:919–23.

Goldman, P. S.; Rosvold, H. E.; and Mishkin, M. 1970. Evidence for behavioral impairment following prefrontal lobectomy in the infant monkey. *J. Comp. Physiol. Psychol.* 70:454–63.

Golub, M. S. 1982. Maze exploration in juvenile rats treated with corticosteroids during development. *Pharmacol. Biochem. Behav.* 17:473–76.

Gordon, W. C. 1981. Mechanisms for cue-induced retention enhancement. In *Information processing in animals: Memory mechanisms*, edited by N. E. Spear and R. R. Miller, 319–39. Hillsdale, N.J.: Lawrence Erlbaum.

Gordon, W. C., and Mowrer, R. R. 1980. An extinction trial as a reminder treatment following electroconvulsive shock. *Anim. Learning Behav.* 8:363–67.

Gormezano, I. 1966. Classical conditioning. In *Experimental methods and instrumentation in psychology*, edited by J. B. Sidowski, 385–420. New York: McGraw-Hill Book Co.

Grant, L. 1976. Research strategies for behavioral teratology studies. *Environ. Health Perspect.* 18:85–94.

Greenhouse, A. H. 1982. Heavy metals and the nervous system. *Clin. Neuropharmacol.* 5:45–92.

Groves, P. M., and Thompson, R. F. 1970. Habituation: A dual-process theory. *Psychol. Rev.* 77:419–50.

Gustavson, C. R.; Garcia, J.; Hankins, W. G.; and Rusiniak, K. W. 1974. Coyote predation control by aversive conditioning. *Science* 184:581–83.

Gustavson, C. R.; Kelley, D. J.; Sweeney, M.; and Garcia, J. 1976. Prey-lithium aversions, I. Coyotes and wolves. *Behav. Biol.* 17:61–72.

Hall, R. D., and Macrides, F. 1983. Olfactory bulbectomy impairs the rat's radial-maze behavior. *Physiol. Behav.* 30:797–803.

Hamilton, G. V. 1911. A study of trial and error reactions in mammals. *J. Anim. Behav.* 1:33–66.

Hane, M.; Axelson, O.; Blume, J.; Hogstedt, C.; Sundell, L.; and Ydreborg, B. 1977. Psychological function among house painters. *Scand. J. Work Environ. Health* 3:91–99.

Hänninen, H.; Eskelinen, L.; Husman, K.; and Nurminen, M. 1976. Behavioral effects of long-term exposure to a mixture of organic solvents. *Scand. J. Work Environ. Health* 4:240–55.

Hänninen, H.; Mantere, P.; Hernberg, S.; Seppäläinen, A.; and Kock, B. 1979. Subjective symptoms in low-level exposure to lead. *Neurotoxicology* 1:333–47.

Harada, Y. 1977. Congenital Minamata disease. In *Minimata disease: Methylmercury poisoning in Minimata and Niigata, Japan,* edited by T. Tsubaki and K. Irukayama, 209–39. New York: Elsevier Scientific Publishing Co.

Härkönen, H.; Lindström, K.; Seppäläinen, A.; Asp, S.; and Hernberg, S. 1978. Exposure-response relationship between styrene exposure and central nervous functions. *Scand. J. Work Environ. Health* 4:53–59.

Harmant, K.; Roucoux, M.; Culee, C.; and Lyon, G. 1983. Vision, attention and discrimination in infants at risk and neurological outcome. *Behav. Brain Res.* 10:203–7.

Harrell, L. E.; Barlow, T. S.; and Davis, J. N. 1983. Sympathetic sprouting and recovery of a spatial behavior. *Exp. Neurol.* 82:379–90.

Harrell, L. E.; Barlow, T. S.; Miller, M.; Haring, J. H.; and Davis, J. N. 1984. Facilitated reversal learning of a spatial-memory task by medial septal injections of 6-hydroxydopamine. *Exp. Neurol.* 85:69–77.

Harvey, J. A.; Gormezano, I.; and Cool, V. A. 1982. Effects of d-lysergic acid diethylamide, d-2-bromolysergic acid diethylamide, d1-2, 5-dimethoxy-4-methylamphetamine and d-amphetamine on classical conditioning of the rabbit nictitating membrane response. *J. Pharmacol. Exp. Ther.* 221:289–94.

Harvey, J. A.; Gormezano, I.; and Cool-Hauser, V. A. 1983. Effects of scopolamine and methylscopolamine on classical conditioning of the rabbit nictitating membrane response. *J. Pharmacol. Exp. Ther.* 225:42–49.

Hawkins, R. D., and Kandel, E. R. 1984. Is there a cell-biological alphabet for simple forms of learning? *Psychol. Bull.* 91:375–91.

Heise, G. A.; Conner, R.; and Martin, R. A. 1976. Effects of scopolamine on variable interval spatial alternation and memory in the rat. *Psychopharmacologia* 49:131–37.

Heise, G. A.; Keller, C.; Khavari, K.; and Laughlin, N. 1969. Discrete trial alternation in the rat. *J. Exp. Anal. Behav.* 12:609–22.

Hirst, W. 1982. The amnesic syndrome: Descriptions and explanations. *Psychol. Bull.* 91:435–60.

Hoffman, H. S.; Selekman, W.; and Jensen, P. 1966. Stimulus aspects of aversive controls: Long-term effects of conditioned suppression procedures. *J. Exp. Anal. Behav.* 9:659–62.

Hogstedt, C.; Hane, M.; Agrell, A.; and Bodin, L. 1983. Neuropsychological test results and symptoms among workers with well defined long-term exposure to lead. *Br. J. Indus. Med.* 40:99–105.

Holmes, J. H., and Gaon, M. D. 1956. Observations on acute and multiple exposure to anticholinesterase agents. *Trans. Am. Clin. Climatol. Assoc.* 6:86–101.

Honig, W. K. 1978. Studies of working memory in the pigeon. In *Cognitive processes in animal behavior,* edited by S. H. Hulse, H. Fowler, and W. K. Honig, 211–48. Hillsdale, N.J.: Lawrence Erlbaum.

Husman, K. 1980. Symptoms of car painters with long-term exposure to a mixture of organic solvents. *Scand. J. Work Environ. Health* 6:19–32.

Husman, K., and Karli, P. 1980. Clinical neurological findings among car painters exposed to a mixture of organic solvents. *Scand. J. Work Environ. Health* 6:33–39.

Inglis, J. 1959. Learning, retention, and conceptual usage in elderly patients with memory disorder. *J. Abnorm. Soc. Psychol.* 59:210–15.

Ingram, D. K.; London, E. D.; and Goodrick, C. L. 1981. Age and neurochemical correlates of radial maze performance in rats. *Neurobiol. Aging* 2:41–47.

Inskip, M. J., and Piotrowski, J. K. 1985. Review of the health effects of methylmercury. *J. Appl. Toxicol.* 5:113–33.

Izquierdo, I.; Vendite, D. A.; Souza, D. O.; Dias, R. D.; Carrasco, M. A.; and Perry, M. L. S. 1983. Some neurochemical effects of behavioral training and their relevance to learning and memory modulation. In *Neural transmission, learning and memory,* edited by R. Caputto and C. Ajmone-Marsan, 221–35. New York: Raven Press.

Jarrard, L. E. 1980. Selective hippocampal lesions and behavior. *Physiol. Psychol.* 8:198–206.

Jarvic, M. E., and Kopp, R. 1967. An improved one-trial passive avoidance learning situation. *Psychol. Rep.* 21:221–24.

Kandel, E. R. 1979. *Cellular insights into behavior and learning*. Harvey Lecture Series, no. 73. New York: Academic Press.

Kandel, E. R., and Schwartz, J. H. 1982. Molecular biology of learning: Modulation of transmitter release. *Science* 218:433–43.

Keppel, G., and Underwood, B. J. 1962. Proactive inhibition in short-term retention of single items. *J. Verb. Learn. Verb. Behav.* 1:153–61.

Kesner, R. P. 1985. Correspondence between humans and animals in coding of temporal attributes: Role of hippocampus and prefrontal cortex. In *Memory dysfunctions*, 122–36. *See* Cohen et al. 1985.

Kesner, R. P.; Hardy, J. D.; and Novak, J. M. 1983. Phencyclidine and behavior: II. Active avoidance learning and radial arm maze performance. *Pharmacol. Biochem. Behav.* 18:351–56.

Kesner, R. P., and Novak, J. M. 1982. Serial position curve in rats: Role of the dorsal hippocampus. *Science* 218:173–74.

Kjellstrand, P.; Lanke, J.; Bjerkemo, M.; Zetterqvist, L.; and Mansson, L. 1980. Irreversible effects of trichloroethylene exposure on the central nervous system. *Scand. J. Work Environ. Health* 6:40–47.

Kleinknecht, R. A., and Donaldson, D. 1975. A review of the effects of diazepam on cognitive and psychomotor performance. *J. Nerv. Ment. Dis.* 161:399–411.

Ksir, C. J., Jr. 1974. Scopolamine effects on two-trial, delayed-response performance in the rat. *Psychopharmacologia* 34:127–34.

Kutscher, C. L.; Yamamoto, B. K.; and Hamburger, J. N. 1979. Increased and decreased preference for saccharin immediately following injections of various agents. *Physiol. Behav.* 23:461–64.

Landauer, M. R.; Lynch, M.; Balster, R. L.; and Kallman, M. J. 1982. Trichloromethane-induced taste aversions in mice. *Neurobehav. Toxicol. Teratol.* 4:305–9

Langolf, G. D.; Smith, P. J.; Henderson, R.; and Whittle, H. 1981. Measurements of neurological functions in the evaluations of exposure to neurotoxic agents. *Ann. Occup. Hyg.* 2:293–96.

Laties, V. G. 1975. The role of discriminative stimuli in modulating drug action. *Fed. Proc.* 34:1880–88.

Laughlin, N. K.; Finger, S.; and Bell, J. 1984. Early undernutrition and later hippocampal damage: Effects on spontaneous behaviors and reversal learning. *Physiol. Psychol.* 11:269–77.

Leander, J. D., and Gau, B. A. 1980. Flavor aversion rapidly produced by inorganic lead and triethyl tin. *Neurotoxicology* 1:635–42.

Leander, J. D., and MacPhail, R. C. 1980. Effect of chlordimeform (a formamidine pesticide) on schedule-controlled responding of pigeons. *Neurobehav. Toxicol. Teratol.* 2:315–31.

———. 1981. Chlordimeform effects on schedule-controlled behavior in rats. *Neurobehav. Toxicol. Teratol.* 3:19–26.

Leaton, R. N. 1976. Long-term retention of the habituation of lick suppression and startle response produced by a single auditory stimulus. *J. Exp. Psychol.: Anim. Behav. Proc.* 2:248–59.

Levin, E. D., and Bowman, R. E. 1983. The effect of pre- or postnatal lead exposure on Hamilton search task in monkeys. *Neurobehav. Toxicol. Teratol.* 5:391–94.

Levin, H. S., and Rodnitzky, R. L. 1976. Behavioral effects of organophosphate pesticides in man. *Clin. Toxicol.* 9:391–405.

Levine, T. E. 1978. Conditioned aversion following ingestion of methylmercury in rats and mice. *Behav. Biol.* 25:489–96.

Levy, A.; Kluge, P. B.; and Elsmore, T. F. 1983. Radial arm maze performance of mice: Acquisition and atropine effects. *Behav. Neural Biol.* 39:229–40.

Lezak, M. D. 1976. *Neuropsychological assessment.* New York: Oxford University Press.

———. 1984. Neuropsychological assessment in behavioral toxicology—Developing techniques and interpretative issues. *Scand. J. Work Environ. Health* 10, suppl. 1: 25–29.

Lindström, K. 1981. Behavioral changes after long-term exposure to organic solvents and their mixtures: Determining factors and research results. *Scand. J. Work Environ. Health* 7:48–53.

Lindström, K.; Härkönen, H.; and Hernberg, S. 1976. Disturbances in psychological functions of workers occupationally exposed to styrene. *Scand. J. Work Environ. Health* 3:129–39.

McCoy, D. F.; Nallan, G. B.; and Pace, G. M. 1980. Some effects of rotation and centrifugally produced high gravity on taste aversion in rats. *Bull. Psychon. Soc.* 16:255–57.

McGaugh, J. L. 1973. Drug facilitation of learning and memory. *Annu. Rev. Pharmacol.* 13:229–41.

Mackay, B. 1974. Conditioned food aversions produced by toxicosis in the Atlantic cod. *Behav. Biol.* 12:347–55.

McKeown-Eyssen, G. E., and Ruedy, J. 1983. Prevalence of neurological abnormality in Cree Indians exposed to methylmercury in northern Quebec. *Clin. Invest. Med.* 6:161–69.

McMillan, D. E. 1981. Effects of chemicals on delayed matching behavior in pigeons I. Acute effects of drugs. *Neurotoxicology* 2:485–98.

———. 1982. Effects of chemicals on delayed matching behavior in pigeons II. Tolerance to the effects of diazepam and cross tolerance to phencyclidine. *Neurotoxicology* 3:138–41.

MacPhail, R. C. 1982. Studies on the flavor aversions incuded by trialkyltin compounds. *Neurobehav. Toxicol. Teratol.* 4:225–30.

MacPhail, R. C., and Leander, J. D. 1980. Flavor aversions induced by chlordime form. *Neurobehav. Toxicol.* 2:363–65.

Mactutus, C. F., and Fechter, L. D. 1984. Prenatal carbon monoxide exposure: Learning and memory deficits in avoidance performance. *Science* 223:409–11.

Mactutus, C. F., and Tilson, H. A. 1984. Neonatal chlordecone exposure impairs early learning and retention of active avoidance in the rat. *Neurobehav. Toxicol. Teratol.* 6:75–83.

Magni, S.; Krekule, I.; and Bureŝ, J. 1979. Radial maze type as determinant of the choice behavior of rats. *J. Neurosci. Methods* 1:342–52.

Maier, N. R., and Schneirla, T. C. 1964. *Principles of animal psychology.* Rev. ed. New York: Dover Publications.

Mair, R. G., and McEntee, W. J. 1983. Korsakoff's psychosis: Noradrenergic systems and cognitive impairment. *Behav. Brain Res.* 9:1–32.

Majkowski, J. 1984. Gothenburg first and second workshop on epilepsy and memory function: Summing up and concluding remarks. *Acta Neurol. Scand.* [suppl.] 69:11–18.

Maki, W. S.; Beatty, W. W.; Hoffman, N.; Bierley, R. A.; and Clouse, B. A. 1984. *Behav. Neural Biol.* 41:1–6.

Maki, W. S.; Brokofsky, S.; and Berg, B. 1979. Spatial memory in rats: Resistance to retroactive interference. *Anim. Learning Behav.* 7:25–30.

Marsh, D. O. 1985. The neurotoxicity of mercury and lead. In *Neurotoxicity of industrial and commercial chemicals*, 159–69. *See* Anger and Johnson 1985.

Martinez, J. L., and Rigter, H. 1983. Assessment of retention capacities in old rats. *Behav. Neural Biol.* 39:181–91.

Matsuzawa, T.; Hasegawa, Y.; Gotoh, S.; and Wada, K. 1983. One-trial long-lasting food-aversion learning in wild Japanese monkeys (*Macaca fuscata*). *Behav. Neural Biol.* 39:155–59.

Melin, K. A., ed. 1984. Third workshop on memory functions. *Acta Neurol. Scand.* 69:11–134.

Menzel, E. W. 1973. Chimpanzee spatial memory organization. *Science* 182:943–45.

Metcalf, D. R., and Holmes, J. H. 1969. EEG, psychological, and neurological alterations in humans with organophosphate exposure. *Ann. N.Y. Acad. Sci.* 160:357–65.

Mewaldt, S. P., and Ghoneim, M. M. 1979. The effects and interactions of scopolamine, physostigmine and methamphetamine on human memory. *Pharmacol. Biochem. Behav.* 10:205–10.

Miczek, K. A. 1973. Effects of scopolamine, amphetamine, and benzodiazepines on conditioned suppression. *Pharmacol. Biochem. Behav.* 1:401–11.

Mikkelsen, S. 1980. A cohort study of disability pension and death among painters with special regard to disabling presenile dementia as an occupational disease. *Scand. J. Soc. Med.* [suppl.] 16:34–43.

Mikulka, P.; Vaughan, P.; and Hughes, J. 1981. Lithium chloride-produced prey aversion in the toad (*Bufo americanus*). *Behav. Neural Biol.* 33:220–29.

Milar, K. S.; Krigman, M. R.; and Grant, L. D. 1981. Effects of neonatal lead exposure on memory in rats. *Neurobehav. Toxicol. Teratol.* 3:369–73.

Miller, D. B. 1984. Effects of early postnatal triethyltin on pre- and postweaning indices of neurotoxicity. *Toxicol. Appl. Pharmacol.* 72:557–65.

Miller, D. B.; Eckerman, D. A.; Krigman, M. R.; and Grant, L. D. 1982. Chronic neonatal organotin exposure alters radial-arm maze performance in adult rats. *Neurobehav. Toxicol. Teratol.* 4:185–90.

Miller, D. B., and Miller, L. L. 1983. Bupropion, d-amphetamine and amitriptyline-induced conditioned taste aversion in rats: Dose effects. *Pharmacol. Biochem. Behav.* 18:737–40.

Miller, D. B., and O'Callaghan, J. P. 1984. Biochemical, functional, and morphological indicators of neurotoxicity: Effects of acute administration of trimethyltin to the developing rat. *J. Pharmacol. Exp. Ther.* 131:744–51.

Miller, R. R.; Ott, C. A.; Berk, A. M.; and Springer, A. D. 1974. Appetitive memory restoration after electroconvulsive shock in the rat. *J. Comp. Physiol. Psychol.* 87:717–23.

Miller, R. R., and Springer, A. D. 1972. Induced recovery of memory in rats following electroconvulsive shock. *Physiol. Behav.* 8:645–51.

Milner, B. 1962. Les Troubles de la memoire accompagnant des lesions hippocampiques bilaterales. In *Physiologie de l'hippocampe*, Colloques internationaur, no. 107, 257–72. Paris: Centre National Recherche Scientifique.

———. 1978. Clues to the cerebral organization of memory. In *Cerebral correlates of conscious experience*, edited by P. A. Buser and A. Rougeul-Buser, 139–53. Amsterdam: Elsevier.

Miranda, S. B., and Fantz, R. L. 1973. Visual preferences of Down's syndrome and normal infants. *Child Dev.* 44:555–61.

———. 1974. Recognition memory in Down's syndrome and normal infants. *Child Dev.* 45:651–57.

Miranda, S. B.; Hack M.; Fantz, R. L.; Fanaroff, A. A.; and Klaus, M. H. 1977. Neonatal pattern vision: A predictor of future mental performance. *J. Pediatr.* 91:642–47.

Mishkin, M., and Delacour, J. 1975. An analysis of short-term visual memory in the monkey. *J. Exp. Psychol.: Anim. Behav. Proc.* 1:326–34.

Mitchell, S. J.; Rawlins, J. N. P.; Steward, O.; and Olton, D. S. 1982. Medial septal area lesions disrupt theta rhythm and cholinergic staining in medial entorhinal cortex and produces impaired radial arm maze behavior in rats. *J. Neurosci.* 2:292–302.

Mizumori, S. J. Y.; Rosenzweig, M.; and Kermisch, M. G. 1982. Failure of mice to demonstrate spatial memory in the radial maze. *Behav. Neural Biol.* 35:33–45.

Moerschbaecher, J. M.; Boren, J. J.; Schrot, J.; and Simoes-Fontes, J. C. 1979. Effects of cocaine and d-amphetamine on the repeated acquisition and performance of conditional discriminations. *J. Exp. Anal. Behav.* 31:127–40.

Mohs, R. C.; Tinklenberg, J. R.; Roth, W. T.; and Kopell, B. S. 1980. Sensitivity of some human cognitive functions to effects of methamphetamine and secobarbital. *Drug Alcohol Depend.* 5:145–50.

Morris, R. G. M. 1981. Spatial localization does not require the presence of local cues. *Learn. Motiv.* 12:239–60.

———. 1983. Modelling amnesia and the study of memory in animals. *Trends NeuroSci.* 6:479–83.

Morris, R. G. M.; Marrud, P.; Rawlins, J. N. P.; and O'Keefe, J. 1982. Place navigation impaired in rats with hippocampal lesions. *Nature* 297:681–83.

Mullin, L. S. and Krivanek, N. D. 1982. Comparison of unconditioned reflex and conditioned avoidance tests in rats exposed by inhalation to carbon monoxide, 1,1,1-trichloroethane, toluene or ethanol. *Neurotoxicology* 3:126–37.

Murdock, B. B., Jr. 1982. A theory for the storage and retrieval of item and associative information. *Psychol. Rev.* 89:609–26.

Murray, E. A., and Mishkin, M. 1985. Amygdalectomy impairs crossmodal association in monkeys. *Science* 228:604–6.

Nelson, B. K.; Brightwell, W. S.; Setzer, J. V.; Taylor, B. J.; Hornung, R. W.; and O'Donohue, T. L. 1981. Ethoxyethanol behavioral teratology in rats. *Neurotoxicology* 2:231–49.

Olton, D. S. 1977. Spatial Memory. *Sci. Am.* 23:82–98.

———. 1978. Characteristics of spatial memory. In *Cognitive processes in animal behavior*, edited by S. H. Hulse, H. Fowler, and W. K. Honig, 341–73. Hillsdale, N.J.: Lawrence Erlbaum.

———. 1979. Mazes, maps and memory. *Am. Psychol.* 2:313–65.

Olton, D. S., and Collison, C. 1979. Intramaze cues and "odor trails" fail to direct choice behavior on an elevated maze. *Anim. Learning Behav.* 7:221–23.

Olton, D. S.; Collison, C.; and Werz, M. A. 1977. Spatial memory and radial arm maze performance in rats. *Learn. Motiv.* 8:289–314.

Olton, D. S., and Papas, B. C. 1979. Spatial memory and hippocampal function. *Neuropsychologia* 17:669–82.

Olton, D. S., and Samuelson, R. J. 1976. Remembrance of places passed: Spatial memory in rats. *J. Exp. Psychol.: Anim. Behav. Proc.* 2:97–116.

Olton, D. S., and Schlosberg, P. 1978. Food-searching strategies in young rats: Win-shift predominates over win-stay. *J. Comp. Physiol. Psychol.* 92:609–18.

Olton, D. S., and Werz, M. A. 1978. Hippocampal function and behavior: Spatial discrimination and response inhibition. *Physiol. Behav.* 20:597–605.

Orr, W. B., and Berger, T. W. 1985. Hippocampectomy disrupts the topography of conditioned nictitating membrane responses during reversal learning. *Behav. Neurosci.* 99:35–45.

Otto, D. A.; Benignus, V. A.; Muller, K. E.; and Barton, C. N. 1981. Effects of age and body lead burden on CNS function in young children. I. Slow cortical potentials. *Electroencephalogr. Clin. Neurophysiol.* 52:229–39.

Pentschew, A. 1965. Morphology and morphogenesis of lead encephalopathy. *Acta Neuropathol.* 5:133–60.

Perlstein, M. A., and Attala, R. 1966. Neurologic sequelae of plumbism in children. *Clin. Pediat.* 5:292–98.

Peterson, L. R., and Peterson, M. J. 1959. Short-term retention of individual verbal items. *J. Exp. Psychol.* 58:193–98.

Petit, T. L.; Alfano, D. P.; and LeBoutillier, J. C. 1983. Early lead exposure and the hippocampus: A review and recent advances. *Neurotoxicology* 4:79–94.

Petit, T. L.; Biederman, G. B.; and McMullen, P. A. 1980. Neurofibrillary degeneration, dendritic dying-back and learning-memory deficits after aluminum administration: Implications for brain aging. *Exp. Neurol.* 67:152–62.

Pico, R. M., and Davis, J. L. 1984. The radial maze performance of mice: Assessing the dimensional requirements for serial order memory in animals. *Behav. Neural Biol.* 40:5–26.

Pollard, G. T.; McBennett, S. T.; Rohrback, K. W.; and Howard, J. L. 1981. Repeated acquisition of three-response chains for food reinforcement in the rat. *Drug Dev. Res.* 1:67–75.

Pryor, G. T.; Dickinson, J.; Howd, R. A.; and Rebert, C. S. 1983. Transient cognitive deficits and high-frequency hearing loss in weanling rats exposed to toluene. *Neurobehav. Toxicol. Teratol.* 5:53–57.

Puff, C. R. 1982. *Handbook of research methods in human memory and cognition.* New York: Academic Press.

Rabe, A.; Lee, M. H.; Shek, J.; and Wisniewski, H. M. 1982. Learning deficits in immature rabbits with aluminum-induced neurofibrillary changes. *Exp. Neurol.* 76:441–46.

Rabin, B. M.; Hunt, W. A.; and Lee, J. 1982. Studies on the role of central histamine in the acquisition of a radiation-induced conditioned taste aversion. *Radiat. Res.* 90:609–20.

————. 1984. Effects of dose and of partial body ionizing radiation on taste aversion learning in rats with lesions of the area postrema. *Physiol. Behav.* 32:119–22.

Rauch, S. L., and Raskin, L. A. 1984. Cholinergic mediation of spatial memory in the pre-weanling rat: Application of the radial arm maze paradigm. *Behav. Neurosci.* 98:35–43.

Reinstein, D. K.; deBoissiere, T.; Robinson, N.; and Wurtman, R. J. 1983. Radial maze performance in three strains of mice: Role of the fimbria/fornix. *Brain Res.* 263:172–76.

Reiter, L. W.; Heavner, G. G.; Dean, K. F.; and Ruppert, P. H. 1981. Developmental and behavioral effects of early postnatal exposure to triethyltin in rats. *Neurobehav. Toxicol. Teratol.* 3:285–93.

Reiter, L. W.; MacPhail, R. C.; Ruppert, P. H.; and Eckerman, D. A. 1980. Animal models of toxicity: Some comparative data on the sensitivity of behavioral tests. In *Proceedings of the eleventh conference on environmental toxicology,* 11–23. AFAMRL-TR-80-125. Springfield, Va.: National Technical Information Services.

Reuhl, K. R., and Chang, L. W. 1979. Effects of methylmercury on the development of the nervous system: A review. *Neurotoxicology* 1:21–55.

Roberts, W. A. 1981. Retroactive inhibition in rat spatial memory. *Anim. Learning Behav.* 9:566–74.

Roberts, W. A., and Dale, R. H. I. 1981. Remembrance of places lasts: Proactive inhibition and patterns of choice in rat spatial memory. *Learn. Motiv.* 12:261–81.

Roberts, W. A., and Smythe, W. E. 1979. Memory for lists of spatial events in the rat. *Learn. Motiv.* 10:313–36.

Rodier, P. M. 1978. Postnatal functional evaluations. In *Handbook of teratology,* edited by J. G. Wilson and F. C. Fraser, 397–428. New York: Plenum Press.

Rodnitzky, R. L.; Levin, H. S.; and Mick, D. L. 1975. Occupational exposure to organophosphate pesticides. *Arch. Environ. Health* 30:98–103.

Roitblat, H. L.; Tham, W.; and Golub, L. 1982. Performance of Betta splendens in a radial-arm maze. *Anim. Learning Behav.* 10:108–14.

Ross, E. D. 1982. Disorders of recent memory in humans. *Trends NeuroSci.* 6:170–73.

Rozin, P. 1967. Specific aversions as a component of specific hungers. *J. Comp. Physiol. Psychol.* 64:237–42.

Ruppert, P. H.; Dean, K. F.; and Reiter, L. W. 1983. Developmental and behavioral toxicity following acute postnatal exposure of rat pups to trimethyltin. *Neurobehav. Toxicol. Teratol.* 5:421–29.

Rusiniak, K. W.; Garcia, J.; Palmerino, C. C.; and Cabral, R. J. 1983. Developmental flavor experience affects utilization of odor, not taste in toxiphobic conditioning. *Behav. Neural Biol.* 39:160–80.

Sahley, C.; Gelperin, A.; and Rudy, J. W. 1981. One-trial associative learning modifies food odor preferences of a terrestrial mollusc. *Proc. Natl. Acad. Sci. U.S.A.* 78:640–42.

Sands, S. F., and Wright, A. A. 1981. Monkey and human pictorial memory scanning. *Science* 216:1333–34.

Schaumburg, H. H.; Spencer, P. S.; and Arezzo, J. C. 1983. Monitoring potential neurotoxic effects of hazardous waste disposal. *Environ. Health Perspect.* 48:61–64.

Schrot, J., and Thomas, J. R. 1983. Alteration of response patterning by d-amphetamine on repeated acquisition in rats. *Pharmacol. Biochem. Behav.* 18:529–34.

Schrot, J.; Thomas, J. R.; and Banvard, R. A. 1980a. Modification of the repeated acquisition of response sequences in rats by low-level microwave exposure. *Bioelectromagnetics* 1:89–99.

———. 1980b. Repeated acquisition of four-member response sequences in rats. *Psychol. Rep.* 47:503–9.

Scoville, W. B., and Milner, B. 1957. Loss of recent memory after bilateral hippocampal lesions. *J. Neurol. Neurosurg. Psychiat.* 20:11–21.

Seppäläinen, A. M. 1981. Neurophysiological findings among workers exposed to organic solvents. *Scand. J. Work Environ. Health 7*, suppl. 4:29–33.

Shepard, G. M. 1983. *Neurobiology.* New York: Oxford University Press.

Sjoden, P. O., and Archer, T. 1977. Conditioned taste aversion to saccharin induced by 2,4,5-trichlorophenoxyacetic acid in albino rats. *Physiol. Behav.* 19:159–61.

Sjoden, P. O.; Archer, T.; and Carter, N. 1979. Conditioned aversion induced by 2,4,5-trichlorphenoxyacetic acid: Dose-response and preexposure effects. *Physiol. Psychol.* 7:93–96.

Smith, P. J., and Langolf, G. D. 1981. The use of Sternberg's memory-scanning paradigm in assessing effects of chemical exposure. *Hum. Factors* 2:701–8.

Smith, P. J.; Langolf, G. D.; and Goldberg, J. 1983. Effects of occupational exposure to elemental mercury on short-term memory capacity. *Br. J. Ind. Med.* 40:413–19.

Smith, S. M.; Glenberg, A.; and Bjork, R. A. 1978. Environmental context and human memory. *J. Exp. Psychol.: Learn. Memory Cognition* 6:342–53.

Snyder, D. R., and Braun, J. J. 1977. Dissociation between behavioral and physiological indices of organomercurial ingestion. *Toxicol. Appl. Pharmacol.* 41:277–84.

Sobotka, T. J.; Brodie, R. E.; and Cook, M. P. 1975. Psychophysiological effects of early lead exposure. *Toxicology* 5:175–91.

Sobotka, T. J., and Cook, M. P. 1974. Postnatal lead acetate exposure in rats: Possible relationship to minimal brain dysfunction. *Am. J. Ment. Defic.* 79:5–9.

Spear, N. E., and Parsons, P. 1976. Analysis of a reactivation treatment: In *Processes of animal memory*, edited by D. Medin, R. Davis, and W. Roberts, 135–65. Hillsdale, N.J.: Erlbaum.

Sperling, G. 1960. The information available in brief visual presentations. *Psychol. Mono.* 74(498).

———. 1963. A model for visual memory tasks. *Hum. Factors* 5:19–31.

Squire, L. R. 1982a. Human memory: Neuropsychological and anatomical aspects. *Annu. Rev. Neurosci.* 5:241–73.

———. 1982b. The neuropsychology of human memory. *Annu. Rev. Neurosci.* 5:241–73.

Staubli, U.; Baudry, M.; and Lynch G. 1984. Leupeptin, a thiol proteinase inhibitor, causes a selective impairment of spatial maze performance in rats. *Behav. Neural Biol* 40:58–69.

Sterman, A. B., and Varma, A. 1983. Evaluation of human neurotoxicity of the pesticide aldicarb: When man becomes the experimental animal. *Neurobehav. Toxicol. Teratol.* 5:493–95.

Sternberg, S. 1966. High speed scanning in human memory. *Science* 153:652–54.

———. 1975. Memory scanning: New findings and current controversies. *Q. J. Exp. Psychol.* 27:1–32.

Stiglick, A., and Kalant, H. 1982. Learning impairment in the radial-arm maze following prolonged cannabis treatment in rats. *Psychopharmacology* 77:117–23.

———. 1983. Behavioral effects of prolonged administration of delta 9-tetrahydrocannabinol the rat. *Psychopharmacology* 80:325–30.

Stross, J. K.; Nixon, R. K.; and Anderson, M. D. 1979. Neuropsychiatric findings in patients exposed to polybrominated biphenyls. *Ann. N.Y. Acad. Sci.* 320:368–69.

Sutherland, R. J., and Linggard, R. 1982. Being there: A novel demonstration of latent spatial learning in the rat. *Behav. Neural Biol.* 36:103–7.

Sutherland, R. J.; Whishaw, I. Q.; and Kolb, B. 1983. A behavioral analysis of spatial localization following electrolytic, kainate- or colchicine-induced damage to the hippocampal formation in the rat. *Behav. Brain Res.* 7:133–53.

Takeuchi, T. 1972. Biological reactions and pathological changes of human beings and animals under the condition of organic mercury contamination. In *Environmental mercury contamination*, edited by R. Hartung and B. D. Dinman, 247–89. Ann Arbor: Ann Arbor Scientific Publication.

———. 1977. Pathology of fetal Minamata disease. *Pediatrician* 6:69–87.

Taylor, J. R.; Selhorst, J. B.; Houff, S. A.; and Martinez, A. J. 1978. Chlordecone intoxication in man. I. Clinical observations. *Neurology* 28:626–30.

Thomas, G. J.; Brits, G. N. O.; Stein, D. P.; and Berko, J. K. 1982. Memory and septo-hippocampal connections in rats. *J. Comp. Physiol. Psychol.* 96:339–47.

Thomas, R. A., and Riccio, D. D. 1979. Forgetting of a CS attribute in a conditioned suppression paradigm. *Anim. Learning Behav.* 7:191–95.

Thompson, D. M. 1973. Repeated acquisition as a behavioral baseline for studying drug effects. *J. Pharmacol. Exp. Ther.* 184:506–14.

———. 1974. Repeated acquisition of behavioral chains under chronic drug conditions. *J. Pharmacol. Exp. Ther.* 188:700–710.

———. 1978. Stimulus control and drug effects. In *Contemporary research in behavioral pharmacology*, edited by D. E. Blackman and D. J. Sanger, 159–207. New York: Plenum Press.

Thompson, D. M., and Moerschbaecher, J. M. 1979. An experimental analysis of the effects of d-amphetamine and cocaine on the acquisition performance of response chains in monkeys. *J. Exp. Anal. Behav.* 32:433–44.

———. 1984. Phencyclidine in combination with d-amphetamine: Differential effects on acquisition and performance of response chains in monkeys. *Pharmacol. Biochem. Behav.* 20:619–27.

Thompson, R. F. 1983. Neuronal substrates of simple associative learning: Classical conditioning. *Trends NeuroSci.* 6:270–75.

Thompson, R. F.; Groves, P. M.; Teyler, T. J.; and Roemer, R. A. 1973. A dual-process theory of habituation: Theory and behavior. In *Habituation*, edited by H. V. S. Peeke and M. J. Herz, 239–71. New York: Academic Press.

Thompson, R. F., and Spencer, W. A. 1966. Habituation: A model phenomenon for the study of neuronal substrates of behavior. *Psychol. Rev.* 73:16–43.

Tilson, H. A., and Mitchell, C. 1984. Neurobehavioral techniques to assess the effects of chemicals on the nervous system. *Annu. Rev. Pharmacol. Toxicol.* 24:425–50.

Townsend, J. T. 1971. A note on the identifiability of parallel and serial processes. *Percept. Psychophysics* 10:161–63.

Tulving, E. 1972. Episodic and semantic memory. In *Organization of memory*, edited by E. Tulving and W. Donaldson, 382–403. New York: Academic Press.

Tulving, E., and Thomson, D. M. 1973. Encoding specificity and retrieval processes in episodic memory. *Psychol. Rev.* 80:352–73.

Valciukas, J. A.; Lilis, R.; Eisinger, J.; Blumberg, W. E.; Fischbein, A.; and Selikoff, I. J. 1978. Behavioral indicators of lead neurotoxicity: Results of a clinical field survey. *Int. Arch. Occup. Environ. Health* 41:217–35.

Vogt, M. B., and Rudy, J. W. 1984. Ontogenesis of learning: I. Variation in the rat's reflexive and learned responses to gustatory stimulation. *Dev. Psychobiol.* 17:11–33.

Vorhees, C. V.; Brunner, R. L.; McDaniel, C. R.; and Butcher, R. E. 1978. The relationship of gestational age to vitamin A–induced postnatal dysfunction. *Teratology* 17:271–76.

Vroom, F. Q., and Greer, M. 1972. Mercury vapour intoxication. *Brain* 95:305–18.

Wallace, J. E.; Krauter, E. E.; and Campbell, B. A. 1980. Animal models of declining memory in the aged: Short-term and spatial memory in the aged rat. *J. Gerontol.* 35:355–63.

Walsh, T. J.; Miller, D. B.; and Dyer, R. S. 1982. Trimethyltin, a selective limbic system neurotoxicant, impairs radial-arm maze performance. *Neurobehav. Toxicol. Teratol.* 4:177–83.

Walsh, T. J.; Tilson, H. A.; DeHaven, D. L.; Mailman, R. B.; Fisher, A.; and Hanin, I. 1984. AF64A, a cholinergic neurotoxin, selectively depletes acetylcholine in hippocampus and cortex, and produces long-term passive avoidance and radial-arm maze deficits in the rat. *Brain Res.* 321:91–102.

Watt, J.; Stevens, R.; and Robinson, C. 1980. Effects on scopolamine on radial maze performance in rats. *Pharmacol. Biochem. Behav.* 12:595–602.

Wechsler, D. 1945. A standardized memory scale for clinical use. *J. Psychol.* 19:87–95.

Weingartner, H.; Grafman, J.; Boutelle, W.; Kaye, W.; and Martin, P. R. 1983. Forms of memory failure. *Science* 221:380–82.

Weiskrantz, L., and Warrington, E. G. 1979. Conditioning in amnesic patients. *Neurophsychologia* 17:187–94.

Weiss, B. 1983a. Behavioral toxicology and environmental health science: Opportunity and challenge for psychology. *Am. Psychol.* 38:1174–87.

Weiss, B. 1983b. Specifying the nonspecific. In *Application of behavioral pharmacology in toxicology*, edited by G. Zbinden, 71–86. New York: Raven Press.

Wesnes, K., and Warburton, D. M. 1984. Effects of scopolamine and nicotine on human rapid information processing performance. *Psychopharmacology* 82:147–50.

Wickens, D. D. 1970. Encoding categories of words: An empirical approach to meaning. *Psychol. Rev.* 77:1–15.

Wilkie, D. M., and Slobin, P. 1983. Gerbils in space: Performance on the 17-arm radial maze. *J. Exp. Anal. Behav.* 40:301–12.

Wilkie, D. M.; Spetch, M. L.; and Chew, I. 1981. The ring dove's short-term memory capacity for spatial information. *Anim. Behav.* 29:639–41.

Williams, H. L., and Rundell, O. H. 1983. Secobarbital effects on recall and recognition in a levels-of-processing paradigm. *Psychopharmacology* 80:221–25.

Winocur, G. 1982. Radial-arm maze behavior by rats with dorsal hippocampal lesions: Effects of cuing. *J. Comp. Physiol. Psychol.* 96:155–69.

Wirsching, B. A.; Beninger, R. J.; Jhamandas, K.; Boegman, R. J.; and el-Defrawy, S. R. 1984. Differential effects of scopolamine on working and reference memory of rats in the radial maze. *Pharmacol. Biochem. Behav.* 20:659–62.

Wirtshafter, D., and Asin, K. E. 1983. Impaired radial maze performance in rats with electrolytic median raphe lesions. *Exp. Neurol.* 79:412–21.

Wise, R. A.; Yokel, R. A.; and DeWitt, H. 1976. Both positive reinforcement and conditioned aversion from amphetamine and from apomorphine in rats. *Science* 191:1273–75.

Witt, E. D., and Goldman-Rakic, P. S. 1983. Intermittent thiamine deficiency in the rhesus monkey. II. Evidence for memory loss. *Ann. Neurol.* 13:396–401.

Wood, R. W.; Rees, D. C.; and Laties, V. G. 1983. Behavioral effects of toluene are modulated by stimulus control. *Toxicol. Appl. Pharmacol.* 68:462–72.

Yoerg, S. I., and Kamil, A. C. 1982. Response strategies in the radial arm maze: Running around in circles. *Anim. Learning Behav.* 10:530–34.

Yokel, R. A. 1983. Repeated systemic aluminum exposure effects on classical conditioning of the rabbit. *Neurobehav. Teratol. Toxicol.* 5:41–46.

———. 1985. Toxicity of gestational aluminum exposure to the maternal rabbit and offspring. *Toxicol. Appl. Pharmacol.* 79:121–33.

Zenick, H.; Padick, R.; Torarek, T.; and Aragon, P. 1978. Influence of prenatal and postnatal lead exposure on discrimination learning in rats. *Pharmacol. Biochem. Behav.* 8:347–50.

Zoladek, L., and Roberts, W. A. 1978. The sensory basis of spatial memory in the rat. *Anim. Learning Behav.* 6:77–81.

Zola-Morgan, S., and Squire, L. R. 1984. Preserved learning in monkeys with medial temporal lesions: Sparing of motor and cognitive skills. *J. Neurosci.* 4:1072–85.

II

Exposure at Critical Periods of Development

*Zoltan Annau and
Christine U. Eccles*

7

Prenatal Exposure

Increasing concern about the effects of environmental chemicals on human health has resulted in massive governmental efforts in most parts of the world to regulate the manufacture, distribution, and disposition of these chemicals. A quick glance at the weekly headlines is sufficient to reveal that toxic chemicals are only too ubiquitous and that the fear of exposure to carcinogens is pervasive. This somewhat one-sided view of the environmental crisis has overshadowed what may be equally health-threatening to much larger populations. This threat could arise from prenatal exposure to neurotoxic chemicals and their effects on fetal brain development, as well as the subsequent irreversibility of the neuronal dysfunction. While there is clear evidence in the animal experimental literature that such irreversible damage can be induced by low-level exposures, the evidence for human studies is either lacking or just becoming strong enough to influence legislation. What evidence there is, however, indicates that the human fetus is at least as sensitive as fetuses of other species to prenatal neurotoxic insult and that under the right conditions similar dysfunctions can be demonstrated. In this chapter we review some of the important concepts that have emerged in this area of research during the past 30 years, as well as deal with specific chemicals in order to illustrate these concepts. In order to limit this review, we ignore the large literature that deals with the effects of pharmacologic agents. The reader is referred to recent excellent reviews of this literature such as those by Hutchings (1978) and Yanai (1984).

Vulnerability of the Developing Nervous System

Even though we deal only with chemicals administered in utero in this chapter, it must be borne in mind that the half-life of many chemicals extends well into the postnatal life of the organism, and thus some of the observed effects are not attributable entirely to prenatal exposure. A distinction arises, therefore, between experimental administration of chemicals that have clearly defined, brief effects on neural tissue and chemicals that have long half-lives. This distinction, as we shall see, can be made in the laboratory but, unfortunately, rarely applies to the human case.

As can be seen from figure 7.1, the development of the brain (in this case, a mouse brain) occurs in spurts, with different nuclei evolving at different periods of

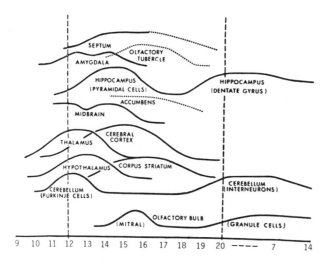

Fig. 7.1 Rates of cell proliferation in various regions of the mouse brain during gestation (days 9–20) and during early neonatal life (days 20–14). (*Source:* data taken from Rodier 1977.)

gestation. While the rodent brain matures more rapidly than the human brain, both undergo extensive development postnatally as well.

The vulnerability of the developing nervous system arises from the fact that cells undergoing mitosis and migrating cells seem to be particularly sensitive to toxic insult (Jacobson 1978). Damage to these cells can result from exposure to a variety of agents, such as 5-azacytidine (Rodier and Reynolds 1977), methylmercury (Chang and Annau 1984), and X-ray irradiation (Altman and Anderson 1972). The evidence that developing cells are more susceptible to injury arises not only from animal studies but from human data as well, as demonstrated by the Minamata episode in Japan, where asymptomatic mothers gave birth to severely retarded children following methylmercury ingestion. Presumably, some functional recovery can occur following the destruction of developing neurons, hence the term *neuronal plasticity,* but as Jacobson (1978) suggests, this term has to be used with caution and perhaps retained only in cases where adaptive responses have occurred. As an example of this adaptation, following viral destruction of granule cells, altered synaptic connections by mossy fibers can be seen in the cerebellum (Llinas, Hillman, and Precht 1973). The functional consequences of such "abnormal" connections are not known, however, and therefore one must bear in mind, perhaps, the difference between physiological and behavioral adaptation.

In the case of rapidly excreted cytotoxic agents, the destruction of specific neuronal populations has been used advantageously by several investigators to relate functional alterations to cellular loss (Langman, Webster, and Rodier 1975). Unfortunately, these studies reveal one of the inherent weaknesses of this approach: neither the chemical lesions nor the behavioral tests are specific enough to arrive at precise conclusions regarding the relationship between structural loss and altered function. As will be seen later, when measures such as open-field activity are taken following brain lesions, the nature of these measures is such that they can only vary in two dimensions (increase or decrease in activity); as a result, both types of effects are seen following lesions induced at different prenatal times. While this type of loose relationship may be useful for diagnostic purposes, it is simply not precise enough to relate morphology to function. Clearly, more precise chemical destruction of selected neuronal populations and more specific behavioral determinations of function are needed.

Damage following exposure to toxic chemicals is not necessarily restricted to neurons but can also occur in neuronal processes. Experimental models of fetal alcohol syndrome (FAS) are characterized by a decrease in the number of synapses and decreased synaptic maturation in the cerebellum, as well as delayed differentiation in the cortex (Volk 1984). At this time it is not clear whether the effects described by Volk can account for the FAS observed in humans, which is characterized by mental retardation as well as growth deficiency.

In all of these examples the effects of the toxic chemicals are on the developing nervous system of the fetus and not on the maternal nervous system. Numerous reasons for this special sensitivity of the fetal nervous system may be given, although each chemical may be unique in its neurotoxic action. Thus, the immature nervous system lacks the protection of the blood-brain barrier until well into the postnatal period (Thornburg and Moore 1976), and chemicals that cross the placental barrier reach the fetal brain with ease. In addition, drug-metabolizing systems develop primarily after birth, and the ability of the fetus to deal with toxic chemicals is very low (Waddell and Marlowe 1976). These factors, in combination with the rapid proliferation of cells during gestation, may result in the continuous exposure of these cells to chemicals such as the heavy metals. As an example, methylmercury administered to the rat during the fetal period is not secreted until approximately three weeks after birth (Ballatori and Clarkson 1982), and presumably, the circulating mercury is bound to the rapidly growing population of neurons in the brain. This continuous exposure of immature neurons to mercury may account for the "congenital" Minamata syndrome, characterized by nonspecific neuronal loss, in contrast to the adult syndrome, in which the visual and motor cortex is specifically targeted by this chemical.

The experimental evidence indicates, therefore, not only that the developing nervous system is more likely to be exposed to toxic chemicals more readily than the adult nervous system but that this exposure tends to be prolonged and more direct because of the lack of a blood-brain barrier and metabolic disposition. As we shall see later, other factors, such as alterations in maternal health owing to the toxic exposure, may profoundly influence the developing fetus as well and further complicate the interpretation of the data.

Animal Models

The use of animal models in research has enabled us to move from phenomenological studies characterizing much of human toxicology into the realm of biological mechanisms. This is especially important in the area of behavioral teratology, where the intent of the prenatal exposure of animals to toxic chemicals is to alter neural function. This alteration could range from a modification of subtle biochemical processes to outright destruction of neurons and glia. Thus, while the behavioral measurements made on the offspring after parturition constitute the primary yardstick of behavioral toxicity, they become only the first step in determining the nature and extent of the neural injury caused by the treatment. Apart from providing a more comprehensive biological picture of toxicity, the use of animal models can provide us with many other approaches that are the basis of the scientific approach. Thus, we can establish (1) dose-response relationships, (2) time-response relationships, (3) control for maternal effects and postnatal exposures by fostering studies, and (4) correlative neurobiological studies to understand mechanisms of toxicity. These experimental approaches lead to a better understanding of the biologic action of each chemical, and it is hoped that they will lead to the establishment of safe exposure levels for human populations.

Dose-Response Relationship

The interest aroused by the Minamata incident led to the beginning of the field of behavioral teratology, not surprisingly with an animal model of methylmercury toxicity. Spyker and Smithberg (1972) treated 129/SvSl pregnant mice with a single intraperitoneal injection of 0.1 mg per 20 gm of body weight of methylmercury dicyandiamide on day 7 or 9 of pregnancy. This dose of mercury did not alter the number or birth weight of pups per litter. At 30 days of age the prenatally treated animals showed abnormal locomotion in an open-field test (backward locomotion), as well as signs of neuromuscular impairment in a swimming task. Although this study did not use more than one dose of mercury, its importance lies in the demonstration that doses of mercury not toxic to the mother and showing no overt toxicity in the offspring can alter behavior in a structured test situation.

A more complete exploration of a series of prenatal mercury doses was undertaken by Hughes and Annau (1976). Pregnant CFW mice were administered 0, 1, 2, 3, 5, and 10 mg/kg methylmercury hydroxide by intubation on the eighth day of gestation. Control mice were intubated with an equivalent volume of saline. The mercury had a dose-related effect on the number of pups born per litter (See table 7.1).

At the highest dose, 10 mg/kg, only 2.53 pups per litter were alive at birth, an effect also noted by others (Su and Okita 1976). The birth weight of the pups was also reduced, with the 10 mg/kg mercury group being significantly lower at 24 hours after birth and the 3, 5, and 10 mg/kg dose groups becoming significantly lower through day 21. At nine weeks of age, however, all groups had reached control weight.

Behavioral testing was started when the offspring were 56 days of age. In a two-way avoidance test the animals treated with 3 and 5 mg/kg doses of mercury

Table 7.1 Mean number of pups of mice treated with methylmercury hydroxide on day 8 of gestation surviving per litter 24 hours after birth

Dosage (mg Hg/kg)	Mean Number of Survivors per Litter (SEM experimental)
0	9.20 ± 0.62 (N = 66)
1	8.55 ± 0.71 (N = 11)
2	8.13 ± 1.33 (N = 8)
3	6.02 ± 0.65 (N = 23)[a]
5	5.54 ± 0.16 (N = 23)[a]
10	2.53 ± 0.94 (N = 12)[a]

Source: Hughes and Annau 1976. Reprinted by permission of the publisher.

Notes: N denotes the number of litters in the group. Since there were no significant differences between the number of survivors in the various saline control groups, the control results have been pooled.

[a] t-score obtained was significant at the 0.05 level (single-tailed test).

showed a significant increase in the number of trials required to reach a criterion of 11 consecutive avoidances. Approximately one third of the mice at these doses failed to meet the criterion even after 800 trials. The shock-escape latency of the mercury-treated animals was not different from that of controls, suggesting that neither motor impairment nor pain-threshold alteration was the cause of the impaired learning. In a passive-avoidance task the 5 mg/kg treated group showed a significantly earlier extinction of the punished response than did the control group. Other behavioral tests, such as the open-field test, conditioned suppression, and a water-escape test, showed no differences between mercury-exposed and control mice.

These experiments were a clear demonstration that a single dose of methylmercury administered on day 8 of gestation could cause a long-term learning deficit. This deficit was dose-related in that the number of trials to reach criterion on the avoidance task increased as a function of the dose of mercury. While the avoidance task indicated an impairment, several of the other behavioral tasks showed no difference between treated and control animals. This finding is not unusual in the behavioral teratology literature and may be an indication that the neuropathology induced by chemical exposures is not all-inclusive in affecting all behavioral expressions of the animal. The relative specificity of behavioral alteration clearly makes it imperative that more than one behavioral test be used in the evaluation of postnatal effects.

The use of behavioral test batteries and strategies such as those described by Tilson, Cabe, and Burne (1980), Adams and Buelke-Sam (1981), and Vorhees (1983) will increase the probability of detecting the consequences of prenatal chemical exposure. This can be enhanced further by testing the animals over a wider span of their lives. Although the range of behaviors in the neonatal rodent is somewhat limited, in the past 10 years a number of tests have been developed that have allowed us to utilize these behaviors as markers of prenatal chemical exposures. The development of locomotor activity in the rat has been characterized well by Campbell and colleagues (Campbell, Lytle, and Fibiger 1969; Campbell and Mabry 1969). Alterations in this pattern have been used to describe early indexes of neurotoxicity. Thus, Eccles and Annau (1982a) have shown that prenatal exposure of rats to 5 or 8 mg/kg methylmercury chloride increases motor activity in the offspring at an earlier age than in controls (day 8). The effect of the higher mercury dose was to make this increase in motor activity last longer (days 8 and 15). By day 21, however, the activity of the rats had returned to control levels, indicating that this was a transient effect. Nevertheless, challenging these animals in adulthood (120+ days of age) with d-amphetamine revealed that their response to this stimulant was different from that of controls in an activity-monitoring device. This is an example of how the same behavioral test can be used from birth to adulthood as a longitudinal test of neurotoxicity.

An interesting behavioral paradigm was explored by Bornhausen, Musch, and Greim (1980) using methylmercury as the toxic chemical. Pregnant rats were administered methylmercury by gavage in doses of 0.005, 0.01, and 0.05 mg/kg on days 6, 7, 8, and 9 of pregnancy. Following birth, both mercury-treated and control pups were reared by foster mothers. At four months of age, the animals were trained on "differential-reinforcement-of-high-rates" schedules. Three schedules were used. In the first the rats had to press the lever twice in one second to obtain reinforcement; in the second, four times in two seconds; and in the third, eight times in four seconds. The lowest dose of mercury had no effect on performance, and there was no deficit in performance at the lowest ratio at any dose. At the higher ratios there was a dose-dependent decrease in performance in both male and female animals. While this experiment is a mixed design in that both dose and duration of treatment are varied simultaneously, the behavioral effects are again demonstrated at 4 months of age in the adult animal. These effects become measurable at the more difficult behavioral task, that is, at the higher ratio, demonstrating again that under simple conditions the prenatally intoxicated animal can cope adequately.

Neonatal alterations in behavior following prenatal chemical exposure may be subtle and brief. Their disappearance with maturity, however, does not necessarily indicate that the apparent functional recovery is total. It is more likely that the recovery allows the animal to mask the underlying neurological alteration under normal circumstances, but when challenged by stress or pharmacological agents, some aspect of the dysfunction reappears. Although common sense would suggest that the dysfunction would be dose-related, that is, that the larger the prenatal dose the greater the postnatal behavioral effect, this may not be a direct relationship. Because the larger doses of mercury (and, presumably, other toxic agents administered prenatally) not only destroy more neurons but possibly alter the function of larger neuronal networks as well, the ultimate behavioral expression of the toxicity may be quite complex. Unfortunately, the careful work required to clarify these important questions still remains to be done.

Time-Response Relationships

The exposure of human populations to toxic chemicals rarely occurs in a single episode. Continuous or repeated exposures are much more common, and therefore a more realistic animal model would have to simulate these exposures. A review of the literature shows that a great variety of exposure models ranging from continuous, throughout gestation, to specific exposures at various time points during gestation have been used. As we pointed out above, the difference between single and continuous exposures may not be as clear-cut as it appears from the experimental protocol if the chemicals in question, such as organomercurials, have a prolonged half-life. Great differences in experimental outcome could also occur if the chemical is accumulated during continuous exposure, in contrast to chemicals excreted or metabolized rapidly by the fetus. These questions are important not only from the point of view of the environmentalist but also from the point of view of the neurotoxicologist who is interested in determining whether interference with neuronal growth at certain stages of development leads to different functional outcomes. Continuous exposures, which presumably will affect all stages of development, therefore may be more real simulations of environmental exposures, while discrete exposures during critical phases of nervous-system development may be more related to fundamental questions of basic science. Clearly, both approaches are needed in order to arrive at a better understanding of behavioral teratology.

Well-documented studies relating morphological alterations to behavioral observations following perinatal chemical insult were carried out by Rodier and colleagues (Langman, Webster, and Rodier 1975; Rodier and Reynolds 1977; Rodier,

Table 7.2 Postnatal behavior measurements of exposure to 5-azacytedene during gestation in mice

Behavioral Measures	Day of Treatment					
	E12	E14	E15	E16	E18	E19
1. Righting tasks	*	—	—	—	—	*
2. Gait rating	o	o	o	—	—	—
3. Grid walking	o	—		—	—	
4. Adult activity	*↓	*↑	*↑	—	*↑	*↓
5. Bolus counts	—	—	*↓	—	—	—
6. Passive avoidance						
Immediate	—	*↓	—	—	*↓	—
24-hour retest	—	*↓	*↑	*↑	*↓	—
7. Active avoidance						
Light-to-dark	—	—		*↓	—	
Dark-to-light	—	*↑		*↓	*↑	
8. Spatial observations	—	—		o	—	
9. Spatial maze	*	*				

Source: Rodier, Reynolds, and Roberts 1979. Reprinted by permission of the publisher.

Note: The mothers were treated with a single administration of the cytotoxic agent on days 12, 14, 15, 16, 18, and 19 of gestation.

o   = Observational data difference.

*   = Different from controls at p < 0.02.

*↓ = Direction of difference on tasks where treated animals may differ in two directions.

—   = No difference between treated animals and controls.

Reynolds, and Roberts 1979). These studies were designed to determine the effects of 5-azacytidine, which is toxic to developing cells, on the development of mice when this agent was administered to the mother on various days of gestation or to the offspring on postnatal day 3. Doses that were not toxic to the mothers were used. The authors reported that all doses of 5-azacytidine caused a significant reduction in weight in the offspring, an indication that the toxicity of this chemical extended to all cells. The behavioral measures used in these studies related to measures of motor activity and measures of cognitive function or learning (see table 7.2). Rodier, Reynolds, and Roberts (1979) point out that the behavioral deficits tended to fall into two categories. Early administration of 5-azacytidine (days E12–E15) tended to affect motor measures and coincided with cerebellar morphological alterations seen in the histological analyses. Later administration of the chemical (E16–E18), which caused hippocampal damage, showed up on the learning tasks, as would be expected. The major anomaly to this separation of the data came from the E14 group of animals, which seemed to show learning deficits that could not be correlated with the anatomical findings to the authors' satisfaction.

    Unfortunately, it is not possible to limit the exposure of the fetus to other toxic agents to short periods of time, and in many cases—for example, with the animal models of the fetal alcohol syndrome—it is not even desirable. Even in this particular case, however, there are differences in the duration of the alcohol exposure of the dams. Fernandez et al. (1983), for example, exposed the dams to 8 g/kg per day in two dosings, on days 10–14 of gestation. These doses gave a mean maternal blood alcohol level of 238.9 mg percent one hour after intubation. The control animals either were fed an isocaloric sucrose solution on the same days or had ad libitum access to food. The birth weights of both the alcohol and the sucrose pups were significantly less than those of the ad libitum group. Behavioral measures were taken on the pups starting within 24 hours after birth. The tests comprised locomotion of a separated pup toward the mother and retrieval of the pup by the mother through postnatal day 10. Prenatal ethanol intake decreased the total distance traveled by the pups, and fewer pups reached the nesting area where the mother was. On postnatal days 31–32 or 53–54, the offspring were tested in an open field. The ethanol-exposed offspring were more active at both ages of testing.

Using a different experimental approach, Driscoll, Chen, and Riley (1982) administered the alcohol as a liquid diet to the pregnant females on days 7–13, 7–20, or 14–20 of gestation. The alcohol provided 35 percent of the calories in the diet and represented a dose of approximately 13 g/kg. As before, the alcohol treatment decreased the birth weight of the offspring, as well as their growth. At 18 days of age the offspring were trained on a passive-avoidance task. The results indicated that those groups treated with ethanol on days 7–20 and 14–20 took significantly more trials to reach criterion (not entering the compartment where they were shocked) than did controls.

In addition to chemicals' being administered intragastrically or through the drinking water, the inhalation route is also commonly used in teratological studies. Fechter and Annau (1977) exposed pregnant rats to 150 ppm carbon monoxide (CO) throughout gestation. This level of CO produces approximately 15 percent carboxy-hemoglobin in the mothers. The CO exposure resulted in a decreased birth weight, and by day 21 the CO-exposed pups weighed significantly less than controls. On days 1, 4, 14, and 21 the motor activity of individual pups was determined in an open-field device. In order to increase the activity of the 1- and 4-day-old pups, they were injected subcutaneously with 100 mg/kg L-dopa immediately prior to testing. Activity was recorded for 60 minutes. The activity of the CO-exposed pups was lower than that of air-exposed controls at all ages of testing.

A second study by these authors (Fechter and Annau 1980), using the same exposure paradigm and CO concentration, examined other behavioral indexes of neuromotor development and simple learning. The negative geotaxis test was used in 3-, 4-, 5-, and 6-day-old pups. In this test the pups are placed nose down on an inclined plane, and the time it takes the pup to turn its body facing nose up is measured. The CO-exposed pups were significantly less successful in performing this task until day 6, when they caught up with controls. Another test, the homing test, showed similar results. Pups prenatally exposed to CO were less successful in orienting toward the mother's cage than controls until day 8, when they reached control performance. Neurochemical analyses showed no alterations in catecholamine levels in the brains of the CO-exposed pups. Mactutus and Fechter (1984) showed that the CO-exposed animals made fewer avoidances in a two-way avoidance task than controls at 30 days of age and showed less retention on retest at 31 days of age, an effect still measurable at 300 days of age (Mactutus and Fechter 1985).

These data indicate that the early delays in the development of motor skills following prenatal insult may be transient, but as in the case of methylmercury intoxication, a challenge in adulthood shows up other deficits. It is difficult to determine whether the continuous low-dose exposure is more potent than single high-dose exposure at critical periods of development. The results of Rodier and colleagues suggest that even rapidly metabolized chemicals, like continuous exposures, can have behavioral effects throughout the animal's lifetime. The time-effect data, therefore, are complementary to the dose-effect data in that presumably when a critical number of neurons and their processes are damaged by the toxic chemical, a behavioral alteration, and most probably a permanent alteration, will arise. In contrast to the prevailing notions of neuronal plasticity and recovery from injury, these data suggest that the injury is only masked and that the recovery is only sufficient to compensate function under normal circumstances. It would be of interest to determine whether more complete recovery could be achieved with specific training early in the animal's life.

The role of nutrition. One of the central issues in many prenatal exposure studies is the nutritional status of the fetus. This has been particularly true of the field of prenatal alcohol exposure, and as can be seen above, in some of these studies isocaloric sucrose diets are administered to the mother to control for that. Recently, Schapiro, Rosman, and Kemper (1984) compared the effects of undernutrition on the developing brain to those of alcohol exposure using Golgi techniques. The outcome of this study suggests that the effects of undernutrition and alcohol are additive in decreasing cortical thickness and brain weight and adversely affect the oblique dendritic extent and density of basal, oblique, and terminal apical dendritic synaptic spines.

Unfortunately, studies dealing with prenatal alcohol intoxication generally report single behavioral tests in the offspring rather than the correlative tests used by Rodier and colleagues. The picture that emerges from the data (for a recent review see Abel 1981) is that the offspring become hyperactive and have learning deficits, sometimes reminiscent of hippocampal damage. The data are not consistent, however, in that animals with hippocampal damage as a rule perform better than controls on two-way avoidance and worse than controls on passive avoidance (O'Keefe and Nadel 1978). As can be seen from the reports cited above, this is only partially confirmed in the prenatal alcohol data. That each experimenter almost inevitably chooses a different treatment regimen possibly contributes to the discrepancy of these results. The morphological data, on the other hand, point to at least hippocampal damage and possibly a cerebral and cerebellar delay in synaptic development as well (Volk 1984). Thus, while we can make some generalizations regarding the effects of prenatal alcohol on the behavior of the offspring and the morphological damage, we are not yet in a position to define with accuracy the dose-response relationships and the threshold effects. The time-consuming nature of these studies prevents most laboratories from undertaking the types of analyses that would lead to such insights.

Fostering

One of the vexing problems of prenatal treatment, as we have seen, is the variable half-life of the chemical in question and the consequent prolonged exposure of the offspring. This prolonged exposure not only occurs during gestation following the administration of the agent to the mother but in many instances will occur during lactation through the mother's milk. A related problem in this area of research is the possibility that the chemical may affect the behavior of the mother during the lactation period, thereby altering her care of the pups and influencing their behavior in turn. These problems have been addressed by many investigators in a variety of ways, as we shall see, but the most common procedure to control for maternal influences has been fostering. Joffe (1969) defines fostering as rearing of the pups by a nonbiological mother who has received the same treatment. Cross fostering, on the other hand, is rearing by a nonbiological mother who is undergoing different treatment. Depending on the number and types of control groups used, these two approaches can lead to rather elaborate experimental designs.

In a simple approach to the problem Hughes and Annau (1976), using only one dose of methylmercury hydroxide diluted in saline, created four groups of animals: (1) mercury-treated mothers rearing their offspring; (2) mercury-treated mothers rearing offspring of saline-treated mothers; (3) saline-treated mothers rearing their offspring; and (4) saline-treated mothers rearing offspring of mercury-treated mothers. At maturity the offspring were trained on a two-way avoidance task to a criterion of 11 consecutive avoidances. An analysis of variance confirmed the apparent difference between the groups, namely, that the increased number of trials required to reach criterion was owing to mercury exposure through the biological mother during gestation, and exposure through the milk of the foster mother had no effect on this late measure of toxicity.

While these experiments do not rule out the toxicity of methylmercury in the neonatal period, they indicate that at the doses used there was not enough mercury in the mother's milk to cause a behavioral effect in the offspring in adulthood. In this case, there did not seem to be a problem with the mother's nutritional status at least as indicated by normal weight gain during gestation. In experiments where the intake of the toxic substance causes a reduction in food intake and a reduced weight gain during gestation, additional controls have to be used. This is illustrated by a study on prenatal alcohol exposure reported by Weinberg and Gallo (1982). Three groups of animals were used. The first group was fed ad libitum a liquid diet containing 5.5 percent w/v ethanol. The second group was fed a control liquid diet, but each animal was given an amount equal to the amount of alcohol consumed by its alcohol-fed pair. The third group was fed a pelleted diet ad libitum. There were no behavioral data recorded in this study, but the effect of stress on plasma corticosterone levels was determined. As can be seen in figure 7.2, at 30 minutes the three groups differed significantly in stress response, and the pair-fed group showed no decline in stress level at 90 minutes. These data may have significant implications for behavioral tests, since, as we described above, many of the latent markers of neurotoxicity are only revealed in a stressed animal. Barlow, Knight, and Sullivan (1978) have shown that stressing the mother will delay in mice several developmental milestones in a manner reminiscent of prenatal toxicity.

In order to control for the fostering procedure itself, Fernandez et al. (1983) added another group of animals. The object of this study was to determine the effects of prenatal alcohol exposure on maternal (pup retrieval) and homing behaviors (see table 7.3). In this instance no pups were reared by natural mothers, since all groups of pups were fostered. Although it would have made the study inordinately complex, it could be argued that these groups should have been added for completeness.

The results of this study indicated that groups EO/PFM and EO/EM (see table 7.3) did not show persistent retrieval behavior. This was taken as an indication that the treatment affected the mothers. The increased mortality of the alcohol-exposed offspring was not affected by the availability of an untreated mother (group

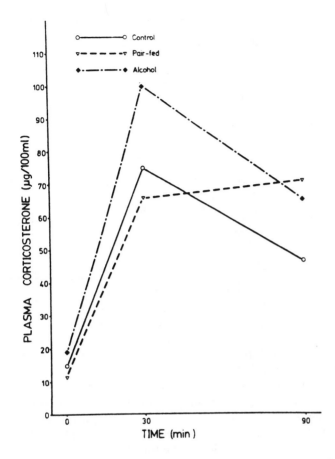

Fig. 7.2 Time course of plasma corticosterone levels in pregnant rats on the 19th day of gestation as a function of diet. Alcohol-exposed animals were given a liquid diet with ethanol 5.5 percent w/v; the pair-fed animals received an equivalent amount of ethanol-free liquid diet; and the controls were fed a pellet diet. Stress comprised handling and anesthesia induced by ether. (*Source*: data taken from Weinberg and Gallo 1982.)

EO/ALM) even though these mothers showed normal retrieval behavior. Thus, the effects of prenatal ethanol exposure apparently cannot be compensated for by postnatal exposure to uncontaminated milk and "normal" mothering.

These examples of fostering techniques illustrate some of the possibilities for controlling experimental variables related to prenatal exposure models. Other methods have also been devised to alter the postnatal environment of the pups, such as the artificial rearing method. In this procedure the pups are separated from their mothers and fed intragastrically, individually by the experimenter. While this method eliminates mother-infant interactions, it raises interesting questions regarding the effect of artificial and asocial conditions on the subsequent behavior of the offspring. This technique has been most useful in short-term studies concerned with the effects of toxic chemicals on biological parameters (see Samson et al. 1982).

Correlative Measures

Behavioral teratology, narrowly defined, determines the behavioral consequences of prenatal exposure to neurotoxic chemicals. Many studies have been done to demonstrate such relationships. It is difficult, though, to stop at this point if one is truly interested in the "toxic" effects of the chemicals under investigation. Some researchers therefore have gone to the next logical step; using the information derived from behavioral studies, they have attempted to correlate these with altera-

Table 7.3 Experimental design of fostering experiments to control for maternal treatments and postnatal conditions

Group Designation	Offspring and Treatment Rearing Condition
EO/EM	Ethanol offspring reared by a different ethanol mother
EO/PFM	Ethanol offspring reared by a pair-fed mother
EO/ALM	Ethanol offspring reared by an ad lib mother
PFO/PFM	Pair-fed offspring reared by a different pair-fed mother
PFO/EM	Pair-fed offspring reared by an ethanol mother
PFO/ALM	Pair-fed offspring reared by an ad lib mother
ALO/ALM	Ad lib offspring reared by a different ad lib mother
ALO/PFM	Ad lib offspring reared by a pair-fed mother
ALO/EM	Ad lib offspring reared by an ethanol mother

Source: Fernandez et al. 1983. Reprinted by permission of the publisher.

tions in nervous-system function (see Chang and Annau 1984). In a review of his work on ionizing radiation, Furchtgott (1975) concluded that the period from day 13 to day 18 during gestation was particularly important for normal development of behavioral function and that damage during this period would lead to severe behavioral dysfunction. Studies illustrating this conclusion showed that pregnant rats irradiated at 14, 16, or 18 days of gestation with 50, 100, 200, or 300 R produced offspring that had altered locomotor capability and impaired maze-learning ability (Furchtgott and Echols 1958; Furchtgott, Echols, and Openshaw 1958). At 300 R both behavioral tasks were affected regardless of age. Learning was disrupted by 100 R at 14 days of age, and locomotion by 50 R at 1 day of age. The authors discuss these differences in terms of differential development of the brain through gestation, with the forebrain developing earlier and the cerebellum later. Despite these findings, the feeling has remained that the relationship between structural damage and function is rather loose, as we saw earlier (Rodier, Reynolds, and Roberts 1979). It seems that at this point we simply do not have sufficiently clear correlative morphological data to understand why, for example, prenatal intoxication leads to either increased or decreased activity postnatally. As we saw earlier, these alterations in fact can be transient, and thus their ultimate functional significance may be less obvious. One possibility, of course, is that it is not sufficient to correlate morphological damage with behavior; one must take into account other biological factors such as neurochemical changes. Campbell and Mabry (1969) suggested that the development of motor activity, for example, correlated with the maturation of catecholaminergic systems. Lesions of these systems with 6-hydroxydopamine will alter the typical pattern of postnatal motor activity (Erinoff et al. 1979).

Most attempts to correlate neurochemical variables with behavioral alterations have been aimed at determining the steady-state levels of catecholamines and other major neurotransmitter pathways. Sobotka, Cook, and Brodie (1974) showed that rats that had received 0, 0.1, 0.5, or 2.5 mg/kg methylmercury on days 6–15 of gestation had subtle alterations in the achievement of certain developmental landmarks. Eye opening and clinging ability occurred earlier in pups treated with the highest dose of mercury. In the neurochemical measures there seemed to be a decline in brain pseudo-cholinesterase levels in the telencephalon and cerebellum, which the authors attributed to possible alterations in glial formation. There was a significant reduction in both serotonin and norepinephrine in the midbrain diencephalon at the 2.5 mg/kg dose of mercury.

A more comprehensive approach was recently undertaken by Cuomo et al. (1984). Pregnant rats were given 8 mg/kg methylmercury on day 8 of gestation. Behavioral measures on the offspring consisted of locomotor activity in a toggle cage, drug-induced stereotyped behavior, and passive avoidance. At 15, 22, 40, and 60 days of age there were no differences in locomotor activity between treated and control groups. Clonidine at 0.025 mg/kg significantly increased activity in all groups equally. On the other hand, 1 mg/kg apomorphine induced stereotyped sniffing in only the mercury-treated rats at 15 days of age, and both 0.5 and 1.0 mg/kg apomorphine enhanced stereotyped behavior at 22 days of age in the mercury-treated animals. There were no differences at later ages. Mercury-treated animals had a significantly shorter avoidance latency than controls on the passive-avoidance task at 60 days of age. The neurochemical measurements showed a significant increase in 3H-spiroperidol binding sites in the striatal membranes of 22-day-old mercury-treated rats. This effect was not seen at other ages. The authors suggest that the enhanced stereotypy seen at 22 days of age was probably owing to dopamine-receptor supersensitivity, but the neurochemical alterations could not account for the altered performance on the avoidance task.

Using a totally different treatment approach, Bartolome et al. (1984) recently have also shown that 1 mg/kg methylmercury given daily to the dam from day 8 of gestation until parturition significantly lowered the brain dopamine levels of the offspring by postnatal day 20. Dopamine turnover was also similarly affected, whereas no changes were observed in norepinephrine levels or turnover.

In addition to neurochemical and neuropathological measurements, neurophysiological data have been collected, although with less regularity. Dyer, Eccles, and Annau (1978) studied visually evoked potentials in female offspring of dams treated with 5 mg/kg methylmercury on day 7 of gestation. At 60 days of age the offspring had cortical recording electrodes implanted over the visual cortex. The prenatal mercury treatment significantly increased the P1 and N1 amplitudes, and both P2 and N2 latencies were significantly shortened by the exposure. The functional significance of these alterations is not entirely clear, but the data confirm other evidence described above of the long-lasting deficits induced by prenatal mercury treatment. Similar findings were reported following prenatal exposure to carbon monoxide by Dyer et al. (1979).

Recently, Kabat, Buterbaugh, and Eccles (1985) described the use of convulsive electroshock thresholds as a measure of postnatal effects of prenatal neurotoxic treatment. The anti-mitotic agent methazoxymethanol (MAM) was administered to rats on gestation days 15 and 19. Measurements of locomotor activity during postnatal development indicated that the day-15 treatment group increased its activity through postnatal day 29, in contrast to the control group, which showed the normal decline following day 15. In contrast, the day-19 treatment group showed a delayed development of locomotor activity. The convulsive threshold of the day-15 treatment group was lower than that for controls, while the threshold of the day-19 treatment group was higher than that of the control group. While locomotor activity and seizure thresholds may not be related in any obvious way, it is interesting that both measures deviated from control in opposite ways as a function of prenatal treatment. It is clear that neurophysiological measures at the present level of our understanding are useful as an index of neurotoxicity but are not yet sufficiently developed to lead to a better understanding of the mechanisms of toxicity.

As the above brief outline of selected portions of the literature indicates, the correlative neurobiological measures used in conjunction with behavioral measures give us a better understanding of the range of the neural alterations induced by toxic chemicals. It is difficult to imagine a situation in which a significant alteration in locomotor activity would not be accompanied by measurable neurochemical alterations. It is not quite so obvious that behavioral alterations are accompanied by readily observable neuropathology, but this is very often owing to the fact that the neuropathological measures are not detailed enough or do not use sufficiently exact methods. When threshold doses of neurotoxic chemicals are used, alterations in the total number of neurons or their processes may not be readily verifiable. Finally, with electrophysiological techniques we can study the activity of large or small neuronal populations in vivo. Data from such studies are just beginning to yield the type of correlative information necessary to understand how the function of neurons and their processes are altered by toxic chemicals.

Conclusions

Behavioral teratology has had a brief history and can be considered to be in its infancy. A great number of techniques have been drawn into this field in order to determine which postnatal behavioral effects can be measured following prenatal exposures. Most of the research has been concerned with just that—demonstrating effects at a single dose. Although there are thousands of potentially neurotoxic chemicals, most of our research has been concerned with the few that have posed the greatest human health hazard. By now most of these chemicals have been described in animal studies to some degree. What is lacking is a thorough description of dose-response relationships, as well as duration of effects. Since behavioral teratology is part of the environmental health field, it has had to respond to urgent human health problems by developing the appropriate animal models of prenatal intoxication. This has led to some haste in providing data for safe exposure levels or no-effect doses, and instead of well-organized research programs, we have had researchers jumping from one chemical to the next as the crisis or the funding of the day required. We now know that most prenatal neurotoxic exposures that cause behavioral alterations in the neonatal period will also cause behavioral alterations in adulthood. We have to go beyond that in order to determine through the lifetime of the animal species whether these alterations remain or whether the injured animal may show a dramatic deterioration during senescence. In other words, we have to extend the range of our observations to cover the life span of each organism that we choose as a model. In addition, we have to learn how to extrapolate better from animals to man. This extrapolation has to be not only in the realm of chemical doses but also in the behavioral methodologies. How do we equate the performance of an animal on a learning task with the performance of a child in school? A thorough study of some of the accidental exposures of human populations to neurotoxic chemicals is badly needed. Finally, we have to improve the experimental approach to the problem with two approaches. First we have to move from the random use of behavioral tests to the systematic use of tests to generate behavioral and neurobiological hypotheses to guide the next test based on the results of the previous tests. Then we have to use multidisciplinary research efforts increasingly in order to gain an understanding of the mechanism of toxicity, as well as simply the phenomenology. These two approaches will help prevent the endless repetition of single-dose, single-behavioral-result experiments. The preliminary data have been collected; now it is time to begin the real experimental work in behavioral teratology.

Acknowledgments

The authors gratefully acknowledge the assistance of Angela James in the preparation of this chapter.

References

Abel, E. L. 1981. Behavioral teratology of alcohol. *Psychol. Bull.* 90:564–81.

Adams, J., and Buelke-Sam, J. 1981. Behavioral assessment of the postnatal animal: Testing and methods development. In *Developmental toxicology,* edited by C. A. Kimmel and J. Buelke-Sam, 233–58. New York: Raven Press.

Altman, J., and Anderson, W. J. 1972. Experimental reorganization of the cerebellar cortex. I. Morphological effects of elimination of all microneurons with prolonged x-irradiation started at birth. *J. Comp. Neurol.* 146:355–406.

Ballatori, N., and Clarkson, T. W. 1982. Developmental changes in the biliary excretion of methylmercury and glutathinone. *Science* 216:61–63.

Barlow, S. M.; Knight, A. F.; and Sullivan, F. M. 1978. Delay in postnatal growth and development of offspring produced by maternal restraint stress during pregnancy in the rat. *Teratology* 18:211–18.

Bartolome, J.; Whitmore, W. L.; Seidler, F. J.; and Slotkin, T. A. 1984. Exposure to methylmercury in utero: Effects on biochemical development of catecholamine neurotransmitter systems. *Life Sci.* 35:657–70.

Bornhausen, M.; Musch, H. R.; and Greim, H. 1980. Operant behavior performance changes in rats after prenatal methylmercury exposure. *Toxicol. Appl. Pharmacol.* 56:305–10.

Campbell, B. A.; Lytle, L. D.; and Fibiger, H. C. 1969. Ontogeny of adrenergic arousal and cholinergic inhibitory mechanisms in the rat. *Science* 166:635–37.

Campbell, B. A., and Mabry, P. D. 1969. The role of catecholamines in behavioral arousal during ontogenesis. *Psychopharmacologia* 31:253–64.

Chang, L. W., and Annau, Z. 1984. Developmental neuropathology and behavioral teratology of methylmercury. In Yanai 1984, 405–32.

Cuomo, V.; Ambrosi, L.; Annau, Z.; Caggiano, R.; Brunello, N.; and Racagni, G. 1984. Behavioral and neurochemical changes in offspring of rats exposed to methyl mercury during gestation. *Neurobehav. Toxicol. Teratol.* 6:249–54.

Driscoll, C. D.; Chen, J.; and Riley, E. F. 1982. Passive avoidance performance in rats prenatally exposed to alcohol during various gestation periods. *Neurobehav. Toxicol. Teratol.* 4:99–103.

Dyer, R. S.; Eccles, C. U.; and Annau, Z. 1978. Evoked potential alterations following prenatal methylmercury exposure. *Pharmacol. Biochem. Behav.* 8:137–41.

Dyer, R. S.; Eccles, C. U.; Swartzwelder, H. S.; Fechter, L. D.; and Annau, Z. 1979. Prenatal carbon monoxide and adult evoked potentials in rats. *J. Environ. Sci. Health* C13(2):107–20.

Eccles, C. U., and Annau, Z. 1982a. Prenatal methylmercury exposure: I. Alterations in neonatal activity. *Neurobehav. Toxicol. Teratol.* 4:371–76.

———. 1982b. Prenatal methylmercury exposure: II. Alterations in learning and psychotropic drug sensitivity in adult offspring. *Neurobehav. Toxicol. Teratol.* 4:377–82.

Erinoff, L.; MacPhail, R. C.; Heller, A.; and Seiden, L. S. 1979. Age-dependent effects of 6-hydroxydopamine on locomotor activity in the rat. *Brain Res.* 64:195–205.

Fechter, L. D., and Annau, Z. 1977. Toxicity of mild prenatal carbon monoxide exposure. *Science* 197:680–82.

———. 1980. Prenatal carbon monoxide exposure alters behavioral development. *Neurobehav. Toxicol. Teratol.* 2:7–11.

Fernandez, K.; Caul, W. F.; Haenlein, M.; and Vorhees, C. 1983. Effects of prenatal alcohol on homing behavior, maternal responding and open-field activity in rats. *Neurobehav. Toxicol. Teratol.* 5:351–56.

Furchtgott, E., and Echols, M. 1958. Locomotor coordination following pre- and neonatal x-irradiation. *J. Comp. Physiol. Psychol.* 51:292–94.

Furchtgott, E.; Echols, M.; and Openshaw, J. W. 1958. Maze learning in pre- and neonatally x-irradiated rats. *J. Comp. Physiol. Psychol.* 51:178–80.

Hughes, J. A., and Annau, Z. 1976. Postnatal behavioral effects in mice after prenatal exposure to methylmercury. *Pharmacol. Biochem. Behav.* 4:385–91.

Hutchings, D. E. 1978. Behavioral teratology: Embryopathic and behavioral effects of drugs during pregnancy. In *Studies on the development of behavior and the nervous system,* vol. 4, *Early influences,* edited by G. Gottlieb, 7–34. London: Academic Press.

Jacobson, M. 1978. *Developmental neurobiology.* New York: Plenum Press.

Joffe, J. M. 1969. *Prenatal determinants of behavior,* 11–12. Oxford: Pergamon Press.

Kabat, K.; Buterbaugh, G. B.; and Eccles, C. U. 1985. Methylazoxymethanol as a developmental model of neurotoxicity. *Neurobehav. Toxicol. Teratol.* In press.

Langman, J.; Webster, W.; and Rodier, P. 1975. Morphological and behavioral abnormalities caused by insults to the CNS in the perinatal period. In *Teratology: Trends and applications,* edited by C. L. Berry and D. E. Poswillo, 188–200. New York: Springer Verlag.

Llinas, R.; Hillman, D. E.; and Precht, W. 1973. Neuronal circuit reorganization in mammalian agranular cerebellar cortex. *J. Neurobiol.* 4:69–94.

Mactutus, C. F., and Fechter, L. D. 1984. Prenatal carbon monoxide exposure: Learning and memory deficits in avoidance performance. *Science* 223:409–11.

———. 1985. Moderate prenatal carbon monoxide exposure produces persistent, and apparently permanent memory deficits in rats. *Teratology.* 31:1–12.

O'Keefe, J., and Nadel, L. 1978. *The hippocampus as a cognitive map,* 291–315. Oxford: Clarendon Press.

Rodier, P. M. 1977. Correlations between prenatally-induced alterations in CNS cell populations and postnatal function. *Teratology* 16:235–46.

Rodier, P. M., and Reynolds, S. S. 1977. Morphological correlates of behavioral abnormalities in experimental congenital brain damage. *Exp. Neurol.* 57:81–93.

Rodier, P. M.; Reynolds, S. S.; and Roberts, W. N. 1979. Behavioral consequences of interference with CNS development in the early fetal period. *Teratology* 19:327–36.

Samson, H. H.; Grant, K. A.; Coggan, S.; and Sachs, V. M. 1982. Ethanols induced microcephaly in the neonatal rat: Occurrence without withdrawal. *Neurobehav. Toxicol. Teratol.* 4:115–16.

Schapiro, M. B.; Rosman, N. P.; and Kemper, T. L. 1984. Effects of exposure to alcohol on the developing brain. *Neurobehav. Toxicol. Teratol.* 6:351–56.

Sobotka, T. J.; Cook, M. P.; and Brodie, R. E. 1974. Effects of perinatal exposure to methylmercury on functional brain development and neurochemistry. *Biol. Psychiatry* 8:307–20.

Spyker, J. M., and Smithberg, M. 1972. Effects of methyl mercury on prenatal development in mice. *Teratology* 5:181–90.

Su, M., and Okita, G. T. 1976. Behavioral effects on the progeny of mice treated with methylmercury. *Toxicol. Appl. Pharmacol.* 38:195–205.

Thornburg, J. E., and Moore, K. E. 1976. Pharmacologically induced modification of behavioral and neurochemical development. In *Perinatal pharmacology and therapeutics,* edited by B. L. Mirkin, 270–345. New York: Academic Press.

Tilson, H. A.; Cabe, P. A.; and Burne, T. A. 1980. Behavioral procedures for the assessment of neurotoxicity. In *Experimental and clinical neurotoxicology,* edited by P. S. Spencer and H. H. Schaumburg, 758–66. Baltimore: Williams & Wilkins.

Volk, B. 1984. Neurohistological and neurobiological aspects of fetal alcohol syndrome in the rat. In Yanai 1984.

Vorhees, C. 1983. Behavioral teratogenicity testing as a method of screening for hazards to human health: A methodological approach. *Neurobehav. Toxicol. Teratol.* 5:469–74.

Waddell, W. J., and Marlowe, G. C. 1976. Disposition of drugs in the fetus. In *Perinatal pharmacology and therapeutics. See* Thornburg and Moore 1976.

Weinberg, J., and Gallo, P. V. 1982. Prenatal ethanol exposure: Pituitary-adrenal activity in pregnant dams and offspring. *Neurobehav. Toxicol. Teratol.* 4:515–20.

Yanai, J., ed. 1984. *Neurobehavioral teratology.* Amsterdam: Elsevier.

Patricia H. Ruppert

8

Postnatal Exposure

Overview

Behavioral teratology is the study of the functional consequences of exposure to toxicants during the period of nervous-system development. These toxicants include therapeutic drugs, food additives, hormones, alcohol, drugs of abuse, heavy metals, pesticides, solvents, and X-irradiation. "Birth defects of the mind" (Kolata 1978) have become a matter of public concern as more has become known about adverse effects of chemicals in our environment (Spyker 1975), as well as adverse effects of drugs to which pregnant women and infants are exposed (Hutchings 1978; Barlow 1982). Organizational principles derived from teratology, neurobiology, and psychology are applicable to the study of behavioral teratology as a scientific discipline (Vorhees and Butcher 1982):

- Psychoteratogenicity is expressed as delayed behavioral maturation, impaired rates of learning, abnormal activity, impaired adaptation and problem solving, and other indexes of compromised behavioral competence.
- The type and magnitude of the response is a function of (1) the type of agent administered; (2) the dose of the agent; (3) the stage of development at which the agent acts; (4) the genetic milieu of the target organism; and (5) the environment of the target organism, i.e., maternal and placental metabolic influences before birth and maternal metabolism, behavior, and living environs after birth.
- Psychoteratogenic agents are those that are CNS teratogens or those that may be classified as psychoactive agents.
- Psychoteratogenesis is a manifestation of abnormal development that is demonstrable at doses of the agent at or below which malformations are induced.
- The period of susceptibility to psychoteratogenesis is isomorphic with the period of CNS development, and the period of maximum susceptibility corresponds to the period of maximum susceptibility to structural and physiological abnormalities of the CNS.
- Not all agents that are capable of producing malformations are psychoteratogens.

The prolonged period of nervous-system development, which begins early in gestation and extends into postnatal life, contributes to the vulnerability of the

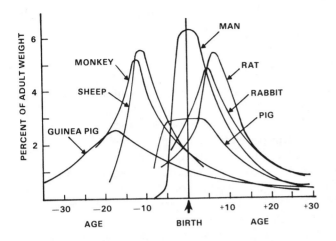

Fig. 8.1 The brain growth spurts of seven mammalian species, expressed as first-order velocity curves of the increase in weight with age. The units of time for each species are as follows: guinea pig, days; rhesus monkey, 4 days; sheep, 5 days; pig, weeks; man, months; rabbit, 2 days; rat, days. Rates are expressed as weight gain as a percentage of adult weight for each unit of time.
(*Source:* Dobbing and Sands 1979. Reprinted by permission of the publisher.)

developing brain. Although teratological studies have focused on prenatal exposure to toxicants, later stages of nervous-system development are also vulnerable to toxic insult. Exposure during this later period, when the complex circuitry of the brain is being established, may produce subtle alterations in brain development that are most easily detected by behavioral assays (Davison and Dobbing 1966).

In order to assess the risk to the human fetus and infant from exposure to potential neurotoxicants during later stages of brain development, i.e., in the perinatal period, a comparable stage of brain growth in an animal model must be evaluated. In the rodent a comparable period occurs postnatally. Donaldson (1908) described the relationship between the growth of the brain in the albino rat and that in man and concluded that the brain of the rat on postnatal day (PND) 5–6 was equivalent to that of the human at birth. Subsequent comparisons of brain growth in several species (Dobbing and Sands 1979) confirmed that the timing of the brain "growth spurt" in the rat and in man was comparable (fig. 8.1): the first week of postnatal life in the rat is equivalent to the stage of development of the human brain at the end of the third trimester of pregnancy. Therefore, early postnatal exposure in the rodent encompasses a time span equivalent to perinatal exposure in the human.

Behavioral evaluation in rats following postnatal exposure to potential neurotoxicants can be a useful strategy for assessing the functional consequences of neurotoxic insult during later stages of brain development. The objectives of this review are: (1) to present the major events of postnatal brain development in the rat, (2) to present some behavioral approaches for assessing postnatal insult, (3) to indicate how postnatal disruption of brain development by X-irradiation or by alterations in the hormonal milieu produces behavioral dysfunction, and (4) to present experimental data on the behavioral effects of postnatal exposure to heavy metals. Animal models of postnatal exposure to metals are particularly relevant given the potential for direct exposure to human infants by transferral through the mother's milk, the use of contaminated water in the preparation of infant formula, and the contamination of either food or containers used for infant and junior food (Schmidt and Hildebrandt 1983). Experimental data on the behavioral effects of heavy metal exposure will include recent research, including published abstracts, whereas literature reviews will be cited as sources for much of the background material presented in this chapter.

Postnatal Development of the Nervous System

In contrast to the recent origin of behavioral teratology as a scientific discipline, elegant studies by Ramon y Cajal and by other early neurobiologists in the late nineteenth century established many fundamental principles of brain organization and development. Following induction of the neural plate, the stages of neurogenesis are: proliferation of cells, migration of cells, aggregation of cells into brain regions, differentiation of immature neurons, formation of synaptic connections, selective cell death, and the elimination and stabilization of synapses (Cowan 1979. See also Jacobson 1978; and Suzuki 1980). The timing of these neural events differs by species, but the sequence of development does not.

In the rat, even the early stage of neurogenesis, the proliferation of neurons, continues postnatally. Allen (1912) reported evidence of mitosis in the cortex and cerebellum of the rat during the first postnatal week. Although the majority of proliferating cells in the postnatal brain are glia, later studies demonstrated that granule cells in the olfactory bulb, cerebellum, and hippocampus continue to proliferate in postnatal life (Altman 1970). Because of this ongoing neurogenesis, X-irradiation and agents that affect dividing cells can disrupt postnatal development. In humans, the time span for nervous-system development is longer than in the rat, yet proliferation of neurons still occurs in bursts separated by periods of inactivity (Rodier 1980). Therefore, even acute insults can have profound consequences in both species during episodes of rapid growth.

Examples of postnatal processes that are susceptible to insult during this period of rapid development in the rat are as follows:

Neuronogenesis. In the hippocampus, 80 percent of the granule cells are formed postnatally, and during the peak of proliferation (PND 5–PND 8) at least 50,000 neurons are generated each day (Schlessinger, Cowan, and Gottlieb 1975).

Synaptogenesis. Less than 1 percent of the adult number of synapses are present in the dentate gyrus of the hippocampus on PND 4, but the number doubles every day between PND 4 and PND 11 (Crain et al. 1973).

Myelinogenesis. During the peak period of myelination (PND 20), each oligodendrocyte synthesizes three times its own weight of myelin each day (Norton and Poduslo 1973).

As these examples illustrate, the brain growth spurt encompasses many developmental events, which occur at different times in different brain regions. The question arises, When is brain development complete? Many neuroanatomical and neurochemical parameters of development attain adult levels in the postweaning period (Ford 1973); others, such as deposition of myelin (Norton and Poduslo 1973) and proliferation of granule cells in the hippocampus (Bayer, Yackel, and Puri 1982), continue to occur well into adult life. These later "developmental" phenomena may be particularly sensitive to toxic insult. For example, brain growth in juvenile rats is reduced by administration of phenobarbital from PND 25 to PND 39 (Diaz 1983), indicating that the developmental neurotoxicity of barbiturates (Reinisch and Sanders 1982; Fishman and Yanai 1983) continues beyond the prenatal and immediate postnatal period.

Postnatal Development of Behavior

Although the development of behavior can be studied prenatally (behavioral embryology), behavioral assessment usually encompasses the period from birth to maturity or old age. Many behavioral test strategies and test batteries have been recommended for assessment of animals exposed to toxicants during development (see Butcher 1976; Grant 1976; Rodier 1978; Buelke-Sam and Kimmel 1979; Zbinden 1981; and Vorhees and Butcher 1982). Most recommendations agree that multiple functions should be assessed, since it is unlikely that any single behavior will be disrupted by all toxicants. Two promising approaches to assessing effects of postnatal toxicant exposure are the development of behavioral function in pups and the development of social behavior in juveniles and adults.

Behaviors that are specific to development, such as homing, suckling, and distress vocalizations, can be indicators of acute toxicity and also predictors of impaired development (Adams and Buelke-Sam 1981; Zbinden 1981). In addition, these species-specific or instinctive behaviors have allowed developmental psychopharmacologists to study the role of neurotransmitter systems in regulating behavior at a very early age. This is particularly true for suckling (Caza and Spear 1982; Spear and Ristine 1982). Thus, these behaviors can be informative because they provide for the study of mechanisms as well as for the detection of toxicity.

Preweaning evaluation of sensory, cognitive, and motor function can be used to assess delays in development and can allow comparison with deficits seen after maturity. For reflexes such as the startle response, more than the presence or absence of a reflex can be assessed; the number of responses, amplitude, latency, habituation, sensitization, and prepulse inhibition (e.g., Parisi and Ison 1979) also can be assessed, and these may be more sensitive indicators of toxicity. Preweaning tests of passive avoidance, taste aversion, runway performance, and so on (see Spear and Campbell 1978) have been adapted to the motor and sensory capacities of the developing animal. A peak in preweaning locomotor activity, which occurs on PND 15 (Campbell, Lytle, and Fibiger 1969), can be useful for assessing acceleration or retardation of development. Also, the daily monitoring of behavior such as emergence of pups from a nest box (Norton, Culver, and Mullenix 1975) can be informative for assessing the development of motor activity of pups within the social unit of dam and siblings.

Social behavior generally has been ignored in behavioral teratology studies (Buelke-Sam and Kimmel 1979), and most laboratories that do investigate social behavior use a criterion of mating success or fertility as the endpoint. Sexually dimorphic behaviors, which depend on the hormonal environment in perinatal life, offer a different perspective in behavioral teratology (Balazs 1981; Larsson and Hard 1982), since alterations in behavior produced by toxicant exposure can reflect damage to the developing neuroendocrine system. Social interactions at different stages of the life span can be assessed in prepubertal play behavior and adult mating behavior.

Juvenile rats are often described as active, playful, and "inattentive" (Altman, Brunner, and Bayer 1973) when compared with either neonates or adults. They may perform better than adults on simple learning tasks, while performance of juveniles can be impaired on more complex tasks (Spear and Brake 1983). Experimental studies have confirmed observational reports of playfulness in juvenile rats and have described the ontogeny of this behavior (see Panksepp 1981), which is characterized by vigorous chasing, pouncing, and wrestling. The presence or absence of androgen (Olioff and Stewart 1978; Meaney and Stewart 1981), brain lesions (Meaney, Dodge, and Beatty 1981; Beatty and Costello 1983), and psychotropic drugs (Beatty et al. 1982; Thor and Holloway 1983) can modify the intensity of juvenile play behavior.

Social behaviors in adults that are related to reproductive function include dominance, aggression, mating behavior, and parental behavior. These behaviors in the postpubertal rat depend not only on the action of gonadal hormones during development, as does play behavior, but also on the action of gonadal hormones in adulthood. The temporal patterning and frequency of these behaviors, such as male sexual behavior, can be altered by hormone withdrawal or replacement, by specific brain lesions, and by alterations of neurotransmitter functioning (see Sachs and Barfield 1976). Tests that evaluate precopulatory behaviors such as approach and contact directed toward a partner (Eliasson and Meyerson 1975, 1981) may indicate behavioral alterations that precede reproductive failure.

Maternal behavior is of interest in behavioral teratology from another perspective, namely in the interactions between the dam, the pups, and littermates following toxicant exposure. A continuing concern in behavioral teratology is that these interactions will confound the interpretation of developmental toxicity. Consequently, in prenatal studies, pair feeding of dams and cross fostering have been used as control procedures. In postnatal studies, comparisons have been made between litters in which pups were reared with dosed littermates and litters in which pups were reared with littermate controls (Pearson et al. 1980; Booze et al., Experimental design comparisons, 1983; Ruppert, Dean, and Reiter 1983a) Also, rearing of pups in an artificial environment (Goldenring et al. 1982) or an enriched environment (Petit and Alfano 1979) can modify the effects of toxicant exposure. Rather than being considered a confounding variable, the preweaning environment can be considered a source of information on how toxicity can be modulated by nutritional, social, and experimental factors.

Experimental Disruption of Postnatal Development

The study of abnormal development often has been used to elucidate processes involved in normal development. Within behavioral teratology, as in other disciplines, a range of interests is represented. Experiments have focused on nervous-system development, behavioral function, the action of a particular agent, or the development of animal models of human disorders. Studies of X-irradiation and hormonal imbalances during postnatal development are relevant to behavioral teratology, since toxicants themselves can affect postnatal neurogenesis and the developing neuroendocrine system.

X-Irradiation

Experiments investigating the effects of ionizing radiation during development have been directed toward several objectives: (1) describing the effects of radiation and analyzing the mechanisms of malformation, (2) using radiation as a technique to produce specific brain damage, (3) using malformed animals to find correlations between the developing brain and behavior, and (4) understanding and preventing radiation hazards in humans (Hicks and D'Amato 1978). Altman and his colleagues have used postnatal X-irradiation of the cerebellum and hippocampus to examine the relationship between abnormal brain development and behavioral function. These studies have described the types of experimental situations in which X-irradiated animals show behavioral deficits.

Focal X-irradiation of the cerebellum beginning on or before PND 4 produced an extensive reduction in the number of granule cells and severe disturbances of motor coordination and balance (Anderson and Altman 1972). When X-irradiation began on PND 8 or PND 12, hyperactivity with only minimal motor impairment was seen (Pellegrino and Altman 1979). Lynch et al. (1976) described a transition between PND 6 and PND 8 for the severity of motor impairment produced by X-irradiation of the cerebellum. These studies emphasize that the type of damage produced within a given brain area and the behavioral changes that result depend on the timing of the insult during the postnatal period.

Destruction of granule cells of the hippocampus resulted in hyperactivity (Bayer et al. 1973; Peters and Brunner 1976) and deficits on learning and memory tasks (Bayer et al. 1973; Gazzara and Altman 1981) that were typical of animals with hippocampal lesions. Learning disabilities in X-irradiated animals were seen more often on tasks that required an animal to inhibit responding and on tasks that involved more difficult discriminations. The level of task difficulty was also an important factor in detecting motor impairment produced by X-irradiation of the cerebellum, which emphasizes that careful behavioral analysis is often needed to detect even gross brain damage.

Because of the extensive postnatal proliferation of granule cells in the cerebellum and hippocampus, these areas might be generally susceptible to postnatal insult and motor incoordination; changes in motor activity and altered learning behavior would be anticipated behavioral outcomes. The postnatal effects of chemical neurotoxicants, e.g., methylazoxymethanol (Lai et al. 1978), are consistent with X-irradiation effects and support the postnatal susceptibility of the cerebellum and hippocampus.

Hormones

Either deficiency or excess of thyroid, adrenal, or gonadal hormones in the postnatal period can have pronounced consequences for brain development and behavior. Areas of the brain such as the hippocampus and cerebellum which are vulnerable to X-irradiation are also vulnerable to alterations in the postnatal hormonal milieu. Lauder (1983) has summarized evidence that in the hippocampus and cerebellum, cell proliferation, cessation of cell division, formation of neurons, axonal and dendritic growth, neuronal migration, and formation of synapses depend on the varying levels of thyroid and corticosteroid hormones in postnatal life. In the hypothalamus, gonadal hormones modify the type of synapse (Raisman and Field 1973) and the volume of a sexually dimorphic nucleus (Gorski, Harlan, and Christensen 1977) within the preoptic area. Toxicants can interact with the developing neuroendocrine system to disrupt function at several levels: chlorinated hydrocarbon insecticides have estrogenic properties (Gellert 1978), and excitatory amino acids produce hypothalamic lesions (Olney 1980).

Behavioral studies exploring effects of hypothyroidism and hyperthyroidism have placed special emphasis on the preweaning period to assess retardation or acceleration of development. A systematic study of the effects of thyroid hormone excess and deficiency on development was begun by Eayrs in the 1950s. To determine the critical period for the effects of triiodothyroxine (T3) stimulation (Eayrs 1964), rat pups were injected either throughout lactation (PND 1–24) or only at the beginning (PND 2–4) or end (PND 14–20) of the preweaning period. Eye opening was accelerated by 4–5 days in pups receiving T3 throughout PND 1–24 or only on PND 2–4. Both groups made more errors than controls on a maze-learning task as adults. No deficits in maze learning were seen in animals injected only at the end of the preweaning period. Therefore, in subsequent studies by other investigators that characterized effects of excess thyroid hormones on development (Schapiro 1968; Schapiro, Salas, and Vukovich 1970; Davenport and Gonzalez 1973; Stone and Greenough 1975; Murphy and Nagy 1976a, 1976b; Sjoden and Soderberg 1976; Kessler and Spear 1980; Brunjes and Alberts 1981), pups were injected during this sensitive period between PND 1 and PND 5. The general conclusion from these studies, in agreement with the work of Eayrs, is that hyperthyroidism during the first week of postnatal life in both rats and mice accelerates behavioral maturation and development in the preweaning period but produces performance deficits in adolescents and adults. Hypothyroidism results in hyperactivity and learning deficits (Eayrs and Lishman 1953; Eayrs and Levine 1963; Davenport and Dorcey 1972; Schalock, Brown, and Smith 1979; Strupp and Levitsky 1983).

Postnatal life is also a critical period for the action of gonadal hormones on sexual differentiation of the brain and behavior in rats. Table 8.1 illustrates the effects of perinatal androgen treatment on sexually dimorphic characteristics in females of several species. There is a striking correspondence between the time of the brain growth spurt in these species (see fig. 8.1) and the time of maximum effect of gonadal hormones on these sexually dimorphic characteristics. Both periods occur prenatally for the guinea pig, the sheep, and the monkey and postnatally for the rat. Like the brain growth spurt, sexual differentiation is not a single process occurring at a single time in postnatal life. Rather, the production of anovulation, masculinization, and/or defeminization depends on the type of hormone, the

Table 8.1 The effect of perinatal administration of androgens to females on the development of sexually dimorphic traits

| | | Dimorphic Characteristic | | |
| | | | Sexual Behavior | |
Species	Critical Period	Ovulation	Female	Male
Guinea pig	Prenatal	− −	− − −	+ +
Sheep	Prenatal	− −	+ +	+ +
Rhesus	Prenatal	Delayed	?	+ +
Dog	Pre + postnatal	?	− −	+ +
Rat	Postnatal	− − − −	− − −	+
Mouse	Postnatal	− − − −	− − −	+ +
Hamster	Postnatal	−	+	+ + + +
Ferret	Postnatal	?	0	+ + +

Source: Goy and McEwen 1980. Copyright 1980 by MIT Press. Reprinted by permission of the publisher.
Note: Symbols indicate the direction and relative ease of obtaining effect: − = defeminization; + = masculinization; 0 = no effect.

amount, and the time within this period when it is present (see MacLusky and Naftolin 1981). In female rats, a single injection of testosterone produces a continuum of effects on ovarian function that are age-dependent: anovulatory sterility is produced by dosing on PND 1–4, while a delayed anovulatory syndrome is produced by dosing on PND 5–6 (Gorski 1968). Male rats castrated on or before PND 5 display high levels of feminine sexual behavior but incomplete masculine sexual behavior when treated with appropriate hormones as adults (Grady, Phoenix, and Young 1965).

Sexually dimorphic behaviors that are not directly related to reproduction may also be influenced by the presence or absence of gonadal hormones in postnatal life. Behaviors for which sex differences have been described in adult rats include motor activity, pain, taste sensitivity, food intake and body weight regulation, learning and retention of certain types of mazes, avoidance responses, taste aversion, and performance on some schedules of reinforcement (see Beatty 1979). The magnitude of these differences is generally small and is critically dependent on test procedures. Therefore, if toxicants affect the contribution of sex differences to these behavioral baselines, this effect might be difficult to detect.

Behavioral Consequences of Postnatal Exposure to Metals

Metals that have been evaluated for behavioral toxicity in animal models following postnatal exposure include cadmium, inorganic lead, triethyl lead, methylmercury, triethyltin, and trimethyltin. In general, the toxicity of these metals is characterized by steep dose-response functions. To provide a framework for interpreting behavioral toxicity, dosages that produce mortality and reduce growth have been reported in most studies. In addition, brain weight has been included in most studies to indicate the relationship between dosages producing behavioral dysfunction and those producing overt CNS toxicity. Reductions in brain weight have been reported following postnatal exposure to cadmium (Rastogi, Merali, and Singhal 1977; Wong and Klaassen 1982), lead (Petit and Alfano 1979), triethyltin (Reiter et al. 1981), and trimethyltin (Ruppert, Dean, and Reiter 1983b). Hippocampal weight was preferentially decreased by inorganic lead (Petit and Alfano 1979) and the organotins (Ruppert, Dean, and Reiter 1983a, 1983b), indicating selective toxicity. Many studies have evaluated behaviors related to neural function in the hippocampus, cerebellum, and olfactory system owing to the extensive postnatal development in these brain areas.

Cadmium

Cadmium (Cd), which produces limited CNS toxicity in adults (Arvidson 1981), is neurotoxic to developing animals, producing gross structural damage to the brain following postnatal exposure (Gabbiani, Baic, and Deziel 1967; Webster and Valois 1981; Wong and Klaassen 1982). Age-related changes have been observed during postnatal life in the profile of neuropathology in both rats (Gabbiani, Baic, and Deziel 1967) and mice (Webster and Valois 1981). Either acute or repeated postnatal exposure produces behavioral toxicity, including alterations in motor activity. Rats exposed to Cd on PND 1–30 were hyperactive in a selective activity meter 24 hours after the last dose (Rastogi, Merali, and Singhal 1977); rats exposed to Cd on PND 6–15 were hyperactive in tilt cages on PND 45–46 (Smith, Pihl, and Garber 1982);

and rats exposed to Cd on PND 4 were hyperactive in figure-eight mazes on PND 23 (Wong and Klaassen 1982). However, mice injected on either PND 1 or PND 8 were hypoactive at 8 weeks in an open field (Webster and Valois 1981). This differential effect of Cd on motor activity could be owing to a difference in species, activity measuring device, age at testing, or age of exposure. In a recent study, the development of locomotor activity (PND 13–21) was assessed in rat pups receiving Cd on PND 5 (Ruppert and Dean 1983). Pups were hypoactive in the initial days of testing but gradually became hyperactive. This biphasic effect on activity may be a characteristic of Cd toxicity that contributes to differences between experiments described above.

Preweaning evaluation of Cd toxicity has recently been reported for pups injected on PND 1 (Newland et al. 1983). Fewer Cd-exposed pups suckled from an anesthetized dam (PND 2) or showed a preference for home bedding (PND 7). For pups injected with Cd on PND 6 (Infurna et al. 1982), homing behavior was altered (PND 7), and deficits in passive-avoidance retention were seen in adults. These acute effects of Cd on behaviors such as suckling and homing, which are regulated by olfactory cues, may be predictive of later behavioral effects of Cd exposure; Smith, Pihl, and Garber (1982) hypothesized that Cd-induced anosmia could account for altered behavior in learning tests.

Inorganic Lead and Triethyl Lead

Effects of inorganic lead exposure on the development of the nervous system in both humans and several animal models have been extensively studied and reviewed (e.g., Bornschein, Pearson, and Reiter 1980a, 1980b). A recent synthesis is that behavioral effects of postnatal lead exposure reflect disruption of hippocampal development (Alfano and Petit 1981; Petit, Alfano, and LeBoutillier 1983). In table 8.2 behavioral deficits seen in lead-exposed rats are compared with deficits produced by hippocampal lesions. The value of this conceptualization is the neural framework that it provides for further research. However, delays in the development of motor activity and deficits in performance of a preweaning learning task have been reported that correspond to delays in metabolic development of the cerebral cortex (Bull et al. 1983), emphasizing that lead toxicity is not restricted to the hippocampus.

Although the majority of studies describing lead toxicity are based on long-term exposures intended to mimic chronic exposure in children, a few studies have compared the effects of acute and chronic exposure. For example, lithium-induced polydipsia was augmented following chronic lead exposure from PND 3 through PND 30 (Mailman et al. 1978). Control animals increased their fluid intake in response to an injection of lithium, and this polydipsic response was augmented in lead-exposed rats. This facilitation has been attributed to an alteration of central catecholaminergic functioning (ibid.) or to damage within the septal area or hippocampus (Dantzer 1980). To determine the critical age for this effect, Mailman, DeHaven, and Krigman (1982) intubated rat pups with lead acetate at different times during the preweaning period. A single dosage of 200 mg/kg on either PND 5 or PND 15 produced an increase in lithium-induced polydipsia similar to that produced by daily dosing from PND 3 to PND 30. Thus, acute exposure to inorganic lead can be toxic during development.

Triethyl lead (TEL) can also be neurotoxic following a single postnatal ex-

Table 8.2 A comparison of the effects of hippocampal dysfunction and postnatal lead exposure in several testing situations

Behavior Class	Hippocampal Damage	Postnatal Lead Exposure	Similar
Avoidance behavior			
Passive avoidance	Impaired	Impaired	✓
1-way active avoidance	Impaired	Impaired	✓
2-way active avoidance	Facilitation	Not clear	
Schedule-controlled behavior			
CRF	No effect	No effect	✓
DRL	Impaired	Impaired	✓
Extinction	Impaired	Impaired	✓
Maze learning			
Hebb-Williams maze	Impaired	No effect	
Eight-arm spatial maze	Impaired	Impaired	✓
Spontaneous alternation	Impaired	Impaired	✓
Visual discrimination			
T-maze	Impaired	Impaired	✓
Y maze	Impaired	Impaired	✓
Operant chamber	Impaired	Impaired	✓
Reversal	Impaired	Impaired	✓
Locomotor behavior			
Open field	Increased	Increased	✓
Running wheel	No effect	No effect	✓
Small cage	No effect	Not clear	

Source: Petit, Alfano, and LeBoutillier 1983. Reprinted by permission of the publisher.

posure. Booze et al. (1983*b*) assessed preweaning and juvenile behavior in rat pups exposed to TEL on PND 5. Preweaning testing indicated impaired olfactory discrimination (PND 7), fewer pups attaching to a nipple (PND 9), and the presence of tremor (PND 10). Juvenile testing (PND 20–29) indicated a decreased number of responses to a startle stimulus, hypoactivity in male pups, and alterations in affective behavior on passive-avoidance retention trials. Long-term evaluation of TEL-exposed pups revealed hyperactivity on several behavioral tests and cell loss in area CA3 of the hippocampus (Booze et al. 1983*a*), indicating that postnatal exposure to TEL, like postnatal exposure to inorganic lead, produces hippocampal dysfunction.

Methylmercury

Methylmercury (MM) intoxication in human populations resulting from poisonings in Japan and Iraq indicated that gestational exposure disrupted nervous-system development more severely than lactational exposure. Therefore, the majority of animal studies describing neurobehavioral sequelae of MM poisoning have used prenatal exposure (see Reuhl and Chang 1979).

To differentiate between the effects of gestational and lactational exposure to MM, Spyker and Spyker (1977) injected dams with MM on day 7, 9, or 12 of gestation and then cross-fostered pups to produce exposure: (1) both prenatally and postnatally, (2) prenatally only, (3) postnatally only, and (4) no exposure. Effects of prenatal exposure to MM on pup survival and growth were twice as great as postnatal effects in cross-fostered pups and were greatest late in organogenesis.

This study provides a valuable contribution in explicitly testing for carry-over effects of prenatal exposure that could be owing to persistence of MM, alterations in maternal behavior, and so on; however, it does not address the question of direct effects of postnatal exposure to pups.

Zenick (1974) used a water-escape T-maze to test groups of rats that had received gestational, lactational, or postweaning exposure to MM. Learning deficits were found following gestational exposure (via the maternal water supply) or postweaning exposure (directly to pups). No deficits were found following postnatal exposure via the dams' milk (PND 1–21). A single dose of mercury to pups on PND 15 or 21 also produced no changes in discrimination learning or open-field behavior (Post et al. 1973).

When younger pups were exposed directly to MM by intubation or injection, both the morphological development (Sager, Doherty, and Rodier 1982) and the biochemical development (Taylor and DiStefano 1976; Bartolome et al., Neonatal methylmercury, 1982; Bartolome et al., Organ specificity, 1982) of the nervous system were disrupted. For example, a single injection of 8 mg/kg MM in mice on PND 2 produced neuropathological changes in the cerebellum 24 hours after dosing (Sager, Doherty, and Rodier 1982). Therefore, behavioral effects of postnatal exposure to MM, especially on behaviors sensitive to cerebellar insult, deserve further consideration.

Organotins

Triethyltin (TET) and trimethyltin (TMT) both produce persistent behavioral toxicity when administered to developing animals either on PND 5 or throughout the preweaning period (PND 3–30). Although the behavioral toxicities produced by TET and by TMT in adults are dissimilar (Reiter and Ruppert 1984), there are similarities in the behavioral toxicities produced by these organotins in developing animals. Behavioral consequences of exposure to TET on PND 5 have been most extensively investigated (Harry and Tilson 1981, 1982; Reiter et al. 1981; Ruppert, Dean, and Reiter 1983a; Miller 1984).

Pups exposed to TET on PND 5 demonstrated motor incoordination, hypoactivity, and a learning deficit in the preweaning period. The ability of pups to descend a rope suspended above the home cage was impaired in pups exposed to TET (Reiter et al. 1981). This deficit in motor coordination may represent cerebellar dysfunction, since cerebellar weight was decreased following TET exposure and postnatal X-irradiation of the cerebellum also produces deficits in rope descent (Anderson and Altman 1972). Motor activity was decreased in two preweaning tests: homing orientation and residential activity in a figure-eight maze (Reiter et al. 1981). Both tests provide olfactory and other sensory cues from the litter that have been shown to modulate the activity of rat pups; open-field testing of pups in the absence of these cues did not detect differences in activity. Miller (1984) reported decreased activity in TET-exposed pups tested over home-cage bedding, but not in the absence of bedding. Therefore, this developmental hypoactivity may reflect hypoarousal to olfactory cues. TET-exposed pups required more trials to acquire an alleyway task in which access to home-cage litter and littermates was the reinforcer (ibid.), which also suggests an altered response to olfactory and other cues from the nest.

Postweaning evaluation of animals exposed to TET on PND 5 demonstrated that behavioral deficits were persistent. Hyperactivity (Harry and Tilson 1981; Reiter et al. 1981; Ruppert, Dean, and Reiter 1983*a*) and decreased startle responsiveness (Harry and Tilson 1981; Ruppert, Dean, and Reiter 1983*a*) were found in TET-exposed animals tested as adults; in figure-eight mazes hyperactivity persisted beyond 200 days of age (Reiter et al. 1981). Harry and Tilson (1982) have shown that stereotypy induced by apomorphine was altered in animals exposed to TET on PND 5, suggesting a persistent functional change in dopaminergic transmission in these animals as adults. Unlike the effects of adult exposure to TET, developmental exposure did not produce neuromuscular impairment in preweaning tests (Reiter et al. 1981) or in grip strength and negative geotaxis tested on PND 21, 28, 60, or 90 (Harry and Tilson 1981).

Since TET is neurotoxic when injected on PND 5, the toxicity of a single exposure to TET was compared at several ages during the brain growth spurt in early postnatal life (Ruppert, Dean, and Reiter 1984). Impaired ability to descend a rope, adult hyperactivity, and decreased brain weight resulted from TET exposure on PND 5 but not from exposure on PND 1, 10, or 15. Figure 8.2 illustrates motor

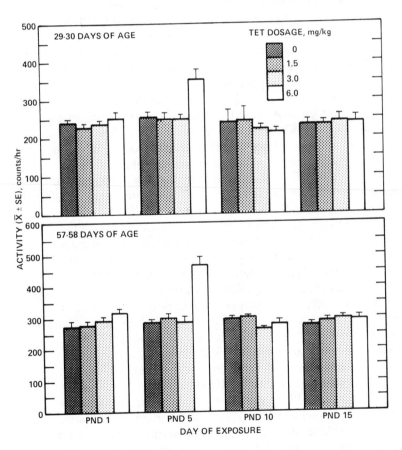

Fig. 8.2 Figure-eight maze activity for control and TET-exposed rats. Data are expressed as photocell interruptions ($\bar{X}$ + SE) during a one-hour test session. Exposure to 6 mg/kg TET on PND 5 produced an increase in motor activity at both times of testing.
(*Source:* Ruppert, Dean, and Reiter 1984. Reprinted by permission of the publisher.)

activity in figure-eight mazes as a function of age at exposure and age at testing. These data demonstrate a differential sensitivity to TET during early postnatal life, with maximum susceptibility on PND 5. TET did produce acute toxicity at other exposure ages, as indicated by reduced preweaning growth, and persistent toxicity, as indicated by deficits in mating behavior in adult males.

TMT is a structurally related trialkyltin compound that is also neurotoxic in adults. Rupport, Dean, and Reiter (1983*b*) evaluated the neurobehavioral toxicity of TMT following exposure on PND 5 and compared these findings with the behavioral toxicity of TET following exposure on PND 5. Impariment of pups' ability to descend a rope, decreased startle response, and adult hyperactivity were found. Acquisition deficits in a preweaning learning task and changes in locomotor activity in the presence of home-cage bedding (Miller and O'Callaghan 1983) were also similar to those produced by TET on PND 5. However, qualitative differences distinguish the developmental toxicity of these organotins; for example, the spatial distribution of motor activity in figure-eight mazes was altered by TET but not by TMT.

In a chronic dosing model, neuropathological changes produced by TET and TMT were different (Mushak, Krigman, and Mailman 1982), yet both organotins produced similar signs of poisoning: tremors and convulsions. Performance on a radial arm maze of animals exposed to TET or TMT on PND 3–29 did not differ; neither TET nor TMT impaired accuracy once the task was acquired (Miller et al. 1982). This is surprising because hippocampal pathology following exposure to TMT on PND 3–29 is similar to morphological changes in the adult (Bouldin et al. 1981), and accuracy of performance was decreased following adult exposure to TMT (Walsh, Miller, and Dyer 1982). The radial arm maze, which requires the use of spatial memory (Olton and Samuelson 1976), provides some interesting comparisons between the developmental toxicities of heavy metals.

Like chronic exposure to TET and TMT, postnatal exposure to inorganic lead increased the number of days required to reach criterion without decreasing the number of correct choices once the task was acquired (Alfano and Petit 1981). However, exposure to either TET (Miller 1984) or TMT (Miller and O'Callaghan 1983) on PND 5 did decrease accuracy of performance in a radial arm maze. All the above metals disrupt hippocampal development, and lesions of the hippocampus reduce accuracy on this task (Olton, Becker, and Handelmann 1979). These divergent results underscore the difficulty in defining relationships between damage to specific brain regions and behavioral changes. The hippocampus is not a homogeneous structure; for example, selective lesions of either the CA1 or the CA3–4 pyramidal cell fields have different behavioral effects (Jarrard 1976). Therefore, differential accuracy of performance may be owing to subtle differences in hippocampal pathology between metals and between dosing models or, alternatively, to disruption in other brain regions (see Miller 1984).

Noland, Taylor, and Bull (1982) used preweaning learning tasks to assess organotin toxicity in rat pups whose dams received either vehicle, monomethyltin (MMT), or TMT in the drinking water 14 days before mating through weaning. In this dosing model, unlike in other models for assessing organotin toxicity, exposure began prior to conception and continued through lactation; therefore, pups were tested during exposure. Pups from dams receiving organotins in the drinking water required more trials both to acquire and to extinguish responding in an

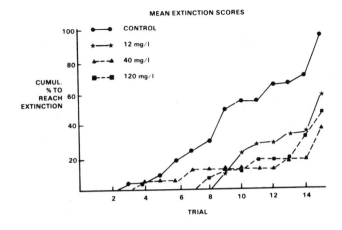

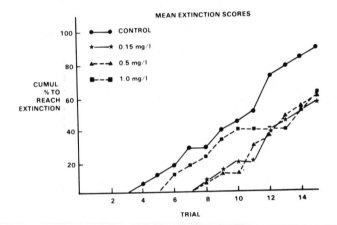

Fig. 8.3 Extinction scores for mono-methyltin- (*top panel*) and tri-methyltin- (*bottom panel*) exposed groups. Each panel shows the cumulative percentage of animals reaching extinction and plotted against trials.
(*Source:* Noland, Taylor, and Bull 1982. Reprinted by permission of the publisher.)

appetitive learning task. Responding during extinction persisted in pups receiving all dosages of both MMT and TMT, and many animals did not reach extinction within the 15-trial criterion (see fig. 8.3). Although the toxicity of monomethyltin compounds is considered to be low (LD50 = 1,370 mg/kg), Noland, Taylor, and Bull calculated that the total dosage of Sn received by the dams at the lowest dose of MMT was 104.1 mg/kg. Thus, the potential toxicity of monoalkyltins during development may be greater than for adults.

Summary

This review has focused on assessment of neurobehavioral function following exposure to toxicants during the early postnatal period in rodents. It was argued—and data were presented for heavy metals—that postnatal exposures can be useful for assessing developmental neurotoxicity. Developmental toxicity can be more persistent than adult toxicity, as shown by triethyltin, and metals that are not overtly neurotoxic in adults, such as cadmium and monomethyltin, can be toxic during development. Given these data, animal models of exposure to potential neurotoxicants during later stages of brain development warrant further emphasis.

Acknowledgments

The viewpoint presented in this chapter was shaped by my graduate training in behavioral endocrinology with Dr. Lynwood Clemens and by my subsequent collaboration in behavioral toxicology with Dr. Lawrence Reiter. I thank Ginger Boncek, Lee Bynum, Janice Israel, and Jerry Tolson for their perseverance in organizing my reprint files. This paper has been reviewed by the Health Effects Research Laboratory, U.S. Environmental Protection Agency, and approved for publication. Mention of trade names or commercial products does not constitute endorsement or recommendation for use.

References

Adams, J., and Buelke-Sam, J. 1981. Behavioral assessment of the postnatal animal: Testing and methods development. In *Developmental toxicology,* edited by C. A. Kimmel and J. Buelke-Sam, 233–58. New York: Raven Press.

Alfano, D. P., and Petit, T. L. 1981. Behavioral effects of postnatal lead exposure: Possible relationship to hippocampal dysfunction. *Behav. Neural Biol.* 32:319–33.

Allen, E. 1912. The cessation of mitosis in the central nervous system of the albino rat. *J. Comp. Neurol.* 22:547–68.

Altman, J. 1970. Postnatal neurogenesis and the problem of neural plasticity. In *Developmental neurobiology,* edited by W. A. Himwich, 197–237. Springfield, Ill.: Charles C Thomas.

Altman, J.; Brunner, R. L.; and Bayer, S. A. 1973. The hippocampus and behavioral maturation. *Behav. Biol.* 8:557–96.

Anderson, W. J., and Altman, J. A. 1972. Retardation of cerebellar and motor development in rats by focal X-irradiation beginning at four days. *Physiol. Behav.* 8:57–67.

Arvidson, B. 1981. Is cadmium toxic to the nervous system? *Trends NeuroSci.* 4:xi–xiii.

Balazs, T. 1981. The delayed long-term effects of chemicals following neonatal exposure in laboratory animals. *Food Cosmet. Toxicol.* 19:533–37.

Barlow, S. M. 1982. Drugs in pregnancy: Effects on post-natal development and behavior. *Trends Pharmacol. Sci.* 3:254–56.

Bartolome, J.; Chait, E. A.; Trepanier, P.; Whitmore, W. L.; Weigel, S.; and Slotkin, T. A. 1982. Organ specificity of neonatal methyl mercury hydroxide poisoning in the rat: Effects on ornithine decarboxylase activity in developing tissues. *Toxicol. Lett.* 13:267–76.

Bartolome, J.; Trepanier, P.; Chait, E. A.; Seidler, F. J.; Deskin, R.; and Slotkin, T. A. 1982. Neonatal methylmercury poisoning in the rat: Effects on development of central catecholamine neurotransmitter systems. *Toxicol. Appl. Pharmacol.* 65:92–99.

Bayer, S. A.; Brunner, R. L.; Hine, R.; and Altman, J. 1973. Behavioral effects of interference with the postnatal acquisition of hippocampal granule cells. *Nature* 242:222–24.

Bayer, S. A.; Yackel, J. W.; and Puri, P. S. 1982. Neurons in the rat dentate gyrus granular layer substantially increase during juvenile and adult life. *Science* 216:890–92.

Beatty, W. W. 1979. Gonadal hormones and sex differences in nonreproductive behaviors in rodents: Organizational and activational influences. *Horm. Behav.* 12:112–63.

Beatty, W. W., and Costello, K. B. 1983. Medial hypothalamic lesions and play fighting in juvenile rats. *Physiol. Behav.* 31:141–45.

Beatty, W. W.; Dodge, A. M.; Dodge, L. J.; White, K.; and Panksepp, J. 1982. Psychomotor stimulants, social deprivation and play in juvenile rats. *Pharmacol. Biochem. Behav.* 16:417–22.

Booze, R. M.; Mactutus, C. F.; Annau, Z.; and Tilson, H. A. 1983a. Increased behavioral reactivity in adult rats following neonatal triethyl lead administration. *Soc. Neurosci. Abs.* 9:1245.

————. 1983*b*. Neonatal triethyl lead neurotoxicity in rat pups: Initial behavioral observations and quantification. *Neurobehav. Toxicol. Teratol.* 5:367–75.

Booze, R. M.; Tilson, H. A.; Annau, Z.; Mitchell, C. L.; and Mactutus, C. F. 1983. Experimental design comparisons in acute neonatal triethyl lead toxicity. *Teratology* 27:32A.

Bornschein, R.; Pearson, D.; and Reiter, L. W. 1980*a*. Behavioral effects of moderate lead exposure in children and animal models: Part 1, clinical studies. *CRC Crit. Rev. Toxicol.* 8:43–99.

————. 1980*b*. Behavioral effects of moderate lead exposure in children and animal models: Part 2, animal studies. *CRC Crit. Rev. Toxicol.* 8:101–52.

Bouldin, T. W.; Goines, N. D.; Bagnell, C. R.; and Krigman, M. R. 1981. Pathogenesis of trimethyltin neuronal toxicity: Ultrastructural and cytochemical observations. *Am. J. Pathol.* 104:237–49.

Brunjes, P. C., and Alberts, J. R. 1981. Early auditory and visual function in normal and hyperthyroid rats. *Behav. Neural Biol.* 31:393–412.

Buelke-Sam, J., and Kimmel, C. A. 1979. Development and standardization of screening methods for behavioral teratology. *Teratology* 20:17–30.

Bull, R. J.; McCauley, P. T.; Taylor, D. H.; and Crofton, K. M. 1983. The effects of lead on the developing central nervous system of the rat. *Neurotoxicology* 4:1–18.

Butcher, R. E. 1976. Behavioral testing as a method for assessing risk. *Environ. Health Perspect.* 18:75–78.

Campbell, B. A.; Lytle, L. D.; and Fibiger, H. C. 1969. Onotogeny of adrenergic arousal and cholinergic inhibitory mechanisms in the rat. *Science* 166:635–37.

Caza, P. A., and Spear, L. P. 1982. Pharmacological manipulation of milk-induced behaviors in three-day-old rat pups. *Pharmacol. Biochem. Behav.* 16:481–86.

Cowan, W. M. 1979. The development of the brain. *Sci. Am.* 241:112–33.

Crain, B.; Cotman, C.; Taylor, D.; and Lynch, G. 1973. A quantitative electron microscopic study of synaptogenesis in the dentate gyrus of the rat. *Brain Res.* 63:195–204.

Dantzer, R. 1980. Effects of postnatal lead exposure on lithium induced polydipsia and glucoprivic feeding in rats. *Neurobehav. Toxicol.* 2:373–77.

Davenport, J. W., and Dorcey, T. P. 1972. Hypothyroidism: Learning deficit induced in rats by early exposure to thiouracil. *Horm. Behav.* 3:97–112.

Davenport, J. W., and Gonzalez, L. M. 1973. Neonatal thyroxine stimulation in rats: Accelerated behavioral maturation and subsequent learning deficit. *J. Comp. Physiol. Psychol.* 85:397–408.

Davison, A. N., and Dobbing, J. 1966. Myelination as a vulnerable period in brain development. *Br. Med. Bull.* 22:40–44.

Diaz, J. 1983. Disruption of the brain growth spurt in adolescent rats by chronic phenobarbital administration. *Exp. Neurol.* 79:559–63.

Dobbing, J., and Sands, J. 1979. Comparative aspects of the brain growth spurt. *Early Hum. Dev.* 3:79–83.

Donaldson, H. H. 1908. A comparison of the albino rat with man in respect to the growth of the brain and the spinal cord. *J. Comp. Neurol.* 18:345–92.

Eayrs, J. T. 1964. Effect of neonatal hyperthyroidism on maturation and learning in the rat. *Anim. Behav.* 12:195–99.

Eayrs, J. T., and Levine, S. 1963. Influence of thyroidectomy and subsequent replacement therapy upon conditioned avoidance learning in the rat. *J. Endocrinol.* 25:505–13.

Eayrs, J. T., and Lishman, W. A. 1953. The maturation of behavior in hypothyroidism and starvation. *Brit. J. Anim. Behav.* 3:17–24.

Eliasson, M., and Meyerson, B. J. 1975. Sexual preference in female rats during estrous cycle, pregnancy and lactation. *Physiol. Behav.* 14:705–10.

————. 1981. Development of sociosexual approach behavior in male laboratory rats. *J. Comp. Physiol. Psychol.* 95:160–65.

Fisherman, R. H. B., and Yanai, J. 1983. Long-lasting effects of early barbiturates on central nervous system and behavior. *Neurosci. Biobehav. Rev.* 7:19–28.

Ford, D. H. 1973. Selected maturational changes observed in the postnatal rat brain. *Prog. Brain Res.* 40:1–12.

Gabbiani, G.; Baic, D.; and Deziel, C. 1967. Toxicity of cadmium for the central nervous system. *Exp. Neurol.* 18:154–60.

Gazzara, R. A., and Altman, J. 1981. Early postnatal X-irradiation of the hippocampus and discrimination learning in adult rats, *J. Comp. Physiol. Psychol.* 95:484–95.

Gellert, R. J. 1978. Kepone, mirex, dieldrin and aldrin: Estrogenic activity and the induction of persistent vaginal estrus and anovulation in rats following neonatal treatment. *Environ. Res.* 16:131–38.

Goldenring, J. R.; Shaywitz, B. A.; Wool, R. S.; Batter, D. K.; Anderson, G. M.; and Cohen, D. J. 1982. Environmental and biologic interactions on behavior: Effects of artificial rearing in rat pups treated with 6-hydroxydopamine. *Dev. Psychobiol.* 15:297–307.

Gorski, R. A. 1968. Influence of age on the response to paranatal administration of a low dose of androgen. *Endocrinology* 82:1001–4.

Gorski, R. A.; Harlan, R. E.; and Christensen, L. W. 1977. Perinatal hormonal exposure and the development of neuroendocrine regulatory processes. *J. Toxicol. Environ. Health* 3:97–121.

Goy, R. W., and McEwen, B. S. 1980. *Sexual differentiation of the brain.* Cambridge: MIT Press.

Grady, K. L.; Phoenix, C. H.; and Young, W. C. 1965. Role of the developing rat testis in differentiation of the neural tissues mediating mating behavior. *J. Comp. Physiol. Psychol.* 59:176–82.

Grant, L. D. 1976. Research strategies for behavioral teratology studies. *Environ. Health Perspect.* 18:85–94.

Harry, G. J., and Tilson, H. A. 1981. The effects of postpartum exposure to triethyl tin on the neurobehavioral functioning of rats. *Neurotoxicology* 2:283–96.

———. 1982. Postpartum exposure to triethyl tin produces long-term alterations in responsiveness to apomorphine. *Neurotoxicology* 3:64–71.

Hicks, S. P., and D'Amato, C. J. 1978. Effects of ionizing radiation on developing brain and behavior. In *Studies on the development of behavior and the nervous system,* vol. 4, *Early influences,* edited by G. Gottlieb, 35–72. New York: Academic Press.

Hutchings, D. E. 1978. Behavioral teratology: Embryopathic and behavioral effects of drugs during pregnancy. In *Studies on the development of behavior and the nervous system,* vol. 4, 7–34. *See* Hicks and D'Amato 1978.

Infurna, R. N.; Stanton, M.; Baggs, R. B.; and Miller, R. K. 1982. Neonatal exposures to cadmium: Behavioral toxicity. *Teratology* 26:48A.

Jacobson, M. 1978. *Developmental neurobiology.* New York: Plenum Press.

Jarrard, L. E. 1976. Anatomical and behavioral analysis of hippocampal cell fields in rats. *J. Comp. Physiol. Psychol.* 90:1035–50.

Kessler, P., and Spear, N. E. 1980. Neonatal thyroxine treatment enhances classical conditioning in the infant rat. *Horm. Behav.* 14:204–10.

Kolata, G. B. 1978. Behavioral teratology: Birth defects of the mind. *Science* 202:732–34.

Lai, H.; Quock, R. M.; Makous, W.; Horita, A.; and Jen, L. S. 1978. Methylazoxymethanol acetate: Effect of postnatal injection on brain amines and behavior. *Pharmacol. Biochem. Behav.* 8:251–57.

Larsson, K., and Hard, E. 1982. Some aspects on behavioral teratology research. *Scand. J. Psychol.* [Supp.] 1:97–103.

Lauder, J. M. 1983. Hormonal and humoral influences on brain development. *Psychoneuroendocrinology* 8:121–55.

Lynch, A.; Dobbing, J.; Adlard, B. P. F.; and Smart, J. L. 1976. Effects of early postnatal X-irradiation on the cerebellum correlated with adult motor performance in rats. *Biol. Neonate* 28:140–52.

MacLusky, N. J., and Naftolin, F. 1981. Sexual differentiation of the central nervous system. *Science* 211:1294–1302.

Mailman, R. B.; DeHaven, D. L.; and Krigman, M. R. 1982. Effects of lead administration on postnatal day 5 or day 15 of life on lithium-induced polydipsia, striatal 3H-spiperone binding and dopamine metabolism in adult rats. *Soc. Neurosci. Abs.* 8:81.

Mailman, R. B.; Krigman, M. R.; Mueller, R. A.; Mushak, P.; and Breese, G. R. 1978. Lead exposure during infancy permanently increases lithium-induced polydipsia. *Science* 201:637–39.

Meaney, M. J.; Dodge, A. M.; and Beatty, W. W. 1981. Sex-dependent effects of amygdaloid lesions on the social play of prepubertal rats. *Physiol. Behav.* 26:467–72.

Meaney, M. J., and Stewart, J. 1981. Neonatal androgens influence the social play of prepubescent rats. *Horm. Behav.* 15:197–213.

Miller, D. B. 1984. Pre- and postweaning indices of neurotoxicity in rats: Effects of triethyltin (TET). *Toxicol. Appl. Pharmacol.* 72:557–65.

Miller, D. B.; Eckerman, D. A.; Krigman, M. R.; and Grant, L. D. 1982. Chronic neonatal organotin exposure alters radial-arm maze performance in adult rats. *Neurobehav. Toxicol.* 4:185–90.

Miller, D. B., and O'Callaghan, J. P. 1983. Behavioral and nervous-system specific protein changes associated with early postnatal exposure to trimethyltin (TMT). *Soc. Neurosci. Abs.* 9:266.

Murphy, J. M., and Nagy, Z. M. 1976*a*. Neonatal thyroxine stimulation accelerates the maturation of both locomotor and memory processes in mice. *J. Comp. Physiol. Psychol.* 90:1082–91.

———. 1976*b*. Neonatal hyperthyroidism alters the development of behavioral arousal and inhibition in the mouse. *Bull. Psychon. Soc.* 8:121–23.

Mushak, P.; Krigman, M. R.; and Mailman, R. B. 1982. Comparative organotin toxicity in the developing rat: Somatic and morphological changes and relationship to accumulation of total tin. *Neurobehav. Toxicol.* 4:209–15.

Newland, M. C.; Ng, W. W.; Baggs, R. B.; Miller, R. K.; Infurna, R. N.; and Gentry, G. D. 1983. Acute behavioral toxicity of cadmium in neonatal rats. *Teratology* 27:65A–66A.

Noland, E. A.; Taylor, D. H.; and Bull, R. J. 1982. Monomethyl and trimethyl tin compounds induce learning deficiencies in young rats. *Neurobehav. Toxicol. Teratol.* 4:539–44.

Norton, S.; Culver, B.; and Mullenix, P. 1975. Development of nocturnal behavior in albino rats. *Behav. Biol.* 15:317–31.

Norton, W. T., and Poduslo, S. E. 1973. Myelination in rat brain: Changes in myelin composition during brain maturation. *J. Neurochem.* 21:759–73.

Olioff, M., and Stewart, J. 1978. Sex differences in the play behavior of prepubescent rats. *Physiol. Behav.* 20:113–15.

Olney, J. W. 1980. Excitatory neurotoxins as food additives: An evaluation of risk. *Neurotoxicology* 2:163–92.

Olton, D. S.; Becker, J. T.; and Handelmann, G. E. 1979. Hippocampus, space and memory. *Behav. Brain Sci.* 2:313–65.

Olton, D. S., and Samuelson, R. J. 1976. Remembrance of places passed: Spatial memory in rats. *J. Exp. Psychol.: Anim. Behav. Proc.* 2:97–116.

Panksepp, J. 1981. The ontogeny of play in rats. *Dev. Psychobiol.* 14:327–32.

Parisi, T., and Ison, J. R. 1979. Development of the acoustic startle response in the rat: Ontogenetic changes in the magnitude of inhibition by prepulse stimulation. *Dev. Psychobiol.* 12:219–30.

Pearson, D. E.; Teicher, M. H.; Shaywitz, B. A.; Cohen, D. J.; Young, J. G.; and Anderson,

G. M. 1980. Environmental influences on body weight and behavior in developing rats after neonatal 6-hydroxydopamine. *Science* 209:715–17.

Pellegrino, L. J., and Altman, J. 1979. Effects of differential interference with postnatal cerebellar neurogenesis on motor performance, activity level, and maze learning of rats: A developmental study. *J. Comp. Physiol. Psychol.* 93:1–33.

Peters, P. J., and Brunner, R. L. 1976. Increased running wheel activity and dyadic behavior of rats with hippocampal granule cell deficits. *Behav. Biol.* 16:91–97.

Petit, T. L., and Alfano, D. P. 1979. Differential experience following developmental lead exposure: Effects on brain and behavior. *Pharmacol. Biochem. Behav.* 11:165–71.

Petit, T. L.; Alfano, D. P.; and LeBoutillier, J. C. 1983. Early lead exposure and the hippocampus: A review and recent advances. *Neurotoxicology* 4:79–94.

Post, E. M.; Yang, M. G.; King, J. A.; and Sanger, V. L. 1973. Behavioral changes of young rats force-fed methyl mercury chloride. *Proc. Soc. Exp. Biol. Med.* 143:1113–16.

Raisman, G., and Field, P. M. 1973. Sexual dimorphism in the neuropil of the preoptic area of the rat and its dependence on neonatal androgen. *Brain Res.* 54:1–29.

Rastogi, R. B.; Merali, Z.; and Singhal, R. L. 1977. Cadmium alters behavior and the biosynthetic capacity for catecholamines and serotonin in neonatal rat brain. *J. Neurochem.* 28:789–94.

Reinisch, J. M., and Sanders, S. A. 1982. Early barbiturate exposure: The brain, sexually dimorphic behavior and learning. *Neurosci. Biobehav. Rev.* 6:311–19.

Reiter, L. W.; Heavner, G. G.; Dean, K. F.; and Ruppert, P. H. 1981. Developmental and behavioral effects of early postnatal exposure to triethyltin in rats. *Neurobehav. Toxicol. Teratol.* 3:285–93.

Reiter, L. W., and Ruppert, P. H. 1984. Behavioral toxicity of trialkyltin compounds: A review. *Neurotoxicology* 5:177–86.

Reuhl, K. R., and Chang, L. W. 1979. Effects of methylmercury on the development of the nervous system: A review. *Neurotoxicology* 1:21–55.

Rodier, P. M. 1978. Behavioral teratology. In *Handbook of teratology*, vol. 4, edited by J. G. Wilson and F. C. Fraser, 397–428. New York: Plenum Press.

———. 1980. Chronology of neuron development: Animal studies and their clinical implications. *Dev. Med. Child Neurol.* 22:525–45.

Ruppert, P. H., and Dean, K. F. 1983. Development of locomotor activity in rat pups is altered by postnatal exposure to cadmium. *Soc. Neurosci. Abs.* 9:668.

Ruppert, P. H.; Dean, K. F.; and Reiter, L. W. 1983a. Comparative developmental toxicity of triethyltin using split-litter and whole-litter dosing. *J. Toxicol. Environ. Health* 12:73–87.

———. 1983b. Developmental and behavioral toxicity following acute postnatal exposure of rat pups to trimethyltin. *Neurobehav. Toxicol. Teratol.* 5:421–29.

———. 1984. Neurobehavioral toxicity of triethyltin in rats as a function of age at postnatal exposure. *Neurotoxicology* 5:9–22.

Sachs, B. D., and Barfield, R. J. 1976. Functional analysis of masculine copulatory behavior in the rat. In *Advances in the study of behavior*, vol. 7, edited by J. S. Rosenblatt, R. A. Hinde, E. Shaw, and C. Beer, 91–154. New York: Academic Press.

Sager, P. R.; Doherty, R. A.; and Rodier, P. M. 1982. Effects of methylmercury on developing mouse cerebellar cortex. *Exp. Neurol.* 77:179–93.

Schalock, R. L.; Brown, W. J.; and Smith, R. L. 1979. Long-term effects of propylthiouracil-induced neonatal hypothyroidism. *Dev. Psychobiol.* 12:187–99.

Schapiro, S. 1968. Some physiological, biochemical, and behavioral consequences of neonatal hormone administration: Cortisol and thyroxine. *Gen. Comp. Endocr.* 10:214–228.

Schapiro, S.; Salas, M.; and Vukovich, K. 1970. Hormonal effects on ontogeny of swimming ability in the rat: Assessment of central nervous system development. *Science* 168:147–50.

Schlessinger, A. R.; Cowan, W. M.; and Gottlieb, D. I. 1975. An autoradiographic study of the time of origin and the pattern of granule cell migration in the dentate gyrus of the rat. *J. Comp. Neurol.* 159:149–76.

Schmidt, E. H. F., and Hildebrandt, A. G., eds. 1983. *Health evaluation of heavy metals in infant formula and junior food.* Berlin: Springer-Verlag.

Sjoden, P.-L., and Soderberg, U. 1976. Effects of neonatal thyroid hormone stimulation and differential preweaning rearing on open-field behavior in adult rats. *Dev. Psychobiol.* 9:413–24.

Smith, M. J.; Pihl, R. O.; and Garber, B. 1982. Postnatal cadmium exposure and longterm behavioral changes in the rat. *Neurobehav. Toxicol. Teratol.* 4:283–87.

Spear, L. P., and Brake, S. C. 1983. Periadolescence: Age-dependent behavior and psychopharmacological responsivity in rats. *Dev. Psychobiol.* 16:83–109.

Spear, L. P., and Ristine, L. A. 1982. Suckling behavior in neonatal rats: Psychopharmacological investigations. *J. Comp. Physiol. Psychol.* 96:244–55.

Spear, N. E., and Campbell, B. A., eds. 1978. *Ontogeny of learning and memory.* Hillsdale, N.J.: Lawrence Erlbaum Associates.

Spyker, D. A., and Spyker, J. M. 1977. Response model analysis for cross-fostering studies: Prenatal versus postnatal effects on offspring exposed to methylmercury dicyandiamide. *Toxicol. Appl. Pharmacol.* 40:511–27.

Spyker, J. M. 1975. Assessing the impact of low level chemicals on development: Behavioral and latent effects. *Fed. Proc.* 34:1835–44.

Stone, J. M., and Greenough, W. T. 1975. Excess neonatal thyroxine: Effects on learning in infant and adolescent rats. *Dev. Psychobiol.* 8:479–88.

Strupp, B. J., and Levitsky, D. A. 1983. Early brain insult and cognition: A comparison of malnutrition and hypothyroidism. *Dev. Psychobiol.* 16:535–49.

Suzuki, K. 1980. Special vulnerabilities of the developing nervous system to toxic substances. In *Experimental and clinical neurotoxicology,* edited by P. S. Spencer and H. H. Schaumburg, 48–61. Baltimore: Williams & Wilkins.

Taylor, L. L., and DiStefano, V. 1976. Effects of methylmercury on brain biogenic amines in the developing rat pup. *Toxicol. Appl. Pharmacol.* 38:489–97.

Thor, D. H., and Holloway, W. R., Jr. 1983. Play soliciting in juvenile male rats: Effects of caffeine, amphetamine and methylphenidate. *Pharmacol. Biochem. Behav.* 19:725–27.

Vorhees, C. V., and Butcher, R. E. 1982. Behavioral teratogenicity. In *Developmental toxicology,* edited by K. Snell, 247–98. London: Croom Helm Press.

Walsh, T. J.; Miller, D. B.; and Dyer, R. S. 19B2. Trimethyltin, a selective limbic system neurotoxicant, impairs radial-arm maze performance. *Neurobehav. Toxicol. Teratol.* 4:177–83.

Webster, W. S., and Valois, A. A. 1981. The toxic effects of cadmium on the neonatal mouse CNS. *J. Neuropathol. Exp. Neurol.* 40:247–57.

Wong, K.-L., and Klaassen, C. D. 1982. Neurotoxic effects of cadmium in young rats. *Toxicol. Appl. Pharmacol.* 63:330–37.

Zbinden, G. 1981. Experimental methods in behavioral teratology. *Arch. Toxicol.* 48:69–88.

Zenick, H. 1974. Behavioral and biochemical consequences in methylmercury chloride toxicity. *Pharmacol. Biochem. Behav.* 2:709–13.

III

The Determination of Mechanisms of Toxicity

The Interactions of Behavior and Neurophysiology

Comprehensive evaluations of potential neurotoxicants often include neurophysiological studies. Depending upon the methods selected, neurophysiological measures may be used to achieve goals as diverse as detecting neurotoxicity, characterizing neurotoxicity (e.g., which neural systems are involved), and unraveling mechanisms of neurotoxicity. A review of the relevant literature produces the disappointing finding that relatively few of many potentially useful neurophysiological methods have ever been employed in a toxicologic context. The purpose of this chapter is threefold: (1) to review the potential application of neurophysiological methods rarely used in toxicology; (2) to describe neurophysiological methods that have been used most often in toxicology, providing examples of data obtained using these methods; and (3) to identify relevant methodological and interpretational issues.

Conceivably, any of several hundred available neurophysiological methods could be applied to problems of neurotoxicology. To avoid beginning a task that could not be finished, some limits were placed upon the scope of the present chapter. Given the nature of this book, a decision was made to concentrate upon measures that are relevant to vertebrate behavior. Specifically excluded from discussion are studies of isolated systems (cell culture, slice, etc.), invertebrate studies, and studies generally considered to require anesthesia for their successful completion (e.g., intracellular studies). There is no intent to place a value judgment upon excluded methods. Rather, they are better suited for investigation of the mechanisms of toxicity at a more molecular level than that implied by the title of this book. A substantial literature of macroelectrode methods remains from which to choose. The remaining methods provide the interface between behavioral studies and more mechanistically directed neurophysiological studies. Some methods such as kindling (Joy 1985) and recovery processes (Dyer and Boyes 1983b) have been reviewed recently and therefore will not be discussed here.

In an effort to provide organization and understanding to such a complex integrated organ, it is convenient to divide the brain into discrete functional systems. Thus, one may refer to the visual system, the somatosensory system, the hippocampal system, the extrapyramidal system, and so on. While few would argue that these systems are not interrelated, they are almost always treated separately. Most such systems are constructed of neurons with similar membrane and axonal properties but differ with respect to connectivity and may differ with respect to transmitters and metabolic activity. Therefore, it is logical to assume that evaluation of any system provides information concerning general CNS effects as well as effects unique to the system under investigation.

Certain systems appear to be more sensitive to neurotoxicants than others. Often, it is not known whether apparent sensitivity or insensitivity of a system reflects (1) sensitivity of the test method; (2) accessibility of the system to the investigator; (3) accessibility of the system to the toxicant; or (4) relative vulnerability to damage of the system or its constituents. While considerable work must be done to address this issue for each case, the real message is that the careful investigator will give these issues thought before adopting or rejecting a particular test method.

In this chapter certain specific systems and methods have been selected for more detailed consideration as general examples of classes of systems (e.g., the visual system as a general example of sensory systems) and methods (e.g., the use of flash-evoked potentials [FEPs] as a general method for assessing the visual system). For any system or method the following questions should be kept in mind: What can we learn from this general approach, that is, what are the behavioral and neurobiological correlates of alterations in the endpoints? How does one do these experiments most effectively? What have we learned about neurotoxicants from studies that have used this approach? What control factors seem to be particularly important? What are the limitations of the approach? Answers to some of these questions will be found in the text; others must await further study.

Evoked potentials are among the oldest tools available to the neurophysiologist. Simply defined, they are alterations in voltage recorded from a particular brain area that are time-locked to an evoking stimulus. The recordings are presumed to reflect graded postsynaptic potentials integrated over a large population of neurons. Because they are often small relative to ongoing ("spontaneous") electrical activity, they are customarily averaged over a number of trials. The averaging process improves the signal-to-noise ratio by a factor of the square root of the number of trials averaged. Much has been written about evoked potentials, and the reader is referred to some extensive treatments for many of the issues that will not be addressed here (Regan 1972; Rebert 1983; Dyer 1985).

Four different classes of evoked potentials will be considered here: those that evaluate sensory systems, those that evaluate hippocampal systems, those that evaluate interhemispheric function, and those that evaluate electrical correlates of cognition. Each of these classes of evoked potentials evaluates a function that has behavioral correlates and that either has been demonstrated or is presumed to be affected by exposure to neurotoxicants.

Sensory evoked potentials are the most commonly recorded. They may be recorded in classically defined sensory systems following either sensory stimulation or electrical stimulation in part of the system. Sensory evoked potentials may also be recorded from brain areas that are not often considered part of sensory systems (e.g., basal ganglia, cerebellum, hippocampus, etc.). The only sensory-system evoked potentials to be considered here are those elicited by sensory stimulation. Further, the most extensive discussion will be reserved for flash-evoked potentials, since these have been used most extensively in neurophysiological assessments of neurotoxicity.

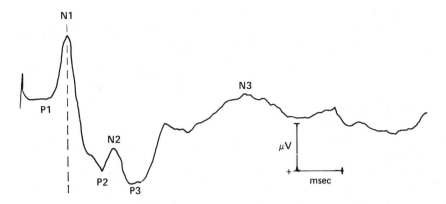

Fig. 9.1 A prototype flash-evoked potential recorded from a Long-Evans hooded rat. The time scale is 30 msec, and the amplitude scale is 100 μV. A 10-μsec flash stimulus occurred at the beginning of the trace.

Flash-evoked Potentials

Flash-evoked potentials are most often elicited by intense but brief (on the order of 10 μsec) flashes of light, usually from a strobe. When recorded from the visual cortex of rats, FEPs take on a characteristic appearance (see fig. 9.1). The primary evoked potential may be defined as comprising 3 positive and 3 negative peaks occurring within about 200 msec of the flash. Under certain conditions, the third negative peak is followed by a series of waves known as the photic afterdischarge (Bigler 1977). FEPs may also be recorded from noncortical structures, including the optic tract, the lateral geniculate nucleus, and the superior colliculus, although such recordings have been less frequently employed in neurotoxicology than those obtained from the visual cortex.

The data obtained from FEP experiments are typically peak latencies, in msec, and either peak-to-peak amplitudes or baseline-to-peak amplitudes, in μvolts. With 3 positive and 3 negative peaks, 6 latencies and 5 peak-to-peak or 6 baseline-to-peak amplitudes may be obtained, or a total of 11–12 variables. Any or all of these variables may change as a function of exposure to a toxicant, and the task is to interpret the meaning of different patterns of change. While few definitive answers are available from FEP studies of the visual cortex, some educated inferences are possible.

Generators of FEP Peaks

Before considering different patterns of change that have been observed, it is important to summarize the current status of our knowledge about the generators of the different peaks of the FEP. Generators may be defined at many different levels. A first and important question concerns whether in fact all of the peaks recorded from electrodes positioned over the visual cortex reflect activity in the visual cortex or whether the potentials are volume-conducted potentials from either subcortical structures or distant cortical structures. This question is best answered by recording FEPs from (a) different cortical loci and (b) different depths (i.e., a laminar analysis) within the cortex. If the recorded potentials are all of local origin, then as the active electrode is lowered through the cortex, the wave-form will either reverse polarity or disappear, depending upon the location and orientation of the generators within the cortex. Furthermore, locally generated potentials will decrease in amplitude as a function of the square of the distance from the source along the cortical surface and, if the source is below the surface, in proportion to the cosine of the angle from the source to the recording point (see Lopes da Silva and Van Rotterdam 1982).

A formal experimental treatment of the reversal of FEPs recorded from an unanesthetized rat visual cortex does not appear in the literature, although several investigators have noted reversal within 1.5 mm from the surface (Ebe, Honma, and Ishiyama 1972; Schwartzbaum, Kreinick, and Levine 1972; Hetzler, personal communication). It is also known that in cats the FEP reverses within the cortex (Creutzfeldt and Kuhnt 1973), and in most reports the assumption that the recorded potentials are of cortical origin is implicit. Furthermore, there is evidence that in the rat, FEPs diminish rapidly with distance from the primary visual areas (Montero 1973). It thus seems likely that FEPs recorded from electrodes located over the rat visual cortex originate in the rat visual cortex.

Knowing that FEPs recorded from the visual cortex originate in the visual cortex is important, but interpretation of alterations in the various components requires further information. The positive and negative waves recorded from the surface could each reflect either excitatory or inhibitory activity, depending upon both the location of the activated cells and the activated portion of them within the cortical layer (Lopes da Silva and Van Rotterdam 1982). In other words, similar wave-forms following widely different patterns of activity could be recorded. Creutzfeldt and Kuhnt (1973) have proposed a cellular model to account for FEPs recorded in the cortex of anesthetized cats, and they provide some correlative data to support the model. However, an adequate test of the model is difficult, since it would require simultaneous intracellular recording from a large number of neurons. Furthermore, identification of the mechanism generating a particular component is of limited value until the connectivity of the responsive cell population is established.

It is possible that the cortically recorded FEP provides a passive reflection of the pattern of input from the lateral geniculate nucleus (LGN). Indeed, some postflash histograms of LGN single-cell activity correlate well with cortically recorded peaks N1 and N3 in the rat FEPs (Bigler 1977). This suggestion is also supported by the work of Verzeano (1973), who suggests that positive and negative FEP waves are correlated with the probability of discharge of different cortical neurons, which in turn could simply reflect patterns of LGN input.

Assuming that cortical waves N1 and N3 of a rat FEP simply reflect the input from the LGN, it is still not certain why the pattern of LGN inputs shows the rhythmicity that it does. Mounting evidence suggests that the pattern of LGN activity is a reflection of recurrent interaction between LGN principal relay neurons and inhibitory interneurons, which may be located within the LGN or in nearby loci, such as the thalamic reticular formation (e.g., Standage, Fleming, and Bigler 1981).

Nor is it certain where cortical wave N2 originates. Several studies in cats have addressed the origins of a secondary cortical response elicited by flash stimulation (e.g., Brazier 1957; and Torres and Warner 1962). Torres and Warner (1962) have described two types of secondary responses. The first type is augmented by pentobarbital anesthesia and brainstem transections at the midcollicular level. The second type is eliminated by pentobarbital anesthesia and intercollicular transections. Since the P2N2P3 complex in rats is eliminated by pentobarbital anesthesia (Hetzler and Oaklay 1981), it seems reasonable to assume that this complex is analogous to the type 2 secondary response of Torres and Warner (1962). Therefore, brainstem or midbrain involvement is implicated as generators of this potential. A major pathway of visual information to the brainstem reticular formation is through the superior colliculus (Burne et al. 1981); thus, it is possible that this component is generated via activity in a collicular-reticular-cortical loop. A further suggestion that this component is derived from collicular activity came from the developmental studies of Rose and Lindsley (1968). In these studies, a portion of the 17-day-old kitten wave-form recorded from the cortex following flashes could be abolished by lesions of the superior colliculus and pretectum. While these data imply an influence of the superior colliculus on this peak, studies by Barnes (1984) demonstrate that massive lesions of the superior colliculus do not abolish the P2N2P3 wave complex in rats. Therefore, the origin of this peak remains elusive.

Interpreting Altered FEPs

While knowing the origin of peaks should assist in determining the locus of dysfunction when peak morphology is disturbed, assessing the nature of the dysfunction requires more information. The physiological significance of an increase or decrease in the latency or amplitude of a particular peak must be understood in order to determine the nature of the dysfunction. Since the same effect may be obtained by different mechanisms, adequate explanation of results in terms of mechanism will always require further experimentation and analysis. While it should also be pointed out that only rarely are such further analyses beyond the capabilities of a resourceful laboratory, each investigator must weigh the importance of such further analyses in the context of their laboratory's effort. In other words, it is often of major interest to simply identify that toxicity exists in a certain system and of secondary interest to know the cellular mechanism. Many applied labs are not afforded the luxury of pursuing secondary interests.

Figure 9.2 illustrates several simple schematic wave-forms which will be used for purposes of discussing toxicant-induced alterations. It must be remembered that even such simple wave-forms represent integrated responses obtained from perhaps millions of postsynaptic potentials. Any process that systematically disrupts the amplitude, duration, or latency of a significant portion of the individual postsynaptic potentials will affect the evoked potential. In the context of an FEB study, we can think of the figure 9.2 wave-form as representing the P1N1P2 complex.

Among the more common findings in FEP studies of neurotoxicity is that peak latencies are increased. A latency increase may or may not be accompanied by an increase or decrease in amplitude. We shall consider each of these cases separately, beginning with the case in which the only observed alteration is an increase in latency of the wave. The most plausible interpretation of such a finding is that the same population of inputs to the visual cortex has been activated as in control conditions but that the onset of activation has been delayed. Other interpretations are possible (e.g., that a different population of inputs has been activated, or the

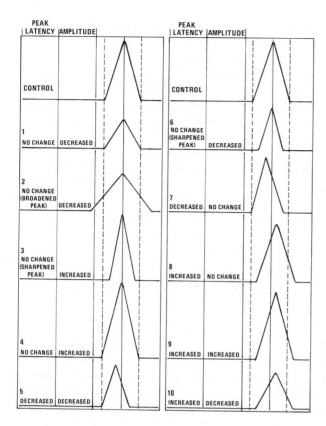

Fig. 9.2 Some possible patterns of evoked potential amplitude and latency changes. The pattern of change in an evoked potential may provide clues to interpretation. This figure shows ten of the possible combinations of amplitude and latency change that can occur in a simple evoked potential as a result of treatment. Not all of these possible changes have been reported in the literature.

durations and magnitudes of some of the inputs have been changed, but the pattern of change is such that it exactly duplicates the control condition in all but latency) but unlikely because of the extraordinary coincidence they require. If the onset and return to baseline of the wave are shifted by the same amount, then a delay in conduction velocity is a most likely explanation. A disruption in myelin such as produced by triethyltin produces such a change (Dyer and Howell 1982*a*).

Another way of evaluating the patterns of change in latency of a wave-form is illustrated in figure 9.3. In this figure the treatment-induced latency change is plotted on the ordinate, and the normal FEP peak latency is plotted on the abscissa. The peaks are separated on the abscissa by a distance corresponding to their normal separation in time from the stimulus. It is evident that the function describing the points for any given treatment can indicate the magnitude of effect, since this is simply a function of distance on the ordinate. This analysis can also describe the extent to which an effect is evenly distributed within the wave. If the function is linear and the slope is 0, then the entire wave has shifted by a constant amount. Constant wave-form shifts are unusual in the literature but have been reported for rats administered daily dosages of 1 mg/kg triethyltin (TET) (Dyer and Howell 1982*a*). The implication of this finding is that the entire effect of treatment occurred at a distant location, probably upon conduction velocity. In the case of TET, it seems most likely that conduction velocity in the optic nerve was affected (Scheinberg et al. 1966). Such an interpretation supports the reports of visual dysfunction in humans exposed to TET (Pruill and Rompel 1970).

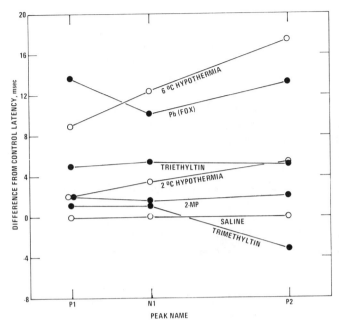

Fig. 9.3 The relationship between treatment and magnitude of latency change in successive flash-evoked potential peaks. Hypothermia (either 2°C or 6°C) produces progressive shifts in latency at successive peaks (Dyer and Boyes 1983a). Triethyltin and 2-methylpyridine (2-MP) produce a shift that is constant at successive peaks (Dyer and Howell 1982a; Dyer et al., in preparation). Trimethyltin and lead (Pb) produce more complex patterns of change in different peak latencies (Fox, Lewkowski, and Cooper 1977; Dyer, Howell, and Wonderlin 1982).

One of the most common patterns of change seen in FEPs following exposure to toxic insult is a progressive shift in latency; each successive peak is shifted by a greater amount than were the preceding peaks. A straightforward example of this type of shift may be seen in the case of hypothermia. Figure 9.3 presents data extrapolated from a recent study in which FEPs were recorded from anesthetized rats at different rectal temperatures (Dyer and Boyes 1983a). The figure illustrates several interesting features. First, all functions appear linear. Second, as extent of hypothermia increases from 2°C below normal to 6°C below normal, the functions shift in both intercept and slope. What this means is that the magnitude of treatment (hypothermia) determines the magnitude of difference between early (P1) and later (P2) peaks. A variety of mechanisms might be invoked to explain this pattern of change. The simplest and most plausible may be found in the work of Westerfield, Joyner, and Moore (1978), who showed that in single nerve fibers progressive hypothermia produces an increase in the duration of an action potential, a decrease in its conduction velocity, and an increase in the length of its relative refractory period. This combination of effects could easily produce the pattern of change produced by hypothermia in the FEP. Hypothermia accompanied by anesthesia also produces an increase in FEP amplitudes (Dyer and Boyes 1983a). While it is tempting to speculate that an increase in amplitude of a population response like the FEP could reflect release of synaptic inhibition, it is noteworthy that increases in amplitude also occur in single-fiber preparations with hypothermia (Westerfield, Joyner, and Moore 1978), thereby rendering synaptic explanations unnecessary (although not necessarily incorrect).

The frequency with which the above pattern of change is seen in FEP latencies following exposure to different agents raises the suspicion that a common underlying mechanism is at work. Similar progressive changes in FEP peak latency are observed with α-methyl para tyrosine (Dyer, Howeel, and MacPhail 1981), chlordimeform (Boyes and Dyer 1984), and sulfolane (Dyer and Boyes 1984*a*).

There are, however, distinctly different patterns in latency change produced by some compounds. One such pattern is evidenced by rats treated with trimethyltin (TMT), an organotin known to produce loss of some retinal ganglion cells (Chang and Dyer 1983). TMT-treated rats have FEPs with slightly longer than normal P1 and N1 latencies and slightly shorter than normal P2 latencies. Such a pattern, coupled with a reduced amplitude of the potential, as occurs in TMT-treated rats (Dyer, Howell, and Wonderlin 1982), is congruent with a reduction in the population of cells responding to the stimulus. Without further studies, however, it would not be possible to determine where the reduction occurred. In the case of TMT, further studies indicated that retinal cells were being lost as a result of exposure (ibid.). Behavioral observations support the interpretation that TMT produces visual dysfunction in hooded rats, since they are noted to collide with walls in an open field (unpublished observations). Decreased latency of N1 and P2 with no change in P1 and no change in amplitude has also been observed in rats exposed pre- or perinatally to lead (Burdette 1983). The latter finding was surprising in light of the report by Fox, Lewkowski, and Cooper (1977) that perinatal exposure to lead produces enormous increases in P1, N1, and P2 latencies. Decreased latency of P2 coupled with increased P1N1 and N1P2 amplitudes has also been observed with prenatal exposure to methylmercury (Dyer, Eccles, and Annau 1978), a treatment that is well known to produce evidence of visual dysfunction in humans (e.g., Rustam and Hamdi 1974).

Very few treatments have been reported to produce amplitude alterations in the absence of latency alterations. However, prenatal administration of carbon monoxide to female rats (Dyer et al. 1979) produces increases in P1N1 and N1P2 amplitudes without changing latencies. Increasing stimulus (flash) intensity produces a more pronounced increase in amplitudes than does a decrease in latencies (Dyer, Eccles, and Annau 1978).

Changes in amplitude, with or without changes in latency, are difficult to interpret. An increase in amplitude may occur at the single-membrane level (as seen in hypothermia, above) as a result of increased synchrony in response to the stimulus (e.g., if spontaneous activity were diminished such that fewer neurons were in the refractory period from spontaneous activity when the stimulus was presented) or as a result of the removal of inhibition (as seen in evoked potentials recorded from dentate gyrus following perforant path stimulation in kainic acid-treated [Sloviter and Damiano 1981] and TMT-treated [Dyer and Boyes 1984*b*] rats). While it also seems likely that increases in amplitude might occur as a result of increased excitability of the neurons, the evidence is conflicting. A study of picrotoxin, strychnine, and pentylenetetrazol failed to reveal any increased amplitudes in the P1N1 or N1P2 of FEPs (Bigler et al. 1978), but pentylenetetrazol did increase the amplitude of the primary auditory-evoked responses (Faingold 1978).

Patterns of change in the P1N1P2 component of the FEP in addition to those discussed above are possible, but those mentioned above have been most commonly observed in FEP studies of neurotoxicity. As the FEP wave discussed becomes further removed from the primary (P1N1P2) component, the interpretation of the different patterns of change becomes progressively more difficult. At present there is little upon which to base explanations of selective alterations in the P2N2P3 component. Interpretation of changes in this wave would be greatly enhanced by an understanding of the origin of the inputs that produce the wave.

More information, particularly in the form of behavioral correlates, is available for interpretation of the P3N3 wave of the FEP than for the P2N2P3 wave. This wave is occasionally considered to be the first wave in the photic afterdischarge, although the evidence to support this contention is contradictory (e.g., Bigler 1975; and Bigler et al. 1978). In any case, alterations in the amplitude of the wave appear related to such variables as arousal, habituation, and excitability. On a continuum from anesthesia to seizures, both extremes seem to depress P3N3 amplitudes. Thus, reduced amplitudes have been observed following administration of the convulsant strychnine (Bigler et al. 1978), the anesthetic sodium pentobarbital (Hetzler and Oaklay 1981), the stimulant amphetamine (Fleming, Shearer, and Creel 1974; Schwartzbaum, Ide-Johanson, and Belgrade 1974), the anticonvulsants sodium valproate (Myslobodsky and Morag 1981a) and dipropylacetic acid (Shearer, Fleming, and Dustman 1978), and the cortical activator physostigmine (Fleming, Shearer, and Creel 1974; Bigler et al. 1978). Rats with a normally high activity level had smaller P3N3 amplitudes than rats with a normally low activity level (Joseph et al. 1981).

On the other hand, P3N3 amplitudes have been increased by procedures that (1) decrease behavioral reactivity to the flash (e.g., Schwartzbaum and Kreinick 1973); (2) tend to promote drowsiness, such as haloperidol administration (Dyer, Howell, and MacPhail 1981); (3) might be related to habituation, such as session number within a series of sessions (e.g., Schwartzbaum and Kreinick 1973, 1974; and Schaefer, Kreinick, and Schwartzbaum 1974; cf. Bartus and Ferris 1974); and (4) produce EEG hypersynchrony, such as gamma-vinyl GABA (Myslobodsky and Morag 1981b). Pentylenetetrazol, a convulsant, has been reported to increase P3N3 amplitudes on some occasions (Bigler 1975) but not others (Bigler et al. 1978).

From the above discussion it should be evident that although interpretation of FEPs is complex, certain patterns emerge, and these tend to characterize certain kinds of changes in neurobehavioral function. In a number of cases these changes may be linked to corresponding behavioral changes. It should be indicated here that while FEPs are still only rarely used in studies of toxicity, at least one major form of neurotoxicity was first described as a result of an FEP study. Trimethyltin (TMT) is an organotin that was known to produce profound damage to neurons in the limbic system and somewhat less damage elsewhere (e.g., Brown et al. 1979; Chang et al. 1982; and Dyer, Deshields, and Wonderlin 1982). As part of the process of validating the FEP, some TMT-treated rats were tested. Although the only existing study describing TMT-induced neuropathology specifically excluded the retina as having TMT-induced damage (Brown et al. 1979), the FEPs recorded from treated animals had a decreased-amplitude P1N1P2 peak, which was narrower than normal (i.e., increased P1 latencies, decreased P2 latencies). Such a pattern would be expected if fewer fibers were contributing to the evoked potential. Subsequent work recording FEPs from the optic tract of TMT-treated rats showed that these changes occurred at the retinal level (Dyer, Howell, and Wonderlin 1982), and a closer look at the retina of TMT-treated rats revealed that there was indeed a loss of retinal ganglion cells (Chang and Dyer 1983). As a result of this study, a series of other studies were performed which indicated that in fact TMT produced widespread damage to other sensory systems as well (ibid.). It is important for behav-

ioral researchers to characterize more fully the nature of these sensory disturbances, thereby strengthening the link between behavioral and physiological
endpoints.

Methodological Considerations

The above discussion has addressed some of the interpretational issues involved in
FEP studies. There are also many methodological issues of concern. In most cases
the optimal conditions under which to perform an FEP study are not known, and
the purpose here is to simply identify the issues. It would be surprising if there
were not particular sets of conditions under which performance of FEP studies
would be more likely to detect toxicity. While on the surface it might appear desirable to systematically manipulate the conditions of recording in routine testing,
thereby obtaining for any given toxicant the most useful set of conditions, the
magnitude of doing such experiments, to say nothing of the complexity of the
subsequent multivariate analyses, is enough to intimidate even the most energetic
of investigators. Furthermore, optimal conditions may vary with the compound
being tested and may be dictated by a specific hypothesis being tested. In identifying these issues, it is hoped that some readers will be tempted to address the
question of which sets of conditions are most likely to detect neurotoxicity.

In performing any evoked-potential study many of the variables that are
important in behavioral studies must be considered. A decision about the modality
and type of stimulus to be used must be followed by a decision about the appropriate stimulus intensity, background stimulus level, and presentation rate, all of
which may be expected to influence recordings. Species, strain, and gender must
be selected carefully. For example, some toxicants produce gender-dependent effects (e.g., Dyer et al. 1979). The size of the animal and the electrode placement may
interact to alter results. Similarly, in the absence of specific controls, the toxicant
under study may interact with peripheral structures (e.g., the pupil) to produce
misleading results.

It is well known that alterations in body temperature affect FEPs (e.g., Dyer and
Boyes 1983a), but it is less well appreciated that many toxicants alter body temperature in a manner that is contingent upon the ambient temperature (e.g., Myers
1981; and Dyer and Howell 1982b). These observations have important implications
for behavioral studies as well, since behavioral endpoints are affected by temperature (Ruppert and Dyer, in preparation).

Two important behavioral variables to consider in evoked-potential studies are
habituation and arousal. While there are few published accounts describing the
influence of habituation upon FEP parameters (e.g., Bartus and Ferris 1974), it is
certain that habituation time affects some of the peaks, especially the amplitude of
late components.

A rat that has not been handled and is placed in the experimental recording
chamber for the first time may be assumed to be in an aroused condition, at least for
a brief period of time. As the test sessions increase in duration, however, or as the
animal gains repeated experience with being handled and/or being placed in the
test chamber, there is an increased probability that sleep will occur. It is known that
evoked potentials differ in sleeping and waking subjects (e.g., Demetrescu, Demetrescu, and Iosif 1965; and Guilbaud, Menetrey, and Oliveras 1972), and therefore rats with fluctuating wakefulness add considerable variability to the data. One

solution to the problem was adopted by Winneke (1979), who recorded only when rats were asleep. If FEPs obtained during one particular stage of sleep or wakefulness are more sensitive to toxicant-induced disruption than those obtained during others, clues to the behavioral effects of the toxicant may be divulged.

Other Sensory Evoked Potentials

While FEPs have been the sensory evoked potentials most studied in the context of neurotoxicology, there are certainly many applications where other methods might be more useful. Even for testing visual function it is easy to argue for more sophisticated methods. One method that has been used extensively in the neurological clinic and is beginning to be used in neurotoxicology is the pattern-reversal evoked potential (PREP). As has been described recently (Dyer 1985), the PREP, the brainstem auditory evoked response (BAER), and the somatosensory evoked potential (SEP) all have unique contributions to make to an electrophysiological evaluation of neurotoxicity. While none of these tests has the extensive background of toxicological and methodological studies enjoyed by the FEP, the recent literature suggests that this will not long be the case (e.g., Rebert 1980; Boyes and Cooper 1981; Arezzo et al. 1982; Rebert et al. 1982; Boyes and Dyer 1983; Janssen, Boyes, and Dyer 1983; Rebert et al. 1983; Boyes and Dyer 1984; and Boyes, Jenkins, and Dyer 1985).

When the goal of a study is to assess the functional integrity of a particular sensory system, it makes most sense to record from either relay or cortical areas presumed to be primary parts of the system. For example, the optic nerve, lateral geniculate, visual cortex, and superior colliculus are logical places from which to record in the visual system. If, however, the experiment is less concerned with determining the functional integrity of a particular system and more concerned with the functional integrity of the whole nervous system, then an alternative strategy is to record the response to sensory stimuli from structures not traditionally considered part of the primary sensory systems. The sensory stimulus is the route into the brain, and in some respects the more polysynaptic the route to the recording electrode, the more likely that alteration of some brain function will be detected by the technique. In this context, one might also record from sensory structures like the visual cortex while delivering stimuli within another modality, such as the auditory modality.

While this approach is logical, there have been few attempts to follow it. Perhaps one reason for the reluctance of investigators to utilize this approach is that recordings from subcortical structures bring with them the onus of demonstrating that the recordings were in fact from the desired area. While histological verification of electrode placement is routine in these studies, this is not always sufficient. For example, the midbrain reticular formation is listed as an often-recorded site. However, given the massive input of sensory information to the overlying superior colliculus, an investigator must demonstrate that his responses are not volume-conducted from above. The same may be said for responses evoked by visual stimuli and recorded in the hippocampal formation overlying the lateral geniculate nucleus or superior colliculus. To date there have been no convincing demonstrations in the toxicological/pharmacological literature that effects reported were not volume-conducted.

Most attempts to use the subcortical and/or nonsensory approach have been in the pharmacological literature (but see Ray 1981). One laboratory that has pursued this approach in a pharmacological context is that of Dafny and coworkers (e.g., Dafny 1978; Dafny and Rigor 1978; Schanzer, Jacobson, and Dafny 1978; and Rabe et al. 1980). In these studies recordings were made from electrodes in structures like the ventromedial hypothalamus, the centromedian, caudate, medial forebrain bundle, and midbrain reticular formation, but there was no convincing demonstration that potentials were not volume-conducted from primary structures. Compounds tested have included ketamine, sodium pentobarbital, prostaglandin E2, and halothane. At present no definitive statement may be made about the relative sensitivity of these recordings compared with that of the more traditional sensory recordings from sensory structures. Further, it is difficult to relate alterations in such recordings to any particular behavioral deficit.

Hippocampal Evoked Potentials

In the last 20 years, it seems that no area of the mammalian brain has attracted more attention from behavioral scientists and neurobiologists than the hippocampus and its connections. There are certainly many reasons for this attention, including its laminar anatomy, its defined input-output pathways, and its apparent involvement in such complex neurobiological processes as memory and epilepsy. The hippocampus is clearly an extremely important brain area and thus is deserving of considerable attention from neurotoxicologists. In addition to being generally important in brain function (or perhaps related to it), the hippocampus also appears to demonstrate an intriguing tendency to (1) accumulate some toxic substances and (2) be damaged more than some other structures by certain toxic insults. For these reasons, it is important to consider the potential utility of hippocampal evoked potentials as measures for detection and characterization of neurotoxicity.

Before considering the few occasions upon which hippocampal EPs have been used in a toxicological assessment, it is important to have a better appreciation for what makes the hippocampus unique. A detailed treatment of these factors is beyond the scope of this chapter, but they will be identified here.

Much of what makes the hippocampal formation unique may be related to its anatomy. While the cross-sectional anatomy of the hippocampus appears simple, the third dimension provides complexity. Many adequate descriptions of hippocampal anatomy exist (e.g., Lorente de No 1934; O'Keefe and Nadel 1978; and Swanson 1979). In cross section the hippocampal formation may be thought of as two thin sheets of tightly packed cells, one in the shape of a partially flattened C, the other in the shape of a backwards, partially flattened C. The two C's face each other, the bottom limb of one entering the opening of the other. The entered C is the sheet of dentate granule (DG) cells; the entering C is the sheet of pyramidal cells, forming what is called Ammon's horn, or the cornu ammonis (CA). The CA is divided into cell fields, depending upon location along the sheet. Those cells at the top of the CA C are the CA1 cells. Most of the other CA cells are CA3 cells, except for a few toward the top of the curvature which are CA2 and a few loose ones inside the DG C which are CA4. The major connections of these cell groups are also quite simple. The primary input to the hippocampal formation (aside from contralateral hippocampal and septal inputs) is from the entorhinal cortex via a pathway known as the perforant path. The perforant path provides excitatory input to the DG cells. The DG cells send axons known as mossy fibers which synapse onto CA3 pyramidal cells. The CA3 pyramidal cells send axons out of the hippocampus via the fornix but also to the CA1 pyramidal cells via the Schaffer collaterals. Both the CA1 and the CA3 are subdivided into three sections, CA1a, CA1b, CA1c, CA3a, CA3b, and CA3c, according to their distance along the sheet of cells from the border between the CA1 and the subiculum. These different sections of the subfields have pyramidal cells with somewhat different properties, some tending to fire in burst discharges, others tending to fire in single spikes (Masukawa, Benardo, and Prince 1982). The DG, CA3, and CA1 cells all have nearby populations of basket cells which provide recurrent inhibition.

As mentioned above, the anatomy of the hippocampus is complex in the third dimension. In fact, the C's described above are really more like two troughs or gutters, extending from the septal area (septal pole) in a posterior-lateral direction at about a 45° angle from the midline. While the lateral shift continues until the end of the hippocampus, the posterior movement stops after several millimeters (in the rat), and the two interlocking C's swing down (ventral) and forward (anterior). Thus, viewed in three dimensions, each of the C's has the shape of a ram's horn. This third dimension is known as the septotemporal axis and is important because at least one toxicant (trimethyltin) produces different types of damage at different locations along the axis (Chang and Dyer 1985). Perhaps not coincidentally, cells at different levels along the septotemporal axis receive input from different areas and with different densities (Gaarskjaer 1978; Ruth, Collier, and Routtenberg 1982).

The anatomical organization of the hippocampus renders it particularly accessible to investigation because it is laminar. That is, if an electrode is placed in a particular layer, the investigator may be assured of knowing the inputs and outputs of that layer. For example, an electrode placed just above the layer of granule cells in the dentate gyrus would record almost exclusively inputs to DG cells. If an input pathway were stimulated, it might be assumed with some certainty that the recorded response arose from dentate dendrites or nearby somas. This anatomy has also opened the way for exploration of recurrent connections. Again, using the DG cells as an example, it is known that collaterals of their axons synapse onto inhibitory basket cells, which in turn inhibit the granule cells via a monosynaptic route. Using a paired-pulse paradigm, it is therefore possible to examine the functional integrity of the recurrent inhibitory pathway. A single shock to the perforant path produces a large EPSP in the granule cells, which contains a spike when stimuli are sufficiently intense. However, since this spike reflects summated action potentials in the granule cells themselves, it may be inferred that the spike produces activity in the basket cells, which in turn inhibit the granule cells. Therefore, a second shock, occurring shortly after the first, should produce a smaller spike response, because some of the granule cells would be inhibited. This recurrent inhibition, first explored physiologically by Anderson, Holmquist, and Voorhoeve (1966), with the paired-pulse paradigm has been recommended as a model system for assessing drugs that affect synapses mediated by GABA, the putative transmitter at the basket cell–granule cell synapse (Matthews, McCafferty, and Setler 1981).

A feature of hippocampal physiology that makes it particularly appealing to those interested in behavior is the extraordinary plasticity of synaptic relationships.

There are at least three types of short-term plasticity—paired pulse potentiation, frequency potentiation, and heterosynaptic potentiation (cooperativity)—and three types of long-term plasticity—post-tetanic potentiation, long-term potentiation, and kindling—in the hippocampus. While the integrity of any of these models of plasticity may be studied as a function of exposure to toxicants, if the investigator is interested, not in plasticity, but in the "normal" synaptic relationships between areas, then extra care must be taken to avoid placing the hippocampus into the "plastic" mode and inadvertently altering its physiology. The simplest way to avoid error is to utilize a low stimulation rate (e.g., 1 pulse/sec or less).

A significant impediment to the use of hippocampal evoked potentials in toxicology is the requirement that electrode placements be absolutely precise if amplitude measurements are to be made and compared across subjects. This requirement is a result of the laminar organization of the structure, which produces large fluctuations in amplitude with small changes in depth. This is not a problem, however, if (1) the design of the study can be a within-subjects design or (2) some form of normalization of the endpoint can occur. An example of the latter is the case in which an investigator is interested in studying recurrent inhibition. In this case, the endpoint is usually the ratio of the second of a pair of responses to the first, a situation that automatically cancels out absolute differences in amplitude of the first response between subjects. Users of in vivo hippocampal evoked potentials in a toxicological context have tended to use a derived measure that normalizes the endpoint across animals.

For example, Abraham et al. (1981) showed that urethane-anesthetized rats tested 8 weeks after cessation of a 20-week chronic ethanol treatment had normal input-output relationships for EPSPs and population spikes recorded from CA1 after stimulation of the Schaffer collateral system; however, treated rats had greater paired-pulse potentiation responses for the population spike than did controls (response measure was response 2 amplitude/response 1 amplitude, or R2/R1). These results were interpreted as a reduction of recurrent inhibition. Jordan and Clark (1983) showed that adult rats undernourished during the prenatal and early postnatal period had reduced magnitude and duration of long-term potentiation produced in the dentate gyrus by stimulation of the perforant path. The response measure was the percentage increase in population spike amplitude compared with the pre-potentiation baseline. Dyer and Boyes (1984b) have demonstrated that within hours of a single acute administration of trimethyltin, there is a reduction of recurrent inhibition in the dentate gyrus, measured by paired-pulse stimulation of the perforant path. In this study the response measure was spike amplitude, R2/R1. In a related investigation of trimethyltin, Hasan, Zimmer, and Woolley (1984) demonstrated altered responses in the dentate gyrus following polysynaptic activation.

While not strictly toxicological, several studies have used in vivo hippocampal evoked potentials as endpoints in studies of aging and senescence. Landfield, McGaugh, and Lynch (1978) recorded from CA1 in aged urethane-anesthetized rats following stimulation of the commissural-Schaffer collateral system. Aged rats did not differ from controls on such measures as stimulus threshold, response latency, response amplitude, or time course of paired-pulse effects. However, compared with controls, aged rats did not show good frequency potentiation at 12 Hz, and they demonstrated a slowed rise of post-tetanic potentiation after a 5-second 100 Hz train of stimuli. Barnes (1979) recorded from the dentate gyrus of senescent rats following stimulation of the perforant path. In this unanesthetized preparation, with recordings taken from different loci than those of Landfield, McGaugh, and Lynch (1978), the outcome was somewhat different. Older rats had smaller EPSPs than did controls. In addition, older rats showed an impaired response to single stimuli after a series of 20 msec bursts of 400 Hz stimuli. Unlike controls, aged rats did not develop an enhanced facilitation with repetition over days. The first day that high frequency stimuli were presented, the responses of both control and aged rats were potentiated by about the same amount and for about the same time period. By the third day of such treatment, however, the potentiation observed in controls was greater and of longer duration than that in aged rats. Paired-pulse stimulation did not differentiate between aged and control rats at interpulse intervals between 7 and 95 msec. These paradigms should achieve even greater utility when the relationships between these forms of synaptic plasticity and the various forms of behavioral plasticity (e.g., learning) are determined.

Interhemispheric Evoked Potentials

Another technique that has been underutilized in toxicological investigation is the interhemispheric-evoked response, or transcallosal response (TCR). If an area of the cerebral cortex is electrically stimulated, the homotopic area on the contralateral side responds with an evoked response (Curtis 1940). The response is presumably mediated via the corpus callosum, although under certain circumstances a late response mediated via a subcortical pathway, the interhemispheric delayed response, may also be observed (Rutledge and Kennedy 1960; Rutledge 1965).

The TCR gives the investigator a measure of the functional integrity of a cortical tract in a monosynaptic system (Pickworth, Sharpe, and Martin 1977). While this tract has been used for a variety of purposes (e.g., Swadlow 1982; and Preston, Waxman, and Kocsis 1983), it has yet to be explored adequately in a toxicologic context. The development of the TCR in rats has been studied (Seggie and Berry 1972), and it has been demonstrated that its development is impaired by thyroidectomy (Hatotani and Timiras 1967) and protein malnutrition (Forbes et al. 1975). Howell has shown that the TCR is impaired by prenatal hexane treatment and prenatal cadmium treatment (Howell 1978).

Recent evidence indicates that a variety of neurobehavioral disturbances, including learning disabilities, may be reflections of a disruption in the normal cerebral lateralization process. Further, it has been suggested that changes in the intrauterine environment, such as may occur following exposure to some toxicants, may initiate the disruption in lateralization (e.g., Geschwind and Galaburda 1985). Physiological studies of the communication channels between the hemispheres may be useful in the prediction and study of these behavioral disorders.

Cognition-related Potentials

If one includes human studies, there is an enormous body of literature dedicated to the search for evoked potentials, or event-related potentials that are in some way related to cognitive processes. Included among these potentials is the contingent negative variation (CNV), a slow potential that develops following an initial stimulus when the initial stimulus is supposed to signal the initiation of a time interval prior to an *imperative* stimulus, one that requires an act, motor or cognitive. These potentials have been recorded in humans and nonhuman primates (Rebert 1972), and similar waves have been reported in rodents (Pirch, Corbus, and Napier 1981). The significance of these waves has been debated for nearly 20 years, but there seems to be some general agreement that they are in some way related to *expectancy*; that is, the subject is expecting the second stimulus.

In contrast to the expectancy wave, others have studied a much more rapid process that seems to be related to surprise or novelty. This wave, generally referred to as the P300 wave, since it occurs at a latency as great or greater than 300 msec, is largest when a stimulus appears that is different from a preceding string of stimuli and has been given some meaning by the experimenter. For example, a subject might be asked to count the number of "rare" stimuli in a series of frequent stimuli in order to correctly complete a task. Evoked potentials recorded to the rare stimuli would have a large positive peak at around 300 msec, whereas evoked potentials recorded to the frequent stimuli would have at best a small peak. Attempts to produce P300 waves in primates have been successful (Arthur and Starr 1984), but there is only a fragile literature on these waves in rodents (O'Brien 1982). Deadwyler, West, and Robinson (1981) have recorded waves with similar properties that appear to originate in the dentate gyrus of the hippocampus, and a few human studies also indicate that the hippocampal formation is a viable candidate for generator of P300 (Halgren et al. 1980; Okada, Kaufman, and Williamson 1983). If this can be demonstrated conclusively, perhaps other tests of hippocampal function, mentioned above, might be more readily implemented in animals and provide similar information.

The CNV and the P300 paradigms, as well as several variants (e.g., Otto et al. 1981), provide potentially useful culture-free indexes of cognitive function in humans, which might be particularly useful in evaluations of neurotoxicity. If these turn out not to be redundant with measures of hippocampal function in rodents, then it would be appropriate for investigators to turn their attention to developing rodent models for them as indexes of neurotoxicity.

Summary

In summary, a wide variety of electrophysiological techniques is available for use in detection and characterization of neurotoxicity and may provide an interface between behavioral and physiological studies. One of these techniques, the flash-evoked potential, or FEP, has been discussed in some detail to provide a forum for raising issues common to many electrophysiological techniques. The issues raised include interpretation of results and methodological variables important for the successful use of the techniques. In addition, several little-used but potentially valuable methods were identified. While the relationship between some of the endpoints discussed and behavioral alterations has been left to the reader's imagination, it is evident that certain of the endpoints are very closely tied to behavior. It is hoped that this chapter will stimulate interest in pursuing the behavioral-neurophysiological interface within the context of toxicology.

Acknowledgments

This manuscript has been reviewed by the Health Effects Research Laboratory, U.S. Environmental Protection Agency, and approved for publication. Mention of trade names or commercial products does not constitute endorsement or recommendation for use.

References

Abraham, W. C.; Hunter, B. E.; Zornetzer, S. F.; and Walker, D. W. 1981. Augmentation of short term plasticity in CA1 of rat hippocampus after chronic ethanol treatment. *Brain Res.* 221:271–87.

Anderson, P.; Holmquist, B.; and Voorhoeve, P. E. 1966. Entorhinal activation of dentate granule cells. *Acta Physiol. Scand.* 66:448–60.

Arezzo, J. C.; Schaumburg, H. H.; Vaughan, H. G., Jr.; Spencer, P. S.; and Barna, J. 1982. Hind limb somatosensory evoked potentials in monkey: The effects of distal axonopathy. *Ann. Neurol.* 12:24–32.

Arthur, D. L., and Starr, A. 1984. Task-relevant late positive component of the auditory event-related potential in monkeys resembles P300 in humans. *Science* 223:186–88.

Barnes, C. A. 1979. Memory deficits associated with senescence: A neurophysiological and behavioral study in the rat. *J. Comp. Physiol. Psychol.* 93:74–104.

Barnes, M. I. 1984. Superior colliculus lesions and the visual evoked response. Master's thesis, North Carolina State University.

Bartus, R. T., and Ferris, S. H. 1974. Neural correlates of habituation and dark adaptation in the visual cortex of the rat. *Physiol. Psychol.* 2:55–59.

Bigler, E. D. 1975. Lateral geniculate multiple-unit activity related to metrazol potentiated after-discharges. *Electroencephalogr. Clin. Neurophysiol.* 39:491–97.

———. 1977. Neurophysiology, neuropharmacology and behavioral relationships of visual system evoked after-discharges: A review. *Biobehav. Rev.* 1:95–112.

Bigler, E. D.; Shearer, D. E.; Dustman, R. E.; and Fleming, D. E. 1978. Differential effects of convulsants on visually evoked responses in the albino rat. *Pharmacol. Biochem. Behav.* 8:727–33.

Boyes, W. K., and Cooper, G. P. 1981. Acrylamide neurotoxicity: Effects on far-field somatosensory evoked potentials in rats. *Neurobehav. Toxicol. Teratol.* 3:467–90.

Boyes, W. K., and Dyer, R. S. 1983. Pattern reversal and flash evoked potentials following acute triethyltin exposure. *Neurobehav. Toxicol. Teratol.* 5:571–77.

———. 1984. Chlordimeform produces profound, selective and transient changes in visual evoked potentials of hooded rats. *Exp. Neurol.* 86:434–47.

Boyes, W. K.; Jenkins, D. E.; and Dyer, R. S. 1985. Chlordimeform produces contrast-dependent changes in visual evoked potentials of hooded rats. *Exp. Neurol.* 89:391–407.

Brazier, M. A. B. 1957. A study of the late response to flash in the cortex of the cat. *Acta Physiol. Pharmacol. Neerlandica* 6:692–714.

Brown, A. W.; Aldridge, W. N.; Street, B. W.; and Verschoyle, R. D. 1979. The behavioral and neuropathologic sequelae of intoxication by trimethyltin compounds. *Am. J. Pathol.* 97:59–82.

Burdette, L. J. 1983. The effects of asymptomatic lead exposure during different developmental stages in rats: Behavior and electrophysiology. Ph.D. diss., Washington University.

Burne, R. A.; Azizi, S. A.; Mihailoff, G. A.; and Woodard, D. J. 1981. The tecto pontine projection in the rat with comments on visual pathways to the basilar pons. *J. Comp. Neurol.* 202:287–307.

Chalupa, L. M.; Anchel, M. N.; and Lindsley, D. B. 1973. Effects of cryogenic blocking of pulvinar upon visually evoked responses in the cortex of the cat. *Exp. Neurol.* 32:112–22.

Chang, L. W., and Dyer, R. S. 1983. Trimethyltin induced pathology in sensory neurons. *Neurobehav. Toxicol. Teratol.* 5:673–96.

———. 1985. Septo-temporal gradients of trimethyltin-induced hippocampal damage. *Neurobehav. Toxicol. Teratol.* 7:43–49.

Chang, L. W.; Tiemeyer, T. M.; Wenger, G. R.; and McMillan, D. E. 1982. Neuropathology of mouse hippocampus in acute trimethyltin intoxication. *Neurobehav. Toxicol. Teratol.* 4:149–56.

Creutzfeldt, O. D., and Kuhnt, U. 1973. Electrophysiology and topographical distribution of visual evoked potentials in animals. In *Handbook of physiology,* edited by R. Jung, vol. 7/3, pp. 595–646. Berlin: Springer-Verlag.

Curtis, H. J. 1940. An analysis of cortical potentials mediated by the corpus callosum. *J. Neurophysiol.* 3:414–22.

Dafny, N. 1978. Neurophysiological approach as a tool to study the effects of drugs on the central nervous system: Dose effect of pentobarbital. *Exp. Neurol.* 59:263–74.

Dafny, N., and Rigor, B. M. 1978. Dose effects of ketamine on photic and acoustic field potentials. *Neuropharmacology* 17:851–62.

Deadwyler, S. A.; West, M. O.; and Robinson, J. H. 1981. Evoked potentials for the dentate gyrus during auditory stimulus generalizations in the rat. *Exp. Neurol.* 71:615–24.

Demetrescu, M.; Demetrescu, M.; and Iosif, G. 1965. The tonic control of cortical responsiveness by inhibitory and facilitatory diffuse influences. *Electroencephalogr. Clin. Neurophysiol.* 18:1–24.

Dyer, R. S. 1985. The use of sensory evoked potentials in toxicology. *Fund. Appl. Toxicol.* 5:24–40.

Dyer, R. S., and Annau, Z. 1977. Flash evoked potentials from rat superior colliculus. *Pharmacol. Biochem. Behav.* 6:453–59.

Dyer, R. S., and Boyes, W. K. 1983a. Hypothermia and chloropent anesthesia differentially affect the flash evoked potentials of hooded rats. *Brain Res. Bull.* 10:825–31.

———. 1983b. Use of neurophysiological challenges for the detection of toxicity. *Fed. Proc.* 42:3201–6.

———. 1984a. Sulfolane impairs visual function. *Toxicologist* 4:184.

———. 1984b. Trimethyltin reduces recurrent inhibition in rats. *Neurobehav. Toxicol. Teratol.* 6:369–72.

Dyer, R. S.; Deshields, T. L.; and Wonderlin, W. F. 1982. Trimethyltin-induced changes in gross morphology of the hippocampus. *Neurobehav. Toxicol. Teratol.* 4:141–47.

Dyer, R. S.; Eccles, C. U.; and Annau, Z. 1978. Evoked potential alterations following prenatal methyl mercury exposure. *Pharmacol. Biochem. Behav.* 8:137–41.

Dyer, R. S.; Eccles, C. U.; Swartzwelder, H. S.; Fechter, L. D.; and Annau, Z. 1979. Prenatal carbon monoxide and adult evoked potentials in rats. *J. Environ. Sci. Health* C13:107–20.

Dyer, R. S., and Howell, W. E. 1982a. Acute triethyltin exposure: Effects on the visual evoked potential and hippocampal afterdischarge. *Neurobehav. Toxicol. Teratol.* 4:259–66.

———. 1982b. Triethyltin: Ambient temperature alters visual system toxicity. *Neurobehav. Toxicol. Teratol.* 4:267–71.

Dyer, R. S.; Howell, W. E.; and MacPhail, R. C. 1981. Dopamine depletion slows retinal transmission. *Exp. Neurol.* 71:326–40.

Dyer, R. S.; Howell, W. E.; and Wonderlin, W. F. 1982. Visual system dysfunction following acute trimethyltin administration. *Neurobehav. Toxicol. Teratol.* 4:191–95.

Ebe, M.; Honma, I.; and Ishiyama, Y. 1972. Laminal analysis of visual evoked potentials and unit discharges on visual cortex of albino rat. *Tohoku J. Exp. Med.* 108:39–54.

Faingold, C. L. 1978. Brainstem reticular formation mechanisms subserving generalized seizures: Effects of convulsants and anticonvulsants on sensory evoked responses. *Prog. Neuro-Psychopharmacol.* 2:401–22.

Fleming, D. E.; Shearer, D. E.; and Creel, D. J. 1974. Effect of pharmacologically induced arousal on the evoked potential in the unanesthetized rat. *Pharmacol. Biochem. Behav.* 2:187–92.

Forbes, W. B.; Resnick, O.; Stern, W. C.; Bronzino, J. D.; and Morgane, P, J. 1975. The effect of chronic protein malnutrition on transcallosal evoked responses in the rat. *Dev. Psychobiol.* 8:503–9.

Fox, D. A.; Lewkowski, J. P.; and Cooper, G. P. 1977. Acute and chronic effects of neonatal lead exposure on development of the visual evoked response in rats. *Toxicol. Appl. Pharmacol.* 40:449–61.

Gaarskjaer, F. B. 1978. Organization of the mossy fiber system in the rat studied in extended hippocampi I. Terminal area related to number of granule and pyramidal cells. *J. Comp. Neurol.* 178:49–72.

Geschwind, N., and Galaburda, A. M. 1985. Cerebral lateralization. Biological mechanisms, associations, and pathology: I. A hypothesis and a program for research. *Arch. Neurol.* 42:428–59.

Guilbaud, G.; Menetrey, D.; and Oliveras, J. L. 1972. Control exerted during sleep by primary cortical areas upon different sensory afferents. *Electroencephalogr. Clin. Neurophysiol.* 33:15–21.

Halgren, E.; Squires, N. K.; Wilson C. L.; Rohrbaugh, J. W.; Bubb, T. L.; and Crandall, P. H. 1980. Endogenous potentials generated in the human hippocampal formation and amygdala by infrequent events. *Science* 210:803–5.

Hasan, Z.; Zimmer, L.; and Woolley, D. 1984. Time course of the effects of trimethyltin on limbic evoked potentials and distribution of tin in blood and brain in the rat. *Neurotoxicology* 5:217–44.

Hatotani, N., and Timiras, P. S. 1967. Influence of thyroid function on the postnatal development of the transcallosal response in the rat. *Neuroendocrinology* 2:147–56.

Hetzler, B. E., and Oaklay, K. 1981. Dose effects of pentabarbital on evoked potentials in visual cortex and superior colliculus of the albino rat. *Neuropharmacology* 20:969–78.

Howell, W. E. 1978. A neurobehavioral evaluation of the prenatal toxicity of n-hexane in rats. Ph.D. diss., University of Cincinnati.

Janssen, R.; Boyes, W. K.; and Dyer, R. S. 1983. Effects of chlordimeform on the brainstem auditory evoked response in rats. In *Developments in the science and practice of toxicology,* edited by A. W. Hayes, R. C. Schnell, and T. S. Miya, 533–36. North Holland: Elsevier.

Jordan, T. C., and Clark, G. A. 1983. Early undernutrition impairs hippocampal long-term potentiation in adult rats. *Behav. Nuerosci.* 97:319–22.

Joseph, R.; Forrest, N. M.; Fiducia, D.; Como, P.; and Siegel, J. 1981. Electrophysiological and behavioral correlates of arousal. *Physiol. Psychol.* 9:90–95.

Joy, R. 1985. The effects of neurotoxicants on kindling and kindled seizures. *Fund. Appl. Toxicol.* 5:41–65.

Landfield, P. W.; McGaugh, J. L.; and Lynch, G. 1978. Impaired synaptic potentiation processes in the hippocampus of aged, memory-deficient rats. *Brain Res.* 150:85–101.

Lopes da Silva, F., and Van Rotterdam, A. 1982. Biophysical aspects of EEG and MEG generation. In *Electroencephalography,* edited by E. Niedermeyer and F. Lopes da Silva, 15–26. Baltimore: Urban & Schwarzenberg.

Lorente de No, R. 1934. Studies on the structure of the cerebral cortex. II. Continuation of the study of the ammonic system. *J. Psychol. Neurol.* 46:113–77.

Masukawa, L. M.; Benardo, L. S.; and Prince, D. A. 1982. Variations in electrophysiological properties of hippocampal neurons in different subfields. *Brain Res.* 242:341–44.

Matthews, W. D.; McCafferty, G. P.; and Setler, P. E. 1981. An electrophysiological model of GABA-mediated neurotransmission. *Neuropharmacology* 20:561–65.

Montero, V. M. 1973. Evoked responses in the rat's visual cortex to contralateral, ipsilateral and restricted photic stimulation. *Brain Res.* 53:192–96.

Myers, R. D. 1981. Alcohol's effect on body temperature: Hypothermia, hyperthermia or poikilothermia. *Brain Res. Bull.* 7:209–20.

Myslobodsky, M. S., and Morag, M. 1981*a*. Pharmacologic analysis of sodium valproate-induced suppression of secondary components of visual evoked potentials in albino rats. *Pharmacol. Biochem. Behav.* 15:681–85.

––––––. 1981*b*. Suppression by sodium valproate of vinyl GABA-induced facilitation of visual evoked potentials in rats. *Electroencephalogr. Clin. Neurophysiol.* 52:445–50.

O'Brien, J. H. 1982. P300 wave elicited by a stimulus-change paradigm in acutely prepared rats. *Physiol. Behav.* 28:711–13.

Okada, Y.C.; Kaufman, L.; and Williamson, S. J. 1983. The hippocampal formation as a source of the slow endogenous potentials. *Electroencephalogr. Clin. Neurophysiol.* 55:417–26.

O'Keefe, J., and Nadel, L. 1978. *The hippocampus as a cognitive map.* Oxford: Clarendon Press.

Otto, D. A.; Benignus, V. A.; Muller, K. E.; and Barton, C. N. 1981. Effects of age and body lead burden on CNS function in young children. I. Slow cortical potentials. *Electroencephalogr. Clin. Neurophysiol.* 52:229–39.

Pickworth, W. B.; Sharpe, L. G.; and Martin, W. R. 1977. Transcallosally evoked potentials and the EEG in the decerebrate dog: Actions of tryptaminergic, dopaminergic and adrenergic agonists. *Electroencephalogr. Clin. Neurophysiol.* 42:809–16.

Pirch, J. H.; Corbus, M. J.; and Napier, T. C. 1981. Auditory cue preceding intracranial stimulation induces event-related potential in rat frontal cortex: Alterations by amphetamine. *Brain Res.* 7:399–404.

Preston, R. J.; Waxman, S. G.; and Kocsis, J. D. 1983. Effects of 4-aminopyridine on rapidly and slowly conducting axons of rat corpus callosum. *Exp. Neurol.* 79:808–20.

Pruill, G., and Rompel, K. 1970. EEG changes in acute poisoning with organic tin compounds. *Electroencephalogr. Clin. Neurophysiol.* 29:215.

Rabe, L. S.; Moreno, L.; Rigor, B. M.; and Dafny, N. 1980. Effects of halothane on evoked field potentials recorded from cortical and subcortical nuclei. *Neuropharmacology* 19:813–25.

Ray, D. E. 1981. Electroencephalographic and evoked response correlates of trimethyltin induced neuronal damage in the rat hippocampus. *J. Appl. Toxicol.* 3:145–48.

Rebert, C. S. 1972. Cortical and subcortical slow potentials in the monkey's brain during a preparatory interval. *Electroenchephalogr. Clin. Neurophysiol.* 33:389–402.

––––––. 1980. The brain stem auditory evoked response as a tool in neurobehavioral toxicology and medicine. *Prog. Brain Res.* 54:458–62.

––––––. 1983. Multisensory evoked potentials in experimental and applied neurotoxicology. *Neurobehav. Toxicol. Teratol.* 5:659–71.

Rebert, C. S.; Houghton, P. W.; Howd, R. A.; and Pryor, G. T. 1982. Effects of hexane on the brainstem auditory response and caudal nerve action potential. *Neurobehav. Toxicol. Teratol.* 4:75–89.

Rebert, C. S.; Sorenson, S. S.; Howd, R. A.; and Pryor, G. T. 1983. Toluene-induced hearing loss in rats evidenced by the brainstem auditory evoked response. *Neurobehav. Toxicol. Teratol.* 5:69–76.

Regan, D. 1972. *Evoked potentials.* London: Chapman & Hall.

Rose, G. H., and Lindsley, D. B. 1968. Development of visually evoked potentials in kittens: Specific and nonspecific responses. *J. Neurophysiol.* 31:607–23.

Rustam, H., and Hamdi, T. 1974. Methylmercury poisoning in Iraq: A neurological study. *Brain* 97:499–510.

Ruth, R. E.; Collier, T. J.; and Routtenberg, A. 1982. Topography between the entorhinal cortex and the dentate septotemporal axis in rats. I. Medial and intermediate entorhinal projectory cells. *J. Comp. Neurol.* 209:69–78.

Rutledge, L. T. 1965. Facilitation: Electrical response enhanced by conditional excitation of cerebral cortex. *Science* 148:1246–48.

Rutledge, L. T., and Kennedy, T. T. 1960. Extracallosal delayed responses to cortical stimulation in chloralosed cat. *J. Neurophysiol.* 23:188–96.

Schaefer, C. F.; Kreinick, C. J.; and Schwartzbaum, J, S. 1974. Behavioral reactivity, appetitive behavior, and visual evoked potentials to photic stimuli following amygdaloid lesions in rats. *J. Comp. Physiol. Psychol.* 86:793–811.

Schanzer, M.; Jacobson, E. D.; and Dafny, N. 1978. A neurophysiological approach as a tool to study the effect of drugs on the central nervous system. III. Effect of prostaglandin on seven brain sites. *Exp. Neurol.* 60:56–67.

Scheinberg, L. C.; Taylor, J. M.; Herzog, I.; and Mandell, S. 1966. Optic and peripheral nerve response to triethyltin intoxication in the rabbit: Biochemical and ultrastructural studies. *J. Neuropathol. Exp. Neurol.* 25:202–13.

Schwartzbaum, J. S.; Ide-Johanson, L.; and Belgrade, J. 1974. Comparative effects of scopolamine and amphetamine upon behavioral reactivity and visual evoked potentials to flashes in rats. *J. Comp. Physiol. Psychol.* 86:1044–51.

Schwartzbaum, J. S., and Kreinick, C. J. 1973. Interrelationships of hippocampal electroencephalogram, visually evoked response and behavioral reactivity to photic stimuli in rats. *J. Comp. Physiol. Psychol.* 85:479–90.

————. 1974. Visual evoked potentials during appetitive behavior after septal lesions in rats. *J. Comp. Physiol. Psychol.* 86:509–22.

Schwartzbaum, J. S.; Kreinick, C. J.; and Levine, M. S. 1972. Behavioral reactivity and visual evoked potentials to photic stimuli following septal lesions in rats. *J. Comp. Physiol. Psychol.* 80:123–42.

Seggie, J., and Berry, M. 1972. Ontogeny of interhemispheric evoked potentials in the rat: Significance of myelination of the corpus callosum. *Exp. Neurol.* 35:215–32.

Shearer, D. E.; Fleming, D. E.; and Dustman, R. E. 1978. Effects of dipropylacetic acid on late components of the photically evoked potential and afterdischarge in rat. *Pharmacol. Biochem. Behav.* 8:501–4.

Sloviter, R. S., and Damiano, B. P. 1981. On the relationship between kainic acid-induced epileptiform activity and hippocampal neuronal damage. *Neuropharmacology* 20:1003–11.

Standage, G. P.; Fleming, D. E.; and Bigler, E. D. 1981. Thalamocortical coupling and component properties of visually evoked afterdischarge *Brain Res. Bull.* 7:89–92.

Swadlow, H. A. 1982. Impulse conduction in the mammalian brain: Physiological properties of individual axons monitored for several months. *Science* 218:911–13.

Swanson, L. W. 1979. The hippocampus—new anatomical insights. *Trends NeuroSci.* 2:9–12.

Torres, F., and Warner, J. S. 1962. Some characteristics of delayed responses to photic stimuli in the cat. *Electroencephalogr. Clin. Neurophysiol.* 14:654–66.

Verzeano, M. 1973. The study of neuronal networks in the mammalian brain. In *Bioelectric recording techniques. Part A. Cellular processes and brain potentials*, edited by R. F. Thompson and M. M. Patterson, 243–72. New York: Academic Press.

Westerfield, M.; Joyner, R. W.; and Moore, J. W. 1978. Temperature-sensitive conduction failure at axon branch points. *J. Neurophysiol.* 41:1–8.

Winneke, G. 1979. Modification of visual evoked potentials in rats after long term blood lead elevation. *Activ. Nerv. Supp.* 21:282–84.

Diane L. DeHaven and
Richard B. Mailman

10

The Interactions of Behavior and Neurochemistry

The recent emergence of neurobehavioral toxicology as a scientific discipline has generated interest in the neurochemical mechanisms of, and sequelae to, toxicant exposure. Attempts are made frequently to correlate behavioral changes with alterations in neuronal function, and neurochemical studies have provided one way of understanding "target sites" for neurotoxicity. This chapter reviews some of the currently available approaches for assessing neurotransmitter function in the central nervous system (CNS) and discusses how these techniques have been applied to the study of model neurotoxicants, as well as to environmentally relevant compounds that have been shown to cause neurochemical or neurobehavioral toxicity. We believe that rather than being an alternative or competitor, neurobehavioral toxicology is a complement to neurochemical approaches. This review acquaints the reader with basic neurochemical strategies and discusses the potential advantages and shortcomings of these approaches. Where possible, the neurochemical effects of toxic compounds will be related to the known neurobehavioral effects in an attempt to present a more complete picture of neurotoxicity. Clearly, the aim of this chapter is not to provide a compendium of all available neurochemical methods or even those that have been applied successfully to studies in neurotoxicology. Rather, specific examples are used to illustrate strategies that have been employed in an attempt to provide a foundation for understanding mechanisms and sequelae of toxicity.

Measurement of Neurochemical Alterations

In Vitro Methods

Steady-state concentrations. Changes in the total amount of neurotransmitter present in neurons may result from destruction of cellular elements in which neurotransmitters reside or from perturbations that profoundly alter neuronal activity or metabolism. These changes in the steady-state concentrations of the transmitters of interest are one way that toxicants affect neuronal function, and examination of discrete brain regions may demonstrate preferential effects on specific pathways. However, steady-state concentrations reveal little about how a toxicant perturbs the CNS, and these techniques will fail to detect major alterations not affecting total transmitter content or concentration.

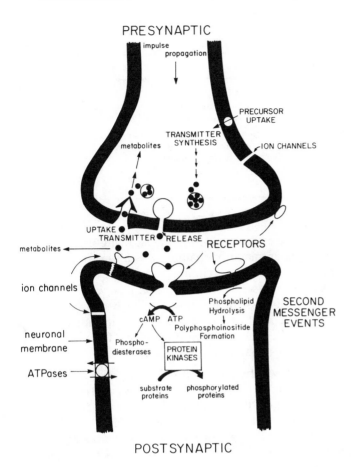

PRESYNAPTIC

impulse
propagation

PRECURSOR
UPTAKE

TRANSMITTER
metabolites   SYNTHESIS

ION CHANNELS

UPTAKE
TRANSMITTER   RELEASE   RECEPTORS

metabolites

ion channels

Phospholipid   SECOND
Hydrolysis   MESSENGER
cAMP ATP   EVENTS
Polyphosphoinositide
Formation
neuronal   Phospho-
membrane   diesterases   PROTEIN
KINASES
ATPases

substrate   phosphorylated
proteins   proteins

POSTSYNAPTIC

Fig. 10.1 Model of a synapse, demonstrating many of the biochemical loci where effects of neurotoxicants have been studied

The advent of high-performance liquid chromatography (HPLC) has simplified the task of accurately measuring neurotransmitters, their precursors, and their metabolites in discrete brain regions and nuclei. The use of HPLC with electrochemical detection was first applied in neurochemistry to the measurement of dopamine (DA) and norepinephrine (NE) (Keller et al. 1976) and later to metabolites and precursors of these compounds (Crombeen, Kraak, and Poppe 1978; Scratchley et al. 1979; Kilts, Breese, and Mailman 1981; Van Valkenburg et al. 1982) and to serotonin (Kilts, Breese, and Poppe 1981; Mefford 1981; Lyness 1982). Excellent HPLC methods are now available for neuroactive alpha-amino acids and GABA (Smith et al. 1975; Lindroth and Mopper 1979; Caudill, Houck, and Wightman 1982), as well as various peptide transmitter candidates (Gruber et al. 1976; Monch and Dehnen 1977; Hancock et al. 1978; Guyon et al. 1979; Meek 1980; Desiderio et al. 1981), although the latter techniques may utilize HPLC for purification prior to radioimmunoassay (Meyer, Phillips, and Eiden 1982). Finally, it is of interest that measurement of acetylcholine, which until recently has required gas chromatography/mass spectroscopy (Hanin and Skinner 1975) or radioenzymatic assays (Goldberg and McCaman 1973), may soon be supplanted by HPLC-electrochemical detection (EC) techniques (Potter, Meek, and Neff 1983).

Table 10.1 Some neurochemical strategies used to assess neuronal function in the central nervous system

In Vitro	In Vivo
Assessment of turnover (injection of labeled precursor or amine; use of enzyme inhibitors, metabolites, etc.)	Brain dialysis
	Push-pull perfusion
	Voltammetry
Uptake and release	Measurement of precursors, transmitters or metabolites in blood, urine, or cerebrospinal fluid
Measurement of enzyme activity	
Receptor properties	
Cyclic nucleotide function	
Protein phosphorylation	

We have asserted that measurement of steady-state transmitter concentrations alone is often of limited value. There are many experiments showing that drugs that markedly perturb neurotransmission may not change transmitter concentrations per se, as has been clearly demonstrated with cholinergic (Cheney and Costa 1978) and dopaminergic systems (Korf, Grasdijk, and Westerink 1976; Umezu and Moore 1979). The following sections discuss means of assessing neurochemical function that complement the measurement of steady-state concentrations, and these approaches are summarized in table 10.1. It will be obvious that the analytical procedures used for both types of studies may be quite similar.

Synthesis and turnover. To avoid some of the pitfalls previously cited, a cogent strategy to pinpoint the effects of a toxicant on CNS function is to examine its effects on the rates of formation and degradation of the neurotransmitter in question (see Weiner 1974). This can be accomplished via several approaches. For example, a radioactive precursor can be injected and the rate of formation of its metabolites measured. Similarly, neuronal pools can be prelabeled with the radioactive neurotransmitter itself, and the decline in specific activity (or rate of decay) can be determined. Although these methods have the theoretical advantage of not perturbing the system being measured, the values derived from the use of these techniques are influenced by many factors. These include diffusion from the site of injection; blood-brain permeability; equilibration with, or alteration of the size of, endogenous pools of amine; metabolism to compounds other than those being studied; uptake into non-neuronal elements; and different rates of turnover for the same neurotransmitter in different brain regions.

Non-steady-state methods involve the use of drugs as enzyme or transport inhibitors, with concurrent measurement of the rate of accumulation or decline of the amine and its metabolites. Several factors may confound these types of studies, including diffusion out of the brain, the possibility of incomplete inhibition of enzyme activity or metabolite efflux, and secondary effects of enzyme blockade on the elevation of precursor concentrations and feedback inhibition.

Because each of these methods may have a particular disadvantage, sound design necessitates the use of two or more of these approaches in a given study. If several techniques result in similar changes, the resulting conclusions are likely to be owing to actual effects on synthesis or turnover.

Uptake and release. Uptake and release procedures are designed to determine whether toxicants alter the release of neurotransmitters (e.g., from synaptic vesicles or brain slices), or transmitter uptake, a major mechanism of inactivation or recycling. A toxicant could affect the packaging or storage of a neurotransmitter in synaptic vesicles, the transport of the vesicle to the synaptic cleft, or uptake mechanisms involved in recycling of the transmitter. In release studies, either membrane or tissue-slice preparations are used, and an uptake inhibitor may be incorporated (Stoof, Den Breejen, and Mulder 1979; Sanders-Bush and Martin 1982; Schoepp and Azzaro 1982). Release can be induced by either electrical stimulation or exposure to buffers with high concentrations of potassium. Electrical stimulation has an advantage in that the frequency of stimulation can be regulated, and under appropriate conditions release seems to represent solely that of the vesicular neurotransmitter. On the other hand, potassium-induced stimulation may cause release of both the vesicular and the nonvesicular transmitter, and the amount of release cannot be adequately controlled (Vargas et al. 1977). Studies using synaptosomal preparations are technically easier to execute but have the disadvantages of using a homogenate of disrupted nerve cells and of being unstable following prolonged incubation. Tissue slices, however, provide an intact preparation of nerve terminals with which one can study release of a given neurotransmitter, as well as the interactions of two or more transmitter systems coexisting in the same brain region (e.g., DA and ACh in the striatum). Release can also be studied in vivo using push-pull perfusion or voltammetry (see below).

Uptake experiments generally use membrane preparations to determine the rate of accumulation of labeled amine (Baldessarini and Vogt 1971; Komiskey et al. 1978; Marquardt, DiStefano, and Ling 1978; Ross 1982). Uptake is dependent upon transport across the neuronal membrane, vesicular storage, rate of release, and presynaptic monoamine oxidase (MAO) activity. The main confounding factor is that the neurotransmitter can be taken up and bound nonspecifically in other cellular compartments; however, with appropriate assay conditions and pharmacological controls, many of these problems can be overcome.

Enzyme activity. Changes in the characteristics of an enzyme that is critical for neurotransmitter activity, synthesis, or degradation may reflect neurotoxicant-induced perturbations in neuronal activity. The enzymes of most interest are usually those at specific regulatory points (e.g., rate-limiting enzymes). For the monoamine transmitters, methods exist for the assessment of tyrosine hydroxylase (McMillen 1982), dopamine-β-hydroxylase (Wallace, Krantz, and Lovenberg 1973), DOPA decarboxylase, 5-HTP decarboxylase (Melamed, Hefti, and Wurtman 1980), tryptophan hydroxylase (Boadle-Biber 1982), and monoamine oxidase (Garrick and Murphy 1980). The best studies usually determine toxicant effects on kinetic parameters of the enzyme (e.g., changes in K_m, V_{max}), or when a toxicant is an enzyme inhibitor, the rate of reaction or determination of K_i is performed. These studies are most logically part of more global investigations that also measure changes in turnover, release, and so on.

Receptor binding. The radioreceptor assay has become one of the most utilized techniques in neurobiology, and its application to toxicological problems has recently been reviewed (Bondy 1982; DeHaven and Mailman 1983). The radioreceptor assay can be used to assess the effects of prior toxicant exposure on receptor characteristics (e.g., density and affinity) or the ability of the toxicant to interact directly with a receptor population and alter the binding of specific ligands (such as the endogenous transmitter). In general, the methods are simple to execute, but one must be certain that the criteria of saturability, specificity, and reversibility of binding are met and that procedures are followed precisely, since small variations in methodology can often have large effects on binding. Briefly, this approach involves homogenization and washing of brain tissue in buffer at physiological pH, and incubation of tissue with radiolabeled ligand until equilibrium is reached. The addition of an excess of unlabeled drug is used to determine nonspecific binding (i.e., binding to receptors or elements other than those under study). In either case, separation of membrane-bound ligand from free ligand is by filtration or centrifugation, thus terminating the reaction. Table 10.2 summarizes the many assays that have been developed to examine receptors for biogenic amines, amino acids, and neuropeptides (see DeHaven and Mailman 1983).

Cyclic nucleotides and protein phosphorylation. Two biochemical changes initiated, at least in part, by receptor interactions and changes in neuronal activity are alterations in cyclic nucleotide metabolism and changes in the rates and types of protein phosphorylation. For DA (Kebabian, Petzold, and Greengard 1972; Clement-Cormier et al. 1974; Kebabian and Saavedra 1976), serotonin (Pagel et al. 1976; Nelson et al. 1980), and NE (Blumberg et al. 1976; Sulser 1978) receptors, the neurotransmitter indirectly activates the enzyme adenylate cyclase, thus causing the conversion of adenosine triphosphate (ATP) to cyclic adenosine monophosphate (AMP). Cyclic AMP can then influence neuronal transmission by altering the permeability of the neuronal membrane to ions (Nathanson 1977) or by activating protein kinases within the cell, which phosphorylate numerous target proteins, ultimately resulting in changes in protein synthesis within the cell (Greengard 1978) as well as affecting a variety of other biochemical responses. In the CNS, protein phosphorylation might influence the synthesis of neurotransmitter receptors, the regulation of enzymes involved in neurotransmitter synthesis (Kuhn and Lovenberg 1983), or the function of microtubules involved in axon transport (Greengard 1976). In addition, it has been proposed that certain receptor subtypes, such as the D_1 for DA (Kebabian 1978; Kebabian and Calne 1979; Creese et al. 1981) and the S_1 for serotonin (Hamon et al. 1980; Peroutka, Lebovitz, and Synder 1981; Peroutka and Synder 1983), may be linked to adenylate cyclase, while other subtypes of these receptors are not. Thus, examination of these processes provides an additional neurochemical probe for assessing neurotoxicity. It should also be noted that changes in phosphoprotein composition have been reported after behavioral training of several sorts (Routtenberg 1982). Extension of these experiments, in concert with in vitro studies, should be useful in the future.

In Vivo Methods

Brain perfusion and dialysis. Recently, technical breakthroughs have permitted the detection of neurochemical changes in freely moving animals. These techniques and their future modifications should permit verification of hypotheses made using the in vitro methods described earlier. The push-pull perfusion techniques described by Tilson and Sparber (1970) and Myers (1974) have been used to examine synthesis, turnover, and release of neurotransmitters and related compounds in vivo (Sparber and Tilson 1972; Kantak et al. 1978; Leviel et al. 1979). Briefly, a concentric push-pull cannula is implanted into the ventricle or brain.

Table 10.2 Some neurotransmitter receptors and ligands proposed for their study

Neurotransmitter/ Modulator	Ligand	Agonist	Antagonist	Reference
Biogenic Amine Receptors				
Acetylcholine				
Nicotinic	^{125}I-α-bungarotoxin		X	Segal, Dudai, and Amsterdam 1978
	^3H-nicotine	X		Romano and Goldstein 1980
Muscarinic	^3H-QNB		X	Yamamura and Snyder 1974
	^3H-oxotremorine	X		Hulme et al. 1983
Dopamine	^3H-dopamine	X		Creese, Burt, and Snyder 1975
	^3H-ADTN	X		Arana, Baldessarini, and Kula 1982; Templeton and Woodruff 1982
Dopamine D_1	^3H-SCH-23390		X	Billard et al. 1984; Schulz, Wyrick, and Mailman 1985
Dopamine D_2	^3H-sulpiride		X	Freedman, Poat, and Woodruff 1982; Zahnister and Dubocovich 1983
Serotonin S_1	^3H-serotonin	X		Fillion et al. 1978
Serotonin S_2	^3H-ketanserin		X	Leysen et al. 1982
Norepinephrine α_1	^3H-prazosin		X	Greengrass and Bremner 1979; Astrachan, Gallager, and Davis 1983
Norepinephrine α_2	^3H-p-aminoclonidine	X		Rouot and Snyder 1979
Norepinephrine β	^3H-dihydroalprenolol		X	Greenberg, Snyder, and U'Prichard 1976
	^{125}I-iodohydroxy-benzylpindolol		X	Minneman, Hegstrand, and Molinoff 1979
Peptide Receptors				
Opioid peptides μ	^3H-dihydromorphine	X		Chang and Cuatrecasas 1979
	^3H-naloxone		X	Chang et al. 1979
	^3H-sufentanyl	X		Leysen, Gommeron, and Niemegeers 1983
Opioid peptides κ	^3H-ethylketocyclazocine	X		Weyhenmeyer and Mack 1985
Substance P	^{125}I-substance P	X		Saria et al. 1980
Angiotensin II	^{125}I-angiotensin II	X		Lin and Goodfriend 1970; Sirett et al. 1977
Cholecystokinin	^{125}I-cholecystokinin	X		Saito et al. 1980
Neurotensin	^{125}I-neurotensin	X		Uhl, Bennett, and Snyder 1977
Somatostatin	^{125}I-somatostatin	X		Epelbaum et al. 1982
Thyrotropin-releasing hormone	^3H-thyrotropin-releasing hormone	X		Burt and Snyder 1975

Table 10.2 (*continued*)

Neurotransmitter/Modulator	Ligand	Agonist	Antagonist	Reference
Amino Acids and Miscellaneous Compounds				
GABA	^{3}H-GABA	X		Zukin, Young and Snyder 1974; Guidotti et al. 1979
"Benzodiazepine"	^{3}H-muscimol ^{3}H-flunitrazepam	X (? unknown)		Beaumont et al. 1978 Braestrup and Squires 1978; Placheta and Karobath 1979
Glutamate	^{3}H-glutamate	X		Baudry and Lynch 1980
Glycine	^{3}H-strychnine	X		Young and Snyder 1974; Snyder 1975
Taurine	^{3}H-taurine	X		Lopez-Colome 1982; Segawa et al. 1982

Tubing connected to a peristaltic pump is then attached, and a fluid or drug is introduced into the brain region via the cannula and removed at the same time. Flow rate is adjusted so that a given area is continually perfused, and the effluent can be collected and assayed for changes in neurotransmitters, precursors, or metabolites. Recently this technique has been refined by the use of dialysis tubing instead of a steel cannula for implantation (Ungerstedt et al. 1982; Hernandez, Paez, and Hamlin 1983). When assessing synthesis or turnover, these methods suffer from some of the same limitations described previously. In addition, appropriate controls must be included to account for possible effects resulting from the lesions caused by cannula implantations. However, brain perfusion does have several advantages. The concentration and time of administration of the compound to which the tissue is exposed can be accurately controlled. Effects of pharmacological manipulation on specific brain structures or nuclei can be examined, and this can be done in the awake animal in conjunction with behavioral experiments (Sparber and Tilson 1972; Loullis et al. 1980).

In vivo voltammetry. In vivo voltammetry also assesses neurotransmitter function in the unanesthetized animal (Kissinger, Hart, and Adams 1973; Adams 1978). A microelectrode similar to the one used in HPLC analysis is implanted in the brain. A small electric potential is applied to the microelectrode, and the current flow is measured. By altering the potential, typically between 0 and +1.0 V, a curve called a voltammogram is generated. Most catecholamines and indoleamines will oxidize within this range. Peaks in the curve indicate that an endogenous compound is being oxidized, and the potential at which this occurs is indicative of the particular compound being oxidized (see Adams 1978; and Hutson and Curzon 1983).

Some of the initial problems encountered in using this method, such as interference from other endogenous compounds that oxidize at similar potentials and overlapping of peaks that oxidize at the same potential, have been resolved by technical advances (Lane et al. 1976; Brazell and Marsden 1982; Ewing, Wightman, and Dayton 1982). Although the contribution of extraneuronal compounds to the electrical signal that is detected must also be considered (Kennett and Joseph 1982), the advantages offered by this method are numerous. As with brain perfusion and dialysis, one can monitor ongoing processes in the awake animal, but unlike in these techniques, the electrode is the only exogenous element introduced into the brain region under study, thus eliminating the need for perfusion fluid or radioactive tracers. Changes seen by in vivo voltammetry can be verified by HPLC analysis and may be correlated with behavioral changes (Yamamoto, Lane, and Freed 1982). It should be noted that the use of several different strategies to resolve the contributions of the electrochemically active compounds that are present may produce results that are not in agreement, and as with neurochemical turnover studies, several strategies together may ultimately be of the greatest value.

Other body fluids. In any discussion of the relationship between neurochemistry and behavior the issue of clinical studies must also be considered. Clearly, it is not possible to perform the types of invasive studies done in lower mammals in humans. In fact, the methods predominantly used have entailed obtaining blood, cerebrospinal fluid (CSF), or urine and measuring the compounds of interest, much as has been discussed earlier. One important issue has been whether the measurements made in these body fluids are representative of neuronal events occurring in the CNS. Thus, the use of 3-methoxy-4-hydroxyphenylglycol (MHPG) as a monitor of central noradrenergic function (Karoum et al. 1977; DeMet and Halaris 1979; Kopin et al. 1982), 3,4-dihydroxyphenylacetic acid (DOPAC) or homovanillic acid (HVA) as monitors of dopaminergic function (Aizenstein and Korf 1978; Bacopoulos, Hattox, and Roth 1979; Kendler, Heninger, and Roth 1981), and 5-hydroxyindoleacetic acid as a monitor of serotonergic function (Aizenstein and Korf 1979) has been suggested. Although direct examination is always preferable in laboratory studies (see above), it is clear that clinically, sampling of body fluids frequently can provide a useful indicator of neuronal function in the CNS. This approach may have special utility in cases of unavoidable, acute exposure to industrial or environmental toxicants.

Applications in Toxicology

Classical Neurotoxicants

Certain chemicals, such as 6-hydroxydopamine (6-OHDA), and 5,6- and 5,7-dihydroxytryptamine (DHT), cause relatively specific lesions of catecholaminergic and serotonergic neurons, respectively. These neurotoxicants act in presynaptic terminals by initiating oxidative events resulting in changes to neuronal proteins and subsequent degeneration of the nerve terminal (Jonsson 1976; Rotman, Day, and Creveling 1976; Creveling and Rotman 1978). As one would expect, these agents cause decreases in the activities of biosynthetic enzymes (Breese and Traylor 1970; Reis and Molinoff, 1972; Baumgarten and Bjorklund 1976), decreased uptake (Uretsky and Iversen 1970; Slotkin et al. 1978), and decreased concentrations of the affected transmitters in most brain regions (Breese and Traylor 1970, 1971; Uretsky and Iversen 1970; Baumgarten and Bjorklund 1976). These compounds may be considered model neurotoxicants owing to these relatively defined actions, and they have been used to study behavioral and neurochemical phenomena related to neurotransmission in the above systems. This has involved administration of the neurotoxicant into the cerebral ventricles to deplete concentrations of neurotransmitters in the whole brain, as well as infusions into specific brain regions to create lesions in neuronal cell bodies or pathways.

Damage to catecholaminergic neurons caused by administration of 6-OHDA produces a variety of behavioral alterations, many of which are attributable to the resultant depletions of DA. Aphagia and adipsia related to disruption of nigrostriatal dopaminergic fibers have been reported (Ungerstedt 1971b; Fibiger, Zis, and McGeer 1973). Subsequent supersensitivity to apomorphine challenge occurs in adults (Ungerstedt 1971a; Creese and Iversen 1975), and hyperactivity occurs in neonates (Erinoff et al. 1979). Deficits in differential reinforcement of low response rates (DRL) performance (Dunnett and Iversen 1982a), active-avoidance acquisition (Cooper et al. 1973), and self-stimulation (Carey 1982; Cooper, Cott, and Breese 1974) are common, and sensorimotor deficits have also been observed (Dunnett and Iversen 1982b). Resistance to extinction in various learning tasks occurs and is related to loss of NE terminals (Mason 1979).

These behavioral alterations are accompanied by postsynaptic neurochemical changes indicative of a supersensitivity of the neuronal system in question. Treatment with 6-OHDA results in an enhancement of DA-stimulated (Parenti et al. 1982) or NE-stimulated (Jonsson, Wiesel, and Hallman 1979) adenylate cyclase activity and increases the B_{max} for DA receptors in the striatum and NE α_1 and α_2 receptors in the cortex (Creese and Snyder 1979; Mishra, Marshall, and Varmuza 1980; Dausse, LeQuan-Bui, and Meyer 1982). Interestingly, the binding of [^{3}H]-DA agonists shows decreases in both adult (Schweitzer and Bacopoulos 1983) and neonatal rats (Mailman et al., Neonatal 6-OHDA treatment, 1983). As expected, 6-OHDA administration results in subsensitivity to the behavioral effects caused by drugs acting presynaptically, such as amphetamine (Creese and Iversen 1975), as well as supersensitivity to drugs acting postsynaptically, such as apomorphine (Ungerstedt 1971a).

Administration of 5,6-DHT or 5,7-DHT induces behavioral changes related to damage of the serotonergic pathways. Destruction of 5-HT terminals results in hyperphagia (Saller and Stricker 1976; Waldbillig, Bartness, and Stanley 1981), increased locomotor activity (Hole, Fuxe, and Jonsson 1976; Mackenzie et al. 1978; Carter and Pycock 1979) and aggression (Breese et al. 1974; Applegate 1980), and facilitated active-avoidance acquisition (Breese et al. 1974). Rats pretreated with 5,7-DHT are also supersensitive to the behavioral effects of serotonergic agonists in producing the *serotonin syndrome*, characterized by tremor, rigidity, Straub tail, head weaving, and forepaw treading (Trulson, Eubanks, and Jacobs 1976). Although treatment with 5,7-DHT results in increases of B_{max} in the hippocampus as determined by [^{3}H]-metergoline and [^{3}H]-5-HT binding, this receptor supersensitivity does not occur in other regions rich in serotonin receptors (Nelson et al. 1978; Hamon et al. 1981). Thus, the evidence for receptor supersensitivity following DHT treatment is not as strong as for 6-OHDA treatment.

Another promising model neurotoxicant is the compound AF64A (ethylcholine mustard aziridinium ion); studies with it should yield new information on central acetylcholine systems. It is selectively taken up into cholinergic neurons and causes a long-term reduction in high-affinity choline transport sites in some brain regions (Mantione, Fisher, and Hanin 1981), resulting in depleted concentrations of ACh (Fisher et al. 1982). The behavioral effects following AF64A administration include a decreased rate of habituation of motor activity, retention deficits in a passive-avoidance task, and impaired performance in a radial arm maze (Walsh et al. 1984). AF64A should be particularly useful in studying cholinergic substrates of learning and memory.

Although the neurotoxicants discussed above selectively produce lesions in presynaptic nerve terminals of particular neurotransmitters, their actions are not limited to the primary lesions they produce. Administration of 6-OHDA in the substantia nigra also increases glutamic acid decarboxylase activity in the caudate nucleus (Saavedra, Setler, and Kebabian 1978). Injection of 5,7-DHT into the median raphe nucleus or the dorsal raphe nucleus results in increased acetylcholine turnover in the cortex alone or in the hippocampus and the cortex, respectively (Robinson 1983). Intraventricular 5,7-DHT administration reduces the affinity of isoproterenol for β-adrenergic receptors (Manier et al. 1983). Even within a given neurotransmitter system, behavioral sub- or supersensitivity is not always paralleled by receptor changes (Mailman et al. 1981). Therefore, the other indexes of neuronal function previously discussed in this chapter, as well as behavioral testing including pharmacological challenge studies, must be employed in the assessment of neurotoxicity.

Heavy Metals

The studies on the neurochemical and behavioral effects of lead are too numerous to discuss in detail. The reader is referred to reviews by Shih and Hanin (1978), Bornschein, Pearson, and Reiter (1980), Govoni et al. (1980), Memo et al. (1980), and Winder (1982). This section focuses on the controversy concerning the effects of lead during development on activity and dopaminergic function.

Sauerhoff and Michaelson (1973) originally reported that neonatal rats from mothers who had been fed a diet of 4 percent lead carbonate during lactation exhibited increased locomotor activity and decreased levels of whole brain dopamine at about 15 weeks of age. This finding generated a great deal of interest concerning the effects of early lead exposure in rodents and their implications for human exposure. Although these investigators subsequently reported that they were unable to replicate their original finding of changes in DA (Golter and Michaelson 1975), a great deal of experimental effort was devoted to investigating lead-dopaminergic interactions.

Silbergeld and Goldberg (1975) reported increased locomotor activity following lead exposure and found paradoxical effects of amphetamine, fenfluramine, and methylphenidate on locomotor activity, with administration of these compounds causing a lesser increase in the activity of lead-treated versus control mice. The suggestion that lead toxicity may be a model for studying hyperactivity and minimal brain dysfunction (Silbergeld and Goldberg 1974) led numerous investigators to attempt replication of these findings, generally without success (see Bornschein, Pearson, and Reiter 1980). At least one factor confounding the early Silbergeld and Goldberg studies was possible undernutrition of the treated animals, which in itself will result in hyperactivity (Castellano and Oliverio 1976).

Lead exposure has been reported to result in altered responding to an amphetamine challenge (Sobotka and Cook 1974; Gray and Reiter 1977; Reiter et al. 1977). In mice, Rafales and coworkers (1979) found that neonatal lead exposure produced an attenuated increase in activity in response to d-amphetamine or apomorphine challenge. This latter group also demonstrated an attenuated d-amphetamine response in rats using a drug-discrimination paradigm (Zenick and Goldsmith 1981). However, in male rats a d-amphetamine challenge increased the activity of lead-treated animals compared with controls (Rafales et al. 1981).

Owing to these findings, attention has focused upon the dopaminergic system as a locus for the effects of lead on the CNS. Decreases in concentrations of DA (on the order of 20 percent) occur in the cortex, the midbrain, and the hypothalamus (Dubas and Hrdina 1978). Decreases in striatal concentrations of DOPAC and HVA (Govoni et al. 1978) and increases in concentrations of DOPAC in the nucleus accumbens (Memo et al. 1981) have been reported. Govoni and coworkers (1979) found decreased striatal DA synthesis and increased DA synthesis in the nucleus accumbens and the frontal cortex, respectively. Neonatal lead exposure has been reported to decrease DA turnover in the striatum at day 35 of life (Jason and Kellogg 1981). Using [^{3}H]-sulpiride as the ligand, an increased B_{max} of DA receptors in the striatum, and a decreased B_{max} of DA receptors in the nucleus accumbens (Lucchi et al. 1981) suggested to these investigators that lead may preferentially affect D_2 receptors. Apomorphine-stimulated activity of the striatal adenylate cyclase was decreased in lead-treated animals (Wince, Donovan, and Azzaro 1980). However, in most cases investigators failed to detect permanent neurochemical consequences after lead exposure had ceased.

Our laboratory has also investigated the effects of lead on dopaminergic systems. We use a dosing paradigm where neonatal rats are intubated from day 2 to day 29 (day of birth = day 0) with 200 mg/kg lead acetate. When these animals are tested as adults for the occurrence of lithium-induced polydipsia (LIP), the lead-treated animals exhibit an exaggerated drinking response compared with controls (Mailman et al. 1978). This effect has been reliably reproduced, is present in the absence of overt toxicity or other effects, and persists for months after cessation of lead administration. A single administration of lead on either day 5 or day 15 of life also results in persistent increased LIP in adult rats (DeHaven et al. 1984). Recent work has shown that contrary to earlier beliefs, LIP is mediated in the CNS, not peripherally (Mailman 1983; Smith and Amdisen 1983), and is dependent upon an intact nigrostriatal dopaminergic pathway (Mailman 1983). This has led us to focus on the striatum as a possible locus for changes in dopaminergic function. We have failed to find alterations in DA or its acidic metabolites DOPAC and HVA following lead exposure in animals not being treated with lithium at time of sacrifice. In addition, we have not found significant changes in the B_{max} of striatal DA receptors using [^{3}H]-spiperone as the radioligand (DeHaven and Mailman, unpublished data). Currently studies are under way to examine neurochemical indexes of dopaminergic function during lithium challenge to elucidate the possible mechanisms underlying this phenomenon. Although the available evidence indicates a role for dopaminergic systems in the neurotoxicity of lead, the exact nature of this dysfunction remains unknown.

The finding that symptoms of manganese poisoning resemble Parkinson's disease (Cotzias et al. 1974) suggested a role for dopaminergic systems in manganese neurotoxicity. Administration of manganese resulted in decreased levels of DA in the brain (ibid.) which occurred selectively in the striatum and were accompanied by a decrease in turnover in this region (Autissier et al. 1982). Treatment of adult rats with 10 mg/kg manganese chloride for 15 days resulted in increased striatal [^{3}H]-spiperone binding (Seth et al. 1981). At 15 mg/kg, decreases were seen in striatal [³H]-QNB binding, frontal cortical [³H]-5-HT binding, and cerebellar [³H]-muscimol binding. Exposure to manganese via the drinking water also increased [³H]-spiperone binding in the striatum and decreased [³H]-muscimol binding in the hippocampus (Gerhart and Tilson 1982). In rats exposed neonatally to manganese, decreases in DA concentrations and tyrosine hydroxylase activity and increases in MAO activity occurred in the hypothalamus (Deskin, Bursian, and Edens 1980). It has been suggested that manganese toxicity in dopaminergic neurons may result in part from its ability to oxidize DA (Donaldson, LaBella, and Gesser 1980), although it clearly affects the function of other neurotransmitter systems as well.

Rats administered cadmium exhibited decreases in serotonin levels in the brainstem and increases in concentrations of DA and ACh in the striatum and the cortex (Singhal, Merali, and Hrdina 1976). Cadmium exposure via the drinking water resulted in decreased [³H]-QNB binding in the striatum and the cerebral cortex (Hedlund, Gamarra, and Bartfai 1979), and this was also reported in rat pups whose mothers were exposed to cadmium (Donaldson et al. 1981). In addition, cadmium has been reported to inhibit [³H]-imipramine binding in the hypothalamus both in vitro and in vivo (Peterson and Bartfai 1983). From the above data, it is evident that exposure to inorganic heavy metals causes a variety of neurochemical alterations that include, but are not limited to, dopaminergic systems. Not surprisingly, these changes are not similar for all toxic metals.

Insecticides and Pesticides

The insecticide chlordimeform belongs to a class of compounds known as the formamidines. Chlordimeform, demonstrated to be an effective inhibitor of MAO, caused marked increases in levels of serotonin, and to a lesser extent NE, in the whole brain (Beeman and Matsumura 1973). Pfister et al. (1978) found similarities between the behavioral effects of chlordimeform and para-chloroamphetamine (pCA), a drug that initially causes 5-HT release, leading to a neurotoxicity owing to depletion of 5-HT (Fuller 1982). Both chlordimeform and pCA induced the serotonin syndrome, as well as circling and backing, salivation, hyperreflexia, hyperactivity, and hyperreactivity. Some of the pCA- and chlordimeform-elicited behaviors were reduced by treatment with the serotonin antagonists cinanserin and methysergide, respectively.

Pyrethroid insecticides characteristically produce seizures, tremor, and choreoathetoid movements upon administration (Ray and Cremer 1979), as well as decreases in motor activity and differential effects on the acoustic startle response (Crofton and Reiter 1984). Deltamethrin or fenvalerate neurotoxicity is attenuated by diazepam (Gammon, Lawrence, and Casida 1982), and diazepam and aminooxyacetic acid attenuate the neurotoxicity of permethrin (Staatz, Bloom, and Lech 1982a). Because pyrethroids affect dihydropicrotoxinin (Leeb-Lundberg and Olsen 1980) and kainic acid (Staatz, Bloom, and Lech 1982b) binding sites in the CNS pyrethroids may act centrally via GABAergic or glutaminergic mechanisms. This view has recently been substantiated by the report of Lawrence and Casida (1983), who found that various pyrethroids inhibited binding of ³⁵S-(+)-butyl-bicyclophosphorothionate to the picrotoxinin site of the GABA receptor complex.

Intoxication with chlordecone (Kepone®) has a variety of effects in the CNS, including decreases in DA in the whole brain and the striatum, increased utilization of serotonin in various brain regions, decreased uptake of catecholamines and GABA in mouse brain synaptosomes, and decreased levels of met-enkephalin in the pituitary and of beta-endorphin in the hypothalamus (Desaiah 1982). The major behavioral effect of chlordecone exposure is a persistent tremor (Taylor et al. 1978), which in rats is antagonized by cholinergic and serotonergic antagonists, suggesting a role for these systems in the expression of this tremor (Gerhart et al. 1982). This idea was supported by the observation that chlordecone administration caused a dose- and time-related increase in striatal 5-HIAA that was correlated with the degree of tremor (Hong et al. 1983).

The ability of organophosphates to inhibit acetylcholinesterase activity has been well documented (see Murphy 1980; and Costa, Schwab, and Murphy 1982b). Several investigators have demonstrated that compounds such as diiso-propylfluorophosphate (DFP) (Schiller 1979; Uchida et al. 1979; Ehlert, Kokka, and Fairhurst 1980), disulfoton (Costa et al. 1981; Schwab et al. 1981; Costa, Schwab, and Murphy 1982a), paraoxon (Smit et al. 1980), and Tetram (Gazit, Silman, and Dudai 1979) caused decreases in B_{max} of the muscarinic receptors. Tolerance to organophosphates develops upon chronic administration, and it has been postulated that this tolerance is due to receptor subsensitivity (Costa, Schwab, and Murphy 1982b). Tolerance to the behavioral changes induced by these compounds also occurs—for example, to the effects of DFP on drinking (Chippendale et al. 1972), fixed-ratio responding (Russell et al. 1975), and single-alternation behavior (Overstreet et al. 1974), as well as to the antinociceptive and hypothermic effects of disulfoton (Costa, Schwab, and Murphy 1982a) and to the effects of paraoxon on two-way-avoidance responding (Giardini et al. 1982). Thus, for organophosphate neurotoxicity, there is a clear correlation between the neurochemical changes in cholinergic systems and the behavioral tolerance resulting from exposure to these compounds.

Organometals

Methylmercury exposure affects catecholaminergic and serotonergic systems. Neonatal exposure to 2.5 or 5 mg/kg methylmercury daily for 21 days resulted in increased DA turnover followed by persistent decreases in synaptosomal [³H]-DA uptake after 20 days of age (Bartolome et al. 1982). Increases in turnover and steady-state levels of NE were also noted. Taylor and DiStefano (1976) administered 5 mg/kg methylmercury to rats on days 5, 6, and 7 postpartum and found decreases in whole-brain concentrations of tryptophan, 5-HT, 5-HIAA, DA, and NE and decreased tryptophan hydroxylase activity and 5-HT turnover at day 8. Increases in 5-HT, 5-HIAA, DA, and NE concentrations were seen at day 15, and the increase in serotonin persisted to day 60. Inhibition of uptake, as well as stimulation of release of DA, 5-HT, and NE, has also been observed following methylmercury exposure (Komulainen and Tuomisto 1981).

Behavioral effects also occur after early exposure to methylmercury. Pregnant rats administered 5 or 8 mg/kg methylmercury on day 8 or 15 of gestation produced offspring that exhibited increased activity within 15 days after parturition (Eccles and Annau 1982a). These investigators also observed deficits in two-way avoidance learning when animals were tested as adults (Eccles and Annau 1982b). Mice treated with 8 mg/kg methylmercury on day 7 or 9 of gestation produced offspring that exhibited differences in open-field behavior, neuromuscular impairment, and abnormal swimming behavior when tested at one month of age (Spyker, Sparber, and Goldberg 1972). Offspring of rat dams exposed to methylmercury during gestation or during the first 9 days after parturition displayed learning deficits in a water-escape T-maze when tested at 4 or 7 weeks of age (Zenick 1974).

Exposure of adult rats to methylmercury resulted in decreased levels of tyrosine in the whole brain at total doses of 5 and 50 mg/kg and decreased DA turnover at 5, 15, and 50 mg/kg (Sharma, Aldous, and Farr 1982). When animals were dosed with 4 mg/kg for 50 days, concentrations of DA were increased in the hypothalamus, the pons-medulla, the brainstem, and the striatum, and there was a corresponding decrease in concentrations of DOPAC in these regions (Tsuzuki 1982). Levels of NE were increased in the brainstem and the striatum, whereas 5-HT and 5-HIAA were decreased in the hypothalamus, the striatum, and the brainstem, with 5-HIAA being lower in the pons-medulla. A single dose of methylmercury also caused changes in benzodiazepine receptors as determined by [^{3}H]-diazepam binding. An increased B_{max} occurred at three days post-dosing in the striatum, the cortex, and the cerebellum, and this increase persisted for up to ten days in the cerebellum (Corda et al. 1981). Because of the variety of neurochemical effects associated with exposure to methylmercury, it is difficult to ascertain those that may be responsible for the behavioral effects caused by methylmercury.

Intoxication with trimethyltin (TMT) affects the neurochemistry of both developing and adult animals. Neonatal rats dosed with TMT hydroxide (1 mg/kg every other day, days 3–30) and sacrificed at 55 days of age showed decreases in hippocampal GABA, with a trend toward decreases in the cerebellum, the brainstem, the hypothalamus, and the striatum. Levels of DA in the striatum were also decreased (Mailman et al., Effects, 1983). In adults, administration of 4.26 mg/kg in mice decreased forebrain synaptosomal GABA and 5-HT uptake at 2 and 14 hours after dosing (Doctor et al. 1982), and dose-dependent effects of TMT on hippocampal [^{3}H]-GABA uptake have also been observed in rats (Valdes et al. 1983). In vitro uptake of GABA and 5-HT as well as NE is inhibited by TMT (Doctor et al. 1982). Acute administration of 7 mg/kg TMT to rats resulted in elevated levels of 5-HIAA and an elevated 5-HIAA/5-HT ratio, suggesting increased 5-HT turnover at 7 days post-dosing in a variety of brain regions (DeHaven, Walsh, and Mailman 1984). These changes also occur to a lesser extent in animals given 3 mg/kg. The alterations in serotonergic function at 7 mg/kg are still present at days 14, 21, and 28 following exposure (DeHaven, Krigman, and Mailman 1983) and may be permanent. Decreases in mesolimbic concentrations of DA at days 7, 14, and 21 are also evident. Further, decreases in protein phosphorylation occur in the hippocampus following exposure of both neonatal and adult rats to TMT (Miller and O'Callaghan 1984; O'Callaghan and Miller 1984).

The behavioral effects of TMT have been extensively investigated and are similar in some respects to those observed after alterations in the GABA, serotonin, and dopamine systems. Acute administration of this compound produces a *behavioral syndrome* characterized by aggression, hyperactivity, hyperreactivity, self-mutilation, and spontaneous seizures (Dyer et al. 1982). Permanent effects include memory deficits (Walsh et al. 1982; Walsh, Miller, and Dyer 1982), increases in open-field (Swartzwelder et al. 1981) and figure-eight maze activity (Ruppert et al. 1982), and increased perseverative responding on a fixed-ratio operant schedule (Swartzwelder et al. 1981). Although these effects may be mediated by the neurochemical changes that occur, some of these behavioral alterations might also be a direct result of the hippocampal lesions produced by TMT (Dyer et al. 1982).

Acrylamide

Investigations into the neurotoxicity of acrylamide have focused upon dopaminergic systems. Dixit et al. (1981) originally observed that administration of 25 mg/kg acrylamide daily for 21 days resulted in decreased levels of DA, NE, and 5-HT in the whole brain and increased MAO activity. Examination of regional changes after administration of 50 mg/kg for 5 days revealed decreased NE content of the basal ganglia and the pons-medulla, decreased 5-HT content of the pons-medulla and the hypothalamus, and decreased DA content of the cerebellum, the pons-medulla, and the hypothalamus. With respect to DA receptors, acrylamide given to pregnant rats (20 mg/kg from days 7 to 16 of gestation) caused decreased striatal [^{3}H]-spiperone binding (Agrawal and Squibb 1981). In adults, 50, 100, or 200 mg/kg acrylamide acutely, or daily doses of 10, 20, or 30 mg/kg for 10 days, increased striatal [^{3}H]-spiperone binding (Agrawal, Squibb, and Bondy 1981). In later studies this increase was also observed after 25 or 50 mg/kg acrylamide, and at 100 mg/kg there occurred increased [^{3}H]-strychnine binding in the medulla and [^{3}H]-5-HT binding in the frontal cortex (Agrawal et al. 1981). With repeated administration of 5, 10, or 20 mg/kg for 2 weeks, there was increased striatal [^{3}H]-spiperone and [^{3}H]-QNB binding at all doses (Bondy, Tilson, and Agrawal 1981). Increases in frontal cortical [^{3}H]-5-HT binding, medullar [^{3}H]-strychnine binding, and cerebellar [^{3}H]-muscimol binding were also observed. In a study by Uphouse and Russell (1981), the changes in [^{3}H]-spiperone and [^{3}H]-5-HT binding following acrylamide exposure were rapid in nature, appearing as soon as a half-hour after dosing. Handling also affected acrylamide toxicity (Uphouse 1981).

In two of these studies (Agrawal et al. 1981; Bondy, Tilson, and Agrawal 1981) attempts were made to correlate the effects of acute and chronic acrylamide on DA receptors with changes in locomotor activity following an apomorphine challenge. Acrylamide pretreatment significantly attenuated the increase in activity seen after apomorphine administration. In the chronic dosing regimen these changes were not evident at 8 days following the last acrylamide dose (Bondy, Tilson, and Agrawal 1981). However, the decreased behavioral sensitivity to the dopaminergic agonist apomorphine does not correlate with the observed up-regulation of dopaminergic receptors. Decreases in nocturnal running-wheel activity were also reported following acrylamide exposure (Rafales, Bornschein, and Caruso 1982). This group noted that the locomotor activity induced by amphetamine was greater in acrylamide-treated rats than in control rats and may be related to the alterations in dopaminergic receptors reported by Bondy and coworkers.

Operant performance is also affected by acrylamide treatment. Responding under a fixed-ratio 30 schedule decreased following a cumulative dose of at least 70 mg/kg acrylamide (Tilson, Cabe, and Burne 1980), and responding returned to control levels following cessation of dosing. Using a variable-interval 15-second schedule of reinforcement, Tilson and Squibb (1982) found that doses of 25, 50, or 100 mg/kg suppressed responding. Decreased responding following an apomorphine or amphetamine challenge was accentuated by pretreatment with 12.5 mg/kg acrylamide, a dose that by itself had no effect on responding. These effects were not observed following clonidine or chlordiazepoxide challenge.

Miscellaneous Compounds

Exposure to carbon disulfide (CS_2) decreased levels of NE and increased levels of DA in the whole brain (Magos 1970; Magos, Green, and Jarvis 1974; McKenna and DiStefano 1977). This apparently resulted from the ability of CS_2 to inhibit dopamine-β-hydroxylase activity (McKenna and DiStefano 1977). The elevated concentrations of DA caused by exposure to CS_2 were linked to increases in amphetamine-induced stereotypy (Magos, Green, and Jarvis 1974) and apomorphine-induced stereotypy (Magos 1976), although the latter data clearly require a different explanation.

Polychlorinated biphenyls (PCBs) also affect brain neurochemistry. Spontaneous release of [^{3}H]-DA, [^{3}H]-NE, [^{3}H]-5-HT, and [^{3}H]-ACh was enhanced as a result of Aroclor 1254 administration (Rosin and Martin 1981), and inhibition of precursor and neurotransmitter uptake was noted. Rosin and Martin also observed decreased spontaneous locomotor activity after a single dose of Aroclor 1254 which subsequently returned to control levels. Mice exposed to 3,4,3',4'-tetra-chlorobiphenyl (TCB) in utero exhibited a "spinning" syndrome characterized by head jerking and bobbing, hyperactivity, and stereotypic circling (Chou et al. 1979). These impairments persisted into adulthood, and mice also displayed decreased forelimb grip strength, decreased ability to traverse a wire rod, and deficits in one-way-avoidance acquisition following TCB exposure (Tilson et al. 1979). Administration of d-amphetamine or apomorphine to these animals resulted in increased spinning at low doses, whereas high doses decreased spinning (Chou et al. 1979). Haloperidol effectively blocked the spinning behavior. Administration of TCB to pregnant mice resulted in decreased DA levels and receptor binding sites in offspring sacrificed at one year of age (Agrawal, Tilson, and Bondy 1981), further supporting a dopaminergic involvement in the action of this compound.

Exposure to toluene has been demonstrated to affect catecholaminergic and serotonergic systems. Studies using catecholamine fluorescence observed that exposure to this solvent caused increased levels of catecholamines in the median eminence and increased turnover in this region, as well as in the periventricular nucleus and the paraventricular hypothalamic nucleus (Andersson et al. 1980). In the caudate nucleus, decreased DA turnover occurred, and decreased levels of DA in the caudate nucleus and the nucleus accumbens were observed (Fuxe et al. 1982). Yamawaki, Segawa, and Sarai (1982) described the appearance of behaviors resembling the serotonin syndrome following toluene exposure. [^{3}H]-5-HT binding was decreased in the hippocampus and the pons-medulla with chronic exposure.

Summary

In the previous sections we have seen that a wide variety of neurochemical techniques for the assessment of neurotoxicity are available, as well as how these techniques have been employed in the study of several neurotoxic compounds. It has been emphasized that neurochemical changes not specific to certain neurotransmitter systems often result from toxicant exposure and that even the so-called specific neurotoxins such as 6-OHDA and 5,7-DHT will cause alterations in other neurotransmitter systems. Owing to this lack of specificity, it has proven difficult to classify neurotoxicants based on their neurochemical sequelae, and, in fact, such an endpoint should not be expected. The ideal approach to the study of neurotoxicity is to combine appropriate neurochemical techniques with tests assessing those behaviors affected by the neurochemical changes observed. The goal of such a direction should be mechanistic rather than simply phenomenological. An especially useful first step is to employ pharmacological challenges that examine the neurotransmitter systems in question. This multifaceted strategy provides important information in evaluating the neurotoxicity of a particular compound, and what is more important, it can provide clues for more detailed biochemical and neurochemical studies. It should be evident from the data outlined in this chapter that almost all of the available neurochemical studies on neurotoxicological problems have been phenomenological rather than hypothesis-oriented (and we include ourselves in this criticism). Although this is sometimes necessary, it seems more rewarding to use available clues (such as from behavioral toxicology) to attempt to elucidate the neurobiological mechanisms of toxicant-induced changes in behaviors. It is hoped that the approaches summarized in this chapter will aid in future efforts in this direction.

Acknowledgments

Research conducted in the laboratory of the authors and cited herein was supported in part by USPHS grants ES-01104, training grants ES-07126 and MH-14277, and EPA Cooperative Agreement CR-809644. The authors thank John Petitto, John Canipe, David Knight, and Emily Halpern for technical assistance, Dr. Jeffrey Gaynor for statistical analysis, and Theresa Brooks for the preparation of this manuscript.

References

Adams, R. N. 1978. *In vivo* electrochemical recording—a new neurophysiological approach. *Trends NeuroSci.* 1:160–63.

Agrawal, A. K.; Seth P. K.; Squibb, R. E.; Tilson, H. A.; Uphouse, L. L.; and Bondy, S. C. 1981. Neurotransmitter receptors in brain regions of acrylamide-treated rats. I: Effects of a single exposure to acrylamide. *Pharmacol. Biochem. Behav.* 14:527–31.

Agrawal, A. K., and Squibb, R. E. 1981. Effects of acrylamide given during gestation on dopamine receptor binding in rat pups. *Toxicol. Lett.* 7:233–38.

Agrawal, A. K.; Squibb, R. E.; and Bondy, S. C. 1981. The effects of acrylamide treatment upon the dopamine receptor. *Toxicol. Appl. Pharmacol.* 58:89–99.

Agrawal, A. K.; Tilson, H. A.; and Bondy, S. C. 1981. 3,4,3'4'-Tetra-chlorobiphenyl given to mice prenatally produces long-term decreases in striatal dopamine and receptor binding sites in the caudate nucleus. *Toxicol. Lett.* 7:417–24.

Aizenstein, M. L., and Korf, J. 1978. Aspects of influx and efflux of rat cerebrospinal fluid. *Brain Res.* 149:129–40.

———. 1979. On the elimination of centrally formed 5-hydroxyindoleacetic acid by cerebrospinal fluid and urine. *J. Neurochem.* 32:1227–33.

Andersson, K.; Fuxe, K.; Toftgard, R.; Nilsen, O. G.; Eneroth, P.; and Gustafsson, J. A. 1980. Toluene-induced activation of certain hypothalamic and median eminence catecholamine nerve terminal systems of the male rat and its effects on anterior pituitary hormone secretion. *Toxicol. Lett.* 5:393–98.

Applegate, C. D. 1980. 5,7-dihydroxytryptamine-induced mouse killing and behavioral reversal with ventricular administration of serotonin in rats. *Behav. Neural Biol.* 30:178–90.

Arana, G. W.; Baldessarini, R. J.; and Kula, N. S. 1982. Differential effects of ascorbate and EDTA on high-affinity binding of ^{3}H-apomorphine and ^{3}H-ADTN to calf caudate membranes. *Neuropharmacology* 21:601–4.

Astrachan, D. I.; Gallager, D. W.; and Davis, M. 1983. Behavior and binding: Desensitization to α_1-adrenergic stimulation of acoustic startle is associated with a decrease in α_1-adrenoreceptor binding sites. *Brain Res.* 276:183–87.

Autissier, N.; Rochette, L.; Dumas, P.; Beley, A.; Loireau, A.; and Bralat, J. 1982. Dopamine and norepinephrine turnover in various regions of the rat brain after chronic manganese chloride administration. *Toxicology* 24:175–82.

Bacopoulos, N. G.; Hattox, S. E.; and Roth, R. H. 1979. 3,4-dihydroxyphenylacetic acid and homovanillic acid in rat plasma: Possible indicators of central dopaminergic activity. *Eur. J. Pharmacol.* 56:225–36.

Baldessarini, R. J., and Vogt, M. 1971. The uptake and subcellular distribution of aromatic amines in the brain of the rat. *J. Neurochem.* 18:2519–33.

Barrett, R. W., and Vaught, J. L. 1983. Evaluation of the interactions of mu and delta selective ligands with [^{3}H]D-Ala^2-D-Leu^5-enkephalin binding to mouse brain membranes. *Life Sci.* 33:2439–48.

Bartolome, J.; Trepanier, P.; Chait, E. A.; Seidler, F. J.; Deskin, R.; and Slotkin, T. A. 1982. Neonatal methylmercury poisoning in the rat: Effects on development of central catecholamine neurotransmitter systems. *Toxicol. Appl. Pharmacol.* 65:92–99.

Baudry, M., and Lynch, G. 1980. Regulation of hippocampal glutamate receptors: Evidence for the involvement of a calcium-activated protease. *Proc. Natl. Acad. Sci. U.S.A.* 77:2298–2302.

Baumgarten, H. G., and Bjorklund, A. 1976. Neurotoxic indoleamines and monoamine neurons. *Annu. Rev. Pharmacol. Toxicol.* 16:101–11.

Beaumont, K.; Chilton, W. S.; Yamamura, H. I.; and Enna, S. J. 1978. Muscimol binding in rat brain: Association with synaptic GABA receptors. *Brain Res.* 148:153–62.

Beeman, R. W., and Matsumura, F. 1973. Chlordimeform: A pesticide acting upon regulatory mechanisms. *Nature* 242:273–74.

Billard, W.; Ruperto, V.; Crosby, G.; Iorio, L. C.; and Barnett, A. 1984. Characterization of the binding of ^{3}H-SCH 23390, a selective D-1 receptor antagonist ligand, in rat striatum. *Life Sci.* 35:1885–93.

Blumberg, J. B.; Vetulani, J.; Stawarz, R. J.; and Sulser, F. 1976. The noradrenergic cyclic AMP generating system in the limbic forebrain: Pharmacological characterization *in vitro* and possible role of limbic noradrenergic mechanisms in the mode of action of antipsychotics. *Eur. J. Pharmacol.* 37:357–66.

Boadle-Biber, M. C. 1982. Biosynthesis of serotonin. In *Biology of serotonergic transmission,* edited by N. N. Osborne, 63–94. New York: John Wiley & Sons.

Bondy, S. C. 1982. Neurotransmitter binding interactions as a screen for neurotoxicity. In *Mechanisms of actions of neurotoxic substances,* edited by K. N. Prasad and A. Vernadakis, 25–50. New York: Raven Press.

Bondy, S. C.; Tilson, H. A.; and Agrawal, A. K. 1981. Neurotransmitter receptors in brain regions of acrylamide-treated rats. II: Effects of extended exposure to acrylamide. *Pharmacol. Biochem. Behav.* 14:533–37.

Bornschein, R.; Pearson, D.; and Reiter, L. 1980. Behavioral effects of moderate lead exposure in children and animal models: Part 2, animal studies. *CRC Crit. Rev. Toxicol.* 8:101–52.

Braestrup, C., and Squires, R. F. 1978. Brain specific benzodiazepine receptors. *Brit. J. Psychiatry* 133:249–60.

Brazell, M. P., and Marsden, C. A. 1982. Differential pulse voltammetry in the anaesthetized rat: Identification of ascorbic acid, catechol and indoleamine oxidation peaks in the striatum and frontal cortex. *Br. J. Pharmacol.* 75:539–47.

Breese, G. R.; Cooper, B. R.; Grant, L. D.; and Smith, R. D. 1974. Biochemical and behavioral alterations following 5,6-dihydroxytryptamine administration into brain. *Neuropharmacology* 13:177–87.

Breese, G. R., and Traylor, T. D. 1970. Effect of 6-hydroxydopamine on brain norepinephrine and dopamine: Evidence for selective degeneration of catecholamine neurons. *J. Pharmacol. Exp. Ther.* 174:413–20.

————. 1971. Depletion of brain noradrenaline and dopamine by 6-hydroxydopamine. *Br. J. Pharmacol.* 42:88–99.

Burt, D. R., and Snyder, S. H. 1975. Thyrotropin releasing hormone (TRH): Apparent receptor binding in rat brain membranes. *Brain Res.* 93:309–28.

Carey, R. J. 1982. Unilateral 6-hydroxydopamine lesions of dopamine neurons produce bilateral self-stimulation deficits. *Behav. Brain Res.* 6:101–14.

Carter, C. J., and Pycock, C. J. 1979. The effects of 5,7-dihydroxytryptamine lesions of extrapyramidal and mesolimbic sites on spontaneous motor behavior and amphetamine-induced stereotypy. *Naunyn Schmiedebergs Arch. Pharmacol.* 308:51–54.

Castellano, C., and Oliverio, A. 1976. Early malnutrition and postnatal changes in brain and behavior in the mouse. *Brain Res.* 101:317–25.

Caudill, W. L.; Houck, G. P.; and Wightman, R. M. 1982. Determination of gamma-aminobutyric acid by liquid chromatography with electrochemical detection. *J. Chromatogr.* 227:331–39.

Chang, K. J.; Cooper, B. R.; Hazum, E.; and Cuatrecasas, P. 1979. Multiple opiate receptors: Different regional distribution in the brain and differential binding of opiates and opioid peptides. *Mol. Pharmacol.* 16:91–104.

Chang, K. J., and Cuatrecasas, P. 1979. Multiple opiate receptors: Enkephalins and morphine bind to receptors of different specificity. *J. Biol. Chem.* 254:2610–18.

Cheney, D. L., and Costa, E. 1978. Biochemical pharmacology of cholinergic neurons. In *Psychopharmacology: A generation of progress*, edited by M. A. Lipton, A. DiMascio, and K. F. Killam, 283–91. New York: Raven Press.

Chippendale, T. J.; Zawolkow, G. A.; Russell, R. W.; and Overstreet, D. H. 1972. Tolerance to low acetylcholinesterase levels: Modification of behavior without acute behavioral change. *Psychopharmacology* (Berlin) 26:127–39.

Chou, S. M.; Miike, T.; Payne, W. M.; and Davis, G. J. 1979. Neuropathology of "spinning syndrome" induced by prenatal intoxication with a PCB in mice. *Ann. N.Y. Acad. Sci.* 320:373–95.

Clement-Cormier, Y. C.; Kebabian, J. W.; Petzold, G. L.; and Greengard, P. 1974. Dopamine-sensitive adenylate cyclase in mammalian brain: A possible site of action of antipsychotic drugs. *Proc. Natl. Acad. Sci. U.S.A.* 71:1113–17.

Cooper, B. R.; Breese, G. R.; Grant, L. D.; and Howard, J. L. 1973. Effects of 6-hydroxydopamine treatments on active avoidance responding: Evidence for involvement of dopamine. *J. Pharmacol. Exp. Ther.* 185:358–70.

Cooper, B. R.; Cott, J. M.; and Breese, G. R. 1974. Effects of catecholamine-depleting drugs and amphetamine on self-stimulation of brain following various 6-hydroxydopamine treatments. *Psychopharmacologia* 37:235–48.

Corda, M. G.; Concas, A.; Rossetti, Z.; Guarneri, P.; Corongiu, F. P.; and Biggio, G. 1981. Methylmercury enhances [^{3}H]-diazepam binding in different areas of the rat brain. *Brain Res.* 229:264–69.

Costa, L. G.; Schwab, B. W.; Hand, H.; and Murphy, S. D. 1981. Reduced [^{3}H]-quinuclidinyl benzilate binding to muscarinic receptors in disulfoton-tolerant mice. *Toxicol. Appl. Pharmacol.* 60:441–50.

Costa, L. G.; Schwab, B. W.; and Murphy, S. D. 1982*a*. Differential alterations of cholinergic muscarinic receptors during chronic and acute tolerance to organophosphorus insecticides. *Biochem. Pharmacol.* 31:3407–13.

————. 1982*b*. Tolerance to anticholinesterase compounds in mammals. *Toxicology* 25:79–97.

Cotzias, G. C.; Papavasiliou, P. S.; Mena, I.; Tang, L. D.; and Miller, S. T. 1974. Manganese and catecholamines. *Adv. Neurol.* 5:235–43.

Creese, I.; Burt, D. R.; and Snyder, S. H. 1975. Dopamine receptor binding: Differentiation of agonists and antagonist states with ^{3}H-dopamine and ^{3}H-haloperidol. *Life Sci.* 17:993–1002.

Creese, I., and Iversen, S. D. 1975. The pharmacological and anatomical substrates of the amphetamine response in the rat. *Brain Res.* 83:419–36.

Creese, I.; Sibley, D. R.; Leff, S.; and Hamblin, M. 1981. Dopamine receptors: Subtypes, localization and regulation. *Fed. Proc.* 40:147–52.

Creese, I., and Snyder, S. H. 1979. Nigrostriatal lesions enhance striatal ^{3}H-apomorphine and ^{3}H-spiroperidol binding. *Eur. J. Pharmacol.* 56:277–81.

Creveling, C. R., and Rotman, A., 1978. Mechanism of action of dihydroxytryptamines. *Ann. N.Y. Acad. Sci.* 305:57–73.

Crofton, K. M., and Reiter, L. W. 1984. Effects of two pyrethroid insecticides on motor activity and the acoustic startle response in the rat. *Toxicol. Appl. Pharmacol.* 75:318–28.

Crombeen, J. P.; Kraak, J. C.; and Poppe, H. 1978. Reversed phase systems for the analysis of catecholamines and related compounds by high-performance liquid chromatography. *J. Chromatogr.* 167:219–30.

Dausse, J. P.; LeQuan-Bui, K. H.; and Meyer, P. 1982. Effect of neonatal 6-hydroxydopamine treatment on α_1- and α_2-adrenoceptors in rat cerebral cortex. *J. Cardiovasc. Pharmacol.* 4:S86–S90.

DeHaven, D. L.; Krigman, M. R.; Gaynor, J. J.; and Mailman, R. B. 1984. The effects of lead administration during development on lithium-induced polydipsia and dopaminergic function. *Brain Res.* 297:297–304.

DeHaven, D. L.; Krigman, M. R.; and Mailman, R. B. 1983. Temporal changes in dopaminergic and serotonergic function caused by administration of trimethyltin to adult rats. *Soc. Neurosci. Abs.* 9:671.

DeHaven, D. L.; and Mailman, R. B. 1983. The use of radioligand binding techniques in neurotoxicology. *Rev. Biochem. Toxicol.* 5:193–238.

DeHaven, D. L.; Walsh, T. J.; and Mailman, R. B. 1984. Effects of trimethyltin on dopaminergic and serotonergic function in the central nervous system. *Toxicol. Appl. Pharmacol.* 75:182–89.

DeMet, E. M., and Halaris, A. E. 1979. Origin and distribution of 3-methoxy-4-hydroxy-phenylglycol in body fluids. *Biochem. Pharmacol.* 28:3043–50.

Desaiah, D. 1982. Biochemical mechanisms of chlordecone neurotoxicity: A review. *Neurotoxicology* 3:103–10.

Desiderio, D. M.; Yamada, S.; Tanzer, F. S.; Horton, J.; and Trimble, J. 1981. High performance liquid chromatography and field desorption mass spectrometric measurement of picomole amounts of endogenous neuropeptides in biologic tissue. *J. Chromatogr.* 217:437–52.

Deskin, R.; Bursian, S. J.; and Edens, F. W. 1980. Neurochemical alterations induced by manganese chloride in neonatal rats. *Neurotoxicology* 2:65–73.

Dixit, R.; Husain, R.; Mukhtar, H.; and Seth, P. K. 1981. Effect of acrylamide on biogenic amine levels, monoamine oxidase, and cathepsin D activity of rat brain. *Environ. Res.* 26:168–73.

Doctor, S. V.; Costa, L. G.; Kendall, D. A.; and Murphy, S. D. 1982. Trimethyltin inhibits uptake of neurotransmitters into mouse forebrain synaptosomes. *Toxicology* 25:213–21.

Donaldson, J.; LaBella, F. S.; and Gesser, D. 1980. Enhanced autoxidation of dopamine as a possible basis of manganese neurotoxicity. *Neurotoxicology* 2:53–64.

Donaldson, J.; McGregor, D.; Gesser, H.; and LaBella, F. S. 1981. Is inhibition of acetylcholine-receptor binding the primary mechanism of cadmium neurotoxicity? *Toxicologist* 1:61–62.

Dubas, T. C., and Hrdina, P. D. 1978. Behavioral and neurochemical consequences of neonatal exposure to lead in rats. *J. Environ. Pathol. Toxicol.* 2:473–84.

Dunnett, S. B., and Iversen, S. D. 1982a. Neurotoxic lesions of ventrolateral but not anteromedial neostriatum in rats impair differential reinforcement of low rates (DRL) performance. *Behav. Brain Res.* 6:213–26.

———. 1982b. Sensorimotor impairments following localized kainic acid and 6-hydroxydopamine lesions of the neostriatum. *Brain Res.* 248:121–27.

Dyer, R. S.; Walsh, T. J.; Wonderlin, W. F.; and Bercegeay, M. 1982. The trimethyltin syndrome in rats. *Neurobehav. Toxicol. Teratol.* 4:127–33.

Eccles, C. U., and Annau, Z. 1982a. Prenatal methylmercury exposure: I. Alterations in neonatal activity. *Neurobehav. Toxicol. Teratol.* 4:371–76.

———. 1982b. Prenatal methylmercury exposure: II. Alterations in learning and psychotropic drug sensitivity in adult offspring. *Neurobehav. Toxicol. Teratol.* 4:377–82.

Ehlert, F. J.; Kokka, N.; and Fairhurst, A. S. 1980. Altered [3H]-quinuclidinyl benzilate binding in the striatum of rats following chronic cholinesterase inhibition with diisopropylfluorophosphate. *Mol. Pharmacol.* 17:24–30.

Epelbaum, J.; Arancibia, L. T.; Kordon, C.; and Enjalbert, A. 1982. Characterization, regional distribution and subcellular distribution of 125I-Tyr-somatostatin binding sites in rat brain. *J. Neurochem.* 38:1515–23.

Erinoff, L.; MacPhail, R. C.; Heller, A.; and Seiden, L. S. 1979. Age-dependent effects of 6-hydroxydopamine on locomotor activity in the rat. *Brain Res.* 164:195–205.

Ewing, A. G.; Wightman, R. M.; and Dayton, M. A. 1982. *In vivo* voltammetry with electrodes that discriminate between dopamine and ascorbate. *Brain Res.* 249:361–70.

Fibiger, H. C.; Zis, A. P.; and McGeer, E. G. 1973. Feeding and drinking deficits after 6-hydroxydopamine administration in the rat: Similarities to the lateral hypothalamic syndrome. *Brain Res.* 55:135–48.

Fillion, G. M. B.; Rousselle, J.-C.; Fillion, M.-P.; Beaudoin, D. M.; Goring, M. R.; Deniau, J.-M.; and Jacob, J. J. 1978. High-affinity binding of [3H]5-hydroxytryptamine to brain synaptosomal membranes: Comparison with [3H]-lysergic acid diethylamide binding. *Mol. Pharmacol.* 14:50–59.

Fisher, A.; Mantione, C. R.; Abraham, D. J.; and Hanin, I. 1982. Long-term central cholinergic hypofunction induced in mice by ethylcholine aziridinium ion (AF64A) in vivo. *J. Pharmacol. Exp. Ther.* 222:140–45.

Freedman, S. B.; Poat, J. A.; and Woodruff, G. N. 1982. Influence of sodium and sulphydryl groups on [3H] sulpiride binding sites in rat striatal membranes. *J. Neurochem.* 38:1459–65.

Fuller, R. W. 1982. Drugs acting on serotonergic neuronal systems. In *Biology of serotonergic transmission*, 221–47. See Boadle-Biber 1982.

Fuxe, K.; Andersson, K.; Nilsen, O. G.; Toftgard, R.; Eneroth, P.; and Gustafsson, J.-A. 1982. Toluene and telencephalic dopamine: Selective reduction of amine turnover in discrete DA nerve terminal systems of the anterior caudate nucleus by low concentrations of toluene. *Toxicol. Lett.* 12:115–23.

Gammon, D. W.; Lawrence, L. J.; and Casida, J. E. 1982. Pyrethroid toxicity: Protective effects of diazepam and phenobarbital in the mouse and the cockroach. *Toxicol. Appl. Pharmacol.* 66:290–96.

Garrick, N. A., and Murphy, D. L. 1980. Species differences in deamination of dopamine and other substrates for monoamine oxidase in brain. *Psychopharmacology* 72:27–33.

Gazit, H.; Silman, I.; and Dudai, Y. 1979. Administration of an organophosphate causes a decrease in muscarinic receptor levels in rat brain. *Brain Res.* 174:351–56.

Gerhart, J. M.; Hong, J. S.; Uphouse, L. L.; and Tilson, H. A. 1982. Chlordecone-induced tremor: Quantification and pharmacological analysis. *Toxicol. Appl. Pharmacol.* 66:234–43.

Gerhart, J. M., and Tilson, H. A. 1982. Manganese chloride exposure alters high affinity receptor binding and drug-induced activity in male rats. *Toxicologist* 2:87.

Giardini, V.; Meneguz, A.; Amorico, L.; DeAcetis, L.; and Bignami, G. 1982. Behaviorally augmented tolerance during chronic cholinesterase reduction by paraoxon. *Neurobehav. Toxicol. Teratol.* 4:335–45.

Goldberg, A. M., and McCaman, R. E. 1973. The determination of picomole amounts of acetylcholine in mammalian brain. *J. Neurochem.* 20:1–8.

Golter, M., and Michaelson, I. A. 1975. Growth, behavior and brain catecholamines in lead-exposed neonatal rats: A reappraisal. *Science* 187:359–61.

Govoni, S.; Memo, M.; Lucchi, L.; Spano, P. F.; and Trabucchi, M. 1980. Brain neurotransmitter systems and chronic lead intoxication. *Pharmacol. Res. Commun.* 12:447–60.

Govoni, S.; Memo, M.; Spano, P. F.; and Trabucchi, M. 1979. Chronic lead treatment differentially affects dopamine synthesis in various rat brain areas. *Toxicology* 12:343–49.

Govoni, S.; Montefusco, O.; Spano, P. F.; and Trabucchi, M. 1978. Effect of chronic lead treatment on brain dopamine synthesis and serum prolactin release in the rat. *Toxicol. Lett.* 2:333–37.

Gray, L. E., and Reiter, L. W. 1977. Lead-induced developmental and behavioral changes in the mouse. *Toxicol. Appl. Pharmacol.* 41:140.

Greenberg, D. A.; Snyder, S. H.; and U'Prichard, D. C. 1976. Alpha-noradrenergic receptor binding in mammalian brain: Differential labeling of agonist and antagonist states. *Life Sci.* 19:69–76.

Greengard, P. 1976. Possible role for cyclic nucleotides and phosphorylated membrane proteins in postsynaptic actions of neurotransmitters. *Nature* 260:101–8.

———. 1978. Phosphorylated proteins as physiological effectors. *Science* 199:146–52.

Greengrass, P., and Bremner, R. 1979. Binding characteristics of [3H]-prazosin to rat brain alpha-adrenergic receptors. *Eur. J. Pharmacol.* 55:323–26.

Gruber, K. A.; Stein, S.; Brink, L.; Radhakrishnan, A.; and Udenfriend, S. 1976. Fluorometric assay of vasopressin and oxytocin: A general approach to the assay of peptides in tissues. *Proc. Natl. Acad. Sci. U.S.A.* 73:1314–18.

Guidotti, A.; Gale, K.; Suria, A.; and Toffano, G. 1979. Biochemical evidence for two classes of GABA receptors in rat brain. *Brain Res.* 172:566–71.

Guyon, A.; Roques, B. P.; Guyon, F.; Foucault, A.; Perdrisot, R.; Swerts, J. P.; and Schwartz, J. C. 1979. Enkephalin degradation in mouse brain studied by a new HPLC method: Further evidence for the involvement of carboxydipeptidase. *Life Sci.* 25:1605–12.

Hamon, M.; Mallat, M.; Herbet, A.; Nelson, D. L.; Audinot, M.; Pichat, L.; and Glowinski, J. 1981. [3H] Metergoline: A new ligand of serotonin receptors in the rat brain. *J. Neurochem.* 36:613–26.

Hamon, M.; Nelson, D. L.; Herbet, A.; and Glowinski, J. 1980. Multiple receptors for serotonin in the rat brain. *Adv. Biochem. Psychopharmacol.* 21:223–33.

Hancock, W. S.; Bishop, C. A.; Prestidge, R. L.; Harding, D. R. K.; and Hearn, M. T. W. 1978. Reversed-phase, high-pressure liquid chromatography of peptides and proteins with ion-pairing reagents. *Science* 200:1168–70.

Hanin, I., and Skinner, R. F. 1975. Analysis of microquantities of choline and its esters utilizing gas chromatography–chemical ionization mass spectrometry. *Anal. Biochem.* 66:568–83.

Hedlund, B.; Gamarra, M.; and Bartfai, T. 1979. Inhibition of striatal muscarinic receptors *in vivo* by cadmium. *Brain Res.* 168:216–18.

Hernandez, L.; Paez, X.; and Hamlin, C. 1983. Neurotransmitters extraction by local intra-cerebral dialysis in anesthetized rats. *Pharmacol. Biochem. Behav.* 18:159–62.

Hole, K.; Fuxe, K.; and Jonsson, G. 1976. Behavioral effects of 5,7-dihydroxytryptamine lesions of ascending 5-hydroxytryptamine pathways. *Brain Res.* 107:385–99.

Hong, J. S.; Tilson, H. A.; Uphouse, L. L.; Gerhart, J. M.; Wilson, W. E.; and Hunter, V. 1983. Possible involvement of brain serotonin in chlordecone-elicited tremor. *Toxicologist* 3:13.

Hulme, E. C.; Berrie, C. P.; Birdsall, N. J. M.; Jameson, M.; and Stockton, J. M. 1983. Regulation of muscarinic agonist binding by cations and guanine nucleotides. *Eur. J. Pharmacol.* 94:59–72.

Hutson, P. H., and Curzon, G. 1983. Monitoring *in vivo* of transmitter metabolism by elec-trochemical methods. *Biochem. J.* 211:1–12.

Jason, K. M., and Kellogg, C. K. 1981. Neonatal lead exposure: Effects on development of behavior and striatal dopamine neurons. *Pharmacol. Biochem. Behav.* 15:641–49.

Jonsson, G. 1976. Studies on the mechanism of 6-hydroxydopamine cytotoxicity. *Med. Biol.* 54:406–20.

Jonsson, G.; Wiesel, F. A.; and Hallman, H. 1979. Developmental plasticity of central nor-adrenaline neurons after neonatal damage—changes in transmitter functions. *J. Neu-robiol.* 10:337–53.

Kantak, K. M.; Wayner, M. J.; Tilson, H. A.; Dwoskin, L. P.; and Stein, J. M. 1978. Synthesis and turnover of ^{3}H-5-HT in the lateral cerebroventricles. *Pharmacol. Biochem. Behav.* 8:153–61.

Karoum, F.; Moyer-Schwing, J.; Potkin, S. G.; and Wyatt, R. J. 1977. Presence of free, sulfate and glucuronide conjugated 3-methoxy-4-hydroxyphenylglycol (MHPG) in human brain, cerebrospinal fluid and plasma. *Brain Res.* 125:333–39.

Kebabian, J. W. 1978. Multiple classes of dopamine receptors in mammalian central nervous system: The involvement of dopamine-sensitive adenylyl cyclase. *Life Sci.* 23:479–84.

Kebabian, J. W., and Calne, D. B. 1979. Multiple receptors for dopamine. *Nature* 277:93–96.

Kebabian, J. W.; Petzold, G. L.; and Greengard, P. 1972. Dopamine-sensitive adenylate cyclase in caudate nucleus of rat brain and its similarities to the dopamine receptor. *Proc. Natl. Acad. Sci. U.S.A.* 69:2145–50.

Kebabian, J. W., and Saavedra, J. M. 1976. Dopamine-sensitive adenylate cyclase occurs in a region of substantia nigra containing dopaminergic dendrites. *Science* 193:683–85.

Keller, R.; Oke, A.; Mefford, I.; and Adams, R. N. 1976. Liquid chromatographic analysis of catecholamines: Routine assay for regional brain mapping. *Life Sci.* 19:995–1004.

Kendler, D. S.; Heninger, G. R.; and Roth, R. H. 1981. Brain contribution to the haloperidol-induced increase in plasma homovanillic acid. *Eur. J. Pharmacol.* 71:321–26.

Kennett, G. A., and Joseph, M. H. 1982. Does *in vivo* voltammetry in the hippocampus measure 5-HT release? *Brain Res.* 236:305–16.

Kilts, C. D.; Breese, G. R.; and Mailman, R. B. 1981. Simultaneous quantification of dopamine, 5-hydroxytryptamine and four metabolically related compounds by means of reversed-phase high performance liquid chromatography with electrochemical de-tection. *J. Chromatogr.* 225:347–57.

Kissinger, P. T.; Hart, J. B.; and Adams, R. N. 1973. Voltammetry in brain tissue—a new neurophysiological measurement. *Brain Res.* 55:209–13.

Komiskey, H. L.; Hsu, F. L.; Bossart, F. J.; Fowble, J. W.; Miller, D. D.; and Patil, P. N. 1978. Inhibition of synaptosomal uptake of norepinephrine and dopamine by conforma-tionally restricted sympathomimetic amines. *Eur. J. Pharmacol.* 52:37–45.

Komulainen, H., and Tuomisto, J. 1981. Interference of methyl mercury with monoamine uptake and release in rat brain synaptosomes. *Acta Pharmacol. Toxicol.* 48:214–22.

Kopin, I. J.; Gordon, E. K.; Jimerson, D. C.; and Polinsky, R. J. 1982. Relation between plasma and cerebrospinal fluid levels of 3-methoxy-4-hydroxyphenylglycol. *Science* 219:73–75.

Korf, J.; Grasdijk, L.; and Westerink, B. H. C. 1976. Effects of electrical stimulation of the nigrostriatal pathway on dopamine metabolism. *J. Neurochem.* 26:579–84.

Kuhn, D. M., and Lovenberg, W. 1983. Hydroxylases. In *Handbook of neurochemistry,* edited by A. Lajtha, 2d. ed., vol. 4, 133–50. New York: Plenum Pub. Corp.

Lane, R. F.; Hubbard, A. T.; Fukunaga, K.; and Blanchard, R. J. 1976. Brain catecholamines: Detection *in vivo* by means of differential pulse voltammetry at surface-modified platinum electrodes. *Brain Res.* 114:346–52.

Lawrence, L. J., and Casida, J. E. 1983. Stereospecific action of pyrethroid insecticides on the gamma-aminobutyric acid receptor-ionophore complex. *Science* 221:1399–1401.

Leeb-Lundberg, F., and Olsen, R. W. 1980. Picrotoxinin binding as a probe of the GABA postsynaptic membrane receptor-ionophore complex. In *Psychopharmacology and biochemistry of neurotransmitter receptors,* edited by H. I. Yamamura, R. W. Olsen, and E. Usdin, 593–606. New York: Elsevier.

Leviel, V.; Cheramy, A.; Nieoullon, A.; and Glowinski, J. 1979. Symmetric bilateral changes in dopamine release from the caudate nuclei of the cat induced by unilateral nigral application of glycine and GABA-related compounds. *Brain Res.* 175:259–70.

Leysen, J. E.; Gommeren, W.; and Niemegeers, C. J. E. 1983. [^{3}H] Sufentanyl, a superior ligand for μ-opiate receptors: Binding properties and regional distribution in rat brain and spinal cord. *Eur. J. Pharmacol.* 87:209–25.

Leysen, J. E.; Niemegeers, C. J. E.; Van Neuten, J. M.; and Laduron, P. M. 1982. [^{3}H]Ketanserin (R 41 468), a selective ^{3}H-ligand for serotonin$_2$ receptor binding sites. *Mol. Pharmacol.* 21:301–4.

Lin, S. Y., and Goodfriend, T. L. 1970. Angiotensin receptors. *Am. J. Physiol.* 218:1319–28.

Lindroth, P., and Mopper, K. 1979. High performance liquid chromatographic determination of subpicomole amounts of amino acids by precolumn fluorescence derivatization with o-phthaldialdehyde. *Anal. Chem.* 51:1667–74.

Lopez-Colome, A. M. 1982. Taurine receptors in CNS membranes: Binding studies. *Adv. Exp. Med. Biol.* 139:293–310.

Loullis, C. C.; Hingtgen, J. N.; Shea, P. A.; and Aprison, M. H. 1980. *In vivo* determination of endogenous biogenic amines in rat brain using HPLC and push-pull cannula. *Pharmacol. Biochem. Behav.* 12:959–63.

Lucchi, L.; Memo, M.; Airaghi, M. L.; Spano, P. F.; and Trabucchi, M. 1981. Chronic lead treatment induces in rat a specific and differential effect on dopamine receptors in different brain areas. *Brain Res.* 213:397–404.

Lyness, W. H. 1982. Simultaneous measurement of dopamine and its metabolites, 5-hydroxytryptamine, 5-hydroxyindoleacetic acid and tryptophan in brain tissue using liquid chromatography and electrochemical detection. *Life Sci.* 31:1435–43.

McKenna, M. J., and DiStefano, V. 1977. Carbon disulfide. II. A proposed mechanism for the action of carbon disulfide on dopamine β-hydroxylase. *J. Pharmacol. Exp. Ther.* 202:253–66.

Mackenzie, R. G.; Hoebel, B. G.; Norelli, C.; and Trulson, M. E. 1978. Increased tilt-cage activity after serotonin depletion by 5,7-dihydroxytryptamine. *Neuropharmacology* 17:957–61.

McMillen, B. A. 1982. Striatal synaptosomal tyrosine hydroxylase activity: A model system for study of presynaptic dopamine receptors. *Biochem. Pharmacol.* 31:2643–47.

Magos, L. 1970. The effects of carbon disulphide exposure on brain catecholamines in rats. *Br. J. Pharmacol.* 39:26–33.

———. 1976. The effect of carbon disulphide on the stereotypic effect of dopamine agonists. *Eur. J. Pharmacol.* 36:257–58.

Magos, L.; Green, A.; and Jarvis, J. A. E. 1974. Half life of CS$_2$ in rats in relation to its effect on brain catecholamines. *Intl. Arch. Arbeitsmed.* 32:289–96.

Mailman, R. B. 1983. Lithium-induced polydipsia: Dependence on nigrostriatal dopamine pathway and relationship to changes in angiotensin-renin system. *Psychopharmacology* 80:143–49.

Mailman, R. B.; Hanin, I.; Frye, G. D.; Kilts, C. D.; and Krigman, M. R. 1983. Effects of postnatal trimethyltin or triethyltin treatment on the neurochemistry of the rat: Studies of catecholaminergic, GABAergic and cholinergic systems. *J. Neurochem.* 40:1423–29.

Mailman, R. B.; Kilts, C. D.; Beaumont, K.; and Breese, G. R. 1981. "Supersensitivity" of dopamine systems: Comparisons between haloperidol withdrawal, intracisternal (IC) and unilateral (UNI) 6-hydroxydopamine (OHDA) treatments. *Fed. Proc.* 40:291.

Mailman, R. B.; Krigman, M. R.; Mueller, R. A.; Mushak, P.; and Breese, G. R. 1978. Lead exposure during infancy permanently increases lithium-induced polydipsia. *Science* 201:637–39.

Mailman, R. B.; Towle, A.; Schulz, D. W.; Lewis, M. H.; Breese, G. R.; DeHaven, D. L.; and Krigman, M. R. 1983. Neonatal 6-OHDA treatment of rats: Changes in dopamine (DA) receptors, striatal neurochemistry and anatomy. *Soc. Neurosci. Abs.* 9:932.

Manier, D. H.; Okada, F.; Janowsky, A. J.; Steranka, L. R.; and Sulser, F. 1983. Serotonergic denervation changes binding characteristics of β-adrenoceptors in rat cortex. *Eur. J. Pharmacol.* 86:137–39.

Mantione, C. R.; Fisher, A.; and Hanin, I. 1981. The AF64A-treated mouse: Possible model for central cholinergic hypofunction. *Science* 213:579–80.

Marquardt, G. M.; DiStefano, V.; and Ling, L. L. 1978. Effects of racemic (S)- and (R)-methylenedioxyamphetamine on synaptosomal uptake and release of tritiated norepinephrines. *Biochem. Pharmacol.* 27:1497–1501.

Mason, S. T. 1979. Noradrenaline: Reward or extinction? *Neurosci. Biobehav. Rev.* 3:1–10.

Meek, J. L. 1980. Prediction of peptide retention times in high-pressure liquid chromatography on the basis of amino acid composition. *Proc. Natl. Acad. Sci. U.S.A.* 77:1632–36.

Mefford, I. N. 1981. Application of high performance liquid chromatography with electrochemical detection to neurochemical analysis: Measurement of catecholamines, serotonin and metabolites in rat brain. *J. Neurosci. Methods* 3:207–24.

Melamed, E.; Hefti, F.; and Wurtman, R. J. 1980. L-3,4-dihydroxyphenylalanine and L-5-hydroxytryptophan decarboxylase activities in rat striatum: Effects of selective destruction of dopaminergic or serotonergic input. *J. Neurochem.* 34:1753–56.

Memo, M.; Lucchi, L.; Spano, P. F.; and Trabucchi, M. 1980. Dose-dependent effects of lead on different neurotransmitter systems in various rat brain areas. In *Advances in neurotoxicology,* edited by L. Manzo, 41–48. New York: Pergamon Press.

———. 1981. Dose-dependent and reversible effects of lead on rat dopaminergic system. *Life Sci.* 28:795–99.

Meyer, D. K.; Phillips, M. I.; and Eiden, L. 1982. Studies on the presence of angiotensin II in rat brain. *J. Neurochem.* 38:816–20.

Miller, D. B., and O'Callaghan, J. P. 1984. Biochemical, functional and morphological indicators of neurotoxicity: Effects of acute administration of trimethyltin to the developing rat. *J. Pharmacol. Exp. Ther.* 231:744–51.

Minneman, K. P.; Hegstrand, L. R.; and Molinoff, P. B. 1979. Simultaneous determination of beta-1 and beta-2 adrenergic receptors in tissues containing both receptor subtypes. *Mol. Pharmacol.* 16:34–46.

Mishra, R. K.; Marshall, A. M.; and Varmuza, S. L. 1980. Supersensitivity in rat caudate nucleus: Effects of 6-hydroxydopamine on the time course of dopamine receptor and cyclic AMP changes. *Brain Res.* 200:47–57.

Monch, W., and Dehnen, W. 1977. High-performance liquid chromatography of peptides. *J. Chromatogr.* 140:260–62.

Murphy, S. D. 1980. Pesticides. In *Toxicology: The basic science of poisons,* 2d ed., edited by J. Doull, C. D. Klaassen, and M. O. Amdur, 357–408. New York: Macmillan.

Myers, R. D. 1974. *Handbook of drug and chemical stimulation of the brain*, 42–77. New York: Van Nostrand Reinhold Co.

Nathanson, J. A. 1977. Cyclic nucleotides and nervous system function. *Physiol. Rev.* 57:157–256.

Nelson, D. L.; Herbet, A.; Bourgoin, S.; Glowinski, J.; and Hamon, M. 1978. Characteristics of central 5-HT receptors and their adaptive changes following intracerebral 5,7-dihydroxytryptamine administration in the rat. *Mol. Pharmacol.* 14:983–95.

Nelson, D. L.; Herbet, A.; Enjalbert, A.; Bockaert, J.; and Hamon, M. 1980. Serotonin-sensitive adenylate cyclase and [^{3}H]-serotonin binding in the CNS of the rat. I. Kinetic parameters and pharmacological properties. *Biochem. Pharmacol.* 29:2445–53.

O'Callaghan, J. P., and Miller, D. B. 1984. Neuron-specific phosphoproteins as biochemical indicators of neurotoxicity: Effects of acute administration of trimethyltin to the adult rat. *J. Pharmacol. Exp. Ther.* 231:736–43.

Overstreet, D. H.; Russell, R. W.; Vasquez, B. J.; and Dalglish, F. W. 1974. Involvement of muscarinic and nicotinic receptors in behavioral tolerance to DFP. *Pharmacol. Biochem. Behav.* 2:45–54.

Pagel, J.; Christian, S. T.; Quayle, E. S.; and Monti, J. A. 1976. A serotonin sensitive adenylate cyclase in mature rat brain synaptic membranes. *Life Sci.* 19:819–24.

Parenti, M.; Gentleman, S.; Olianas, M. C.; and Neff, N. H. 1982. The dopamine receptor adenylate cyclase complex: Evidence for post recognition site involvement for the development of supersensitivity. *Neurochem. Res.* 7:115–24.

Peroutka, S. J.; Lebovitz, R. M.; and Snyder, S. H. 1981. Two distinct central serotonin receptors with different physiological functions. *Science* 212:827–29.

Peroutka, S. J., and Snyder, S. H. 1983. Multiple serotonin receptors and their physiological significance. *Fed. Proc.* 42:213–17.

Peterson, L. L., and Bartfai, T. 1983. *In vitro* and *in vivo* inhibition of [^{3}H]-imipramine binding by cadmium. *Eur. J. Pharmacol.* 90:289–92.

Pfister, W. R.; Noland, V.; Lowy, M. T.; Nichols, D. E.; and Yim, G. K. W. 1978. Comparison of the behavioral effects of para-chloroamphetamine, chlordimeform, quipazine, and intraventricular serotonin in the rat. *Commun. Psychopharmacol.* 2:287–96.

Placheta, P., and Karobath, M. 1979. Regional distribution of Na$^+$-independent GABA and benzodiazepine binding sites in rat CNS. *Brain Res.* 178:580–83.

Potter, P. E.; Meek, J. L.; and Neff, N. H. 1983. Acetylcholine and choline in neuronal tissue measured by HPLC with electrochemical detection. *J. Neurochem.* 41:188–94.

Rafales, L. S.; Bornschein, R. L.; and Caruso, V. 1982. Behavioral and pharmacological responses following acrylamide exposure in rats. *Neurobehav. Toxicol. Teratol.* 4:355–64.

Rafales, L. S.; Bornschein, R. L.; Michaelson, I. A.; Loch, R. K.; and Barker, G. F. 1979. Drug-induced activity in lead-exposed mice. *Pharmacol. Biochem. Behav.* 10:95–104.

Rafales, L. S.; Greenland, R. D.; Zenick, H.; Goldsmith, M.; and Michaelson, I. A. 1981. Responsiveness to d-amphetamine in lead-exposed rats as measured by steady state levels of catecholamines and locomotor activity. *Neurobehav. Toxicol. Teratol.* 3:363–67.

Ray, D. E., and Cremer, J. E. 1979. The action of decamethrin (a synthetic pyrethroid) on the rat. *Pestic. Biochem. Physiol.* 10:333–40.

Reis, D. J., and Molinoff, P. B. 1972. Brain dopamine-β-hydroxylase: Regional distribution and effects of lesions and 6-hydroxy-dopamine on activity. *J. Neurochem.* 19:195–204.

Reiter, L. W.; Anderson, G. E.; Ash, M. E.; and Gray, L. E. 1977. Locomotor activity measurements in behavioral toxicology: Effects of lead administration on residential maze behavior. In *Behavioral toxicology: An emerging discipline*, edited by H. Zenick and L. W. Reiter, 6-1–6-18. Washington, D.C.: Government Printing Office.

Robinson, S. E. 1983. Effect of specific serotonergic lesions on cholinergic neurons in the hippocampus, cortex and striatum. *Life Sci.* 32:345–53.

Romano, C., and Goldstein, A. 1980. Stereospecific nicotine receptors on rat brain membranes. *Science* 210:647–49.

Rosin, D. L., and Martin, B. R. 1981. Neurochemical and behavioral effects of polychlorinated biphenyls in mice. *Neurotoxicology* 2:749–64.

Ross, S. B. 1982. The characteristics of serotonin uptake systems. In *Biology of serotonergic transmission*, 159–95. See Boadle-Biber 1982.

Rotman, A.; Daly, J. W.; and Creveling, C. R. 1976. Oxygen-dependent reaction of 6-hydroxydopamine, 5,6-dihydroxytryptamine and related compounds with proteins *in vitro*: A model for cytotoxicity. *Mol. Pharmacol.* 12:887–99.

Rouot, B. R., and Snyder, S. H. 1979. [^{3}H]Para-aminoclonidine: A novel ligand which binds with high affinity to α-adrenergic receptors. *Life Sci.* 25:769–74.

Routtenberg, A. 1982. Memory formation as a post-translational modification of brain proteins. In *Mechanisms and models of neural plasticity*, edited by C. A. Marsan and H. Matthies, 17–24. New York: Raven Press.

Ruppert, P. H.; Walsh, T. J.; Reiter, L. W.; and Dyer, R. S. 1982. Trimethyltin-induced hyperactivity: Time course and pattern. *Neurobehav. Toxicol. Teratol.* 4:135–39.

Russell, R. W.; Overstreet, D. H.; Cotman, C. W.; Carson, V. G.; Churchill, L.; Dalglish, F. W.; and Vasquez, B. J. 1975. Experimental tests of hypotheses about neurochemical mechanisms underlying behavioral tolerance to the anticholinesterase, diisopropylfluorophosphate. *J. Pharmacol. Exp. Ther.* 192:73–85.

Saavedra, J. M.; Setler, P. E.; and Kebabian, J. W. 1978. Biochemical changes accompanying unilateral 6-hydroxydopamine lesions in the rat substantia nigra. *Brain Res.* 151:339–52.

Saito, A.; Sankaran, H.; Goldfine, I. D.; and Williams, J. A. 1980. Cholecystokinin receptors in the brain: Characterization and distribution. *Science* 208:1155–60.

Saller, C. F., and Stricker, E. M. 1976. Hyperphagia and increased growth in rats after intraventricular injection of 5,7-dihydroxytryptamine. *Science* 192:385–87.

Sanders-Bush, E., and Martin, L. L. 1982. Storage and release of serotonin. In *Biology of serotonergic transmission*, 95–118. See Boadle-Biber 1982.

Saria, A.; Mayer, N.; Lembeck, F.; and Pabst, M. 1980. Regional distribution and biochemical properties of ^{125}I-Tryp-substance P binding sites in synaptic vesicle. *Naunyn Schmiedebergs Arch. Pharmacol.* 311:151–57.

Sauerhoff, M. W., and Michaelson, I. A. 1973. Hyperactivity and brain catecholamines in lead-exposed developing rats. *Science* 182:1022–24.

Schiller, G. D. 1979. Reduced binding of [^{3}H]-quinuclidinyl benzilate associated with chronically low acetylcholinesterase activity. *Life Sci.* 24:1159–64.

Schoepp, D. D., and Azzaro, A. J. 1982. Role of type A and type B monoamine oxidase in the metabolism of released [^{3}H] dopamine from rat striatal slices. *Biochem. Pharmacol.* 31:2961–68.

Schulz, D. W.; Wyrick, S. D.; and Mailman, R. B. 1985. [^{3}H]SCH23390 has the characteristics of a dopamine receptor ligand in the rat central nervous system. *Eur. J. Pharmacol.* 106:211–12.

Schwab, B. W.; Hand, H.; Costa, L. G.; and Murphy, S. D. 1981. Reduced muscarinic receptor binding in tissues of rats tolerant to the insecticide disulfoton. *Neurotoxicology* 2:635–47.

Schweitzer, B. I., and Bacopoulos, N. G. 1983. Reversible decrease in dopaminergic ^{3}H-agonist binding after 6-hydroxydopamine and irreversible decrease after kainic acid. *Life Sci.* 32:531–40.

Scratchley, G. A.; Masoud, A. N.; Stohs, S. J.; and Wingard, D. W. 1979. High-performance liquid chromatographic separation and detection of catecholamines and related compounds. *J. Chromatogr.* 169:313–19.

Segal, M.; Dudai, Y.; and Amsterdam, A. 1978. Distribution of an α-bungarotoxin-binding cholinergic nicotinic receptor in rat brain. *Brain Res.* 148:105–19.

Segawa, T.; Inoue, A.; Ochi, T.; Nakata, Y.; and Nomura, Y. 1982. Specific binding of taurine in central nervous system. *Adv. Exp. Med. Biol.* 139:311–24.

Seth, P. K.; Hong, J. S.; Kilts, C. D.; and Bondy, S. C. 1981. Alteration of cerebral neurotransmitter receptor function by exposure of rats to manganese. *Toxicol. Lett.* 9:247–54.

Sharma, R. P.; Aldous, C. N.; and Farr, C. H. 1982. Methylmercury induced alterations in brain amine syntheses in rats. *Toxicol. Lett.* 13:195–201.

Shih, T. M., and Hanin, I. 1978. Chronic lead exposure in immature animals: Neurochemical correlates. *Life Sci.* 23:877–88.

Silbergeld, E. K., and Goldberg, A. M. 1974. Lead-induced behavioral dysfunction: An animal model of hyperactivity. *Exp. Neurol.* 42:146–57.

———. 1975. Pharmacological and neurochemical investigations of lead-induced hyperactivity. *Neuropharmacology* 14:431–44.

Singhal, R. L.; Merali, Z.; and Hrdina, P. D. 1976. Aspects of the biochemical toxicology of cadmium. *Fed. Proc.* 35:75–80.

Sirett, N. E.; McLean, A. S.; Bray, J. J.; and Hubbard, J. I. 1977. Distribution of angiotensin II receptors in rat brain. *Brain Res.* 122:299–312.

Slotkin, T. A.; Seidler, F. J.; Whitmore, W. L.; Lau, C.; Salvaggio, M.; and Kirksey, D. F. 1978. Rat brain synaptic vesicles: Uptake specificities of [^{3}H] norepinephrine and [^{3}H] serotonin in preparations from whole brain and brain regions. *J. Neurochem.* 31:961–68.

Smit, M. H.; Ehlert, F. J.; Yamamura, S.; Roeske, W. R.; and Yamamura, H. I. 1980. Differential regulation of muscarinic agonist binding sites following chronic cholinesterase inhibition. *Eur. J. Pharmacol.* 66:379–80.

Smith, D. F., and Amdisen, A. 1983. Central effects of lithium in rats: Lithium levels, body weight and water intake. *Acta Pharmacol. Toxicol.* 52:81–85.

Smith, J. E.; Lane, J. D.; Shea, P. A.; McBride, W. J.; and Aprison, M. H. 1975. A method for concurrent measurement of picomole quantities of acetylcholine, choline, dopamine, norepinephrine, serotonin, 5-hydroxytryptophan, 5-hydroxyindoleacetic acid, tryptophan, tyrosine, glycine, aspartate, glutamate, alanine and gamma-aminobutyric acid in single tissue samples from different areas of rat central nervous system. *Anal. Biochem.* 64:149–69.

Snyder, S. H. 1975. The glycine synaptic receptor in the mammalian central nervous system. *Br. J. Pharmacol.* 53:473–84.

Sobotka, T. J., and Cook, M. P. 1974. Postnatal lead acetate exposure in rats: Possible relationship to minimal brain dysfunction. *Am. J. Ment. Defic.* 79:5–9.

Sparber, S. B., and Tilson, H. A. 1972. Schedule controlled and drug induced release of norepinephrine-7-^{3}H into the lateral ventricle of rats. *Neuropharmacology* 11:453–64.

Spyker, J. M.; Sparber, S. B.; and Goldberg, A. M. 1972. Subtle consequences of methylmercury exposure: Behavioral deviations in offspring of treated mothers. *Science* 177:621–23.

Staatz, C. G.; Bloom, A. S.; and Lech, J. J. 1982a. A pharmacological study of pyrethroid neurotoxicity in mice. *Pestic. Biochem. Physiol.* 17:287–92.

———. 1982b. Effect of pyrethroids on [^{3}H] kainic acid binding to mouse forebrain membranes. *Toxicol. Appl. Pharmacol.* 64:566–69.

Stoof, J. C.; Den Breejen, E. J. S.; and Mulder, A. H. 1979. GABA modulates the release of dopamine and acetylcholine from rat caudate nucleus slices. *Eur. J. Pharmacol.* 57:35–42.

Sulser, F. 1978. Functional aspects of the norepinephrine receptor coupled adenylate cyclase system in the limbic forebrain and its modification by drugs which precipitate or alleviate depression: Molecular approaches to an understanding of affective disorders. *Pharmakopsychiatr.* [*Neuropsychopharmacol.*] 11:43–52.

Swartzwelder, H. S.; Dyer, R. S.; Holahan, W.; and Myers, R. D. 1981. Activity changes in rats following acute trimethyltin exposure. *Neurotoxicology* 2:589–93.

Taylor, J. R.; Selhorst, J. B.; Houff, S. A.; and Martinez, A. J. 1978. Chlordecone intoxication in man. I: Clinical observations. *Neurology* 28:626–30.

Taylor, L. L., and DiStefano, V. 1976. Effects of methylmercury on brain biogenic amines in the developing rat pup. *Toxicol. Appl. Pharmacol.* 38:489–97.

Templeton, W. W., and Woodruff, G. N. 1982. Binding of [3H] ADTN to rat striatal membranes. *Biochem. Pharmacol.* 31:1629–32.

Tilson, H. A.; Cabe, P. A.; and Burne, T. A. 1980. Behavioral procedures for the assessment of neurotoxicity. In *Experimental and clinical neurotoxicology,* edited by P. S. Spencer and H. H. Schaumburg 758–66. Baltimore: Williams & Wilkins.

Tilson, H. A.; Davis, G. J.; McLachlan, J. A.; and Lucier, G. W. 1979. The effects of polychlorinated biphenyls given prenatally on the neurobehavioral development of mice. *Environ. Res.* 18:466–74.

Tilson, H. A., and Sparber, S. B. 1970. On the use of the push-pull cannula as a means of measuring biochemical changes during on-going behavior. *Behav. Res. Meth. Instrum.* 2:131–34.

Tilson, H. A., and Squibb, R. E. 1982. The effects of acrylamide on the behavioral suppression produced by psychoactive agents. *Neurotoxicology* 3:113–20.

Trulson, M. E.; Eubanks, E. E.; and Jacobs, B. L. 1976. Behavioral evidence for supersensitivity following destruction of central serotonergic nerve terminals by 5,7-dihydroxytryptamine. *J. Pharmacol. Exp. Ther.* 198:23–32.

Tsuzuki, Y. J. 1982. Effect of methylmercury exposure on different neurotransmitter systems in rat brain. *Toxicol. Lett.* 13:159–62.

Uchida, S.; Takeyasu, K.; Matsuda, T.; and Yoshida, H. 1979. Changes in muscarinic acetylcholine receptors of mice by chronic administrations of diisopropylfluorophosphate and papaverine. *Life Sci.* 24:1805–12.

Uhl, G. R.; Bennett, J. P.; and Snyder, S. H. 1977. Neurotensin, a central nervous system peptide: Apparent receptor binding in brain membranes. *Brain Res.* 130:299–313.

Umezu, K., and Moore, K. E. 1979. Effects of drugs on regional brain concentrations of dopamine and dihydroxyphenylacetic acid. *J. Pharmacol. Exp. Ther.* 208:49–56.

Ungerstedt, U. 1971a. Postsynaptic supersensitivity after 6-hydroxydopamine induced degeneration of the nigro-striatal dopamine system. *Acta Physiol. Scand.* [Suppl.] 367:69–93.

———. 1971b. Adipsia and aphagia after 6-hydroxydopamine-induced degeneration of the nigrostriatal dopamine system. *Acta. Physiol. Scand.* [suppl.] 367:95–122.

Ungerstedt, U.; Herrera-Marschitz, M.; Jungnelius, U.; Stahle, L.; Tossman, U.; and Zetterstrom, T. 1982. Dopamine synaptic mechanisms reflected in studies combining behavioral recordings and brain dialysis. *Adv. Biosci.* 37:219–31.

Uphouse, L. L. 1981. Interactions between handling and acrylamide on the striatal dopamine receptor. *Brain Res.* 221:421–24.

Uphouse, L., and Russell, M. 1981. Rapid effects of acrylamide on spiroperidol and serotonin binding in neural tissue. *Neurobehav. Toxicol. Teratol.* 3:281–84.

Uretsky, N. J., and Iversen, L. L. 1970. Effects of 6-hydroxydopamine on catecholamine-containing neurons in the rat brain. *J. Neurochem.* 17:269–78.

Valdes, J. J.; Mactutus, C. F.; Santos-Anderson, R. M.; Dawson, R.; and Annau, Z. 1983. Selective neurochemical and histological lesions in rat hippocampus following chronic trimethyltin exposure. *Neurobehav. Toxicol. Teratol.* 5:357–61.

Van Valkenburg, C.; Tjaden, U.; Van der Krogt, J.; and Van der Leden, B. 1982. Determination of dopamine and its acidic metabolites in brain tissue by HPLC with electrochemical detection in a single run after minimal sample pretreatment. *J. Neurochem.* 39:990–97.

Vargas, O.; deLorenzo, M. C. D.; Saldate, M. C.; and Orrego, F. 1977. Potassium-induced release of [3H] GABA and of [3H] noradrenaline from normal and reserpinized rat brain cortex slices: Differences in calcium-dependency, and in sensitivity to potassium ions. *J. Neurochem.* 28:165–70.

Waldbillig, R. J.; Bartness, T. J.; and Stanley, B. G. 1981. Increased food intake, body weight, and adiposity in rats after regional neurochemical depletions of serotonin. *J. Comp. Physiol. Psychol.* 95:391–405.

Wallace, E. F.; Krantz, M. J.; and Lovenberg, W. 1973. Dopamine-β-hydroxylase: A tetrameric glycoprotein. *Proc. Natl. Acad. Sci. U.S.A.* 70:2253–55.

Walsh, T. J.; Gallagher, M.; Bostock, E.; and Dyer, R. S. 1982. Trimethyltin impairs retention of a passive avoidance task. *Neurobehav. Toxicol. Teratol.* 4:163–67.

Walsh, T. J.; Miller, D. B.; and Dyer, R. S. 1982. Trimethyltin, a selective limbic system neurotoxicant, impairs radial-arm maze performance. *Neurobehav. Toxicol. Teratol.* 4:177–83.

Walsh, T. J.; Tilson, H. A.; DeHaven, D. L.; Mailman, R. B.; Fisher, A.; and Hanin, I. 1984. AF64A, a cholinergic neurotoxin, selectively depletes acetylcholine in hippocampus and cortex, and produces long-term passive avoidance and radial-arm maze deficits in the rat. *Brain Res.* 321:91–102.

Weiner, N. 1974. A critical assessment of methods for the determination of monoamine synthesis turnover rates in vivo. In *Neuropsychopharmacology of monoamines and their regulatory enzymes*, edited by E. Usdin, 143–59. New York: Raven Press.

Weyhenmeyer, J. A., and Mack, K. J. 1985. Binding characteristics of kappa opioids in rat brains: A comparison of *in vitro* binding paradigms. *Neuropharmacology* 24:111–15.

Wince, L. C.; Donovan, C. A.; and Azzaro, A. J. 1980. Alterations in the biochemical properties of central dopamine synapses following chronic postnatal PbCO$_3$ exposure. *J. Pharmacol. Exp. Ther.* 214:642–50.

Winder, C. 1982. The interaction between lead and catecholaminergic function. *Biochem. Pharmacol.* 31:3717–21.

Yamamoto, B. K.; Lane, R. F.; and Freed, C. R. 1982. Normal rats trained to circle show asymmetric caudate dopamine release. *Life Sci.* 30:2155–62.

Yamamura, H. I., and Snyder, S. H. 1974. Muscarinic cholinergic binding in rat brain. *Proc. Natl. Acad. Sci. U.S.A.* 71:1725–29.

Yamawaki, S.; Segawa, T.; and Sarai, K. 1982. Effects of acute and chronic toluene inhalation on behavior and (³H)-serotonin binding in rat. *Life Sci.* 30:1997–2002.

Young, A. B., and Snyder, S. H. 1974. Strychnine binding in rat spinal cord membranes associated with the synaptic glycine receptor: Cooperativity of glycine interactions. *Mol. Pharmacol.* 10:790–809.

Zahnister, N. R., and Dubocovich, M. L. 1983. Comparison of dopamine receptor sites labeled by [³H]-S-[sulpiride and [³H]-spiperone in striatum. *J. Pharmacol. Exp. Ther.* 227:592–99.

Zenick, H. 1974. Behavioral and biochemical consequences in methylmercury chloride toxicity. *Pharmacol. Biochem. Behav.* 2:709–13.

Zenick, H., and Goldsmith, M. 1981. Drug discrimination learning in lead-exposed rats. *Science* 212:569–71.

Zukin, R. S.; Young, A. B.; and Snyder, S. H. 1974. Gamma-aminobutyric acid binding to receptor sites in the rat central nervous system. *Proc. Natl. Acad. Sci. U.S.A.* 71:4802–7.

Thomas J. Walsh and
Hugh A. Tilson

11

The Use of Pharmacological Challenges

Pharmacological challenges are being used with increasing frequency in behavioral toxicology as a method of assessing alterations in nervous-system function following toxicant exposure or physical insult. A basic rationale inherent in this approach is that subtle or latent deviations in neural processes might not be observed with commonly utilized behavioral methodologies. This contention was borne out by the classic studies of Karl Lashley demonstrating that under the appropriate circumstances, even complex behavior can occur within normal limits despite extensive damage to the central nervous system (CNS) (Lashley 1929). Recent anatomical, physiological, and behavioral studies have demonstrated that the CNS exhibits more plasticity following injury than previously suspected. Processes such as axonal sprouting, neural reorganization and remodeling, and behavioral adaptation all contribute to functional recovery following neural trauma (see Finger and Stein 1982).

The nervous system also adapts to perturbations induced by chemical agents. For example, a basic tenet of modern pharmacology is that repeated exposure to some drugs can result in a diminution of the expected effect, that is, tolerance or tachyphylaxis (Goodman and Gilman 1975). Administration of morphine produces analgesia in both laboratory animals and humans. With repeated administration, however, the drug seems to lose potency and more of it is required to produce the desired effect. The organism is said to have become "tolerant" to its effects (see Martin 1968).

The mechanisms underlying the adaptive processes described in the preceding paragraphs are not well understood. These examples do, however, illustrate that the CNS can dynamically adapt to both chemical and physical insults. One explanation for the resistance of the nervous system to repeated perturbation is that homeostatic or compensatory mechanisms are initiated by injury.

The cardiovascular system provides a concrete example of how homeostatic mechanisms contribute to a maintenance of normal physiology. For example, increases in arterial blood pressure activate a set of pressure-sensitive receptors known as baroreceptors which are located at various nodal points in the vasculature. Activation of these receptors initiates a set of neural impulses to the vasomotor center in the brain stem that acts to inhibit vasomotor tone and decrease both the rate and the force of contractility of the heart and thus averts the potentially catastrophic effects of uncontested hypertension. In contrast, hypotension inhibits the output of these receptors, which results in increased (i.e., disinhibited) cardiac performance. The baroreceptors are activated by the imposition of an appropriate stressor (e.g., rapidly rising or falling arterial pressure). The cardiovascular system utilizes a variety of physiological "safeguards" to regulate itself within limits that are compatible with survival (see Guyton 1971 for other examples of homeostatic mechanisms). Several potential neural counterparts of these processes have been proposed and will be discussed below.

C. P. Richter applied the concept of homeostasis to behavior (Cofer and Appley 1965). In effect, behavioral and neurological functioning may be viewed as operating within upper and lower limits. Exposure to a neurotoxicant alters the dynamic equilibrium of the system, which is compensated for by existing homeostatic mechanisms. If the system has a finite capacity, it is assumed that at some point during exposure the system will exceed this capacity, and impairments will be observed; that is, the "functional reserve" of the system will be depleted, and function will deteriorate.

Norton (1982) has proposed two types of homeostatic mechanisms—structural redundancy and tolerance—that might contribute to normal CNS function following injury. Processes may continue to operate within normal limits despite the death of a certain number of neurons owing to sufficient anatomical, physiological, or behavioral redundancy inherent in the system which permits function to continue, at least up to a certain point. Tolerance is conceptualized as some form of learning in which the toxicant-exposed organism "learns" to compensate for its neurobehavioral impairments.

The neurobiological substrates of structural redundancy and tolerance are not well understood. One homeostatic process that occurs at the molecular level, however, is the change in neurotransmitter receptor binding that can accompany exposure to toxicants (see DeHaven and Mailman 1983 for a review of receptor binding methodology and its utility for studies of neurotoxicity). For example, repeated exposure to a chemical that increases the activation of postsynaptic receptor sites results in a molecular alteration known as receptor *down-regulation*, which is evidenced as a decrease in the number (B_{max}) of receptors or in their affinity (K_d) for their endogenous ligands (i.e., neurotransmitters, peptides, or other neuromodulators). In contrast to this effect, agents that chronically decrease activity at the postsynaptic site increase the number or affinity of specific receptor types, a phenomenon termed *up-regulation*. Animals exposed to chemicals that chronically activate a given receptor population, resulting in a down-regulated system, should exhibit differential sensitivity to agents that act directly at the postsynaptic receptor. An animal that is up-regulated should be more sensitive (i.e., supersensitive) to agents that activate the receptor (i.e., agonist), while a down-regulated animal should be less sensitive. Such differential sensitivities are manifested as shifts in the dose-response curve for agonists or antagonists. A toxicant should shift the dose-response curve to the left (i.e., less compound needed for effect X) for a receptor agonist if there is supersensitivity, and to the right (i.e., more compound required for effect X) if there is subsensitivity.

Alterations in receptor sensitivity have been observed following repeated administration of various psychoactive compounds (Reisine 1981; Kurlan and Shoulson 1982). For example, chronic exposure to neuroleptics and tricyclic antidepressants alters receptor properties. These phenomena will be described and used to illustrate the concepts of up- and down-regulation. Repeated administration of haloperidol, a dopamine receptor antagonist used for a variety of neuropsychiatric disorders, results in an increased number and affinity of dopamine receptors in both striatal and mesolimbic areas of the brain, together with an enhanced bio-chemical and behavioral response to dopamine agonists such as apomorphine (see Muller and Seeman 1978). Thus, persistent blockade of the dopamine receptor by haloperidol "fine-tunes," or up-regulates, the receptor to maximize the efficacy of its interaction with agonistlike substances. In contrast, repeated administration of tricyclic antidepressants such as imipramine, which increase the probability of neurotransmitter-receptor interactions by preventing the reuptake of transmitter molecules released at the synapse, down-regulate receptors (Bergstrom and Kellar 1979; Segawa, Mizuta, and Nomura 1979). Stated simply, too much or too little receptor activation can result in predictable alterations in the sensitivity of the receptor to its appropriate ligands.

Compensatory changes in receptor populations have also been observed in both the peripheral and the central nervous system following exposure to a diverse array of toxic chemicals (DeHaven and Mailman 1983). Therefore, these adapta-tions in neural sensitivity might be a pervasive response to neural insult. While receptor binding methodology has been used to investigate the neurochemical effects of numerous toxicants, a complementary and noninvasive approach for assessing the integrity of transmitter systems uses specific pharmacological chal-lenges.

The use of pharmacological challenges offers several advantages to neurotox-icologists. Given that exposure to a toxicant results in a compromised system, responsiveness to certain pharmacological agents should be altered. The phar-macological-challenge approach could permit detection of a change in an otherwise "normal" animal and might provide a rationale for the study of the mechanism or site of action of the neurotoxicant. Modern neuropharmacology has provided us with a variety of compounds that selectively interact with specific neurotransmitter systems and affect behavior in predictable ways. Table 11.1 provides a list of agents commonly used to investigate the physiology and function of noradrenergic, dopaminergic, serotonergic, and cholinergic processes in the central and the pe-ripheral nervous system. The judicious use of these pharmacological tools together with sensitive behavioral endpoints can provide information about the integrity of various neurochemical processes. In addition, appropriate use of pharmacological challenges has the advantage of providing a noninvasive and reversible probe that can be used at any time during the course of toxicant exposure or during the life of the animal. In the rest of this chapter we discuss examples of how pharmacological challenges have been used by behavioral toxicologists and some of the advantages and problems inherent in their use.

The Use of Pharmacological Agents to Detect the Presence of Toxicity

Pharmacological challenges have been used routinely in both toxicology and clinical medicine for many years. Pulmonary toxicologists, for instance, use drug challenges to unmask hidden respiratory problems (Coffin, Gardner, and Blommer 1976). Neurological disorders such as epilepsy and neuromuscular disease can also

Table 11.1 Pharmacological agents that selectively interact with specific neurotransmitter systems

Increase Synaptic Activity	Decrease Synaptic Activity
A. DOPAMINE	
Agonists	*Antagonists*
Apomorphine	Chlorpromazine
Amphetamine (indirect)	Haloperidol
Lergotrile	Sulpiride
Bromocriptine	Pimozide
Piribedil	α-flupenthixol
	Tyrosine hydroxylase inhibitor
	α-methyl-p-tyrosine
Reuptake inhibitors	*Cytotoxin*
Bupropion	6-hyroxydopamine
B. NOREPINEPHRINE	
Amphetamine	
Alpha agonists	*Alpha antagonists*
Clonidine	Phentolamine
Epinephrine	Phenoxybenzamine
	Yohimbine
Beta agonists	*Beta antagonists*
Isoproterenol	Propranolol
Norepinephrine	
	Dopamine-β-hydroxylase inhibitors
	Diethyldithiocarbamate (DDC)
	FLA-63
	Cytotoxin
	6-hydroxydopamine
	DSP-4
C. SEROTONIN	
Agonists	*Antagonists*
Quipazine	Methysergide
5-methoxydimethyltryptamine	Cyproheptadine
	Pizotifen
	Cinanserin
	Metergoline
Reuptake inhibitors	*Tryptophan hydroxylase inhibitor*
Fluoxetine	Para-chlorophenylalanine (PCPA)
Chlorimipramine	
	Cytotoxin
	5,7-dihydroxytryptamine (5,7-DHT)
D. ACETYLCHOLINE	
Muscarinic agonists	*Muscarinic antagonists*
Carbachol	Scopolamine
Pilocarpine	Atropine
Arecholine	
Oxotremorine	
Nicotinic agonists	*Nicotinic antagonists*
Nicotine	d-tubocurarine
	Curare
Cholinesterase inhibitors	*Choline uptake inhibitors*
Physostigmine	Hemicholinium-3
Diisopropylfluorophosphate (DFP)	
Neostigmine (peripherally active)	
	Cytotoxin
	AF64A

be diagnosed by administering compounds that either promote or attenuate specific symptomatology associated with the disease process. One method of determining whether a patient has myasthenia gravis, a neurological disorder characterized by impaired cholinergic transmission at the neuromuscular junction, is to assess whether he is inordinately sensitive to the paralytic properties of the cholinergic antagonist curare. In contrast, muscular disorders of cholinergic origin are typically improved by the administration of compounds such as physostigmine, which prevent the breakdown of endogenous acetylcholine. Thus, pharmacological challenges can both induce deficits and attenuate preexisting functional impairments. Utilized in this manner, drug challenges can provide valuable information regarding the substrates of neurological dysfunction, as well as give clues to potentially useful therapeutic strategies.

The Russian neurotoxicologist Pavlenko (1975) was among the first to suggest the routine use of pharmacological challenges to determine the presence of underlying neurobehavioral toxicity. This investigator proposed a three-tier approach for the screening of potential neurotoxicants. The initial assessment of a substance involves evaluating the integrity of various orienting and defensive responses, as well as unconditioned reflexes, to noxious stimuli. The second level of testing concerns higher-order nervous-system processes, which are assessed by conditioned reflexes. The information derived from this second tier of testing is subsequently used to determine threshold and subthreshold levels of potentially harmful agents. The third level proposed by Pavlenko utilizes stress tests to better characterize the toxicity and to determine the concentration of a toxicant required to produce functional deficits. Among the tests proposed by Pavlenko for uncovering neurobehavioral impairments were muscular exertion, exposure to cold and noise, and electroconvulsive seizures. Chemical stressors including ethanol, hexobarbital, and chemical convulsants and challenging the toxicant-exposed animal with additional doses of the substance to assess potential changes in sensitivity to its toxic effects were also suggested as useful adjuncts in determining latent toxicity.

Fouts (1963) reported the use of hexobarbital sleeping times to evaluate liver function following exposure to xenobiotics such as DDT and other chlorinated hydrocarbons. These agents have been shown to induce enzymes involved in the metabolism of chemicals such as hexobarbital. Animals exposed repeatedly to DDT have shorter sleeping times than do controls owing to a more rapid metabolism of barbiturates. A similar approach was used by Tilson and Cabe (1979) to study possible latent effects of polybrominated biphenyls (PBBs), which are also known to induce hepatic metabolic enzymes. In this study rats were trained to press a lever to postpone the presentation of electric foot shock on a continuous-avoidance schedule. Once a stable baseline of responding had been established, they were challenged with various doses of phenobarbital or d-amphetamine. While PBB exposure did not alter baseline responding, there was a significant decrease in the behavioral suppressant effects of phenobarbital, possibly owing to an enhanced metabolism of the barbiturate resulting from induction of hepatic enzymes responsible for its degradation (fig. 11.1). Exposure to PBBs, however, did not affect the increased response rate produced by d-amphetamine on this schedule. These data indicate that pharmacological challenges can be used in conjunction with quantifia-

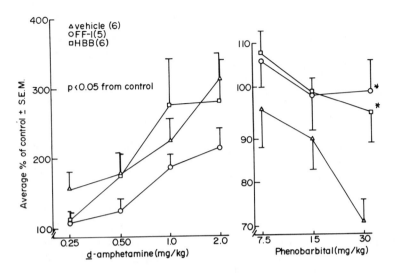

Fig. 11.1 The effect of repeated exposure to PBBs (Firemaster FF-1 or 2,4,5,2′,4′,5′-hexabromobiphe-nyl) on the responsiveness of rats to d-amphetamine and phenobarbital. Data represent the mean ± SEM percentage of response rates observed on the day prior to the drug challenges. Asterisks indicate a significant (p < 0.05) difference from vehicle-injected rats.
(*Source:* Tilson and Cabe 1979. Reprinted by permission of the publisher.)

ble behavioral endpoints to detect the presence of functional toxicity in organ systems other than the CNS.

Drug challenges have frequently been used to assess the effects of toxicants on development; many of these studies will be discussed below. One study that illustrates that pharmacological challenges can be used to detect the presence of toxicity in rats exposed to a toxicant during development and throughout adulthood is that of Reiter and colleagues (1978). Undernutrition comparable to that experienced by lead-exposed animals shifted the amphetamine dose-response curve to the left. In contrast, lead exposure during development shifted it to the right. Therefore, animals exposed to lead exhibited an attenuated drug response, while the undernourished controls were more sensitive to amphetamine. Leander (1980) also found that adult pigeons receiving low daily doses of lead were less sensitive to the rate-increasing effect of d-amphetamine on a food-reinforced fixed-interval task. Moreover, this effect was observed in animals without any sign of systemic toxicity such as weight loss or crop dysfunction (see Laties and Cory-Slechta 1979). These studies, demonstrating a decreased effectiveness of d-amphetamine in lead-exposed animals, prompted investigation of the potential neurochemical and pharmacokinetic mechanisms responsible for this altered sensitivity. Some of these reports will be discussed below.

Several other laboratories have used d-amphetamine to examine possible changes in drug responsiveness in animals exposed to neurotoxic agents during development. Amphetamine is frequently chosen as a pharmacological probe because its neurochemical mechanism and its neuroanatomical sites of action are relatively understood. Amphetamine promotes the release of newly synthesized dopamine from nerve terminals located in both the caudate nucleus and mesolimbic areas such as the nucleus accumbens and the frontal cortex (Besson et al. 1971; Moore 1977). The behavioral effects of amphetamine have been well characterized and consist of dose-related alteration in locomotor behavior, with low doses increasing ambulation and rearing and higher doses inducing motor stereotypes (Segal 1975; Fray et al. 1980). The release of dopamine from mesolimbic sites is believed to mediate the increased activity, while dopamine release in the caudate nucleus appears to be essential for the expression of stereotypy (Creese and Iversen 1975; Kelly, Seviour, and Iversen 1975; Iversen and Koob 1977). Thus, a change in responsiveness to d-amphetamine could reflect altered catecholaminergic function in discrete regions of the nervous system. An alternative hypothesis is that changes in sensitivity are due to a more general change in CNS arousal.

Altered responsiveness to d-amphetamine or any other pharmacological challenge following toxicant exposure is an intriguing observation in and of itself. However, subsequent studies examining the nature and potential mechanisms of the altered dose-response are required to delineate the processes disrupted by the neurotoxicant. The use of d-amphetamine as a routine pharmacological probe in studies involving developmental exposures has gained some degree of acceptance by behavioral toxicologists (Reiter et al. 1977; Adams et al. 1982). An example of this approach can be found in a study in which neonatal rats were dosed with benzene on days 9, 11, and 13 and assessed in a battery of neurobehavioral tests at 45, 60, and 100 days of age; no effects on behavior were seen during these tests (Tilson et al. 1980). When the animals were subsequently tested for spontaneous motor activity in an open field at 100–103 days of age, it was found that the benzene-exposed animals were more active under control conditions. Administration of various doses of d-amphetamine (0.3–3.0 mg/kg) increased motor activity of the rats in a dose-related way, and inspection of the absolute counts gave no indication that the benzene-exposed animals were differentially affected. However, as can be seen in figure 11.2, when the data are expressed as a percentage of the pre-drug baseline, decreased sensitivity of the benzene-treated rats to the highest dose of amphetamine is apparent. These results serve to illustrate one consideration in experiments using pharmacological challenges, namely, that it is imperative to take into account the behavioral baseline before concluding that a treatment has altered sensitivity to a pharmacological probe. Furthermore, when a baseline measure such as locomotor activity is elevated, an apparent decreased response to motor stimulants might actually reflect a system that has reached its maximum output capacity. That is, behavioral as well as pharmacological factors can contribute to changes in drug sensitivity.

In the study reported in the preceding paragraph, the use of a pharmacological challenge successfully demonstrated a change in sensitivity in the absence of other changes in neurobehavioral function (e.g., grip strength, startle responsiveness, negative geotaxis). However, altered drug responsiveness is not a necessary adjunct to other signs of behavioral toxicity. Squibb and colleagues (1981) exposed rats to various concentrations of monosodium glutamate (MSG), a commonly used food additive, on postnatal days 1–5. MSG produced several neurobehavioral and morphometric changes that persisted into adulthood. For example, MSG altered body weight, startle responsiveness, and hindlimb grip strength and also induced self-mutilation. However, when challenged with 0.3–3.0 mg/kg d-amphetamine, MSG-exposed rats had a dose-response curve similar to that of the controls. Thus,

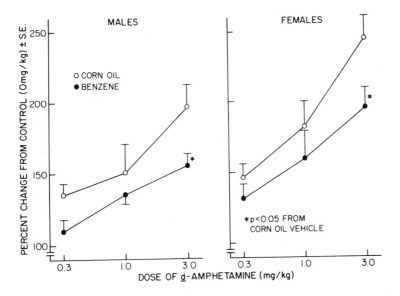

Fig. 11.2 The effect of neonatal benzene exposure on the motor-stimulant effect of d-amphetamine assessed in adulthood. Data given represent the percentage of baseline motor activity. Asterisks represent a significant (p < 0.05) difference from controls.
(*Source:* Tilson et al. 1980. Reprinted by permission of the publisher).

if pharmacological challenges are used in a screening context, they should be used in combination with other tests of neurobehavioral function.

There are several obvious difficulties in interpreting the results of studies using pharmacological challenges. Prior administration of a neurotoxicant can alter the metabolism, accumulation, or biological disposition of various drugs, which could result in a diminished effective concentration at the site of action. Hughes and Sparber (1978) exposed rats in utero to methylmercury and tested their responsiveness to amphetamines during adulthood. Animals exposed to mercury acquired a discrete-trial, autoshaped bar-press response as rapidly as controls and exhibited similar rates of responding. When mercury-exposed animals were challenged with d-amphetamine, their operant performance was affected less than that of the controls. A similar observation was made by Eccles and Annau (1982), who dosed rats in utero with methylmercury and assessed their behavior in adulthood. These investigators found that mercury-exposed rats had similar response rates and obtained the same number of reinforcements as controls on a DRL 10-second schedule for food reinforcement. While control performance was markedly disrupted by 0.5 and 1.0 mg/kg d-amphetamine, the behavior of the mercury-exposed animals was only affected by the 0.5 mg/kg dose. Sparber and colleagues subsequently investigated the possibility that the change in responsiveness to d-amphetamine might be due to the effects of mercury on hepatic enzymes responsible for the metabolism of d-amphetamine. For example, mercury-treated animals could be less sensitive to amphetamine's effects due to an enhanced metabolism and/or elimination of the compound. Robbins and coworkers (1978), on the other hand, found that developmental exposure to methylmercury *decreased* the activity of microsomal enzymes responsible for the metabolism of amphetamine. Therefore, it was likely that more, and not less, amphetamine was gaining access to the CNS. Therefore, developmental exposure to methylmercury alters the sensitivity of the CNS to the effects of d-amphetamine instead of affecting the pharmacokinetics or biological efficacy of the compound.

Pharmacological agents other than d-amphetamine also have been used as probes in behavioral toxicology experiments. Thomas, Burch, and Yeandle (1979) trained rats to press a lever on a fixed-interval schedule of reinforcement, and once a stable baseline was established, they determined the effects of various doses of chlordiazepoxide (1–40 mg/kg) on FI responding. Then the dose-response curve was redetermined while the animals were concurrently exposed to a 1 mW/cm^2 irradiation. The dose-response curve for chlordiazepoxide was altered by the presence of the microwaves in that the magnitude of the effects was increased but the actual shape of the curve remained the same. Microwave exposure has also been reported to change the shape of the dose-response curve for amphetamine on a DRL schedule of reinforcement (Thomas and Maitland 1979) but not for chlorpromazine or diazepam on an FI schedule (Thomas, Schrot, and Bayard 1980).

The Use of Pharmacological Challenges to Study Mechanism of Action

Pharmacological agents can be used to address several different types of mechanistic questions. For example, on many occasions previous experiments have provided information concerning the effects of a neurotoxicant on some neurochemical, neurophysiological, or neuroanatomical parameter, and it is desirable to determine the functional significance of the observed effect. Another use of pharmacological challenges is in drug-interaction studies. For example, much of what is known about the behavioral and biochemical effects of psychoactive drugs has been obtained by attempting to antagonize or exacerbate the effects of an unknown compound by coadministering or pretreating with a pharmacological agent having a known neuropharmacological mechanism of action. Finally, results of an experiment in which a neurotoxicant affects behavior frequently suggests the use of a pharmacological challenge to aid in the interpretation of the original finding. In this section, several specific examples of the use of pharmacological agents to study mechanisms of action are discussed.

Carbon Disulfide

Carbon disulfide (CS$_2$) is an organic solvent that is used in a variety of industrial applications and has been shown to produce both neurobehavioral and systemic effects in exposed populations (see Wood 1981). Studies investigating the toxic mechanisms of CS$_2$ have demonstrated that it inhibits the activity of dopamine-β-hydroxylase (McKenna and DiStefano 1977), the enzyme responsible for the conversion of dopamine to norepinephrine. The immediate neurochemical effects of CS$_2$ include a marked and persistent reduction in whole-brain norepinephrine content (35 percent), together with a transient increase in dopamine concentrations (16 percent) (Magos 1972). To examine the functional consequences of CS$_2$ exposure on brain catecholamine systems Magos (1972, 1976) challenged CS$_2$-exposed rats with either apomorphine, a direct dopamine receptor agonist, or d-amphetamine, an indirect agonist that releases catecholamines, and measured the intensity and duration of motor stereotypy. Relatively short-term CS$_2$ exposure (two daily four-hour exposure periods) increased the intensity of stereotypy induced by both apomorphine and amphetamine and prolonged its duration in the latter group. These data suggested an enhanced dopamine release or increased receptor sensitivity in the exposed animals. A subsequent study using chronic exposure (daily four-hour exposure for six weeks), however, demonstrated that rats exposed to this regimen were less sensitive to the effects of d-amphetamine on spontaneous motor activity and acoustic startle (Tilson et al. 1979). Unfortunately, the long-term effects of this dosing regimen on brain catecholamine systems were not evaluated. Based upon these two conflicting reports, it might be hypothesized that short-term CS_2 exposure enhances sensitivity to amphetamine by increasing the amount of dopamine available for release, while prolonged exposure downregulates the receptor owing to this increased availability, resulting in an attenuated behavioral response to amphetamine. Neurochemical correlates of these alterations in drug sensitivity, as well as a better understanding of the time course of the biochemical changes, will be necessary in order to determine whether the altered sensitivity to dopaminergic drugs is due to alterations in catecholamine synthesis, metabolism, or receptor sensitivity.

Acrylamide

Acrylamide is a commonly used vinyl monomer (see Tilson 1981 for a review) that has been shown to produce a "central-peripheral dying-back axonopathy" and neuromotor impairments (Spencer and Schaumburg 1975). Agrawal and colleagues (Agrawal et al. 1981; Agrawal, Squibb, and Bondy 1981) reported that dopamine receptors in the striatum were increased by 24–44 percent 24 hours following acute exposure to 25, 50, or 100 mg/kg acrylamide. Benzodiazepine, GABA, and muscarinic cholinergic receptors were not affected by any dose of acrylamide, but glycine and serotonin receptors were significantly increased (25 percent) by the highest dose. Scatchard plot analysis of the binding data indicated that acrylamide increased both the affinity (K_d) of the dopamine receptor for the ligand and the number of available receptors (B_{max}).

   In an attempt to determine the functional significance of the receptor binding changes (i.e., an apparent up-regulation), the motor stimulant effects of apomorphine were measured in acrylamide-treated rats. Surprisingly, a significant decrease in the responsiveness to apomorphine was seen 24 hours after a single high dose (100 mg/kg) or after exposure to 10 mg/kg/day for 10 days (Agrawal et al. 1981; Bondy, Tilson, and Agrawal 1981). This effect was unexpected, since an increased receptor affinity or number of receptors should be behaviorally manifested as an increased sensitivity to a receptor agonist (see above). However, the neuromotor impairments produced by this high dose of acrylamide (100 mg/kg) might have contributed to a general decrease in the kind of motor output used to quantify the stereotypic effects of apomorphine. Thus, in a follow-up experiment (Tilson and Squibb 1982), the effects of lower doses of acrylamide were studied alone and in combination with apomorphine and other pharmacological agents on a well-established operant baseline. In this study, animals were trained to press a lever to obtain food reinforcement on a variable-interval (VI) 15-second schedule of reinforcement. Once a stable baseline was established, the effects of pharmacological agents on responding of rats previously treated with a behaviorally ineffective dose of acrylamide (12.5 mg/kg) were determined. As can be seen in

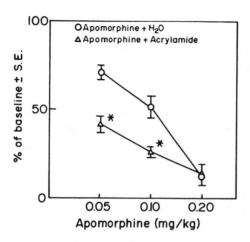

Fig. 11.3 The effect of apomorphine alone or in combination with acrylamide on VI 15-second responding. Rats were dosed with either distilled water or 12.5 mg/kg acrylamide 24 hours prior to apomorphine challenge. Data are mean ± SEM percentage of baseline activity. Asterisks represent a significant ($p < 0.05$) difference between groups.
(*Source:* Tilson and Squibb 1982. Reprinted by permission of the publisher.)

figure 11.3, pretreatment with acrylamide resulted in an increased response to the behaviorally disruptive effects of apomorphine. Similar effects were seen with d-amphetamine. The rate-decreasing effects of the alpha-adrenergic agonist clonidine and the benzodiazepine agonist chlordiazepoxide were similar in acrylamide-treated and control rats, indicating a preferential effect of this compound on dopaminergic systems, which corroborates the radioreceptor binding data. Besides showing that pharmacological challenges can be useful and relatively selective in determining the functional significance of an observed neurochemical effect, these studies illustrate the need to consider the possibility that neurotoxicants may differentially affect behavioral baselines (i.e., locomotor behavior versus operant performance), which could interfere with the ability to see a change in drug sensitivity.

Further studies, using a different dosing regimen, however, have also found that acrylamide increases the sensitivity of animals to amphetamine (Rafales, Bornschein, and Caruso 1982). In these studies, rats were exposed to 100 ppm acrylamide via their drinking water for a period of six weeks. While this dosing regimen induced signs of neuromotor impairment, the spontaneous activity and operant performance of these animals were not altered. These investigators found that acrylamide-exposed rats were more sensitive to the effects of d-amphetamine on locomotor activity in an open field and that they also exhibited an enhanced rotational response to this compound, suggesting a change in the sensitivity of central dopaminergic processes. The results of these studies provide a good example of how an integrative biochemical, pharmacological, and behavioral approach to the problem of neurotoxicity can contribute to an understanding of the sites and mechanisms of action of a given toxicant.

Chlordecone

Chlordecone (Kepone) is an organochlorine insecticide that produces a variety of neurobehavioral effects in both laboratory animals and humans (see Tilson and Mactutus 1982). Neurochemical studies demonstrated that ^{3}H-spiroperidol binding in the corpus striatum of male rats exposed to chlordecone during gestation and for the first twelve days of lactation was increased at 30 days of age (Seth, Agrawal, and Bondy 1981). The effect appeared to be reversible, since animals sacrificed at

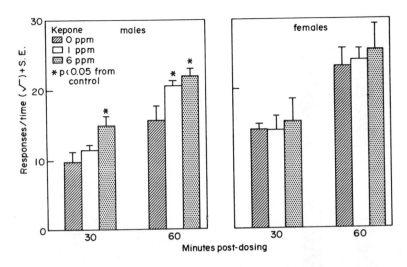

Fig. 11.4 The effect of 1 mg/kg apomorphine on 30 and 60 minutes of spontaneous motor activity of rats exposed to 0, 1, or 6 ppm chlordecone during gestation and for the first 12 days of lactation. Animals were tested at 114 days of age. The data represent the mean activity counts per minute (square root transformed) + SEM. Asterisks indicate a significant difference ($p < 0.05$) from controls. (*Source:* Squibb and Tilson 1982. Reprinted by permission of the publisher.)

100 days of age exhibited a dopamine receptor function comparable to that of the controls. Squibb and Tilson (1982) subsequently examined the potential long-term functional alterations in the responsivity of the dopaminergic system in animals perinatally exposed to chlordecone by challenging them with apomorphine or amphetamine. When challenged with 1 mg/kg apomorphine, chlordecone-exposed male rats exhibited more motor activity than did controls (fig. 11.4); however, they were not differentially sensitive to the indirect dopamine agonist d-amphetamine (not shown). These data suggest that presynaptic events such as dopamine release and turnover probably were unaffected by chlordecone but receptor-mediated processes were enhanced.

In a follow-up study, Tilson, Squibb, and Burne (1982) dosed animals with chlordecone on day 4 neonatally and examined drug responsiveness in adulthood. Rats were trained to respond for food reinforcement on a VI 15-second schedule of reinforcement, and once a stable baseline of responding was established, they were challenged with various doses of d-amphetamine (0.25–2.0 mg/kg) or apomorphine (0.025–0.1 mg/kg). Chlordecone-exposed animals showed little change in sensitivity to the rate-decreasing effects of d-amphetamine or apomorphine. These data appear inconsistent with the work of Squibb and Tilson (1982), in which there was an altered response to a relatively high dose of apomorphine (1 mg/kg) but no change in responsiveness to d-amphetamine. To the extent that the behavioral effects of low doses of apomorphine are mediated by presynaptic activation of dopaminergic receptors and higher doses affect postsynaptic sites (DiChiara et al. 1978), these data could indicate that chlordecone preferentially affects postsynaptic dopamine receptors.

Another series of studies conducted in our laboratory concerns the tremorigenic effects of chlordecone. In these experiments, animals were dosed with chlor-

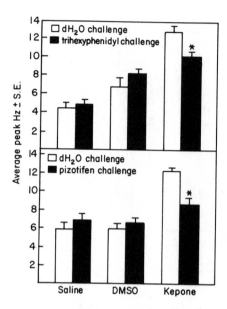

Fig. 11.5 The effect of trihexyphenidyl or BC-105 on chlordecone-induced tremor. The data represent the average peak (+ SEM) of the spectrally analyzed tremor recorded over 2.5 minutes. Asterisks indicate a significant (p < 0.05) difference between distilled water–injected controls and the drug-challenged groups.
(*Source:* Gerhart, Hong, and Tilson 1983. Reprinted by permission of the publisher.)

decone and then treated with various pharmacological agents in an attempt to attenuate or exacerbate the tremor produced by this compound (Gerhart et al. 1982; Gerhart, Hong, and Tilson 1983). Animals treated with the serotonergic antagonist pizotifen (BC-105) or the cholinergic antagonist trihexyphenidyl exhibited significantly less tremor than did rats exposed to chlordecone alone (fig. 11.5). Morever, most catecholaminergic agents were ineffective in altering the tremorigenic effects of chlordecone.

Tremor produced by a related organochlorine pesticide, DDT, has also been studied using pharmacological challenges. These studies indicate that DDT alters the disposition of 5-HT and that p-chlorophenylalanine, a compound that blocks the conversion of 5-hydroxytryptophan to serotonin, suppresses DDT-induced tremor (Peters et al. 1972; Hrdina et al. 1973). Inhibition of catecholamine synthesis with α-methyltyrosine had no effect on DDT-induced tremor. These studies, together with the chlordecone work, indicate that organochlorines might produce their tremorigenic effects via activation of serotonergic and perhaps cholinergic processes. Furthermore, these reports demonstrate that integrated neurochemical and pharmacological investigation of a given phenomenon (i.e., tremor) can help to define the functional consequences of biochemical perturbations induced by a toxicant.

Lead

The prevalence of inorganic lead in the environment and the numerous reports of lead poisoning have made this compound a major focus of research in behavioral toxicology. Coordinated behavioral and biochemical studies have examined various aspects of lead toxicity, in particular the alteration in drug sensitivity following both perinatal and adult exposure to inorganic lead. Despite myriad ambiguities and irreproducible results, the consensus derived from these studies is that perinatal lead exposure attenuates the behavioral effects of dopaminergic agonists such as d-amphetamine and apomorphine (see Bornschein, Pearson, and Reiter 1980). Although the results of these studies have been inconsistent and experimental approaches have differed, this literature dramatically illustrates the utility of using pharmacological challenges and the necessary considerations in evaluating studies of this kind.

Silbergeld and Goldberg (1974, 1975) were the first to report that mice exposed to lead during development were hyperactive as adults. Furthermore, this hyperactivity was paradoxically suppressed by motor-stimulant doses of amphetamine and methylphenidate and augmented by the barbiturate phenobarbital. These compelling observations of hyperactivity, together with altered sensitivity to pharmacological challenges, resembled the clinical picture of minimal brain dysfunction (MBD) or hyperkinesis in children (Wender 1971), and thus lead exposure was proposed as a potential etiological factor in the development of this disorder (see also Sobotka and Cook 1974). In subsequent experiments, Silbergeld and Goldberg investigated several other pharmacological agents and concluded that lead-induced hyperactivity was attenuated by cholinergic agonists (physostigmine) or catecholaminergic antagonists (α-methyl-para-tyrosine) and exacerbated by cholinergic antagonists (atropine) and catecholaminergic agonists (amphetamine, apomorphine, benztropine, 1-dopa, methylphenidate). In their review of the literature concerning the behavioral effects of perinatal lead exposure in animals, Bornschein, Pearson, and Reiter (1980) point out that Silbergeld and Goldberg (1) used only one dose of each pharmacological challenge, (2) inadequately described their statistical analyses, and (3) failed to take into account the weight differential between lead-exposed and control animals, thereby compromising the generality of their data and conclusions.

Experiments performed in other laboratories have tended to confirm the observation that perinatal exposure to inorganic lead attenuates the effects of amphetamine and apomorphine (Gray and Reiter 1977; Rafales et al. 1979). However, altered reactivity to other pharmacological agents (methylphenidate, phenobarbital) has not been replicated (Rafales et al. 1979). In addition, several questions concerning other aspects of their original work have prompted controversy and further study. For example, the observation that developmental exposure to lead produces hyperactivity in adulthood was not found to be a robust phenomenon (see Bornschein et al. 1981 for a review of this literature). Gray and Reiter (1977) and Rafales et al. (1979) exposed mice to lead during development and did not see hyperactivity when animals were tested as adults, although they were less responsive to an amphetamine challenge. However, these investigators used a different apparatus to measure activity, and direct comparisons with Silbergeld and Goldberg may not be appropriate.

A second problem concerns the fact that developmental exposure to lead can result in undernutrition. Using Silbergeld and Goldberg's exposure protocol (5 mg/ml lead acetate in mother's drinking water until weaning and in the pups' water thereafter), other investigators observed a 24–33 percent growth retardation (Sauerhoff and Michaelson 1973). Several studies (Loch et al. 1978; Michaelson 1980) have indicated that early undernutrition can alter responsiveness to d-amphetamine. Loch and colleagues (1978) reported that animals suffering undernutrition comparable to that induced by postnatal lead exposure as a result of being raised in a large litter exhibited a decreased and sometimes "paradoxical" response to amphetamine. Rafales et al. (1979) systematically studied the influence of lead-induced malnutrition on drug sensitivity by using a lower level of lead exposure and concluded that decreased responsiveness to d-amphetamine can, in fact, still be observed in lead-exposed animals not suffering from retarded growth.

Zenick and Goldsmith (1981) used a novel approach to determine the sensitivity of perinatally lead-exposed animals to the "internal cue" produced by d-amphetamine. Animals were exposed to lead acetate (0.2 or 0.5 percent) in their drinking water immediately following parturition until weaning or beyond. Animals were then trained at 90 days of age in a two-lever operant chamber to respond on one lever for sweetened condensed milk when they were injected with d-amphetamine (1 mg/kg) and on the other lever following a saline injection. Once the animals were accurately discriminating the two drug states (i.e., amphetamine versus saline), they were administered different doses of amphetamine (0.07–1.00 mg/kg) to determine the threshold at which amphetamine was no longer discriminable. The data revealed that animals exposed to lead during development required more amphetamine to discriminate this compound from a saline injection. For example, while control animals readily discriminated 0.175 mg/kg (but not 0.07 mg/kg) amphetamine from saline, the lead-treated rats required 0.35 mg/kg amphetamine for accurate discrimination. This study is important in that it shows decreased sensitivity in lead-exposed animals to d-amphetamine using a behavioral procedure other than drug-elicited motor activity. Furthermore, this altered sensitivity was evident in adult animals of normal stature without elevated blood lead levels. Therefore, the data generated by pharmacological challenge studies suggest that perinatal lead exposure decreases sensitivity to d-amphetamine. Neurochemical and pharmacokinetic hypotheses have been proposed to account for this observation, and several of these are discussed below.

The altered response to d-amphetamine has led several investigators to propose that developmental exposure to lead may alter the development of catecholaminergic systems, which mediate the behavioral effects of amphetamine. While perinatal lead exposure has been shown to alter the dynamics of various neurotransmitter systems, the most consistently affected neurochemical processes relate to catecholaminergic and cholinergic function (see Shih and Hanin 1978a for a review). Levels of the catecholamine metabolites homovanillic acid and vanilyl-mandelic acid have been found to be increased in animals exposed neonatally to lead (Silbergeld, Carroll, and Goldberg 1975; Silbergeld and Chisolm 1976), suggesting an enhancement of catecholaminergic function. More recent studies have observed region- and receptor-specific effects of neonatal lead exposure on dopaminergic parameters. For example, Memo and Trabucchi and their colleagues observed that developmental exposure to lead increased dopamine synthesis in the nucleus accumbens and the frontal cortex but decreased it in the striatum (Govoni et al. 1979; Memo et al. 1980). Their dosing regimen did not alter dopamine-stimulated adenylate cyclase or spiroperidol binding in either region. Pharmacological data indicate that there are at least two subtypes of the dopamine receptor. D1 receptors functionally coupled to adenylate cyclase and D2 receptors not coupled to cyclase activity (Kebabian and Calne 1979). Recognizing this multiplicity of dopamine receptor types, Lucchi and colleagues (1981) investigated the influence of lead on these receptor subtypes and observed a 50 percent increase in the number of receptors for sulpiride, a putative D2 antagonist, in the striatum, together with a 35 percent decrease in the nucleus accumbens. Again there were no alterations in dopamine-stimulated adenylate cyclase (i.e., an index of D1 receptors) or spiroperidol binding in either region. Furthermore, these investigators reported that lead-exposed rats were more sensitive than controls to the motor-suppressant effects of sulpiride but not to those of haloperidol (a mixed D1-D2 antagonist). These observations suggest that developmental lead exposure might alter select aspects of dopaminergic function. A problem associated with these reports is that the exposure regimen is likely to have resulted in weight differences between control and exposed animals (i.e., growth rate was not reported in these studies). Several lines of evidence indicate that neonatal undernutrition can alter various aspects of catecholaminergic function, thereby making the conclusions derived from these studies tentative (Shoemaker and Wurtman 1973; Parvez, Ismahan, and Parvez 1980). A well-designed study by Wince, Donovan, and Azzaro (1980) utilizing appropriate pair-fed controls, a wide dose range of pharmacological challenges, and biochemical measures of both pre- and postsynaptic dopaminergic function demonstrated specific alterations in this transmitter system following perinatal exposure to lead. Pups continuously exposed to dietary lead from birth exhibited an attenuated locomotor response to both d-amphetamine (0.5–2.0 mg/kg) and apomorphine (0.5–5.0 mg/kg) when challenged at 25–35 days of age. The biochemical studies demonstrated a diminished KCl-evoked release of exogenous dopamine from forebrain slices and a decreased dopamine- or apomorphine-induced activation of adenylate cyclase in the striatal homogenates. No alteration of synthesis, accumulation, or d-amphetamine-induced release of dopamine was observed. These data indicate that postnatal exposure to inorganic lead can affect various aspects of dopaminergic transmission.

Acetylcholine turnover also appears to be decreased 35–55 percent in various regions (cortex, hippocampus, midbrain, striatum) of lead-exposed animals (Shih and Hanin 1978b), and a recent report indicates that perinatally lead-exposed mice were more susceptible to the behavioral effects of the cholinergic antagonist atropine when tested as adults (Silbergeld and Goldberg 1975).

Another explanation for the differential effects of d-amphetamine in lead-exposed animals is that lead interferes with some pharmacokinetic factor that interferes with the distribution or elimination of amphetamine. To test this hypothesis, Zenick et al. (1982) exposed rats to lead during development and tested them at 90 days of age. This dosing paradigm did not alter body weight or baseline levels of motor activity, but a challenge dose of 1 mg/kg d-amphetamine was found to be less effective in lead-exposed rats. Between 110 and 120 days of age, the rats were injected with ^{3}H-d-amphetamine, and the time course of the appearance and relative distribution of ^{3}H-amphetamine in various regions of the brain was measured. Although the time course of the appearance and regional distribution of d-amphetamine in the brain was the same in lead-treated and control animals, less ^{3}H-amphetamine appeared in the pons-medulla, the hypothalamus, the striatum, and hippocampus of lead-exposed rats. Plasma concentrations of amphetamine in the groups were not different. This experiment illustrates the need to consider pharmacokinetic factors such as metabolism, distribution, and elimination in studies using pharmacological challenges.

The data reported here indicate that developmental exposure to inorganic lead attenuates the behavioral effects of d-amphetamine. While several hypotheses have been proposed to account for this altered sensitivity, it is likely that several mechanisms participate. Zenick and colleagues (1982) suggest that to further define the nature of the lead-induced alterations in drug sensitivity, two separate but interrelated phenomena must be addressed: (1) the concentration of amphetamine reaching sites involved in the mediation of its behavioral effects and (2) the responsiveness of specific neurotransmitter systems to the concentrations attained.

The effect of repeated exposure to low levels of lead has also been studied in adult animals. Carter and Leander (1980) trained pigeons to respond on a multiple fixed-ratio 30, fixed-interval 5-minute schedule of food reinforcement and treated them daily with 6.25 mg/kg lead acetate once a steady baseline of responding was established. The pigeons were subsequently challenged with a battery of pharmacological agents. Lead-exposed animals were less sensitive to catecholaminergic drugs (d-amphetamine, protriptyline) but not to other agents (pentobarbital, hydroxyamphetamine, pentylenetetrazol, quipazine, 5-HTP, scopolamine, physostigmine, and nicotine). Subtle alterations in CNS function occurred in adult animals exposed to inorganic lead, and these changes could be detected only by the appropriate use of drug challenges. In addition, by using several pharmacological agents, the specificity of the change (i.e., the altered response to catecholaminergic drugs) could be determined and correlated with the neurochemical effects induced by the compound.

All of the effects discussed thus far concern the inorganic form of lead. The organic forms of lead, notably triethyl and trimethyl lead, produce behavioral effects that are qualitatively different from those produced by the inorganic forms (Pryor et al. 1983; Walsh and Tilson 1984). A prominent observation following either acute or short-term repeated administration of triethyl lead to adult rats is an increased latency to respond to noxious stimuli (hot plate, tail flick, electric shock to tail). In an attempt to study the mechanism of this "analgesia," animals exposed to 1.75 mg/kg triethyl lead (TEL) for five days were challenged two weeks later with naloxone (an opiate antagonist) or chlordiazepoxide (an anxiolytic benzodiazepine) prior to testing on the hot plate. Both chlordiazepoxide and a high dose of naloxone attenuated the "analgesia" produced by triethyl lead (fig. 11.6). These data suggest that the triethyl lead–induced antinociception may be due to enhanced emotional responsiveness to the noxious testing situation (stress-induced analgesia), mediated through benzodiazepine and/or opiate processes.

Diisopropylflorophosphate (DFP)

DFP is an organophosphate pesticide that is a potent inhibitor of acetylcholinesterase, the enzyme that metabolizes acetylcholine released at the synapse. DFP therefore prevents the breakdown of acetylcholine and promotes the interaction of this neurotransmitter with its postsynaptic receptor. Repeated exposure to this compound results in tolerance to its behavioral and physiological effects. Russell and colleagues (1979) proposed four hypotheses to account for the development of tolerance following chronic DFP exposure: (1) nonspecific metabolic changes, (2) end-product inhibition involving reduction in acetylcholine synthesis, (3) neurochemical redundancy in which another neurotransmitter system compensates for alterations in cholinergic processes, and (4) changes in the sensitivity of postsynaptic cholinergic receptors (i.e., down-regulation). Pharmacological chal-

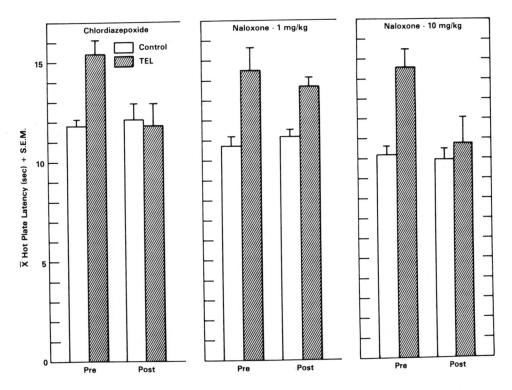

Fig. 11.6 The effect of naloxone and chlordiazepoxide on triethyl lead–induced antinociception. Rats received daily injections of TEL (1.75 mg/kg/day subcutaneously) or distilled water for 5 consecutive days. Two weeks after the last injection, hot-plate latencies were measured before and after the drug challenges. Chlordiazepoxide and the 10 mg/kg dose of naloxone significantly attenuated the increase induced by TEL.

lenges have been used in conjunction with other approaches to study these four possibilities.

Russell et al. (1971) trained rats to lever press for water and then dosed them repeatedly with DFP to produce tolerance to the initial suppression of responding. Once tolerance had developed, the rats were challenged with various doses of atropine, a muscarinic receptor antagonist. DFP-tolerant rats were more susceptible to the behavioral suppressant effects of this agent. In contrast, DFP-treated rats were not sensitive to methylatropine, the peripherally active form of atropine that fails to cross the blood-brain barrier, indicating that alterations in the central rather than the peripheral cholinergic processes were responsible for the development of tolerance.

Chippendale et al. (1972) expanded the number of pharmacological challenges used in DFP-tolerant rats to include scopolamine, methylscopolamine, and α-methyltyrosine (an inhibitor of catecholamine synthesis). Rats chronically treated with DFP were more suppressed following scopolamine, while they did not differ from controls in their response to methylscopolamine and α-methyltyrosine. Since α-methyltyrosine was equally effective in control and DFP-exposed rats, the authors concluded that neurochemical redundancy, at least involving the catecholamine system, was not likely to account for the development of tolerance.

Both Russell et al. (1971) and Chippendale et al. (1972) used behavioral base-lines consisting of suppression of water drinking or responding for a water reward. Overstreet, Kozar, and Lynch (1973) extended their work by measuring DFP-induced hypothermia. Tolerance to the hypothermia developed following repeated exposure to DFP, and when challenged with pilocarpine, a muscarinic agonist, the hypothermia normally produced by this agent was reduced. Again, the effect seemed to be of central origin, since intrahypothalamic injection of carbachol did not produce hypothermia in DFP-tolerant rats. Overstreet et al. (1974) also examined the effects of both muscarinic and nicotinic agonists and antagonists and observed a decreased sensitivity to both types of compounds.

Russell et al. (1975) studied the end-product-inhibition hypothesis by measuring changes in the activity of choline acetyltransferase, the enzyme that synthesizes acetylcholine from choline and acetyl CoA, following chronic DFP exposure. It was hypothesized that the accumulation of acetylcholine due to the inhibition of its breakdown might depress the activity of this synthetic enzyme. It was observed, however, that while DFP increased acetylcholine concentrations (140 percent increase) and decreased cholinesterase activity (28.5 percent of control), the activity of choline acetyltransferase was not diminished. Moreover, adenosine triphosphate, alkaline phosphatase, and cytochrome oxidase were not changed in DFP-tolerant rats, suggesting that nonspecific metabolic changes were not responsible for the development of tolerance. Thus, these data and those from the pharmacological experiments indicated that tolerance to DFP involves a change in the sensitivity of the postsynaptic receptor. Recent studies using radioreceptor binding have observed that chronic exposure to DFP does, in fact, decrease the number of muscarinic cholinergic receptors without changing the affinity of these receptors for their ligands in the cortex, the hippocampus, and the striatum (Schiller 1979; Yamada et al. 1983). Similar receptor changes (i.e., down-regulation), behavioral tolerance, and enhanced response to cholinergic antagonists have been observed after repeated dosing with a related anticholinesterase inhibitor, disulfoton (see Costa et al. 1982a, 1982b for details).

Taken together, the studies reviewed here indicate that a behavioral observation (i.e., tolerance) can lead to the generation of testable hypotheses regarding the mechanisms of a given phenomenon. The work of Russell and his collaborators highlights the utility of combining behavioral measures, pharmacological challenges, and neurochemical procedures to define the molecular mechanisms responsible for toxicant-induced behavioral alterations.

Summary and Conclusions

The literature reviewed here illustrates that exposure to a variety of neurotoxic compounds can produce altered sensitivity to pharmacological challenges. Changes in drug sensitivity can reflect a variety of behavioral and biochemical events. For example, increased or decreased sensitivity to psychostimulants such as amphetamine could reflect alterations in catecholamine function induced by a toxicant or, more simply, the effect of a toxicant on hepatic enzymes, blood-brain-barrier permeability, or neuronal uptake, processes that determine the absorption, distribution, and elimination of drugs. The work of Zenick and collaborators indicates that the decreased sensitivity of perinatally lead-exposed rats to d-amphetamine might be due to alterations in the accumulation of this compound at brain loci that mediate its behavioral effects. In contrast, Russell and coworkers have shown that the tolerance that develops to the behavioral effects of chronically administered organophosphate insecticides is dependent upon alterations in discrete neurochemical elements. Tolerant animals exhibit an enhanced sensitivity to cholinergic antagonists and a compensatory decrease in the number of muscarinic cholinergic receptors (down-regulation) in the central nervous system. These two examples demonstrate that altered sensitivity to pharmacological probes can reflect the involvement of both central and peripheral processes.

The studies reviewed here demonstrate that the appropriate use of pharmacological challenges can provide valuable information regarding the functional integrity of neurotransmitter systems. The utilization of sensitive behavioral baselines together with drugs known to selectively interact with discrete neurochemical systems and to alter behavior in a predictable manner offer the neurotoxicologist a noninvasive approach for assessing the presence of a toxicant-induced biochemical lesion.

In conclusion, the quantitative use of pharmacological probes (i.e., dose- and time-response analysis) together with appropriate behavioral methodologies and correlative neurochemical studies should prove to be an important strategy for determining mechanisms of neurotoxicity.

Acknowledgments

The authors are grateful for the typing assistance of Bonnie Highsmith and for the technical assistance of John N. Peterson and Ronnie McLamb, who helped perform many of the experiments described in this review.

References

Adams, J.; Buelke-Sam, J.; Kimmel, C. A.; and LaBorde, J. B. 1982. Behavioral alterations in rats prenatally exposed to low doses of d-amphetamine. *Neurobehav. Toxicol. Teratol.* 4:63–70.

Agrawal, A. K.; Seth, P. K.; Squibb, R. E.; Tilson, H. A.; Uphouse, L. L.; and Bondy, S. C. 1981. Neurotransmitter receptors in brain regions of acrylamide-treated rats. I: Effects of a single exposure to acrylamide. *Pharmacol. Biochem. Behav.* 14:527–31.

Agrawal, A. K.; Squibb, R. E.; and Bondy, S. C. 1981. The effects of acrylamide treatment upon the dopamine receptor. *Toxicol. Appl. Pharmacol.* 58,89–99.

Bergstrom, D. A., and Kellar, K. J. 1979. Adrenergic and serotonergic receptor binding in rat brain after chronic desmethylimipramine treatment. *J. Pharmacol. Exp. Ther.* 209:256–61.

Besson, M. J.; Cheramy, A.; Feltz, P.; and Glowinski, J. 1971. Dopamine: Spontaneous and drug-induced release from the caudate nucleus in the cat. *Brain Res.* 32:407–24.

Bondy, S. C.; Tilson, H. A.; and Agrawal, A. K. 1981. Neurotransmitter receptors in brain regions of acrylamide-treated rats. II: Effects of extended exposure to acrylamide. *Pharmacol. Biochem. Behav.* 14:533–37.

Bornschein, R.; Pearson, D.; and Reiter, L. 1980. Behavioral effects of moderate lead exposure in children and animal models: Part 2, animal studies. *CRC Crit. Rev. Toxicol.* 8:101–52.

Bornschein, R.; Rafales, L. S.; Hastings, I.; Loch, R. K.; and Michaelson, I. A. 1981. Does lead produce hyperactivity in rats or mice? In *Environmental lead*, edited by D. R. Lyman, L. G. Piantanida, and J. F. Cole, 45–65. New York: Academic Press.

Carter, R. B., and Leander, J. D. 1980. Chronic low-level lead exposure: Effects on schedule-controlled responding revealed by drug challenge. *Neurobehav. Toxicol. Teratol.* 2:345–53.

Chippendale, T. J.; Zawolkow, G. A.; Russell, R. W.; and Overstreet, D. H. 1972. Tolerance to low acetylcholinesterase levels: Modification of behavior without acute behavioral change. *Psychopharmacologia* 26:127–39.

Cofer, C. N., and Appley, M. H. 1965. *Motivation: Theory and research.* New York: Wiley.

Coffin, D. L.; Gardner, D. E.; and Blommer, E. J. 1976. Time-dose response for nitrogen dioxide exposure in an infectivity model system. *Environ. Health Perspect.* 13:11–15.

Costa, L. G.; Schwab, B. W.; and Murphy S. D. 1982a. Differential alterations of cholinergic muscarinic receptors during chronic and acute tolerance to organophosphorus insecticides. *Biochem. Pharmacol.* 31:3407–13.

———. 1982b. Tolerance to anticholinesterase compounds in mammals. *Toxicology* 25:79–97.

Creese, I., and Iversen, S. D. 1975. The pharmacological and anatomical substrates of the amphetamine response in the rat. *Brain Res.* 83:419–36.

DeHaven, D. L., and Mailman, R. B. 1983. The use of radioligand binding techniques in neurotoxicology. *Rev. Biochem. Toxicol.* 5:193–238.

DiChiara, G.; Corsini, G. V.; Mereu, G. P.; Tissari, A.; and Gessa, G. L. 1978. Self-inhibition of dopamine receptors: Their role in the biochemical and behavioral effects of low doses of apomorphine. *Adv. Biochem. Psychopharmacol.* 19:275–92.

Eccles, C. U., and Annau, Z. 1982. Prenatal methylmercury exposure: II. Alterations in learning and psychotropic drug sensitivity in adult offspring. *Neurobehav. Toxicol. Teratol.* 4:377–82.

Finger, S., and Stein, D. G. 1982. *Brain damage and recovery: Research and clinical perspectives.* New York: Academic Press.

Fouts, J. R. 1963. Factors influencing the metabolism of drugs in liver microsomes. *Ann. N.Y. Acad. Sci.* 104:875.

Fray, P. J.; Sahakian, B. J.; Robbins, T. W.; Koob, G. F.; and Iversen, S. D. 1980. An observational method for quantifying the behavioral effects of dopamine agonists: Contrasting effects of *d*-amphetamine and apomorphine. *Psychopharmacology* 69:253–59.

Gerhart, J. M.; Hong, J. S.; and Tilson, H. A. 1983. Studies on the possible sites of chlordecone-induced tremor in rats. *Toxicol. Appl. Pharmacol.* 70:382–89.

Gerhart, J. M.; Hong, J. S.; Uphouse, L. L.; and Tilson, H. A. 1982. Chlordecone-induced tremor: Quantification and pharmacological analysis. *Toxicol. Appl. Pharmacol.* 66:234–43.

Goodman, L. S., and Gilman, A. 1975. *The pharmacological basis of therapeutics.* New York: Macmillan.

Govoni, S.; Memo, M.; Spano, P. F.; and Trabucchi, M. 1979. Chronic lead treatment differentially affects dopamine synthesis in various rat brain areas. *Toxicology* 12:343–49.

Gray, L. E., and Reiter, L. W. 1977. Lead-induced developmental and behavioral changes in the mouse. *Toxicol. Appl. Pharmacol.* 41:140.

Guyton, A. C. 1971. *Textbook of medical physiology.* Philadelphia: W. B. Saunders.

Hrdina, D. D.; Singhal, R. L.; Peters, D. A.; and Ling, G. M. 1973. Some neurochemical alterations during acute DDT poisoning. *Toxicol. Appl. Pharmacol.* 25:276–88.

Hughes, J. A., and Sparber, S. B. 1978. *d*-amphetamine unmasks postnatal consequences of exposure to methylmercury in utero: Methods for studying behavioral teratogenesis. *Pharmacol. Biochem. Behav.* 8:365–75.

Iversen, S. D., and Koob, G. F. 1977. Behavioral implications of dopaminergic neurons in the mesolimbic system. *Adv. Biochem. Psychopharmacol.* 16:209–14.

Kebabian, J. W., and Calne, D. B. 1979. Multiple receptors for dopamine. *Nature* 277:93–96.

Kelly, P. H.; Seviour, P. W.; and Iversen, S. D. 1975. Amphetamine and apomorphine responses in the rat following 6-OHDA lesions of the nucleus accumbens, septi and corpus striatum. *Brain Res.* 94:507–22.

Kurlan, R., and Shoulson, I. 1982. Up and down regulation: Clinical significance of nervous system receptor-drug interactions. *Clin. Neuropharmacol.* 5:345–50.

Lashley, K. 1929. *Brain mechanisms and intelligence.* Chicago: University of Chicago Press.

Laties, V. G., and Cory-Slechta, D. A. 1979. Some problems in interpreting the behavioral effects of lead and methyl mercury. *Neurobehav. Toxicol.* 1, suppl. 1:129–35.

Leander, J. D. 1980. Low-level lead exposure: Attenuation of *d*-amphetamine's rate-increasing effects. *Neurotoxicology* 1:551–59.

Loch, R. K.; Rafales, L. S.; Michaelson, I. A.; and Bornschein, R. L. 1978. The role of under nutrition in animal models of hyperactivity. *Life Sci.* 22:1963–70.

Lucchi, L.; Memo, M.; Airaghi, M. L.; Spano, P. F.; and Trabucchi, M. 1981. Chronic lead treatment induces in rat a specific and differential effect on dopamine receptors in different brain areas. *Brain Res.* 213:397–404.

McKenna, M. J., and DiStefano, V. 1977. Carbon disulphide. II. A proposed mechanism for the action of carbon disulfide on dopamine β-hydroxylase. *J. Pharmacol. Exp. Ther.* 202:253–66.

Magos, L. 1972. Toxicity of carbon disulphide. *Ann. Occup. Hyg.* 15:303–9.

————. 1976. The effect of carbon disulphide on the stereotypic effect of dopamine agonists. *Europ. J. Pharmacol.* 36:257–58.

Martin, W. R. 1968. A homeostatic and redundancy theory of tolerance to and dependence on narcotic analgesics. *Proc. Assoc. Res. Nerv. Ment. Dis.* 46:206–25.

Memo, M.; Lucchi, L.; Spano, P. F.; and Trabucchi, M. 1980. Dose-dependent effects of lead on different neurotransmitter systems in various rat brain areas. In *Advances in neurotoxicology,* edited by L. Manzo, 41–48. New York: Pergamon Press.

Michaelson, I. A. 1980. An appraisal of rodent studies on the behavioral toxicity of lead: The role of nutritional status. In *Lead toxicity,* edited by R. L. Singhal and J. A. Thomas, 301–66. Baltimore and Munich: Urban & Schwarzenberg.

Moore, K. E. 1977. The actions of amphetamine on neurotransmitters: A brief review. *Biol. Psychiatry* 12:451–62.

Muller, P., and Seeman, P. 1978. Dopaminergic supersensitivity after neuroleptics: Time course and specificity. *Psychopharmacology* 60:1–11.

Norton, S. 1982. Methods in behavioral toxicology. In *Principles and methods of toxicology,* edited by A. W. Hayes, 353–73. New York: Raven Press.

Overstreet, D. H.; Kozar, M. D.; and Lynch, G. S. 1973. Reduced hypothermic effects of cholinomimetic agents following chronic anticholinesterase treatment. *Neuropharmacology* 12:1017–32.

Overstreet, D. H.; Russell, R. W.; Vasquez, B. J.; and Dalglish, F. W. 1974. Involvement of muscarinic and nicotinic receptors in behavioral tolerance to DFP. *Pharmacol. Biochem. Behav.* 2:45–54.

Parvez, S.; Ismahan, G.; and Parvez, H. 1980. Role of nutritional factors in the development of catecholamine synthesis and metabolism. In *Biogenic amines in development*, edited by H. Parvez and S. Parvez, 441–90. Amsterdam: Elsevier.

Pavlenko, S. M. 1975. Methods for the study of the central nervous system in toxicological tests. *Methods used in the USSR for establishing biologically safe levels of toxic substances,* 86–108. Geneva: World Health Organization.

Peters, D. A. V.; Hrdina, P. D.; Singhal, R. L.; and Ling, G. M. 1972. The role of brain serotonin in DDT-induced hyperpyrexia. *J. Neurochem.* 19:1131–36.

Pryor, G. T.; Uyeno, E. T.; Tilson, H. A.; and Mitchell, C. L. 1983. Assessment of chemicals using a battery of neurobehavioral tests: A comparative study. *Neurobehav. Toxicol. Teratol.* 5:91–117.

Rafales, L. S.; Bornschein, R. L.; and Caruso, V. 1982. Behavioral and pharmacological responses following acrylamide exposure in rats. *Neurobehav. Toxicol. Teratol.* 4:355–64.

Rafales, L. S.; Bornschein, R. L.; Michaelson, I. A.; Loch, R. K.; and Barker, G. F. 1979. Drug-induced activity in lead-exposed mice. *Pharmacol. Biochem. Behav.* 10:95–104.

Reisine, T. 1981. Adaptive changes in catecholamine receptors in the central nervous system. *Neuroscience* 6:1471–1502.

Reiter, L. W.; Anderson, G. E.; Ash, M. E.; and Gray, L. E. 1977. Locomotor activity measurements in behavioral toxicology: Effects of lead administration on residential maze behavior. In *Behavioral toxicology: An emerging discipline*, edited by H. Zenick and L. W. Reiter, 6-1-6-18. Washington, D.C.: Government Printing Office.

Robbins, M. S.; Hughes, J. A.; Sparber, S. B.; and Mannering, G. J. 1978. Delayed teratogenic effects of methylmercury on hepatic cytochrome p-450-dependent monooxygenase systems of rats. *Life Sci.* 4:287–94.

Russell, R. W.; Carson, V. G.; Jope, R.; Booth, R. A.; and Macri, J. 1979. Development of behavioral tolerance: A search for subcellular mechanisms. *Psychopharmacology* 66:155–58.

Russell, R. W.; Overstreet, D. H.; Cotman, C. W.; Carson, V. G.; Churchill, L.; Dalglish, F. W.; and Vasquez, B. J. 1975. Experimental tests of hypotheses about neurochemical mechanisms underlying behavioral tolerance to the anticholinesterase, diisopropyl fluorophosphate. *J. Pharmacol. Exp. Ther.* 192:73–85.

Russell, R. W.; Vasquez, B. J.; Overstreet, D. H.; and Dalglish, F. W. 1971. Effects of cholinolytic agents on behavior following development of tolerance to low cholinesterase activity. *Psychopharmacologia* 20:32–41.

Sauerhoff, M. W., and Michaelson, I. A. 1973. Hyperactivity and brain catecholamines in lead-exposed developing rats. *Science* 182:1022–24.

Schiller, G. D. 1979. Reduced binding of [³H]-quinuclidinyl benzilate associated with chronically low acetylcholinesterase activity. *Life Sci.* 24:1159–64.

Segal, D. S. 1975. Behavioral characterization of *d-* and *l-*amphetamine: Neurochemical implications. *Science* 190:475–77.

Segawa, T.; Mizuta, T.; and Nomura, Y. 1979. Modifications of central 5-hydroxytryptamine binding sites in synaptic membranes from rat brain after long-term administration of tricyclic antidepressants. *Eur. J. Pharmacol.* 58:75–83.

Seth, P. K.; Agrawal, A. K.; and Bondy, S. C. 1981. Biochemical changes in the brain consequent to dietary exposure of developing and mature rats to chlordecone (Kepone). *Toxicol. Appl. Pharmacol.* 59:262–67.

Shih, T. M., and Hanin, I. 1978a. Chronic lead exposure in immature animals: Neurochemical correlates. *Life Sci.* 23:877–88.

———. 1978b. Effect of chronic lead exposure on levels of acetylcholine and choline and on acetylcholine turnover rate in rat brain areas *in vivo*. *Psychopharmacology* 58:263–69.

Shoemaker, W. J., and Wurtman, R. J. 1973. Effect of perinatal undernutrition on the metabolism of catecholamines in the rat brain. *J. Nutrition* 103:1537–47.

Silbergeld, E. K.; Carroll, P. T.; and Goldberg, A. M. 1975. Monoamines in lead-induced hyperactivity. *Pharmacologist* 17:212.

Silbergeld, E. K., and Chisolm, J. J. 1976. Lead poisoning: Altered urinary catecholamine metabolites as indicators of intoxication in mice and children. *Science* 192:153–55.

Silbergeld, E. K., and Goldberg, A. M. 1974. Lead-induced behavioral dysfunction: An animal model of hyperactivity. *Exp. Neurol.* 42:146–57.

———. 1975. Pharmacological and neurochemical investigations of lead-induced hyperactivity. *Neuropharmacology* 14:431–44.

Sobotka, T. J., and Cook, M. P. 1974. Postnatal lead acetate exposure in rats: Possible relationship to minimal brain dysfunction. *Am. J. Ment. Defic.* 79:5–9.

Spencer, P. S., and Schaumburg, H. H. 1975. Nervous system degeneration produced by acrylamide monomer. *Environ. Health Perspect.* 11:129–33.

Squibb, R. E., and Tilson, H. A. 1982. Effects of gestational and perinatal exposure to chlordecone (Kepone®) on the neurobehavioral development of Fischer-344 rats. *Neurotoxicology* 3:17–26.

Squibb, R. E.; Tilson, H. A.; Meyer, O. A.; and Lamartiniere, C. A. 1981. Neonatal exposure to monosodium glutamate alters the neurobehavioral performance of adult rats. *Neurotoxicology* 2:471–84.

Thomas, J. R.; Burch, L. S.; and Yeandle, S. S. 1979. Microwave irradiation and chlordiazepoxide: Synergistic effects on fixed-interval behavior. *Science* 203:1357–58.

Thomas, J. R., and Maitland, G. 1979. Microwave radiation and *d*-amphetamine: Evidence of combined effects of fixed-interval behavior of rats. *Radio Sci.* 14:253–58.

Thomas, J. R.; Schrot, J.; and Bayard, R. B. 1980. Behavioral effects of chlorpromazine and diazepam combined with low-level microwaves. *Neurobehav. Toxicol. Teratol.* 2:131–35.

Tilson, H. A. 1981. The neurotoxicity of acrylamide: An overview. *Neurobehav. Toxicol. Teratol.* 3:445–61.

Tilson, H. A., and Cabe, P. A. 1979. Studies on the neurobehavioral effects of polybrominated biphenyls in rats. *Ann. N.Y. Acad. Sci.* 320:325–36.

Tilson, H. A.; Cabe, P. A.; Ellinwood, E. H.; and Gonzalez, L. P. 1979. Effects of carbon disulfide on motor function and responsiveness to *d*-amphetamine in rats. *Neurobehav. Toxicol.* 1:57–63.

Tilson, H. A., and Mactutus, C. F. 1982. Chlordecone neurotoxicity: A brief overview. *Neurotoxicology* 3:1–8.

Tilson, H. A., and Squibb, R. E. 1982. The effects of acrylamide on the behavioral suppression produced by psychoactive agents. *Neurotoxicology* 3:113–20.

Tilson, H. A.; Squibb, R. E.; and Burne, T. A. 1982. Neurobehavioral effects following a single dose of chlordecone (Kepone®) administered neonatally to rats. *Neurotoxicology* 3:45–58.

Tilson, H. A.; Squibb, R. E.; Meyer, O. A.; and Sparber, S. B. 1980. Postnatal exposure to benzene alters the neurobehavioral functioning of rats when tested during adulthood. *Neurobehav. Toxicol. Teratol.* 2:101–6.

Walsh, T. J., and Tilson, H. A. 1984. Neurobehavioral toxicology of the organoleads. *Neurotoxicology* 5:67–86.

Wender, P. H. 1971. *Minimal brain dysfunction in children.* New York: Wiley-Interscience.

Wince, L. C.; Donovan, C. A.; and Azzaro, A. J. 1980. Alterations of the biochemical properties of central dopamine synapses following chronic postnatal $PbCO_3$ exposure. *J. Pharmacol. Exp. Ther.* 214:642–50.

Wood, R. W. 1981. Neurobehavioral toxicity of carbon disulfide. *Neurobehav. Toxicol. Teratol.* 3:397–405.

Yamada, S.; Isogai, M.; Okudaira, H.; and Hayashi, E. 1983. Regional adaptation of muscarinic receptors and choline uptake in brain following repeated administration of diisopropylfluorophosphate and atropine. *Brain Res.* 268:315–20.

Zenick, H., and Goldsmith, M. 1981. Drug discrimination learning in lead-exposed rats. *Science* 212:569–71.

Zenick, H.; Lasley, S. M.; Greenland, R.; Caruso, V.; Succop, P.; Price, D.; and Michaelson, I. A. 1982. Regional brain distribution of *d*-amphetamine in lead-exposed rats. *Toxicol. Appl. Pharmacol.* 64:52–63.

Gary L. Wenk and
David S. Olton

12

Lesion Analysis

Neurobehavioral toxicology studies the behavioral effects of toxicants that alter central-nervous-system function. Behavioral neuroscience often studies the behavioral effects of selective lesions. In this chapter we demonstrate how the conceptual frameworks and experimental procedures basic to neuropsychological research can be adapted to toxicological studies. This chapter outlines an approach that may be useful to the neuroscientist interested in understanding the actions of a particular toxicant on the brain by examining its effects on behavior.

Both neurobehavioral toxicology and behavioral neuroscience study the functional disruptions of the central nervous system (CNS) and their effects on behavior. The substances that produce this damage, however, may be very different in the two disciplines. The toxicants studied by the neurobehavioral toxicologist are chosen because of their importance in our everyday lives rather than because of their mode of action on the CNS. In contrast, the lesions studied by the basic neuroscientist are chosen because of their action in the CNS rather than because of their likelihood of occurrence in the world. Indeed, one of the major advances in behavioral neurosciences has come through the development of specific neurotoxicants (Coyle 1983). In spite of these differences, however, the two areas still share the same general problems. While neurobehavioral toxicology is a relatively new field, behavioral neuroscience is a well-established one. Consequently, many of the issues relevant to the neurobehavioral toxicologist have already been addressed by the behavioral neuroscientist. This chapter reviews these principles and shows how they can help make research more productive in neurobehavioral toxicology.

The Functional Specificity of Neurotoxicants

Toxicants can affect the brain both directly and indirectly. Directly, a toxicant can act on some part of the CNS and disrupt it. Indeed, the term *neurotoxicant* implies that the toxicant has its major effect directly on the CNS. Normal brain function requires careful homeostatic control of many different metabolic processes. If a toxicant interferes with one of these metabolic processes, then that toxicant may indirectly change brain function and, subsequently, behavior.

Even a neurotoxicant that acts directly on the brain may not be functionally specific; that is, it may not affect a single behavioral system. Consider, for example, two directly acting neurotoxicants that have a discrete mechanism of action. Colchisine affects the microtubules involved in axonal transport (Dustin 1963), while triethyltin produces demyelination (Jacobs, Cremer, and Cavanagh 1977). Thus, both of these substances selectively disrupt one aspect of the CNS. The functional effects are widespread, however, with the result that many different behaviors are affected. The criterion of functional specificity must be determined by a behavioral analysis rather than a neural one. In contrast, some directly acting neurotoxicants are relatively selective for functional systems. Examples of these kinds of toxicants include manganese and phencyclidine (these neurotoxicants are discussed in detail below).

Toxicants that act indirectly inevitably will have widespread effects on functional systems. Because lesion analyses in the behavioral neurosciences have been developed mainly to deal with functionally specific disruptions, the considerations discussed here probably do not apply very well to these types of toxicants. Even within the class of directly acting neurotoxicants the question of functional specificity still holds. For colchisine and triethyltin, discussed above, lesion analyses have less to contribute than for more functionally specific neurotoxicants. Consequently, we emphasize functionally specific neurotoxicants rather than functionally diverse ones.

Behavioral Tests: Selectivity and Sensitivity

A selective test is one in which performance is severely impaired by disruption of some functional systems but not others. Thus, for example, performance in a behavioral test that requires a fine discrimination of visual stimuli should be markedly impaired by alterations in the visual system but not by alterations in the auditory system. Similarly, performance in a behavioral task that places a strong emphasis on short-term memory should be markedly impaired by lesions that disrupt the brain systems involved in this memory but not so much by lesions in other systems. Thus, a selective test emphasizes one psychological function to a much greater extent than it does any other. A nonselective test, on the other hand, involves many psychological functions equivalently.

In reality, of course, performance in any behavioral test requires the integration of many psychological functions. Thus, in any kind of discrimination procedure, for example, the animals must be sensitive to the discriminative stimuli, learn to associate them with the appropriate reinforcement consequences, make the appropriate motor response, and so on. Thus, an impairment of performance must be carefully interpreted to determine why it occurred (see below). Nonetheless, behavioral tasks can still be organized so that performance is influenced more by changes in some variables than by changes in others.

A sensitive task is one in which sizable changes in performance occur as a result of small changes in the CNS. In essence, a sensitive task is one that magnifies the underlying changes. As described below, sensitivity is always desired in a behavioral test. However, depending on the goal of the research, selectivity may or may not be desired. In particular, in the initial phases of an examination of a toxicant a nonselective test may be the most efficient means to determine whether or not the toxicant has a behavioral effect (even if the reason for that effect is difficult to determine).

Lesion Analyses

At an empirical level, lesion analyses examine the behavioral changes produced by destruction of a component of the CNS. At a theoretical level, lesion analyses are the only means by which the behavioral neuroscientist can determine the types of functions and behaviors that depend on the integrity of a brain structure.

Dissociations between performance on different tasks are necessary for drawing conclusions about the functional organization of neuronal systems. In essence, the logic is the same as that used for troubleshooting any defective system. The pattern of responses on sensitive and selective tests can identify which of the functions are spared and which are disrupted. An animal may fail to make a response in a given task because of impairments in many different psychological processes: sensory input, memory, motivation, arousal, motor output. Simply observing that behavior is altered in a single task is not the same as identifying which of these components is really affected. Only by comparison of performance on different tests can the functions responsible for the observed impairments be identified (Olton 1985). The procedures of strong inference (Platt 1964), converging operations (Garner, Hake, and Erickson 1956), and deductive logic are used in this analysis. A list of possible explanations is produced for the observed behavioral change. Then a series of critical tests is designed to evaluate the validity of each of these hypotheses. Inappropriate explanations are rejected by demonstrating that the function that might have been impaired is actually intact.

For example, consider an animal who fails to perform appropriately in a task of short-term memory. The stimuli are presented to the animal, a delay period then ensues, and the animal is asked to respond on the basis of the memory of the stimulus presented at the beginning of the trial. One possible reason for the impairment is a failure of sensory input. A rat that does not perceive a stimulus clearly cannot remember it. One way to test this hypothesis is to use the same discriminative stimuli in a task that does not require short-term memory. If the impairment in the initial task was due to a failure to perceive the stimuli, then performance in the new task should also be impaired. If, however, the performance in the original task was impaired owing to the memory requirement, then without this type of memory in the new task, performance should be normal.

In a similar way, tests that are sensitive to and selective for other particular functions are designed. As when diagnosing any defective system, the object is to specify which components of the system are intact and which ones are impaired.

Behavioral Neurotoxicology: Two Levels of Analysis

In behavioral neurotoxicology, the researcher's level of analysis depends on the amount of information available about the functional effects of the toxicant being examined. When little information is available, the optimal strategy for determining the functional effects of the neurotoxicant is to use tests that are very sensitive but not selective. The sensitivity ensures that small pathological changes produced by the neurotoxicant will produce large alterations in behavior. The lack of selectivity ensures that disruption of any one of many different systems will produce changes in performance of the task. With nonselective, very sensitive tasks, screening for a functional effect of a toxicant can take place very rapidly.

A second level of analysis begins when more information is desired about the functional effects of a toxicant on the CNS. As indicated previously, sensitivity is still desired; however, selectivity is also important. As described above, selectivity is required if diagnostic troubleshooting is to proceed effectively. To determine whether a neurotoxicant has an effect on short-term memory, a behavioral test in which performance strongly reflects defects in short-term memory and only weakly reflects impairments in other types of functions is needed. In contrast to the first level of analysis, which is designed to determine whether the neurotoxicant produces any kind of behavioral change without regard to the reason that the change occurred, this second level of analysis has as its primary goal the determination of the exact type of function altered by the neurotoxicant.

This second level of analysis is useful for two reasons. First, of course, as described above, it allows some statement as to the psychological mechanism disrupted by the toxicant. One is able to go from the empirical level of the lesion analysis (when a behavior is changed by the neurotoxicant) to the functional level of analysis (when an impairment shows up in a particular psychological process). An accurate characterization of the behavioral effects of a neurotoxicant clearly requires some statement about the functional specificity of its effects.

A second reason for carrying out an analysis of function using selective tests is to identify the pathological changes in the brain that are responsible for the observed behavioral effects. A neurotoxicant may produce many different kinds of pathological changes in the brain. Some of these may cause profound functional alterations, while others may not. The only way to determine the extent to which pathological changes in the brain have functional consequences is to conduct behavioral testing.

The Power of Behavioral Testing

Behavioral testing adds several very important contributions to neurotoxicology. First, it provides some information that can not be obtained in any other way. Other scientific methods can demonstrate whether or not pathological changes take place in the brain as a result of exposure to a neurotoxicant, but they can not indicate whether these changes have any functional (i.e., behavioral) significance. Some relatively small and discrete pathological changes, such as the degeneration of the substantia nigra in the midbrain, which is responsible for Parkinson's disease, have significant behavioral consequences. Other relatively large pathological changes may have small consequences. Thus, the assessment of the functional significance of the pathological changes requires behavioral testing.

Behavioral testing has the advantage of observing simultaneously the results of the brain's integration of many forms of sensory, motor, and emotional information. Using a relatively sensitive but nonselective test, one can examine many different systems simultaneously. Thus, a change in any of them should be detected, allowing parallel assessment of many different systems rather than assessment of only one at a time. Behavioral testing can also focus on certain well-defined aspects of the brain's functioning. Tasks can examine various memory capabilities, mood changes, loss of appetite, altered aggressiveness, and many other simple and complex cognitive functions. These approaches are particularly useful because toxic damage often occurs at all levels of the brain's organization.

Comparisons of Specific Lesions and Specific Neurotoxicants

Neurotoxicants generally produce dysfunction or destruction of the brain region within which they are contained. This destruction, when it is local and discrete, has a parallel with lesion analysis. Lesions may be considered as a general class of manipulations of the brain, of which the actions of a neurotoxicant represent a single specific example. The similarities between experimentally produced lesions and the effects of neurotoxicants suggest that lesion analysis is a valid and useful model for studying the possible mechanism and location of a toxicant's effect upon the brain. In this chapter we do not attempt an exhaustive compilation of all neurotoxicants and their possible counterparts in lesion analyses. Rather, we outline a general framework for studies that use lesion analyses to investigate which brain regions are affected by a specific neurotoxicant and how this effect may lead to observable behavioral alterations.

Manganese

An excellent example of an environmental toxicant that affects the brain in a highly specific manner is manganese (Mn). The mining of Mn and its widespread industrial use have given rise to frequent episodes of neurological poisoning. The poisoning syndrome is characterized by an initial psychiatric phase, including a general mental excitement, with aggresive behavior and incoherent talk (Chandra 1983). This early phase has been correlated in rodents with an increased turnover of two endogenous neurotransmitters, norepinephrine and dopamine, in the striatum. Increased turnover indicates increased activity of the anatomical systems using these transmitters.

The initial phase of this poisoning is followed by a more chronic behavioral disturbance very similar to that seen in patients with Parkinson's disease. The pathological changes in this disease involve the dopaminergic fiber system connecting the substantia nigra with the striatum (Mustafa and Chandra 1971). These neurochemical changes in patients with Parkinson's disease are similar to those described in the brains of experimental animals exposed to Mn (Pentschew, Ebner, and Kovatch 1963). Dopamine and its metabolites in the basal ganglia are deficient, reflecting a decrease in the activity and functional integrity of this system (Chandra and Shukla 1981). The correlation between the dysfunction and degeneration of neurons containing dopamine in the substantia nigra and basal ganglia and the presence of mania and behavioral symptoms similar to those of Parkinson's disease suggests that a destruction of these dopaminergic cells in the substantia nigra and basal ganglia is responsible for the behavioral changes seen shortly after Mn poisoning takes place.

A lesions analysis confirmed the conclusions of these researchers. Cells in the substantia nigra were destroyed; rats with these lesions had a decrease in striatal dopamine and marked locomotor dysfunctioning. Thus, a lesion analysis was able to identify the pathological site responsible for this behavioral syndrome.

Trimethyltin

A second example of a specific neurotoxicant that influences the brain directly is trimethyltin (TMT). TMT is a neurotoxic organometal that produces a neurological syndrome consisting of spontaneous seizures, anorexia, and learning and memory impairments (Fortemps et al. 1978; Ross et al. 1981; Walsh, Miller, and Dyer 1982) TMT produces a fiarly discrete pattern of damage in the limbic system, involving the pyriform cortex, the amygdala, and the hippocampus. Within the hippocampus, it appears that the pyramidal cells in area CA3 are particularly vulnerable to TMT (Walsh, Miller, and Dyer 1982). TMT's toxic effects on the hippocampus are comparable to experimentally produced lesions in this structure (Walsh et al. 1982). The impairment in the performance of a task that requires short-term memory, such as the radial arm maze, following TMT exposure is similar to that seen following experimental destruction of certain neurons within the hippocampus (Handelmann and Olton 1981). These results are consistent with the hypothesis that TMT is a relatively specific neurotoxicant. At an anatomical level it affects primarily the hippocampus; at a behavioral level, primarily performance in tasks that require a working memory.

Previous studies of the behavioral effects of selective lesions of the hippocampal system provide well-documented procedures for testing both of these hypotheses. First, performance in the radial arm maze has been examined following a variety of different specific brain lesions, so that the behavioral effects of pathological changes in several different brain areas have been documented. Second, the effects of hippocampal lesions in a number of different tasks, each relatively selective for a different type of memory, have described the behavioral profile following this type of damage. Thus, if the behavioral neurotoxicologist is interested in analyzing the functional changes produced by TMT in different brain structures or the psychological effects of the damage produced by TMT, reference to the lesion literature will provide ready access to the appropriate kinds of tests.

An essential part of the approach we have outlined is to compare the literature on specific effects of lesions in discrete brain regions upon behavior with reports on the effects of specific neurotoxicants upon behavior. Ultimately, some of the information that lesion analysis provides about the brain may offer insight into questions being asked about the actions of specific toxicants.

Phencyclidine

Thus far we have discussed the link between the effects of well-studied toxicants and specific brain lesions produced experimentally. Next let us consider the neurotoxicant phencyclidine (PCP), which acts as a general nervous-system depressant at toxic doses and provides a psychic "high" at sublethal doses. This euphoric state has made PCP a popular item on the illicit market. Clinically, the drug was initially used as an anesthetic, owing to its properties as a CNS depressant. Its side effects, such as confusion and prolonged stupor, prevented its widespread use. The toxic effects of this compound on the brain can be best discovered by sophisticated testing involving learning and memory tasks. Interestingly, the effects of PCP on selected behaviors are very similar to those of TMT. This does not imply that both produce identical pathologies with related etiologies, only that the behavioral endpoints in certain tasks are similar. The acquisition and performance of a spatial-discrimination radial arm maze and the acquisition of active avoidance are disrupted (Kesner, Hardy, and Novak 1983), following exposure to PCP. Specific lesions produced in the hippocampus or related limbic structures induce a similar impairment of performance in the radial arm maze and active-avoidance learning (Bar, Gispen, and Isaacson 1981).

Correlation of the findings on the effects of PCP and TMT upon behavior with a prior knowledge of the influence of certain experimentally produced lesions may suggest a mechanism of action of these neurotoxicants. The behavioral changes induced by the lesion compare directly with changes in behavior induced during lesion analysis of the brain.

Caveats of the Model

In order for the lesion analysis to apply to the study of behavioral toxicology, the variables that influence the lesions and toxicants must be known, considered, and compared. For example, the recovery of the organism must be predictable and fairly similar in nature and time with regard to both the lesion and the toxicant. Also, the immunological, anatomical, and behavioral adjustments made by the animal must be similar. The validity of the model rests upon the assumption that a particular behavior that is affected by exposure to the toxicant will be affected in the same manner by the production of a lesion in some discrete region of the brain.

The above discussion has generally emphasized the similarities between the effects of neurotoxicants and those of specific lesions. However, toxicants and lesions may differ in many ways, and the extent of these differences may compromise the effectiveness of the analysis described here. A few of the important considerations are outlined below.

The lesions used in basic neurosciences usually have a very distinct onset, so that the lesion is completed within from just a few seconds to perhaps 24 hours. In contrast, toxicants often act more slowly, taking days or even years to produce their effects. The length of time during which a lesion is produced may have significant effects on the behavioral outcomes. In particular, lesions that are gradual and take place over a long period of time may be followed by more recovery of function than lesions that are completed in a much shorter period of time. Thus, a given behavioral task may be much more sensitive to the functional changes produced by an experimentally induced lesion than by exposure to a toxicant.

As indicated previously, toxicants may have a much more widespread affect on the brain than do experimentally induced lesions. Thus, the likelihood of a toxicant's producing complete damage to one structure while sparing all other structures is very small. If the effects of damage in different areas are simply additive, evaluation of the contribution of the different pathologies may proceed without too much difficulty. If, however, the impairments produced by the different lesions interact with each other, then the combination of the various pathologies may produce an outcome that is not easily predictable on the basis of knowledge of each individual component.

The above difficulties are not insurmountable. Indeed, they suggest a number of issues that the basic neuroscientist may wish to pursue. Discrete lesions with an acute onset may be valuable in investigating some aspects of brain function. On the other hand, if many of the insults received by the brain have a more gradual onset and a wider distribution of pathological changes, a number of issues remain to be addressed by the behavioral neuroscientist. Indeed, the information obtained by the behavioral neurotoxicologist concerning the mechanisms of action of various toxicants should provide the behavioral neuroscientist with a whole set of issues that deserve fundamental investigation.

Summary

As mentioned, the usefulness of the protocol for lesion analyses is evident when the toxicant being studied has a well-circumscribed effect on the brain and behavior. Toxicants with broad effects can not be easily compared with any simple lesion. When the effects on behavior are nonspecific and obscure, a lesion analysis may not be as valuable as a tool. The usefulness of a lesion analysis within the context of a specific problem depends on the ability to interrelate the neural and behavioral effects of the toxicant in question.

The logic of the lesion analysis has been developed in the context of behavioral neurosciences that emphasizes identification and analysis of discrete functional systems. Consequently, the application of a lesion analysis to neurobehavioral toxicology occurs most readily when the toxicant is also relatively selective for a single functional system. The emphasis here is not only on a discrete mechanism of action but on a mechanism of action that selectively involves a particular functional system.

Acknowledgments

The authors thank D. Hepler, C. Wible, and M. Shapiro for their critical comments during the preparation of this chapter and E. Picken for typing the manuscript. Funding was provided by grant #DAMD-17-82-8225.

References

Bar, P. R.; Gispen, W. H.; and Isaacson, R. L. 1981. Behavioral and regional neurochemical sequelae of hippocampal destruction in the rat. *Pharmacol. Biochem. Behav.* 14:305–12.

Chandra, S. V. 1983. Psychiatric illness due to manganese poisoning. *Acta Psychiat. Scand.* 67:49–54.

Chandra, S. V., and Shukla, G. S. 1981. Concentrations of striatal catecholamines in rats given manganese chloride through drinking water. *J. Neurochem.* 36:683–87.

Coyle, J. T. 1983. Neurotoxic action of kainic acid. *J. Neurochem.* 41:1–11.

Dustin, P. 1963. New aspects of the pharmacology of anti-mitotic agents. *Pharmacol. Rev.* 15:449–80.

Fortemps, E.; Amand, G.; Bomboir, A.; Lauwerys, R.; and Laterre, E. C. 1978. Trimethyltin poisoning: Report of two cases. *Int. Arch. Occup. Environ. Health* 41:1–6.

Garner, W. R.; Hake, H. W.; and Eriksen, C. W. 1956. Operationism and the concept of perception. *Psychol. Rev.* 63:149–59.

Handelmann, G. E., and Olton, D. S. 1981. Recovery of function after neurotoxic damage to the hippocampal CA3 region: Importance of postoperative recovery interval and task experience. *Behav. Neural Biol.* 33:453–64.

Jacobs, J. M.; Cremer, J. E.; and Cavanagh, J. B. 1977. Acute effects of triethyltin on the rat myelin sheath. *Neuropathol. Appl Neurobiol.* 3:169–81.

Kesner, R. P.; Hardy, J. D.; and Novak, J. M. 1983. Phencyclidine and behavior: II. Active avoidance learning and radial arm maze performance. *Pharmacol. Biochem. Behav.* 18:351–56.

Mustafa, S. J., and Chandra, S. V. 1971. Levels of 5-hydroxytryptamine, dopamine and norepinephrine in whole brain of rabbits in chronic manganese toxicity. *J. Neurochem.* 18:931–33.

Olton, D. S. 1985. Animal models of human amnesia. In *Neuropsychology of memory,* edited by L. R. Squire and N. Butters. New York: Guilford Press.

Pentschew, A.; Ebner, F. F.; and Kovatch, R. M. 1963. Experimental manganese encephalopathy in monkeys. *J. Neuropathol. Exp. Neurol.* 22:488–99.

Platt, J. R. 1964. Strong inference. *Science* 146:347–53.

Ross, W. D.; Emmett, E. A.; Steiner, J.; and Tureen, R. 1981. Neurotoxic effects of occupational exposure to organotins. *Am. J. Psychiatry* 138:1092–95.

Walsh, T. J.; Gallagher, M.; Bostock, E.; and Dyer, R. S. 1982. Trimethyltin impairs retention of a passive avoidance task. *Neurobehav. Toxicol. Teratol.* 4:163–67.

Walsh, T. J.; Miller, D. B.; and Dyer, R. S. 1982. Trimethyltin, a selective limbic system neurotoxicant, impairs radial-arm maze performance. *Neurobehav. Toxicol. Teratol.* 4:177–83.

IV

The Exposure of Humans to Neurotoxic Chemicals

Herbert L. Needleman   **13**

Epidemiological Studies

While studies in celullar systems and in intact animals are necessary to identify toxic mechanisms and then define dose-response relationships, epidemiological investigations of human populations are required in order to set appropriate standards. Neurotoxicants are usually identified first in the workplace, where exposures are high and clusters of unequivocal and often unusual illnesses are recognized. Attention then shifts to the community surrounding the factory, which often shares the toxic exposures of the laborer, if at a lower dose. With the development of more refined toxicological and epidemiological techniques, studies of exposures of the general population become possible. When these studies are undertaken, awareness grows that some of these agents may produce unrecognized health effects and that thresholds for adverse outcome cannot be defined on the basis of stark symptoms alone. Because children are more vulnerable than adults in many cases and because they may live near the workplace and thus encounter the same toxicants as their parents, they become the logical candidates for study of low-level exposure.

In many circumstances, there are clear advantages to having children as subjects for the study of neurotoxicants. Their nervous systems have been subject to fewer risk factors that could confound the effect of the toxicant of interest; their past medical histories are briefer and therefore subject to less distortion under recall; and because of their greater vulnerability, the demonstration of a suspected effect at a lower dose is more likely.

Epidemiologists who study children operate under certain fixed and unavoidable constraints: they cannot administer controlled doses of toxicants to subjects, and they cannot chose littermates as controls. Studies of populations must therefore be observational and rely on careful design and biostatistical analysis to separate out and measure the effects of the independent variables of interest. In this chapter, I attempt to identify the more common difficulties encountered in observational studies of children, to specify some techniques that have proven useful, and to offer, as examples, work on the study of one common neurotoxicant, lead, conducted by my colleagues and myself.

Design Issues in the Study of Neurotoxicants

Seven design problems account for many, if not most, difficulties encountered in the conduct of epidemiological studies.

1. Selection bias. Few studies can evaluate the entire population of interest. In those circumstances where individuals are invited to participate in a study, the reasons for refusal may be related to the outcome under study. If, for example, parents were asked to enroll their children in a study of neurobehavioral development, those who were worried that their child's development was lagging might reject participation at a rate greater than that of other parents. Such a study would necessarily be biased against finding a relationship between the toxicant and the deficit. Some parents might, on the other hand, seek admission to the study because they wanted to find out if their concerns about their child were warranted. If this form of bias predominated, the study would overestimate the relation between the toxicant and the deficit. There is no way of knowing a priori the direction in which this bias operates. Attempts to estimate the direction and magnitude of the bias are therefore required if the conclusions are to be valid. Similarly, studies that derive their samples from psychiatric or medical clinics cannot provide generalizations applicable to the population at large.

2. Classification of exposure. Many studies of neurotoxicity rely on toxicant levels in other tissues than the brain to estimate and classify exposure. These indirect measures may not accurately reflect the concentration of the agent at the critical site and may thus lead to Type I errors. Some investigations, in lieu of any biochemical measure of exposure, are forced to use such surrogate measures as job type and duration or level of the suspected agent at the work site or near the subject's residence. If environmental measures are used to classify subjects, those measures that estimate personal exposure are better classifiers than are more global indexes such as regional level of the pollutant.

3. Outcome measurement. As the study of behavioral toxicology has matured, attention has shifted from measuring unequivocal, stark effects such as death, seizures, and coma to looking for early changes at lesser doses. To do this requires the application of appropriate and sensitive measures of outcome. The standard neurological examination, sensitive to only large deficits in function, is unsatisfactory in the search for low-dose effects. Unsatisfactory for the same reasons are group tests or screening tests of neuropsychological function. The discovery of early damage requires the application of appropriate and sensitive instruments. For example, a specifically designed tremor-detection device has been used to track the course of mercurialism when clinical criteria were wanting (Weiss 1983). Similarly, the use of quantitative electroencephalograms (EEGs) combined with multivariate analysis of the data revealed changes at levels of lead exposure well below those that are encephalopathic (Burchfiel et al 1980). Until this study, the conventional wisdom held that only with frank encephalopathy did one find changes in the EEG.

4. Control of covariates and confounding. Many of the developmental deficits associated with pollutant exposure can be associated with other risk factors that affect development. In general, children of lower socioeconomic status are exposed to higher levels of pollutants; the economically fortunate in general do not live near heavy traffic or factories. Many of the other risk factors, such as malnutrition, poor prenatal care, and inferior schooling, are thus correlated with socioeconomic status and may confound the effect of the pollutant of interest. Identification and control of the salient variables either by matching or by statistical analysis are required to properly evaluate the effect of the agent under study.

5. Inadequate sample size. Many studies choose their samples based upon budgetary or logistical considerations, with no consideration of the number of subjects needed to reduce the Type II error rate to acceptable size. Calculation of the power that a given sample gives will avoid the possibility of not finding an existing significant effect simply because the sample is too small (Schlesselman 1974).

6. Inadequate choice of models. Causal models that are veridical to the phenomenon under examination are necessary to avoid either controlling for the wrong variables or assigning to a control variable a portion of the variance that properly belongs to the independent variable. In a recent study, Winneke and colleagues (1983) measured the relationship between tooth lead levels and IQ in children and found a significant effect on univariate analysis. The investigators then controlled for "sociohereditary" factors by using an index consisting of parental occupation and school placement. After they controlled for this factor, the difference was no longer significant at the $p = 0.05$ level. The conclusion that they drew was that the apparent lead effect was owing to confounding social or hereditary factors. The authors failed to recognize that this "control" factor could be considered an outcome variable, since school placement is a function of academic performance and is thus related to and dependent upon neuropsychological function, the outcome under examination. Similarly, measuring a large number of variables and incorporating them into the model without cognizance of whether this makes biological sense runs the risk of overcontrol and subsequent loss of precision.

7. Multiple comparisons. In studying an agent with little a priori knowledge of the nature of its toxic expression, an investigator is tempted to examine multiple outcome measures in order not to miss any effect that might be present. In doing this, he runs the risk of finding spurious relationships on the basis of chance—roughly 1 in 20 at the $p = 0.05$ level of significance. To minimize this difficulty, the examiner should reduce the number of measures to the number necessary to scan the outcome space. Here, independent replication of positive findings is the strongest arbiter of validity of the relationships found.

Choice of Outcome Measures

Investigators of pollutants at low dose in children find themselves pulled in two directions: they desire to be comprehensive and thereby not miss any area of deficit, but they need to keep the testing time within reasonable bounds. In addition, the application of too many outcome measures risks the possibility of encountering positive findings on the basis of chance.

The number of outcome measures employed should be limited to the minimum needed to cover the field of performances that previous work has shown to be likely targets for the neurotoxicant under study. Standard neuropsychological instruments, which have the advantage of possessing normative data and generally have been validated against other performances, generally are preferable to untried or ad hoc measures of outcome. There is need, of course, for improved measures of specific function, but the question of the validity of any differences found using unstandardized measures will necessarily be raised.

Areas of neuropsychological performance that should be evaluated include general psychometric intelligence, perception, visual-motor integration, speech and language competence, attention, vigilance, classroom behavior, and academic achievement.

Studies of Lead at Low Doses in Children

Lead is the best-studied neurotoxicant. Yet, 40 years after Byers and Lord (1943) first suggested that low-level lead exposure may be responsible for some of the disordered neuropsychological behavior of school children, considerable controversy continues to simmer over whether these low doses were in fact neurotoxic. My colleagues and I set out to systematically address the design questions listed above in a cohort study of children attending public school. In the last few years, our attention has shifted to the study of the effects of lead exposure during pregnancy.

Because we were convinced that the use of blood lead could misclassify children after exposure had ended, we sought a tissue that could read back into the child's history of exposure. Lead is concentrated in bone, but bone biopsies obviously cannot be obtained in screening studies. The shed deciduous tooth is a spontaneous biopsy of bone that does reflect past exposure (Needleman, Tuncay, and Shapiro 1972; Needleman et al. 1974). This offered us a promising opportunity to study the concentration of lead in bony tissue. We collected shed deciduous teeth from 70 percent of all children attending ordinary, nonremedial first and second grades in two towns neighboring Boston, Massachusetts. Teeth were cleansed and sectioned, and the concentration of lead in the dentine was measured by anodic stripping voltammetry (Needleman et al. 1979).

After the analysis of 3,325 teeth, a distribution curve was drawn on which children from the highest and the lowest deciles were identified, and their mothers were contacted. If English was the first language of the home and the child was born at term and had no noteworthy history of head injury and no history of lead exposure, the parents and the child were invited into the neuropsychological follow-up study. Children received a comprehensive neuropsychological battery administered in fixed order by trained psychometricians who were blind to the subject's lead burden. Included and excluded subjects were compared according to their distribution of dentine lead levels and their rating on an 11-item forced-choice teacher's rating scale. Subjects did not differ from the excluded students in either category.

High- and low-lead subjects were compared in terms of 39 nonlead covariates that could affect development. Five covariates were found to differ between groups at p = 0.1 or less (table 13.1). These 5 covariates—mother's age at subject's birth, mother's educational level, father's socioeconomic status, number of pregnancies, and parent IQ—were controlled by analysis of covariance. It is pertinent that these variates are recognized to affect developmental outcome. After control of covariates, the following outcomes were found to differ significantly between lead-exposure groups: full-scale and verbal IQ (WISC-R), three measures of auditory and language performance, and attention as measured by reaction time at varying intervals of delay (table 13.2). All other outcomes measured but one favored the low-lead group, but not at the 0.05 level of significance.

When teachers' ratings were compared between exposure groups, high-lead subjects were significantly more distractible and less organized, and their overall

Table 13.1 Covariates that differed between high and low lead samples at p ≤ 0.1 and that were controlled in preanalysis

| Non-Lead Covariates | Lead-Exposure Group | | p Value |
	Low Lead	High Lead	
Mother's age at subject's birth	26.2 ± 5.5	24.5 ± 5.8	0.07
Mother's educational level (grade)	11.9 ± 2.0	11.4 ± 1.7	0.08
Father's socioeconomic status (2 factor Hollingshead)	3.8 ± 1.0	4.1 ± 0.8	0.02
Number of pregnancies	3.3 ± 1.8	3.8 ± 2.3	0.10
Parent IQ	111.8 ± 14.0	108.7 ± 14.5	NS

Note: Covariates that did not differ at p ≤ 0.1 include marital status of the parents; height, weight, and head circumference; birth weight; length of hospital stay after birth; and number of admissions to hospital.

function was below that of their peers. When teachers' ratings for the entire sample were plotted against the dentine lead levels, a monotonic increase of the proportion of bad ratings was seen in dose-dependent relation to lead level (fig. 13.1).

While the mean difference in IQ scores between groups was only six points, because of the sigmoid nature of the distribution, a shift of the curve of this magnitude resulted in a threefold, increased risk of severe deficit (IQ < 80) (Needleman, Leviton, and Bellinger 1983).

Table 13.2 Outcomes that differed between high- and low-lead groups at p ≤ 0.05

| Test | Lead-Exposure Group | | p Value (2 tail) |
	Low Lead (x̄)	High Lead (x̄)	
WISC-R			
Full-scale IQ	106.6	102.1	0.03
Verbal IQ	103.9	99.3	0.03
Performance IQ	108.7	104.9	0.08
Seashore-rhythm test			
Subtest A	8.2	7.1	0.002
Subtest B	7.5	6.8	0.03
Subtest C	6.0	5.4	0.07
Sum	21.6[a]	19.4[a]	0.002
Token test			
Block 1	2.9	2.8	0.37
Block 2	3.7	3.7	0.90
Block 3	4.1	4.0	0.42
Block 4	14.1	13.1	0.05
Sum	24.8	23.6	0.09
Sentence-repetition test	12.6	11.3	0.04
Reaction time under varying intervals of delay	(x̄ ± S.D.)	(x̄ ± S.D.)	
Block 1 (3 sec)	0.35 ± 0.08 sec	0.37 ± 0.09 sec	0.32
Block 2 (12 sec)	0.41 ± 0.09	0.47 ± 0.12	0.001
Block 3 (12 sec)	0.41 ± 0.09	0.48 ± 0.11	0.001
Block 4 (3 sec)	0.38 ± 0.10	0.41 ± 0.12	0.01

[a]Rounded to the nearest tenth.

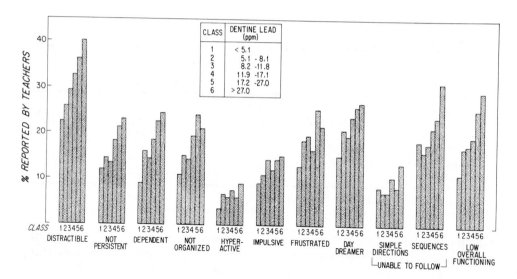

Fig. 13.1 The proportion of negative teachers' ratings on an 11-item forced-choice scale in relation to the dentine lead level. A dose-dependent response is seen. Dentine lead levels were chosen so as to achieve a symmetrical distribution around the mean.

Burchfiel et al. (1980) studied a subsample of these subjects using quantitative EEG analysis and found that significantly less midline alpha, and more midline delta, was associated with lead exposure.

Three groups whose studies were modeled to resemble ours to a greater or lesser degree have reported similar results. Yule et al. (1981) studied London schoolchildren, whom they classified by blood lead level, and found differences in IQ scores of the same magnitude as those we found. This group also used the teachers' rating scale and found relationships between teachers' ratings and lead levels similar to those we found. Winneke et al. (1983) studied two groups of children whom they classified by whole-tooth lead level and found similar differences on the German version of the WISC-R. In the second study, the results did not reach significance after adjusting for "socioeconomic factors." We discussed the problematic nature of this adjustment above. In any event, the difference, after adjusting, was of the same degree as the other studies, although it did not reach the 0.05 level of significance.

This raises the question of the ontological implications of a finding that differs at a level somewhat above the traditional 0.05 level. While it is self-evident that the meaning of p = 0.05 is that a 5 percent chance exists that the differences observed could have occurred because of chance, practice has served to distort the implications of the p value. Many investigators take as evidence of no effect an outcome whose p value is 0.06 or 0.07. This is, of course, incorrect, and a group of independent studies whose reported significance levels are in the range of 0.05 to 0.1 may be considered strong evidence for an effect. This was the interpretation of Smith et al. (1983), who evaluated the relationship between tooth lead level and neuropsychological outcome. While an effect was found, after controlling for covariates, the p value was greater than 0.05. They concluded that lead was not related to outcome. The investigators went further and asserted that had they entered other (unnamed) social variables into the model, they would have further reduced the amount of variance associated with lead. In making this judgment, they treated their study as isolated, unrelated to other work showing effects of the same order.

Prenatal Studies of Lead Exposure

Lead crosses the placenta and has been shown to be embryotoxic in many experimental studies. Deficits in learning have been demonstrated after fetal lead exposure in the lamb, the rodent, and the subhuman primate. No studies of the human infant had been reported as of 1983.

To investigate this route of exposure, we measured the umbilical-cord blood lead levels of 11,834 consecutive births at the Boston Hospital for Women. Over the two-year period of measurement we found a reduction in concentration of 7 percent per year. We then obtained the figures for the monthly sales of gasoline lead additives in the state of Massachusetts and found a correlation of 0.75 between the monthly mean blood lead level and the monthly sales of alkyl lead (Rabinowitz and Needleman 1983).

For 5,000 consecutive births we obtained a detailed interview with the mother on the first postnatal day. This questionnaire measured past health history, medication history, and intake of alcohol, tobacco, and drugs. Blood lead level was cross-tabulated against a number of birth outcomes (weight, infection, jaundice, major and minor anomalies) and was found to be significantly related to the incidence of minor malformations. We then cross-tabulated blood lead level against the relevant covariates in order to select those that could be confounding. Those that did covary with lead were entered into a stepwise logistic regression model. Alcohol, tobacco, and caffeine use were also entered into the model and controlled. The model was reduced by removing those terms with the least weight until the most parsimonious model was achieved (table 13.3). The relative risk of bearing a minor malformation was then calculated, adjusting for the pertinent covariates. The risk of malformation rose in dose-dependent fashion from the referent group to almost

Table 13.3 Logistic models predicting malformations

	BETA ($\pm$ SE)	
Variable	With Lead	Without Lead
Log_{10} lead (μg/dl)	0.66 $\pm$ 0.27	
Maternal age (years)	−0.014 $\pm$ 0.010	−0.013 $\pm$ 0.010
Birth weight (oz.)	0.0036 $\pm$ 0.0021	0.0036 $\pm$ 0.0021
Gestational age (weeks)	−0.040 $\pm$ 0.025	−0.037 $\pm$ 0.024
Race (Black)	0.31 $\pm$ 0.15	0.33 $\pm$ 0.15
Goodness of Model Fit to Data		
−2 log likelihood	2,457.25	2,463.14
Model chi^2	17.61	11.71
Degrees of freedom	5.0	4.0
p	0.004	0.020

Note: Maternal age, gestational age, birth weight, race and blood lead are the significant predictors in this most terse model, shown with and without blood lead terms. Information about lead significantly ($p = 0.015$) improves the model's predictive power.

Table 13.4 The covariate-adjusted relative risk of malformation at selected blood lead levels

Blood Lead (μg/dl)	Relative Risk[a]	Percentage of Neonates at Greater Lead Levels
0.7	1.0	98.7
6.3	1.87 (1.44–2.42)	50.0
15.0	2.39 (1.66–3.43)	1.7
24.0	2.73 (1.80–4.16)	0.2

Note: Beta = 0.655 ± 0.273 (SE).
[a]Mean ± 95 percent confidence interval.

twofold for the median group (6.3 μg/dl) and almost threefold for those subjects with blood lead levels of 24 μg/dl (table 13.4) (Needleman et al. 1984).

From the population of 12,000 births, we selected 250 subjects equally divided among high, medium, and low umbilical blood lead levels. We followed these subjects at six-month intervals, evaluating a large number of control and outcome variables. When relevant covariates were controlled by multiple regression analysis, lead was found to be related to the mental-development index of the Bayley Scales of Infant Development (Needleman et al. 1983).

Taken in sum, these findings indicate that at doses well below those formerly accepted as toxic, lead is associated with evidence of impaired neurotoxic function. The application of appropriate tactics designed to meet the problems listed earlier—selection bias, inadequate classification of exposure, inadequate control of covariates, insensitive outcome measures, and improper model specification—can allow the effects of a pollutant to emerge from the crowded welter of effects that condition the development of the infant and child.

References

Burchfiel, J.; Duffy, F.; Bartels, P. H.; and Needleman, H. L. 1980. Combined discriminating power of quantitative electroencephalopathy and neuropsychologic measures in evaluating CNS effects of lead at low levels. In *Low level lead exposure: The clinical implications of current research,* edited by H. Needleman. New York: Raven Press.

Byers R. K., and Lord, E. E. 1943. Late effects of lead poisoning on mental development. *Am. J. Dis. Child* 66:471–94.

Needleman, H. L.; Bellinger, D.; Leviton, A.; Rabinowitz, M.; and Nichols, M. 1983. Umbilical cord blood lead levels and neuropsychological performance at 12 months of age. *Pediatr. Res.* 17:179A.

Needleman, H. L.; Davidson, I. O.; Sewell, E. M.; and Shapiro, I. M. 1974. Subclinical lead exposure in Philadelphia schoolchildren: Identification by dentine lead analysis. *N. Engl. J. Med.* 290:245–48.

Needleman, H. L.; Gunnoe, C.; Leviton, A.; Reed, R.; Peresie, H.; Maher, C.; and Barrett, P. 1979. Deficits in psychologic and classroom performance of children with elevated dentine lead levels. *N. Engl. J. Med.* 300:689–95.

Needleman, H. L.; Leviton, A.; and Bellinger, D. C. 1983. Lead-associated intellectual deficit. *N. Engl. J. Med.* 306:367.

Needleman, H. L.; Rabinowitz, M.; Leviton, A.; Linn, S.; and Schoenbaum, S. 1984. The relationship between prenatal exposure to lead and congenital anomalies. *JAMA.* In press.

Needleman, H. L.; Tuncay, O. C.; and Shapiro, I. M. 1972. Lead levels in deciduous teeth of urban and suburban American children. *Nature* 235:111–12.

Rabinowitz, M., and Needleman, H. L. 1983. Petrol lead sales and umbilical cord blood lead levels in Boston, Massachusetts. *Lancet* 1:63.

Schlesselman, J. C. 1974. Sample size requirements in cohort and care control studies. *Am. J. Epidemiol.* 99:381–84.

Smith, M.; Delves, T.; Lansdown, R.; Clayton, B.; and Graham, P. 1983. The effects of lead exposure on urban children: The Institute of Child Health/Southampton study. *Dev. Med. Child Neurol.* 25, suppl. 47:1–54.

Weiss, B. 1983. Behavioral toxicology and environmental health science: Opportunity and challenge for psychology. *Am. Psychol.* 38:1174–87.

Winneke, G.; Kramer, G.; Brockhaus, A.; Ewers, U.; Kujanek, G.; Lechner, H.; and Janke, W. 1983. Neuropsychological studies in children with elevated tooth lead concentration. *Int. J. Occup. Environ. Health* 51:231–52.

Yule, W.; Lansdown, R.; Millar, I.; and Urbanowicz, M. 1981. The relationship between blood lead concentrations, intelligence, and attainment in a school population: A pilot study. *Dev. Med. Child Neurol.* 23:567.

Christina M. Gullion and
David A. Eckerman

14

Field Testing

The past decade has seen growing concern about the effects of occupational and environmental exposure to toxicants. An accumulation of clinical reports and neurobehavioral studies has contributed to our increased awareness of these dangers, sometimes confirming effects at exposure levels once taken for granted. The enormous increase in the numbers and prevalence of toxic substances and the seemingly insoluble problem of long-term storage of toxic waste have made the detection and characterization of toxic health effects a matter of urgency. While field studies of toxic impairment provide exceedingly difficult methodological problems which limit the information that can be derived from them, they also provide information that cannot be obtained in laboratory studies. It would be very unfortunate to overlook what lessons an accidental exposure might provide. We have undertaken this chapter in hopes that we might improve the information provided by future evaluations.

In the present chapter, we first briefly review methods currently available or under development for field testing of neurotoxic impairments. We also point to methods currently used in the relevant pharmacology and environmental-factors literatures. This brief review of current methods is intended to set a context for discussion of methodological issues and is not intended as a thoroughgoing review. Several excellent reviews that summarize the current literature on the field testing of neurobehavioral toxicity are now available or in preparation: Bornschein, Pearson, and Reiter (1980); Feldman, Ricks, and Baker (1980); Johnson and Anger (1983); Weiss (1983); Anger and Johnson (1985); Maurissen (1985); Sanes, Colburn, and Morgan (1985); Smith (1985); and Anger (chap. 15 in this volume). The major goal of the chapter, however, is to address the methodological issues that have presented themselves as the literature on field testing has accumulated. Test selection and scoring and issues of data analysis are highlighted in hopes of appropriately complementing matters raised by Anger in this volume.

Assessing subclinical neurobehavioral effects resulting from unintended and uncontrolled exposures is exceedingly elusive. What can be learned from these evaluations is limited. Detection of effects requires precise, sensitive measures, sophisticated analyses, and judicious interpretation. Were we to miss the lessons that accidental exposures can teach, however, we would miss the chance to correct the tragedies they represent.

Current Approaches to Testing for Neurotoxicity

Longstanding programs of field evaluation are found in several European countries and the United States. Over the last several years, communication among these programs has grown, and a consensus is emerging regarding appropriate testing methods. Perhaps a review of this evolution is best begun with a review of some common points of departure for these programs and a description of several of them.

Neurological and Neuropsychological Background for Field Testing

The traditional role for the neurologist or neuropsychologist is to help a client determine the cause of distressing symptoms. A person might request aid, for example, following development of unusual sensations, movement difficulties, or, more rarely, emotional or cognitive changes. The goal of the assessment is to determine the locus of damage and its etiology, possible therapy, and prognosis. The presence of functional impairment is usually assumed—distress brought the individual to ask for aid. The client is often assumed to be a willing confederate, also wishing for a correct diagnosis. Tests developed in such a setting have been refined and are now of proven usefulness (Lezak 1983). Diagnostic procedures developed for this clinical setting, however, may not be optimal for field screening of a population in order to determine whether symptoms of toxic impairment are or are not present. On the other hand, the extensive development of diagnostic tests in neurology and neuropsychology is a resource that those planning field screening should study carefully, selecting what does apply.

The neurological examination typically consists of a structured interview and close observation of the client to characterize symptoms of dysfunction. The time for the exam is usually 20–30 minutes. (Sterman and Schaumburg 1980; and Lezak 1983 review the typical examination approach and give further references for elaboration of methods used.) Considerable training and skill are required of the examiner; even when examiners have considerable training there is concern regarding the reliability of observations across examiners and across examinations (e.g., Tuttle, Wood, and Grether 1977).

The questions and observations are designed to screen for

1. mental status (see below);

2. cranial nerve function (olfaction; taste; visual acuity; color vision; light reflexes; extraocular muscles; facial skin senses; facial, neck, and tongue muscles; hearing; speech and swallowing; gag reflex; and heart slowing);

3. motor function (atrophy; tone, e.g., spasticity or rigidity; involuntary movements, e.g., tremor; reflexes; autonomic activity; coordination; gait; station; and

4. other sensory function (pinprick, warm and cold, passive movement of limbs, vibration, light touch, two-point discrimination, double simultaneous stimulation, object recognition, numbers written on palm).

The mental-status examination includes assessment of demeanor, ability to state the current time and review recent events, ability to state location and show an appreciation of direction and distance, and ability to name and describe the roles of individuals with whom the patient is involved. The examiner judges speech rate and patterns, quality of thinking and thought associations, long-term and recent memory (digit span, delayed word recall), concentration (e.g., serial subtraction of seven, reversed digit recall), general information and reasoning, and emotional state and range and addresses special concerns for the particular individual (Lezak 1983).

While many of the approaches reviewed below may be used as adjuncts to the neurological exam, two approaches seem especially germane. Arezzo and Schaumburg have been especially innovative in developing potentially useful tests for sensory evaluations. They report improved measurement methods for field testing vibratory sensitivity (Arezzo and Schaumburg 1980). They have also developed an approach for evaluating thermal sensitivity. Since long axons are frequently subject to toxic damage, as well as the relatively more commonly tested visual and auditory neurons, the ability to evaluate these sensory channels is an important addition to field screening for early effects of exposure. Second, electrophysiological recording may augment clinical evaluation of sensory and motor ability. Evoked potentials resulting from stimulation of skin, visual, or auditory receptors demonstrate sensory reactivity; electromyography can show motor impairments; and electroneurography (measurement of nerve conduction) can reveal variation in neuron reactivity. Use of these measures is reviewed by Seppäläinen (1983) and Otto (1983). Use of slow-wave brain potentials to evaluate cognitive functioning is less well established as an adjunct to clinical evaluations, though several measures are being developed that seem promising as field tests for impairments once issues of reliability and validity are clarified and resolved (Otto, Bauman, and Robinson 1985).

In clinical practice, the neurological exam is frequently supplemented by neuropsychological assessment. Neuropsychologists have a great many standard tests and observation schedules available to them. In the interests of matching the assessment to the client's needs, it is common for a practitioner to select assessment tools individually for each client, though a core set of tools is usually included. For assessment of adults, this core set is likely to include the Wechsler Adult Intelligence Scale (WAIS), a memory assessment battery (e.g., the Wechsler Memory Scale [WMS]), and additional tests to determine motor control, perceptual capacity, and personality (Smith 1975; Lezak 1983). Unfortunately, for a wide variety of neuropsychological questions there are no standardized batteries that satisfy criteria of suitability, practicality, and usefulness (Lezak 1983).

The best known of the formalized batteries for clinical neuropsychological assessment is the Halstead-Reitan battery (Reitan and Davison 1974). Subtests include (1) the Category Test (an automated test of concept formation and reformation on the basis of stimulus size, shape, number, intensity, color, and location); (2) the Critical Flicker Fusion Test of visual-integration time; (3) the Tactual Performance Test (tactile memory is tested by having blindfolded subjects manipulate several forms and then draw them from memory); (4) the Rhythm Test (discrimination between like and unlike pairs of tone rhythms); (5) the Speech Sounds Perception Test (discrimination between similar consonants); (6) the Finger Tapping Test (rapid tapping of a key with preferred and nonpreferred hand); (7) the Time Sense Test (reaction time and time estimation); (8) the Trail Making Test (connecting drawn items in serial order); (9) the Aphasia Screening Test (copying, naming, spelling, repeating, etc.—over 30 items); and (10) sensory examination for tactile, auditory, and visual modalities. The WAIS and the Minnesota Multiphasic Personality Inventory (MMPI) are also given as part of the battery. A full administration requires six to eight hours of testing by a skilled neuropsychologist (Lezak 1983). The subject's score is compared, in each of the 10 Halstead-Reitan tasks, to a "cutting score" to determine whether performance is subnormal. The Impairment Index is then the number of subnormal scores, with 5 (of these 10) being considered to represent a clinically significant impairment. Patterns of test scores have been statistically related to particular sites and types of lesions (diffuse or focal, static or changing), an approach that encourages computer-aided interpretation of protocols (ibid.).

Though respected as an approach to assessment, the Halstead-Reitan battery is not consistently more effective than other tests in detecting neurological impairments. It also takes substantial time to administer and is not suitable for patients with sensory or motor handicaps. Lezak (1983) notes that "its greatest contribution may not be to diagnostic efficiency, but rather to the practice of neuropsychological assessment, for Reitan undoubtedly has been singularly instrumental in making psychologists aware of the need to test many different kinds of behavior when addressing neuropsychological questions" (p. 566).

An alternate approach to neuropsychological assessment was developed by Luria (1973). The tests in Luria's battery are supposed to measure several classes of function: arousal, sensory input and integration, and behavioral planning and execution. The 285 observations suggested by Luria and formalized by Golden, Hammeke, and Purisch (1978) require about 2.5 hours of testing by a skilled evaluator for full administration. In their formalization of these measures, Golden and colleagues have taken a step toward developing an objective scoring system for these observations: raw scores (usually ratings of quality of verbal and motor performances) are converted to a 0–2 scale, with 0 representing normal performance. The degree of impairment is then measured as a sum of individual converted scores. Unfortunately, Golden, Hammeke, and Purisch failed to carry out an appropriate evaluation of their scoring system (see below). In addition, the Luria battery is quite dependent on the clinical skill and judgment of the examiner and does not seem optimal as a standardized field-screening instrument.

The prior work of neurologists and neuropsychologists should have a major impact on further development of neurotoxic assessment. Though establishing a standard battery for all neurotoxic assessments is not a realistic goal, inclusion of a core set of tests is a useful strategy for quickly developing normative data in neurotoxicological assessment and for assuring a comprehensive evaluation (see below). In selecting such a set of measures, we might look to the set of tests arrived at for clinical neuropsychological assessment.

Representative Field Tests Used in Europe and Australia

Hänninen (1971) provided a seminal report assessing the effects of carbon disulfide on worker health in Finland. She presented data from 150 workers at the same plant—50 who had had sufficiently acute dosing of carbon disulfide to be poisoned (though 38 of them still worked); 50 who had received occupational exposure to carbon disulfide for 5–20 years but had not been acutely poisoned and had no observable clinical symptoms; and 50 of comparable age, educational background, and type and duration of work at the plant who had had only very occasional exposure to carbon disulfide. Workers were given a series of tests for perceptual, motor, and cognitive abilities (see table 14.1). Hänninen concluded that the first

Table 14.1 Batteries of neurobehavioral tests used in representative studies in Europe and Australia

Function[a]	Studies							
	Hänninen 1971; Hänninen et al., Psychological tests, 1978	Hänninen et al. 1976	Hane et al. 1977	Arlien-Søborg et al. 1979	Gamberale, Annwall, and Olson 1976, automated version	Knave et al. 1978	Grandjean, Arnvig, and Beckmann 1978	Williamson Teo, and Sanderson 1982
Sensory		Figure Identification	Figure Classification Figure Identification					Critical Flicker Fusion threshold
Motor	Santa Ana Mira Drawing Symmetry (1971)	Santa Ana Mira Drawing Finger Tapping Simple/choice RT	Rivet test Mirror tracing Simple/choice RT		Simple/choice RT	Simple RT Santa Ana	Finger Tapping	Hand steadiness Simple visual RT Pursuit rotor
Cognitive Attention	Bourdon-Wiersma Digit Symbol	Digit Symbol	Vigilance	Vigilance (continuous RT)		Bourdon-Wiersma	Digit Symbol Graphic continuous performance	Vigilance
Memory	Digit Span[b] Visual Retention Logical Memory (1978)	Digit Span Visual Retention/ Reproduction Logical Memory Associative Learning	Claeson-Dahl Visual Retention	Digit Span Visual gestalts Pair association	Digit Span	Digit/Letter span Syllable recognition	Digit Span Digit learning Sentence recall Word pairs Story recall	Memory scanning Paired associate learning (immediate and delayed) Iconic memory
Other	Similarities Picture Completion Block Design Rorschach	Similarities Picture Completion Block Design Rorschach	Block Design	Similarities Cube test	Mental addition	Mental addition	Visual gestalts Remaining WAIS subtests	
Affective Symptoms	Yes (1978)	No	Medical exam	Medical exam	No	Interview	No	No
Neurophysiological	No	No	No	Nerve conduction	No	EEG/NCV	No	No

[a]The sorting of tasks by function is somewhat arbitrary, as tasks usually tap several functions.
[b]Digit Span is included under Memory, though there is evidence that it might be considered a measure of attention instead (Erickson and Scott 1977).

and third groups were distinguishable on the basis of vigilance (Bourdon-Weirsma speed and variability), manual dexterity (Mira test, Santa Ana), one measure of the Rorschach performance (Originality), and the Picture Completion and Digit Symbol tests ($p < 0.01$ for these tests by t-test). The second group was distinguishable from controls on the basis of slight motor disturbances (Mira test, Santa Ana) and poor visual performance (Picture Completion and Block Design). A discriminant function was developed that correctly classified 75 percent of the subjects in the three groups. The value of this function was confirmed when two subjects first tested as part of the control group subsequently were reassigned work duties and were poisoned. Shifts in their performance were clearly detected, and the discriminant-function classification for them was correct both before and after the poisoning. This report stands as an early success for neurobehavioral testing of toxicity, for subclinical effects were detected and characterized. Follow-up work using a different group of subjects confirmed the effects shown (Hänninen et al., Psychological tests, 1978; Tolonen and Hänninen 1978). In the follow-up study the most discriminating variables were (1) Bourdon-Wiersma speed, (2) Santa Ana (preferred hand), (3) Mira test straight lines, (4) emotional adaptability measured by the Rorschach as well as (5) questionnaire scores for reduced extraversion and (6) symptoms of fatigue.

Investigators at the Finnish Institute of Occupational Health (FIOH) have used the series of tests they recommend in a substantial number of studies (Hänninen 1979; Hänninen and Lindström 1979). For instance, investigators at the institute have used the same battery to evaluate the effects of exposure to paints (Hänninen et al. 1976), solvents (Lindström 1980), styrene (Lindström, Härkönen, and Hernberg 1976), and lead (Hänninen et al., Psychological performance, 1978). Visual/motor problems are a consistent theme in the impairments determined in this series of studies. An exemplary aspect of the Hänninen et al. (1976) study was that a measure of intelligence taken in young adulthood was available. A subsample of 33 pairs of subjects matched according to age and prior intelligence was used to confirm the group differences between exposed and nonexposed groups and to develop a discriminant function that predicted group membership.

A disadvantage of using the FIOH battery for field testing, however, is that both administration and scoring require considerable expertise and training. Care is, of course, always required to ensure that tests are administered in a manner that yields appropriate performance measures. Even when tests are computer-administered, care must be exercised to ensure that the participant is motivated and understands the tasks at hand. Use of drawing and "free interview" tests such as the Rorschach, however, makes the outcome even more dependent on the clinical expertise of the examiner.

Several Scandinavian groups have developed batteries of neurobehavioral tests to evaluate occupational health. Hane et al. (1977), for example, found that performance on figure classification, choice reaction time, eye-hand coordination (rivet test), and a visual-retention test were correlated with exposure to paints (see table 14.1). Again, a prior measure of intelligence was available; in this case it was used to ensure that exposed and control groups were comparable. Arlien-Søborg et al. (1979) evaluated 70 painters with a series of tests (see Table 14.1). Again, visual/motor problems were detected, though measures of memory and learning (visual gestalts, digit span, paired associate learning), as well as reports of forgetfulness, were the predominant symptoms. Neuroradiological examination confirmed cerebral atrophy in 31 patients. Gamberale and colleagues (1976) took a further step by developing an automated battery of tests for toxicity evaluation. Their battery includes reaction time, number manipulation, and Digit Span. In one application of this battery (Gamberale, Annwall, and Olson 1976), they determined that experimental exposure of up to 1,080 mg/m³ of trichloroethylene (yielding about 225 mg/m³ in alveolar air) slowed number manipulation but left the other tested functions unchanged. A second application, with several other measures added to their automated battery (Knave et al. 1978), showed that jet-fuel workers were slowed in the Bourdon-Wiersma test, were variable in reaction time in the mental-addition test, and showed a greater progressive increase in reaction time over trials than did nonexposed controls. Depression, sleep disturbances, and headache were also more common in the exposed subjects. Grandjean, Arnvig, and Beckmann (1978; see table 14.1) found the Digit Symbol, Block Design, Digit Span, Similarities, and Comprehension subtests of the WAIS to be correlated with blood lead, as were the graphic-continuous-performance test and the learning measure from the visual-gestalts test. Finally, the work of Williamson, Teo, and Sanderson (1982) confirmed the finding by Smith, Langolf, and Goldberg (reviewed below) that exposure to mercury leads to impairment of short-term memory. In their study, other functions were apparently unaffected.

Representative Field Tests Used in the United States

Of the many field studies initiated by the National Institute of Occupational Safety and Health (NIOSH) four are reviewed here as representative. Tuttle, Wood, and Grether (1977) studied 139 individuals, 114 of whom had been exposed to carbon disulfide, 25 of whom had not. Six alternative measures of degree of exposure were developed using work histories and interviews. Of the 16 behavioral test scores examined (see table 14.2), Tuttle, Wood, and Grether found that the largest correlations were between exposure indexes (with age partialed out, but see comments later in this chapter regarding this analysis) and (a) simple, choice, and drop reaction time, (b) Santa Ana Dexterity (right hand), (c) the Neisser letter-search task, and (d) the Digit Symbol test of the WAIS. The Block Design test of the WAIS was significantly related to two of the indexes of exposure. Nerve-conduction speed was also significantly correlated with exposure. When participants were grouped on the basis of total neurological score, it was determined that reaction-time measures, the Santa Ana Dexterity measure for the right hand, and the Block Design tests produced significantly different results in distinguishing the most neurologically impaired from unimpaired subjects. Tuttle, Wood, and Grether (1977) considered their "most significant result" to be cross-validation of a regression equation for predicting the neurological examination score from neurobehavioral test scores. In a prior study of the effects of perchloroethylene (PCE), Tuttle et al. (1977) developed two regression models to correlate neurobehavioral to neurological measures. One model was derived from measures of behavior taken in the morning, the other from measures taken in the afternoon. Each correlated 0.73 with the neurological score in the PCE study. When applied to the data of the carbon disulfide study, they correlated with the neurological scores 0.53 (A.M.) and 0.32 (P.M.), respectively (both significant at $p < 0.01$). This degree of consistency in

Table: ...of neuropsychological tests used in representative studies in the United States

Function[a]	Tuttle, Wood and Grether 1977	Repko et al. 1978	Baker et al. 1984	Johnson et al. 1974	Valciukas et al., central nervous system dysfunction, 1978	Brown and Nixon 1979	Smith and Langolf 1981; Smith, Langolf, and Goldberg 1983
Sensory	Critical Flicker Fusion threshold, Farnsworth color vision	Auditory threshold, Tone decay		Critical Flicker Fusion threshold, Letter identification, Time estimation	Embedded Figures	Finger agnosia, Graphesthesia	
Motor	Simple/choice RT, Santa Ana	Choice RT, Dynamometer, Eye-hand coordination, Tremor	Santa Ana	Simple/choice RT, Eye-hand coordination	Santa Ana	Grip strength, Eye-hand coordination, Finger Tapping	Tremor, Myotatic reflexes, Finger Tapping, Eye-hand coordination, Critical tracking
Cognitive Attention	Letter search, Digit Symbol		Continuous performance		Dual monitoring/foot tapping		
Memory	Digit Span[b]		Digit Span, Digit Symbol (recall), Logical Memory, Visual Reproduction, Paired Associate			Digit Span, Logical Memory, Visual Reproduction, Paired Associate, Facial recognition	Memory scanning, Memory distraction, Digit Span (standard and improved)
Other	Block Design		Block Design, Similarities, Vocabulary, Information/ Orientation, Digit Symbol, POMS	Mental Arithmetic	Digit Symbol, Block Design	WAIS (all subtests), Trail-Making Test	
Affective	Feeling Tone checklist	Clinical-analysis questionnaire, Marlowe-Crowne scale				MMPI	
Neurophysiological		Nerve conduction	Nerve conduction				

[a] The sorting of tasks by function is somewhat arbitrary, as tasks usually tap several functions.
[b] Digit Span is included under Memory, though there is evidence that it might be considered a measure of attention instead (Erickson and Scott 1977).

models confirms that similar patterns of functional impairment are produced by these two substances.

Repko et al. (1978) assessed the effects of lead on the sensory/motor functions of 85 storage-battery-industry workers who had blood lead levels close to the recommended maximum (average of 46.0 μg/100 ml) by comparing their performance with that of 55 matched workers with much lower blood lead levels (average of 18.0 μg/100 ml) (see table 14.2). Auditory functioning was found to differ between exposed and unexposed groups, as did visual reaction time and perhaps some personality measures. Strength and coordination did not differ. This study represents a partial replication of work by Repko, Morgan, and Nicholson (1975), who also found that hearing was impaired. In this prior (less well controlled) study, hand steadiness and coordination, strength, and mood (hostility, aggression, and general dysphoria) were also apparently affected.

Baker et al. (1984) reported evaluations of 171 workers from a lead foundry and an adjacent assembly plant. Nerve-conduction speed and a number of neurobehavioral measures were taken (see table 14.2). Blood lead concentrations were obtained as well, showing blood lead levels ranging from 10 to 80 μg/100 ml (mean of 32.75). Since there was considerable overlap in blood lead levels of foundry and assembly plant workers, a correlational approach was used in data analysis. Nerve-conduction speed showed a modest slowing and reduction of response amplitude (sural nerve) as blood lead level increased (several indexes). The neurobehavioral tests found to be sensitive to blood lead concentration were Vocabulary, Similarities, and Digit Span (backwards) subtests of the WAIS; Santa Ana Dexterity; the Mental Control, Visual Reproduction, and Paired Associate Learning subtests of the WMS; and most scales of the Profile of Mood States (POMS). Baker et al. utilized test scores corrected for various demographic characteristics of subjects (age, education, gender) based on a regression equation developed in prior work with unexposed individuals (Baker et al. 1983). This study not only confirmed the effects of lead on psychomotor speed and dexterity and on mood reported by others but also found a previously unconfirmed relation with short-term memory and verbal intelligence. Such cognitive effects had been noted in symptom lists (e.g., Repko, Morgan, and Nicholson 1975) but had not been clearly shown in performance tests for individuals with blood levels below 80 μg/100 ml. A two-year follow-up study of the same population was also undertaken (Baker et al., Occupational lead neurotoxicity, 1985). Considerable reduction of lead-exposure levels had occurred prior to this follow-up evaluation (the highest blood levels fell to 50 μg/100 ml by year 3). A number of individuals were, of course, unavailable for follow-up study, reducing the numbers to 73 in year 2 and 50 in year 3. The highest test-retest correlations in the follow-up were obtained for the Vocabulary, Digit Symbol, Block Design, and Paired Associate Learning subtests. Again, Paired Associate Learning and dexterity measures were found to be linked to lead levels, as were some of the POMS scales. Further, POMS scores improved for individuals whose blood levels were reduced but whose other neurobehavioral scores did not show improvement.

Johnson et al. (1974) conducted a repeated-measurement study of six toll-booth operators exposed to vehicle exhaust during their work shift (carbon monoxide [CO] was judged to be the principal component responsible for the measured short-term toxic effects). After training on each of the tasks, participants were given the battery of tests prior to and immediately following their work shift on six days (they were tested every other day) (see table 14.2). The time-shared task was most clearly related to blood levels of CO. Putz (1979) followed up on this observation by evaluating the effects of controlled laboratory exposure to CO on a dual tracking-monitoring task. He found that low-level exposure to CO (5 percent carbox-yhemoglobin [COHB]) produced a decrement in tracking and a slowed detection of visual stimuli after extended exposure to the test conditions (confounded with exposure level) when the tracking task was sufficiently difficult. This laboratory work nicely confirmed the field-test data and showed that obtaining an effect of CO was highly dependent on test difficulty and length of testing.

Investigators at the Mount Sinai Environmental Sciences Laboratory recommend a battery of tests consisting of the Block Design and Digit Symbol subtests of the WAIS, an Embedded Figures test of their own design (Valciukas and Singer 1982), and the Santa Ana Dexterity test (see table 14.2). With this battery, Valciukas et al. (Central nervous system dysfunction, 1978) reported that age-corrected scores on the first three of these were significantly correlated with blood lead levels (measured using zinc protoporphyrin levels, which allows approximately a four-month average exposure to be determined). Because all three tasks were found to be sensitive to lead level, a composite index of lead effects has been proposed by this group (Valciukas and Lilis 1980).

When this battery was applied in a field evaluation of the effects of accidental exposure to polybrominated biphenyls (PBBs), the performance scores did not differentiate clearly between exposed (Michigan) and unexposed (Wisconsin) groups of farmers (Valciukas et al., Comparative neurobehavioral study, 1978), though there was a suggestion of a correlation between serum PBB and performance (since males in the exposed group scored more consistently below females than did males in the control group, and females in the exposed group had lower levels of serum PBB). Subsequent evaluations of this accidental exposure also revealed that neurobehavioral effects of this accidental exposure were tenuous (though it is clear that at sufficient dosage PBB is neurotoxic). Symptom lists from exposed individuals in Michigan did include concerns regarding concentration and short-term memory, and some field testing suggested that memory deficits were present (Brown and Nixon 1979) (see table 14.2). Brown and Nixon noted, however, that the performance deficits were of a type and degree often found in depressed individuals and that poor memory among exposed farmers was correlated with measures of anxiety and depression on the MMPI and not with body burden of PBBs. In a subsequent study reported by Brown et al. (1981) chemical workers, who had higher PBB levels, did not differ from farmers on memory tests. Further, there was no clear dose-dependent relation between PBB and cognitive or performance measures. On these bases, Brown et al. concluded that the apparent memory deficits in farmers were secondary to crisis-related depression.

In an extended series of evaluations of chlor-alkali workers, Smith, Langolf, and colleagues found the body burden of mercury to be correlated with several aspects of behavior. Langolf et al. (1978) found that workers with a high mercury level in their urine sample showed tremor, faster myotatic reflexes, a decreased mean finger-tapping rate (with increased variability), an increase in variability of hole-to-hole time in the Michigan maze test, and a marginal trend toward reduced critical tracking performance. These effects were detectable but were not felt by the investigators to be functionally significant. Retesting 6–10 months after impaired workers were removed from exposure confirmed that these effects were reversible. Using a task based on Sternberg's (1966) memory-scanning paradigm, Smith and Langolf (1981) found that slowed scanning time was a significant predictor for increased body burden of mercury. Since the overall speed of reaction was not affected except in this scanning measure, the effect seemed quite specific to short-term-memory processing. This effect resembled that which occurs with aging (Anders, Fozard, and Lillyquist 1972). The effect of an increase in 12-month average urinary mercury of only 0.1 mg/l was functionally comparable to the predicted increase in scanning time produced by 9 years of aging (p. 707).

Screening Batteries Developed for Neurobehavioral Field Testing

In May 1983, NIOSH and the World Health Organization (WHO) gathered experts to recommend test methods appropriate for Third World nations interested in undertaking health-hazard evaluations to monitor developing industries. The neurobehavioral tests selected by their panel (Seppäläinen et al. 1983) are shown in table 14.3. Tests were selected that the panel determined (*a*) to have proven sensitivity to neurotoxic agents, (*b*) to be relatively less demanding of examiner skill for administration and scoring, (*c*) to be brief, (*d*) to require little equipment, and (*e*) to be relatively culture-free. The core battery (tests marked with asterisks) should provide a fairly comprehensive description of subject abilities within 40–50 minutes of testing.

Baker and colleagues at the Harvard School of Public Health (Baker et al., Computer-based neurobehavioral testing, 1985) have developed a computer-administered series of tests for field testing of neurotoxic impairment. Their battery can be administered by IBM PC–compatible computers, including the highly portable varieties, and therefore can be quite easily transported to the field-testing site. The tests included in their current battery are listed in table 14.3. There is considerable overlap between the tests that they have included and those proposed by the NIOSH/WHO panel, though motor functions are underrepresented in their set. Their battery also requires approximately 40–50 minutes to complete.

Selection of tests for the NIOSH/WHO and Baker-Letz batteries was considerably influenced by the neuropsychological testing tradition. Such input is important, since neuropsychologists have been at the forefront of neurotoxic evaluations. A group of us at the University of North Carolina, in contrast, have developed a battery of computer-administered tests that derive as much from the experimental-psychology laboratory and from analyses of factors of cognitive abilities as from the neuropsychological testing tradition. In developing this battery of tests, we utilized the Microcomputer Testing System (Foree, Eckerman, and Elliott 1984). This hardware/software system provides the UCSD Pascal language on an Apple II series computer with hardware enhancements (headphones, touch screen, attached buttons) and software routines for handling time-critical functions such as the timing of screen events, reaction times, and so on. Also provided are standard data-handling routines to facilitate standardized data management across tasks. Using this system, we have implemented the tasks shown in the rightmost column of table 14.3. In selecting these tasks, we have tried to provide a broad range of relatively function-specific tests that assess factors identified by Carroll (1980) as covering the range of cognitive abilities. Carroll arrived at this set of proposed factors on the basis of factor-analytic studies of elementary cognitive

Table 14.3 Some developing batteries for field testing for toxicity

Function[a]	Neurobehavioral Testing System (NBTS)		
	WHO Battery[b]	Baker-Letz Battery	Microtox Battery[c]
Sensory			Visual masking (1)
			Choice RT (distract) (2)
			Müeller-Lyer (4)
Motor	Santa Ana*	Simple RT	Simple auditory RT (2)
	Aiming*		Choice auditory RT (2)
	Simple RT*		
	Finger Tapping		
	Flanagan coordination		
	Choice RT		
	Pegboard		
	Rate of manipulation		
Cognitive			
Attention	Digit Symbol*	Digit Symbol	Switching attention (3)
	Bourdon-Wiersma	Continuous performance	Stroop interference (5)
	Letter search		
	Test d-2		
	Auditory serial attention		
	Continuous performance		
	Stroop interference		
Memory	Benton Retention*	Paired Associate learning	Memory scanning (6)
	Digit Span*	Paired Associate recall	Simon Sez (6)
	Visual Retention (WMS)	Digit Span	Digit Span (6)
	Benton Reproduction	Visual Retention	Supra-span learning (6)
	Logical Memory	Memory scanning	Objects in house (6)
	Associate memory		Which first/last? (6)
			Continuous recognition (6)
			Items in categories (6)
Other	Block Design	Mill Hill vocabulary	"Fuzzy set" bounds (3)
	Similarities	Armed Forces Qualification	
Affective	POMS*	Mood scales	
	Eysenck P.I.		

Sources: For WHO Battery, Seppäläinen et al. 1983; for Baker-Letz Battery, Baker et al., Computer-based neurobehavioral testing, 1985; and for Microtox Battery, Eckerman et al. 1984 and Eckerman et al. 1985.

[a]The sorting of tasks by function is somewhat arbitrary, as tasks usually tap several functions.

[b]The WHO Battery is divided into core tests, making up a brief, 40–50-minute battery (marked with an asterisk); additional tests, requiring more time or resources and recommended where a fuller account is desired; and tests-in-development, which require still more elaborate apparatus or training and are as yet not validated for toxic assessments. This listing includes the core and additional tests.

[c]The number in parentheses indicates tthe cognitive-task paradigm (Carroll 1980; see table 14.4) that the task represents.

tasks. He identified experimental studies that included tasks from more than one of the eight paradigms he identified from the literature and carried out factor analyses on data from these investigations to determine the isolatable sources of individual differences in performance on these tasks. On the basis of these analyses, he proposed ten factors that represent the range of cognitive abilities (table 14.4). We believe that assessing these factors will ensure that an evaluation is comprehensive, and we have selected tasks accordingly. The battery has had some evaluation for sensitivity in detecting the effects of carbon monoxide and alcohol (Eckerman et al. 1985).

Table 14.4 Carroll's elementary cognitive tasks and cognitive factors

Paradigms	Example Tasks	Factors
1. Perceptual apprehension	Recognizing objects Single-letter threshold *Visual-duration threshold*	1. Monitor process (e.g., instructions, strategies)
2. Reaction time and movement	Simple reaction time *Choice reaction time* Fitt's tapping task	2. Attention process (focus, stimuli expected)
3. Evaluation/decision	*Word or nonword* Dichotic-order judgment Picture or nonpicture	3. Apprehension (sensory buffer representation)
4. Stimulus matching/comparison	Letter search Letter matching Letter rotation *Same/different pictures*	4. Perceptual integration (matching with prior buffer representations)
5. Naming/reading/association	Stroop task Word naming Naming pictures	5. Encoding process (formation of a mental representation, abstraction)
6. Episodic-memory read-out	*Memory span* *Probed memory scanning* *Running recognition*	6. Comparison of mental representations
7. Analogical reasoning	People-piece analogy Miller Analogies test	7. Co-representation formation (a new representation of a pair of representations)
8. Algorithmic manipulation	Mental arithmetic Sunday + Tuesday Raven's Matrices	8. Co-representation retrieval from memory
		9. Transformation of representation (e.g., rotation, transposition)
		10. Response-execution planning (cognitive process preceding the overt response)

Source: Carroll 1980.

Note: Tasks given in italics represent Carroll's proposed experiment to estimate process parameters (Carroll 1980, pp. 71–73).

Batteries Developed for Assessing Drug Effects

The drug-evaluation literature provides many examples of effective assessment of neurobehavioral functioning which should suggest appropriate measures for neurotoxic assessment. Tasks that have been used by five notable research groups in their drug evaluations are listed in table 14.5. The work of Weingartner, Sitram, and colleagues (see sources with these individuals as first author) offers an especially thorough coverage of memory effects. The work of Mohs, K. Davis, and colleagues (see sources with these individuals as first author) provides assessment of a somewhat broader range of functions. Like Smith, Langolf, and Goldberg, this group has also focused on the memory-scanning task, which attempts to provide a measure of specific components of memory processing rather than memory capacity.

For another instructive use of this task in drug-toxicity evaluation see MacLeod, Dekaban, and Hunt (1982). The set of tasks utilized by Branconnier and Cole (e.g., Branconnier 1985) represents an especially thorough literature-based selection that is commercially available as a portable hardware/software package. The tasks selected by Ferris, Crook, and colleagues (see sources with these individuals as first author) are notable, since they represent tasks that derive from common laboratory measures of cognitive processing and yet have high face validity to both young and old subjects from a broad range of the population. By arranging the learning of grocery lists, phone numbers, faces, and names, they are able to recruit subject cooperation and motivation more readily than by use of nonsense syllables. These tests have been found to be sensitive to drug manipulations. Finally, the study of Squire et al. (1980) broadly sampled cognitive performance using more traditional neuropsychological tests; it is included here as an example of the use of these instruments in evaluating the effect of a pharmacological agent (here the effect of lithium carbonate on the performance of psychiatric patients).

Batteries Developed for Assessing Unusual Working Environments and Conditions

Table 14.6 lists tasks selected for inclusion in several recently developed batteries seeking to assess the effects of work environments and conditions on behavior. These include tasks that have been selected to be sensitive to work-cycle and shift-duration variables (Walter Reed PAB), tasks currently implemented in the automated battery being evaluated by the Navy for testing unusual work environments (see Harbeson et al. 1983 for a bibliography of the evaluation studies of the Navy's PETER project that have been used in selecting tasks for this battery), a battery under development by the Air Force for use in selecting recruits with good potential for high-level training (Allen and Morgan 1985), and the classic battery of Alluisi (Alluisi et al. 1973). This last battery is referenced through a study on the toxic effects of viral disease on performance. In general, the tasks selected for Alluisi's battery tap more complex skills than those represented in the toxicity- and drug-evaluation literatures.

Methodological Issues

The balance of this chapter discusses methodological issues in the use of tests for field evaluation of the effects of known or suspected neurotoxicants. Some of these issues are also discussed in Valciukas and Lilis (1980), which serves as a useful adjunct to this chapter. This section is closer to being a tutorial than a review of the state of the art, though recent reports of field-testing results are cited as examples. We have tried to be heuristic rather than complete, since sufficient detail to apply the methods mentioned here is beyond the scope of a single chapter; sufficient detail *can* be found in the references cited.

Overview

In the quasi-experimental designs typical of neurobehavioral field testing the quality and characteristics of both the dependent (behavioral measures) and independent (exposure indexes) variables can have substantial effects on the power of an

Table 14.5 Test batteries used in example drug evaluations

Function[b]	Weingartner, Sitram	Mohs, K. Davis	Branconnier, Cole	Ferris, Crook	Squire
			Research Groups[a]		
Sensory	Detect tone in noise Detect gap of silence Tonal-order judgment		Iconic memory		
Motor				Finger Tapping Simple RT	Porteus maze
Cognitive					
Attention	Detect repeated words	Time production Visual search Divided attention (digit transformation, detect letter)		Visual search (digit) Visual search (word)	Visual search (letter pairs) Visual search (word) Digit symbol Delayed target detection
Learning	Serial learning Selective reminding	Selective reminding	Selective reminding Supra-span digits	Shopping-list learning First/last names	Number learning Pair Associate
Episodic memory	Distracted forgetting Consistent recall Visual-pattern recall Delayed recall (10 min) Free vs. categorized cued recall Recall, given different encodings	Memory scanning Digit Span (forward/ backward) Delayed recall Story recall Consistent recall	Memory scanning Cued recall, semantic and phonetic Recognition memory, learned/ incidental	Digit span (dialing) Running digit span Face recognition Misplaced objects Paragraph recall Category retrieval Design recall Paired associate recall	Recognition of items (immediate) Recognition of item (10 min delay) Paragraph recall Design recall Self-rating scale for memory complaints

Semantic memory	Recall words by first letter		Squire Television test	Remote-event recall
	Recall words by category		Category/instance fluency	
Other		Trail map	Spatial-rotation time	Trails A and B
		Serial sevens subtraction	Simple visual RT	
		Picture Arrangement	National Adult Reading	
			Road-map test	
Affective		Bunny-Hamburg Scale	NIMH mood scales	
			Mood scale—elderly	
			Psychic/somatic complaints	

[a] Designated by principal investigators. See sources with these individuals as first author.
[b] The sorting of tasks by function is somewhat arbitrary, as tasks usually tap several functions.

303

Table 14.6 Batteries for testing unusual work environments

Function[a]	Walter Reed PAB	Navy Biodynamics	Air Force	Alluisi Battery
Sensorimotor	4-choice RT	Choice RT (auditory, visual) Spoke test		
Cognitive Attention	2-letter search 6-letter search	Pattern comparison		Warning lights Blinking lights Probability monitoring
Learning/memory	Missing digit Pattern recognition (two levels of difficulty)	Memory scanning Auditory digit span Letter recognition	Coded messages (12 pairs) Emergency procedures (ordered set) Time check (compare analog & digital clocks) Security check (spatially ordered pair associates) Communication control (hierarchically structured verbal material) Strategic decision (object/number pairing and mental arithmetic) Direction judgment (map learning)	
Other	Letter-map coding Mental arithmetic (2-column addition and serial addition/subtraction) Logical reasoning	Code substitution Serial addition Mental arithmetic (4 functions) Manikin (figure rotation) Grammatical reasoning (auditory, visual)		Mental arithmetic Code-lock solving Target identification
Affective	Mood-activation scale			

Sources: For Walter Reed PAB, Thorne et al. 1985; for Navy Biodynamics, Irons and Rose 1985; for Air Force, Allen and Morgan 1985; for Alluisi Battery, Alluisi et al. 1973.

[a]The sorting of tasks by function is somewhat arbitrary, as tasks usually tap several functions.

investigation to detect a relationship between the two classes of variables, as well as set limits on the generality (or external validity) of any findings.

For example, Tuttle, Wood, and Grether (1977) limited the validity of part of their data analysis by using the outcome of a neurological exam (total neurological score) for assignment to "exposure" groups when they undertook a replication of the effects of carbon disulfide found by Hänninen (1971). A neurological examination is at best an indirect and nonspecific measure of exposure. Factors that may reduce the validity of this type of examination as a marker for exposure include (a) the sensitivity of the test to neuropsychological deficits that are completely unrelated to exposure to carbon disulfide and (b) the presence of deficits associated not only with carbon disulfide exposure but with other kinds of neurological insults as well, such as chronic alcohol abuse or physical trauma. Either type of confounding undermines the validity of the test as a measure of exposure and consequently weakens the chain of evidence linking cognitive-test performance with exposure to carbon disulfide. The only justification for interpreting a score on this test as a measure of exposure would be empirically demonstrated validity for that purpose. Since Tuttle, Wood, and Grether reported average correlations of about 0.23 (age not partialed) between the exam score and various measures of years of exposure, the test in fact does not appear to be sufficiently valid.

Measures with adequate reliability and validity are necessary but not sufficient to achieve sufficient power to detect relationships among them. To actually achieve the needed power, the study as a whole must also be adequately designed. Other factors contributing toward adequate power are sufficient sample size, controls for extraneous sources of variance, and the use of appropriate analytic techniques.

In the following sections we discuss a selected set of psychometric methods and problems relevant to the success of field-testing studies of the behavioral effects of toxic substances. We give particular priority to those about which there appears to be limited awareness. In doing so, we add our voices to reiterated calls by others for improvements in practice (e.g., Feldman, Ricks, and Baker 1980; Valciukas and Lilis 1980; Schaumburg et al. 1981; Seppäläinen et al. 1983; Smith 1985; and Anger, chap. 15 in this volume).

The primary emphasis in the discussion below is on methods for improving the power of field-testing studies to detect subtle effects, principally by decreasing the magnitude of error variance and increasing the systematic component of variance in the measures used. The principal issues and methods addressed here include

1. Rationales and strategies for assembling a test battery and developing a scoring system, including issues of validity and sensitivity;
2. Considerations in the evaluation of reliability, including a brief overview of generalizability theory;
3. Use of exploratory data analysis, particularly nonlinear transformations and functions of variables; and
4. Considerations in controlling for confounded factors.

We are well aware of the presence in the behavioral toxicology literature of inappropriate statistical analyses (e.g., multiple univariate tests instead of the appropriate multivariate test, failure to adjust α levels in repeated tests and *post hoc* tests, overinterpretation of results). We have chosen, however, to limit the discussion here to psychometric concerns. Kirk (1968) provides an excellent general discussion of hypothesis testing and the factors affecting Type I and Type II errors. In addition, Muller, Barton, and Benignus (1984) provide a useful discussion of the properly conservative use of statistics in experimental toxicology. Our one reservation regarding their discussion is that they assert that "α and power are antagonistic in that improving one worsens the other" (p. 114). The probability of a Type II error in fact is a function not only of α but of the distance between means in the population, the size of error variance, and the sample size (Kirk 1968); power can be improved without affecting α at all. We discuss methods for doing exactly that in the pages that follow.

Assembling a Test Battery

In a review of the effects of industrial toxicants, Feldman, Ricks, and Baker (1980) noted that "the principal difficulty in evaluating behavioral effects is the relative lack of available standardized neuropsychological tests which can be administered to exposed workers in a practical period of time, and which can then be scored or interpreted with reliability, accuracy, and reproducibility" (p. 224). Other major problems they noted were methodological inconsistencies, which limit the possibility of generalizing across studies, and the failure to establish convergent and discriminant evidence of effects.

The situation has not changed substantially since 1980. As Anger (chap. 15 in this volume) notes, no standardized batteries yet exist in the United States, despite the longstanding example of the FIOH and the clear need for continuity and consistency of methods in order to build a coherent picture of the effects of industrial and environmental toxicants.

Convergent and discriminant validation. Given the state of the art, there is a pressing need to approach battery development with the objective of bringing the field to a stage of development at which evaluation of the effects of toxicants can proceed on a solid basis of reliable evidence. This larger goal need not conflict with the usual immediate goal in assembling a test battery, which is to find an effective and trustworthy way to detect and quantify the performance of a particular set of functions that appear to be affected by a particular neurotoxicant. The need for standardized procedures and for investigation of confounding factors, construct validity, and reliability exists in both cases. Thus, a strategy for development of a battery that meets the immediate objectives of a particular study can also respond to the larger need for a web of convergent and discriminant evidence in terms of which the generality and practical significance of individual studies can be evaluated. The elements of such a strategy are the following:

1. Replicate previous findings by using tests (called *effective tests* below) that were significantly related to the effects of a toxicant in earlier studies of that substance; use the same form of each as was used previously and administer each under the same standardized conditions.

2. Extend the range of functions measured to others for which effects have not been demonstrated but which it is reasonable to infer might be affected, based on the nature of signs and symptoms observed in connection with exposure to the target substance.

3. Add tests that are hypothesized to measure the same functions as the effective

tests and *should* show the same effects and be highly correlated with them; this is a basis for testing the generality of the observed effect.

4. Add tests expected to measure functions other than those inferred to be measured by effective tests to delineate what the latter tests are *not* measuring.

5. Explore the domain of measures that might potentially serve as calibrating or baseline markers in cross-study comparisons (e.g., longitudinal research or meta-analysis) (Feldman, Ricks, and Baker 1980).

6. Include measures of aspects of functioning that are particularly important in the subject's life, such as those affecting ability to work, ability to maintain social and family life, and sense of well-being.

In deciding whether a test is effective or not (1), the quality of the empirical evidence needs to be taken into consideration. Particularly important aspects include (*a*) the reliability and validity of both independent and dependent variables; (*b*) the power of the earlier studies to detect an effect, which is a function of sample size, the relative sizes of error and systematic-variance components, and whether the assumptions of the statistical tests were met; and (*c*) whether appropriate statistical and design controls were used to minimize Type I errors and threats to external validity (such as confounded variables or biased subject selection) (Cook and Campbell 1979).

When the purposes of testing include extending the range of demonstrated relationships (2), a previous nonsignificant result may not be a sufficient reason not to renew investigation of a hypothesized relationship unless the null result has been verified across alternate measures and subject samples and the studies involved met standards for quality such as those sketched in the previous paragraph.

The choice of tests for convergent and discriminant validation (3 and 4) may be guided by either empirical findings or theory. For instance, empirical studies of cognitive and sensorimotor functioning in areas other than toxicology research (e.g., aging, psychopharmacology, human factors, cognitive psychology) may be a source of useful measures, particularly if the population being studied (e.g., the aging) or a treated group (e.g., in pharmacological research) displayed signs and symptoms similar to those seen with neurotoxicant exposure.

As suggested by Smith (Smith and Langolf 1981; Smith 1985), cognitive-process theories (Pellegrino and Glaser 1979; Carroll 1980) can guide selection of tests as well as development of completely new test tasks. As was mentioned above, theories about the "elementary cognitive tasks" required in various experimental paradigms, based on an extensive study of the literature on individual differences in abilities (Carroll 1980), guided selection of the tasks in the Microtox Battery (see tables 14.3 and 14.4). As noted below, however, the relevance of these theories needs to be evaluated before they are used to justify test development.

With regard to (5), there appear to be no well-established baseline measures of stable functions at present. Intelligence-test scores obtained prior to exposure have been used to demonstrate that exposed and control groups were comparable in intelligence prior to exposure (Hänninen et al. 1976; Hane et al. 1977). The WAIS is sometimes given at the time of a study of neurotoxic effects and used as a covariate or a matching variable for blocking; however, there is accumulating evidence that performance on many of the subscales of the WAIS is affected by exposure or body burden (e.g., Block Design, Digit Span, Digit Symbol, and Picture Completion).

There is also evidence that vocabulary, which has been considered a stable component of intelligence, is affected by lead (Baker et al., Occupational lead neurotoxicity, 1985). This area needs much further work.

The practical significance of behavioral effects of neurotoxicants (6) is important because their effects on daily functioning are relevant to setting exposure standards, to workmen's compensation, and to latent-disease litigation. In addition, effects that can be shown to impair functioning in a job may move a labor union or industrial firm to seek improved working conditions and/or to institute a systematic exposure-monitoring program.

Deficits that affect the individual's sense of well-being and family and social functioning, such as subtle memory deficits or a personality change, are not easily quantified; however, since they can be devastating to the quality of life of the individual, the effort to develop ways of measuring these aspects seems well justified. Another difficulty in evaluating the practical significance of observed deficits is that of determining how much (if any) deficit attributable to a toxic substance is acceptable. One suggested benchmark is normal aging (Smith 1985). However, it is not clear what should be considered normal, since individuals in the general population differ drastically in life history (e.g., diet, accidents, disease, drug abuse, alcohol use) and genotype (e.g., vulnerability to degenerative diseases). In addition, there is reason to believe that the risk-benefit analysis underlying the individual's determination of what is an unacceptable level of deficits is weighted by seemingly extraneous factors such as perception of control over exposure and economic needs (Peterson 1985).

The *scope* of the battery used in a particular study should reflect the state of knowledge, as well as practical constraints such as budget and time. At an early stage of investigation, elaborate evaluation procedures seem warranted; these include (*a*) measurement of a wider array of functions than is apparently affected, (*b*) inclusion of measures for discriminant and convergent validation of observed relationships between exposure and test results (Campbell and Fiske 1959; Cook and Campbell 1979; Smith 1985), (*c*) detailed clinical evaluation, including qualitative observations and extensive exploratory work (Lezak 1983), and (*d*) design of studies specifically to develop norms (Baker et al. 1983) and carry out a full evaluation of reliability (Cronbach et al. 1972).

Accumulating knowledge about the nature of neurotoxic effects and the best measures of these effects provides a basis for reducing the scope of a test battery to those tests that have been found to be sensitive and reliable measures of the effect. Once this later stage of development is reached, the use of a " 'shotgun' approach would be most likely classed as naive by the active researchers in the area" (Alluisi 1975).

Sensitivity. A sensitive test provides sufficiently fine discrimination between levels on a trait within the critical region to meet the objectives of the testing program. In behavioral toxicology, the *trait* is commonly some aspect of CNS functioning (see tables 14.1 and 14.2), and the *critical region* typically is at the level of subclinical symptoms of adverse effects of an industrial or environmental toxicant. Sensitivity is a test characteristic distinct from reliability or validity. A neuropsychological or cognitive-abilities test may be reliable and valid over a wide range of levels of the trait measured and yet not be sufficiently sensitive to variation within the restricted range of subclinical effects to be useful for a monitoring or screening program.

Maximizing the sensitivity of tests in a field-testing program is important in minimizing Type II errors (missing an effect that is there) and increasing the precision of predictions (e.g., in modeling a dose-response relationship) (Poulton 1965; Feldman, Ricks, and Baker 1980). Because of small subject samples, short tests, and the substantial effects of confounding factors, many field studies of the effects of neurotoxicants have low power to detect an effect. In this situation, methods for improving sensitivity, which in turn can improve reliability, validity, and power, merit particular attention.

A strategy for maximizing sensitivity involves selection of both appropriate content and an optimal scoring plan. Two views have been expressed in the literature regarding the best rationale for selecting sensitive tests. Smith (1985) emphasizes the importance of psychological theory for the development of sufficiently precise, "ability-specific" tests, while others (Baker et al. 1983; Seppäläinen et al. 1983; Anger, chap. 15 in this volume) stress the importance of basing further work on previous positive findings in field testing (for summaries of these findings see Feldman, Ricks, and Baker 1980; and Johnson and Anger 1983).

Smith and Langolf (Smith and Langolf 1981; Smith 1985) argue that detecting subtle neurotoxic effects calls for "precise behavioral tests that are well grounded in cognitive theory . . . gross performance measures may not pose a sufficiently severe test to detect the impaired system" (Smith and Langolf 1981, p. 701), because compensatory mechanisms or strategies can mask a deficit when tested by a multi-process (complex) task. They conclude that "ability-specific" tests are needed, the development of which rests, in turn, on "well-developed cognitive theories" that "can provide insight into the processing stages or systems involved in a task and can supply measures sensitive to the performance of a single stage" (ibid.).

An additional consideration when weighing the relevance of theory to test development is that despite immediate pressures for finding the most sensitive measures as quickly as possible, in the long run maximizing the efficiency of a testing program may depend on achieving a good understanding of the phenomenon. In addition, the credibility of test results ultimately rests on the ability of the test user to interpret the results in terms of a coherent, empirically validated theory, in this case one that relates psychological test scores to the effects of toxic substances on the nervous system.

On the other hand, cognitive-psychology theories should not be used without first carefully evaluating their validity and relevance. We see four ways in which cognitive theory may not be appropriate for use in test development in behavioral toxicology. Since Smith and colleagues chose short-term memory as the process domain in which to operationalize their approach (Smith and Langolf 1981; Smith, Langolf, and Goldberg 1983), we draw on research in that area to illustrate our remarks.

First, cognitive-process theories may not be relevant to neurotoxicity assessment. These theories are generally developed and tested using data collected in the laboratory on healthy, literate young adults who have had extensive practice with the tasks used to generate data. Their physical and neurological health, their attitude toward the task at hand, and their status as practiced performers of the task contrast markedly with the characteristics of most groups coping with chronic exposure to toxic substances. Just as observation of lesion effects may not be a valid basis for theories about normal brain function, observations of cognitive functioning in the "average" college student in the cognitive-psychology lab may not generalize to the study of effects of neurotoxicants (Smith 1985).

Second, research in process-oriented cognitive psychology is often characterized by lack of convergent and discriminant validation, by few replications, and by underdetermined research designs which may support alternative theories equally well (Theios 1973, 1977; Townsend 1974; Anderson 1978; Townsend and Ashby 1978; Snow 1979; Cooper and Regan 1982). In many studies, the conclusion that a model accounts adequately for the data is based on the failure to find a significant difference between the predicted and estimated parameters of the model. If a model makes weak predictions and the experimental test of it is poorly designed, with insufficient power to detect a significant difference (e.g., a small sample, too many parameters given the number of subjects), these failings favor *accepting* the model. As a consequence, these theories are frequently the subject of controversy among cognitive psychologists and may be under constant revision. For example, Sternberg's (1966) serial, exhaustive search model of short-term memory, which was the original rationale for developing and interpreting the memory-scanning task used by Smith and Langolf (1981), was challenged some years ago by the superior account of data from that task provided by a self-terminating, parallel-processing model (Townsend, 1974; Kintsch 1977; Theios 1977), and debate continues in this area.

Third, the tasks developed to test cognitive theories are rarely evaluated for construct validity or reliability (but see Smith 1979 for an exception). Construct-validity research on some widely used memory tests suggests that some of these tests actually measure something else (Erickson and Scott 1977). For instance, the Digit Span test of the WMS (used by Smith, Langolf, and Goldberg 1983) appears to be a measure of attention rather than memory (Davis and Swenson 1970; Kear-Colwell 1973; Wang, Kaplan, and Rogers 1975; Baker et al. 1983). This suggests that the appearance of validity (i.e., face validity) is not necessarily supported in empirical validation studies; such studies are a necessity whenever a test is to be used to make decisions affecting people's lives.

In addition, performance on many cognitive tasks may be affected by "extraneous" variables (with respect to the exposure-behavior relationship) such as motivation or mood; these represent confounded factors that may be identified only through the use of appropriate validation strategies. For example, Brown and Nixon (1979) found a significant deficit in memory performance following exposure to PBBs that was reduced to nonsignificance when depression was controlled for. To sort out the roles of depression and PBBs in memory performance, a follow-up study (Brown et al. 1981) was carried out on chemical workers with higher body burdens of PBBs than the original group. This study failed to find worsening memory performance as PBB level increased. The results of extending the range of exposure, as well as the pattern of evidence among multiple measures (both cognitive and personality), were needed to delineate the relationship between mood, memory, and PBB effects in this case. Other strategies for validation include using dose-response relationships rather than group differences and (where exposure levels are high enough) corroboration from physiological or laboratory tests (Smith 1985).

Finally, there is evidence in the neurotoxicology literature (Putz 1979) suggesting that in some cases a dual-process task is more likely to reveal deficits than are tests designed to measure the functioning of a single process. Though one description of this is that complex tasks are more sensitive than simple, ability-specific ones, the distinction between ability-specific and complex may be less relevant than a distinction between complicated, poorly focused tasks (which are likely to be multiprocess) and tasks that are well targeted, in both difficulty and required capacities, to detect a behavioral deficit. The latter features could be found both in the ability-specific tasks advocated by Smith and in more complex, dual- or multi-process tasks that have been well designed to stress a particular capacity.

To summarize, cognitive theories should be carefully evaluated for empirical status and relevance before they are used as a rationale for test development or selection. The test developer might raise the following questions: (1) Is the theory under consideration sufficiently validated, through empirical tests and replications, to warrant interpretation of field-testing data in terms of the model and to serve as a basis for decisions affecting public health? (2) Are parameters estimated on data collected in the field consistent with those seen in the laboratory? What happens to these parameters when subject characteristics such as age, education, and culture differ from those found in the cognitive-psychology laboratory? (3) Are model parameters reliable under field conditions? Can one obtain stable estimates, using small numbers of trials and unpracticed subjects, of model parameters estimated in the laboratory using large numbers of trials and well-practiced subjects?

In addition to the choice of content, a variety of choices made during implementation of a test task can affect sensitivity. The following list of some of these is adapted from Poulton (1965):

1. When accuracy or success is scored, adjust the difficulty of the task to match the level of performance in the subclinical range, since maximum sensitivity is found in the middle of the distribution of scores on a homogeneous test (Lord and Novick 1968, p. 329);

2. Saturate channel capacity (e.g., by making the test part of a dual-task situation), which may increase the difficulty sufficiently to achieve (1) and may get past automaticity or compensatory strategies that mask a deficit (Putz 1979);

3. Use an unfamiliar task (another way of getting around automaticity or compensatory strategies);

4. Use as a score the part of the variation in performance that is most affected by exposure (e.g., use the variance rather than the mean; when latency is measured, a method of scoring the variable part of the latency is to divide the frequency distribution over trials into quintiles and use the mean of the slowest quintile as the score) (Alluisi 1975);

5. Score performance in conjunction with specific events instead of cumulating over varying conditions within a task (e.g., in a switching-attention task use the mean RT—over all switches—on the first trial after each switch);

6. In cases where trade-offs or interactions between aspects of performance pro-

duce two sources of variability (Pachella 1974), try to hold one constant and channel all the variation into the other (e.g., induce subjects doing an RT task to respond at a speed that allows perfect accuracy and use RT as the score, or conversely, pace responding at a fixed rate and use errors as the score).

A particular problem in targeting the sensitivity of a test battery in studying the effects of neurotoxicants is that the nature of observable symptoms, as well as the underlying clinical picture of neuropathies, appears to change as the level of exposure changes (Feldman, Ricks, and Baker 1980; Seppäläinen et al. 1983; Smith 1985). For instance, Tuttle, Wood, and Grether (1976) report that the earliest manifestations of chronic carbon disulfide poisoning are nonspecific psychological changes (insomnia, fatigue, labile mood) and that "slowed peripheral nerve conduction velocity and abnormal electromyographic tracings are observed prior to onset of other clinical symptoms of neurological damage" (p. 5). As cumulative exposure increases, abnormal reflexes are seen, along with lesions in the visual system and accompanying visual deficits and an array of metabolic and enzymatic disturbances (such as diabetes) that can also affect sensorimotor functioning and other behavior.

In another study of carbon disulfide effects, Hänninen (1971) found that different tests distinguished groups at different levels of exposure—unexposed from poisoned and exposed from poisoned—while two tests (Digit Symbol and Santa Ana) distinguished all three groups. Subjects in the poisoned group displayed deficits also seen in the exposed, subclinical group plus others not seen in the latter group. The difference in the pattern of deficits in these two exposed groups may result from either the insensitivity of the tests to deficits that do exist at the subclinical level or the fact that these deficits have not yet developed at that level of exposure. Inability to differentiate insufficient test sensitivity from absence of an effect is a serious impediment to determining when and how toxicants start causing deficits in functioning. If a given test fails to detect a deficit when other evidence suggests that a deficit *does* exist, then an attempt to develop a more sensitive test for the affected function seems warranted.

While sufficient sensitivity is needed, a test can be *too* sensitive. Lezak (1983) comments that tests that are very sensitive to individual differences in the general population may be too sensitive for evaluating gross losses: "Using a finely scaled vocabulary test to examine an aphasic patient, for example, is like trying to discover the shape of a flower with a microscope: the examiner will simply miss the point" (p. 133). In addition, Seppäläinen et al. (1983) caution that overly sensitive tests may result in false positives, with costly emotional, political, and social consequences for the population involved.

Another aspect of achieving an adequate level of sensitivity to the effects of a toxicant is a research design that permits sorting out different types of effects, such as distinguishing chronic from acute effects and short-latency from long-latency effects. Both are functions of time—either length of or interval since exposure. Time-series research (Cook and Campbell 1979) would be valuable in this area to relate processes such as metabolism and excretion, neural regeneration, and the development of compensatory mechanisms to observable physiological, histological, and behavioral abnormalities at the time of testing. For instance, Xintaras and Burg (1980) note that "exposure to *n*-hexane may result in a peripheral neuropathy *and* degeneration of the central nervous system" (p. 671). However, if testing is done only shortly after acute exposure, the symptoms of the former, the more likely of the two to heal, may mask the presence of the latter, more permanent loss.

Scoring

The usefulness of a test depends on whether its content is appropriate and on whether a valid, replicable scoring method is used. As was indicated in the discussion of sensitivity, scoring can be central to achieving the needed level of sensitivity. Even when published standardized tests are used in a battery, development of an optimal scoring strategy may be needed. For instance, it may be possible to use a composite score—that is, a linear combination of scores on related tests—to obtain a better measure of an aspect of behavior than any single test will give (Valciukas and Lilis 1980).

Development of a scoring procedure involves deciding which variables to include in scoring and how to handle these mathematically in order to obtain an optimal score or set of scores. For instance, in a test in which speed and accuracy of responses are measured, the best score may be an aspect of reaction time (e.g., variability over trials) or a joint function of accuracy and speed information, such as the increase in latency following an error trial. These choices should be guided by the goals of maximizing reliability and sensitivity and by evidence regarding the multivariate structure of the measures in a battery. (Sensitivity was discussed above; reliability and multivariate structure are covered below.)

Because field studies of neurobehavioral toxicology typically involve a *measured* rather than an assigned independent variable, the independent variables used in a study should undergo the same kinds of psychometric evaluation as those applied to the dependent measures. A measured independent variable also often offers a choice between classification and continuous scaling on it, with consequences for the choice of analytic method (correlational versus analysis of variance) and for the power to detect a relationship between independent and dependent variables (these topics are discussed more fully below).

Level of measurement. The choice of a scoring system determines the level of measurement of the scores. The level of measurement is the amount and type of information about variation in the measured behavior that is preserved in the scores. Binary and categorical scores contain information about group membership; if the categories are ordered, an ordinal level of measurement is achieved. Scores that provide information about the distance between pairs of levels on a trait (in addition to their rank order) are considered to be at a quantitative (interval or ratio) level of measurement. In many cases, it is not clear whether test scores should be considered ordinal or truly interval. Young (1986) argues that some types of data may fall between ordinal and interval, containing some distance information but not consistently enough to be considered strictly interval-level; scores on many tests seem to fit this case.

There are several reasons why level of measurement should be a concern in behavioral toxicology. A major reason is that in those cases where the level can be changed (often true of test scores), reliability can sometimes be improved by changing the level of measurement (Cochran 1983), with a consequent increase in the power to detect an effect (Sutcliffe 1980). For instance, since a quantitative score *appears* to contain the maximum information that can be had about variation in a trait, it seems highly desirable to achieve that level. However, if a quantitative scale has low reliability, a substantial proportion of the apparent distance information is actually random error; ranks or categories might be just as informative.

In quasi-experimental research (such as field studies in behavioral toxicology), the reliability of the *independent* variable is of particular concern. Hypothesis tests (such as the F-test) are based on the implicit assumption that both independent and dependent variables are perfectly reliable; that is, no provision is made for sorting out error of measurement from other sources of error. In group-oriented analyses (analysis of variance, t-tests) error of measurement in the dependent variable is taken into account, though not separately, as part of within-group error. On the other hand, errors of classification into groups as a result of the unreliability of the *independent* variable are completely hidden in the analysis but do reduce the power of the test (Cochran 1970).

Strategies for dealing with an unreliable independent variable are not discussed in experimental statistics texts, since these assume assignment to predefined (and thus perfectly reliable) levels on the independent variable. Cochran filled this void with a thoughtful discussion of the problem in his book on observational research (1983). In particular, he examined the effect on the power of a statistical test of shifting from a continuous scale to ordered categories in the independent variable. Cochran found that if there is a relationship between independent and dependent variables, grouping results in a loss of power when the distribution on the independent variable is reasonably symmetric and unimodal; this is because the covariance between the independent and dependent variables is reassigned from systematic, "true" variance to within-group error. The loss of power may be completely offset if there is a substantial component of random error of measurement in scores on the continuous independent variable, most of which would be discarded in the categorization. If, in addition, the independent variable has a multimodal distribution, and grouping occurs around these modes, there may even be a *gain* in power.

In general, increasing the number of groups increases power, as does increasing the distance between group means (computed on the continuous variable underlying the categories). The former makes available to the analysis more information about systematic differences in the continuous independent variable, while the latter decreases errors by decreasing misclassification at the boundaries between groups. For instance, taking the highest and lowest 40 percent on a distribution is more powerful than using the upper and lower halves of a distribution, since fewer subjects are likely to be misclassified in the former than in the latter approach.

A second reason for paying attention to the level of measurement is that it determines the best approach to statistical evaluation of the data. Whether it makes sense to use a particular statistical technique to analyze a variable depends in part on the match between distance and order information available in the variable and that used in computing the statistic. For example, both the rank-order and product-moment methods of computing correlations will give the same results on an ordinal-level variable, since only ordinal information is available in the data. In contrast, if a rank-order correlation is computed on a quantitative-level variable, the distance information in the variable is ignored, with a possible loss of power to detect a relationship if one exists.

To summarize, level of measurement, power, and reliability are all interrelated. Choice of level of measurement can affect both of the latter, in part because improving reliability improves power but also because the appropriate level of measurement maximizes the amount of valid information available to the statistical analysis.

Issues in using multiple scores. Another consideration in deciding how to score test performance—in addition to level of measurement—is the amount of differential information about distinct aspects of functioning that it is desirable to retain in the resulting data. The amount can range from a single score representing a global evaluation of overall functioning up to a multiscore profile in which each score represents a distinct domain of functioning.

The choice of optimal level of differential information depends on the purposes for which the battery is being developed. For screening, a single score recording presence or absence of any deficit may suffice. However, unless the aspects are highly correlated, combining separate aspects of performance in a single score reduces the validity of that score as a measure of any specific deficit. Thus, for diagnostic testing and dose-response studies, separate scores for distinct dimensions of behavior are needed. Another situation in which a profile of distinct scores is particularly needed is that in which a toxicant appears to have multiple effects, with individuals differing in the pattern of effects.

When the profile approach is chosen for scoring a battery, in the optimal case each score contributes information not contained in the others (Lord and Novick 1968; Nunnally 1978). This implies both that each score is a reliable measure of a relevant aspect of functioning and that it is not redundant with another score in the profile. As understanding of the relationship between a neurotoxicant and psychological functioning grows, scores (and possibly tests) that are consistently uninformative can be eliminated. In addition, redundancy between scores can be reduced either by dropping all but one of a set of redundant scores or by combining the redundant measures to obtain a more reliable composite score. The objective is to have the smallest number of distinct and useful measures possible. Achieving this goal maximizes efficiency in the use of resources (staff, time) as well as in the statistical power of the data. Power is increased both by reducing the degrees of freedom used in multivariate tests and by increasing the proportion of total variance that is systematically related to the effects being studied.

Identification of the best subset or best composite score is based on multivariate data analysis (Morrison 1967; Mulaik 1972; Nunnally 1978). Alternative methods (with examples of their use in the neurotoxicity literature) include principal-components analysis, factor analysis (Lindström 1980; Baker et al. 1983), canonical correlation (Brown et al. 1981), discriminant-function analysis (Hänninen 1971; Hane et al. 1977), and multiple regression (Tuttle, Wood, and Grether 1977; Tuttle et al. 1977).

Appropriate use of multivariate methods requires a fairly sophisticated understanding of what these methods do with data and how they may be interpreted properly. This is an area in which working with an experienced psychometrician is definitely an advantage. Factor analysis provides an example of some of the pitfalls of analyzing multivariate structures; it appears to be particularly appropriate for development of optimal scoring systems, but as Carroll (1978) notes, "factor analysis is a very tricky technique; in some ways it depends more . . . on intuition and judgment than on formal rules of procedure" (p. 91).

The variety of information required for an adequate report of a factor analysis indicates the number of choice points involved in a complete analysis. Humphreys (1967; see also Carroll 1978) points out that "the techniques of factor analysis are not sufficiently objective that a reader can accept final rotated matrices without question" (p. 129). At a minimum, the factor analyst should report the criterion for number of factors (or components), the method of factoring, the initial estimates of communalities (if common-factor analysis is used), the kind of rotation that was done, and, if the rotation was oblique, the factor intercorrelations. In addition, reliability estimates, mean and variance of scores, and the number of subjects all help to evaluate how stable the correlations are.

Lindström (1980) provided an instance of an appropriate description of a factor analysis: "The factorization was performed with the principal-axes method, the biggest correlations of variables being used as communality estimates; and the solutions chosen for interpretration were rotated by the Varimax method" (p. 73). He omits the number-of-factors criterion but provides enough information in the accompanying table to support an educated guess as to how this was decided; the only thing completely missing is the rotation matrix, which is not crucial in an orthogonal rotation. In contrast, Baker et al. (1983) say only that they performed "a factor analysis" (p. 127), which leaves far too much to the fevered imagination of skeptics.

A multivariate analysis produces coefficients (or weights) that can be used to obtain a weighted combination of scores that is optimal vis-à-vis one of three criteria. The criterion in principal components and factor analysis is maximal *discrimination among individuals* on each factor or component. Multiple regression and canonical correlation are used to obtain the maximum *multiple correlation* between combinations of predicted and predictor variables, respectively, while the criterion in discriminant-function analysis is to maximize the *difference between the two groups*.

The magnitude of the weights used to form linear composites cannot be interpreted as indicating the importance of a particular variable; these linear combinations all work on the principle (familiar to users of multiple-regression analysis) of partialing out variance accounted for by previously entered variables before computing the weight on the next variable entered. Thus, if two variables have a substantial intercorrelation, the more discriminating variable in the pair will be entered first and assigned the higher weight, while the second variable may have a weight close to zero, since after being partialed by the first variable, it does not add new information to the composite score.

An alternative to using weighted combinations of scores (such as factor scores or discriminant scores) as a means of obtaining a set of nonredundant scores is to select a subset of the scores, each of which has a high loading on a distinct factor (e.g., Baker et al. 1983). Scores that have their highest loading on the same factor are inferred to measure the same latent variable and thus to be redundant, while scores loading on separate factors are inferred to be measuring distinct aspects of the domain.

Since the multivariate methods discussed in this section are designed to maximize variance accounted for in the specific data set to which they are applied, they can return results that are unique to a particular data set and not replicable. Multivariate analysis in particular calls for the use of very conservative statistical standards (Muller, Barton, and Benignus 1984), such as Bonferroni-adjusted significance levels and strict application of assumptions of linearity and homogeneity of variance (see below).

In addition, the results of any of these optimizing techniques should be validated before composite scores or subsets of measures based on the analysis are used in formal hypothesis testing or decision making. This is a major reason why development of standardized, validated batteries outside the context of any single study is needed. It is particularly important that selection of an optimal set of tests for a battery or the development of a composite scoring method be done on a sample different from that on which subsequent hypothesis testing will be undertaken; carrying out an optimizing analysis and then drawing conclusions based on statistical tests of optimal data in the same group (as was done, for example, by Golden, Hammeke, and Purisch 1978) carries a high risk of being misled by sampling error. Cross-validation is one method of checking replicability (e.g., Tuttle, Wood, and Grether 1977); this approach involves developing optimal scoring equations independently on two randomly assigned groups of subjects and then checking the validity of each scoring equation in the group on which it was not developed.

Reliability

Reliability is a concern in criterion-oriented research such as behavioral toxicology because errors of measurement obscure the relationship between dependent and independent variables. A reliable score is relatively insensitive to variation in irrelevant characteristics of subjects and the conditions of test administration (e.g., alternate forms, different examiners) and thus has a favorable ratio of systematic, or "true," variance to total variance (including that due to irrelevant factors). While the immediate outcome of reliability evaluation is an estimate of the relative magnitude of error in observed scores, in the longer run a systematic analysis of the sources of error variance (as in generalizability analysis, described below) can pinpoint where improvements are needed in the test, testing conditions, or sampling plan.

A systematic reliability evaluation starts with an attempt to identify all of the factors in the design for testing that are likely to contribute to variation in scores. Stanley (1971, p. 364) provides a useful framework for identifying sources of variance generally encountered in behavioral testing. Stanley classifies characteristics of subjects that affect their test performance along two primary dimensions: lasting versus temporary and general versus specific (to the test and testing conditions). Additional categories in his taxonomy are systematic biases and random errors in test administration and scoring.

As sources of variance are identified, they are assigned to either true or error variance. What determines whether a source of variance is assigned to true or error variance is not intrinsic to the source of variance itself but depends on whether the variation is trait-related (true) or irrelevant (error); the assignment must be decided by the test user in accordance with the purposes of testing and the design of the study. For instance, if the ability to profit from practice is highly related to neurological status after exposure to a neurotoxicant, then effects of practice on scores constitute part of true variance. If, on the other hand, practice effects are unrelated to neurological status, then these effects are assigned to error variance.

The treatment of affective factors in reliability evaluation is particularly complicated. When an affective state such as euphoria or depression is attributable to neuropathy caused by a neurotoxicant, it constitutes a source of true variance (Hänninen 1971; Feldman, Ricks and Baker 1980). On the other hand, emotional reactions such as anxiety about being exposed or being tested (Lawrence 1962; Tryon 1980) should be classified as error variance, since they interfere with test performance and may result in an overestimate of deficits in nonaffective aspects of behavior. Teasing out the relationships between exposure, affective state, and test performance may require use of a well-rationalized array of cognitive, personality, and mood measures, as discussed above in the section on sensitivity.

Erratic performance (e.g., wide variation in RTs from trial to trial) or an unlikely pattern of responses (e.g., easy items incorrect, difficult items correct) suggests that the resulting score may not be a valid measure of level of functioning. This may be due to a lack of motivation (particularly in control subjects). For instance, Repko et al. (1978) comment that there were unusual features in the performance of control subjects in the study reported by Repko, Morgan, and Nicholson (1975) and that "variability in performance . . . suggests not only inconsistent test behavior but also an overall group shift in a criterion of what constitutes appropriate test behavior" (p. 2). Another reason for a random or unexpected pattern of responses is that the subject misunderstood the instructions, indicating a need for revision of test-administration procedures. Finally, an *increase* in the number of incorrect or erratic responses in tests given later in a session may indicate that the examinee was too fatigued or discouraged to respond adequately. This may be attributable to neuropathy, lack of motivation, or tests that are too difficult; this pattern of errors demands further investigation.

Limitations of reliability theory. A substantial gap stands between the assumptions about test scores made in "classical" reliability theory (e.g., Lord and Novick 1968) and the characteristics of real data. Cronbach, Rajaratnam, and Gleser (1963) summarized the limitations of classical reliability theory as follows:

> The heart of classical reliability theory is the concept of "parallel" measures . . . in content, in mean, in variance, and in intercorrelations. In internal-consistency analysis, it is further supposed that half-tests or even separate items satisfy these (or slightly weaker) equivalence assumptions. For standardized tests, parallel forms can be constructed that very nearly satisfy the equivalence conditions; but test items are usually heterogeneous, and half tests may likewise fall short of equivalence.
>
> For many other types of measurements, parallel observations are hard to obtain and sometimes the very concept of parallel observations is obscure, . . . one rater is rarely identical to the next in what he attends to, in the variance of the ratings he gives or in his correlations with other raters. . . . In the field . . . different situations in which the subject is observed are rarely equivalent. (P. 137)

Other assumptions of classical reliability theory are (*a*) that error variance and true variance are uncorrelated and (*b*) that error variance is unidimensional, that is, affected by only one factor. These assumptions provided the formal basis for deriving methods of estimating reliability such as test-retest, split halves, and internal consistency. Unfortunately, these assumptions are rarely met in real data; when they are not, estimates of reliability are biased.

In order to bring reliability theory closer to reality, a number of alternative theoretical bases for evaluating reliability have been developed that make less stringent assumptions than classical test theory, with generalizability theory having the least stringent assumptions.

Generalizability theory. In generalizability theory, the objective of the evaluation is to determine whether measures are "generalizable" across the variety of testing conditions in which they may be obtained. The concept of generalizability is analogous to the concept of external validity in experimental research (Cook and Campbell 1979; Fyans 1983). If the results of an experiment have external validity, "we can infer that the presumed causal relationship can be generalized to and across alternate measures of the cause and effect and across different types of persons, settings, and times" (Cook and Campbell 1979, p. 37).

Generalizability theory (Cronbach et al. 1972; Van der Kamp 1976; Shavelson and Webb 1981; Brennan 1983) permits the evaluation of multiple sources of true and error variance, called *facets*. In addition, the assumption (in classical test theory) of equivalent measures is weakened (in generalizability theory) to that of sampling from a "universe" of equally acceptable conditions.

In a field-testing program, testing conditions may vary on several facets; for example, several examiners (facet 1) may be using several alternate forms of a test (facet 2) to examine, on several occasions (facet 4), a group of subjects who differ in exposure level (facet 4), age (facet 5), and education (facet 6). What the investigator wants to know is whether scores reliably measure variation in exposure level (facet 3) over all of the other facets, and if not, which facets are the locus of the largest components of error variance and need to be changed to improve reliability.

In actually carrying out a generalizability analysis, the expected magnitude of various sources of variance and an estimated generalizability index analogous to a reliability index are computed from estimates of variance components obtained using analysis of variance (Winer 1971, pp. 244–51).

Recent work in generalizability theory has sought to extend the analysis to the multivariate case, allowing simultaneous evaluation of a profile of scores such as would be obtained using a test battery (Cronbach et al. 1972; Joe and Woodward 1976; Webb, Shavelson, and Maddahian 1983).

Quantitative estimates of reliability. The final step in reliability evaluation is a quantitative analysis that may alternatively yield (*a*) a reliability coefficient, (*b*) an estimate of the standard error of measurement, and/or (*c*) (in the case of generalizability analysis) information on the expected magnitude of variance components in the data-collection design.

Some designs for reliability estimation that are probably familiar to most users of tests are test-retest, alternate forms, interrater, and internal-consistency reliability. In each of these, *one* source of error variance is assumed—occasions, forms, examiners, and item sampling, respectively. These are simple cases of the more general situation in reliability evaluation, in which multiple sources of error variance affect the measurements, thus requiring a more complex research design for reliability evaluation (American Psychological Association, American Educational Research Association, and National Council on Measurement in Education 1974).

Generalizability analysis is the method of choice for evaluating the reliability of a score in the more complex case of multifaceted error.

The appropriateness of an index of reliability depends on the level of measurement, as well as the intended use of a measure. When the reliability of an individual's score is of interest (i.e., as an estimate of his "true" score for use in diagnosis or comparison to norms), the most informative index is the *standard error of measurement*. When the stability of *relative position* among subjects is of interest in a correlation analysis (e.g., in a study of dose-response relationships), a correlational index, such as test-retest or split-half, provides an estimate of the theoretical ceiling on correlations between the test and other variables. This index is not an unbiased estimate of reliability unless the assumption of parallel measures is met. Finally, when reliability of classification into groups is the concern (e.g., for screening or analysis of variance designs), it is more appropriate to evaluate the reliability of the classifications rather than that of the scores used to do the classification, since it is the classification that will be used in subsequent analyses or decision making (see Kane and Brennan 1980).

The estimated communality from a factor analysis is sometimes treated as an estimate of reliability (e.g., Tuttle, Wood, and Grether 1977, p. 39), but it is actually an indeterminate combination of the reliability of the variable (which places a ceiling on its correlation with other variables) and the amount of common variance that it shares with the other variables in the data set. The relation of communalities to reliabilities is unpredictable but *can* be a gross overestimate in an underdetermined factor model (e.g., when a Heywood case occurs).

Exploratory Data Analysis

Working with data is like working with any material one might use to build a solid, functional structure, whether it be a house, a microscope, or an empirically verified scientific model: it is essential that the user know the qualities of the material, what its irregularities are, how far it can be trusted to bear the weight to be put on it. Exploratory data analysis (EDA) provides a repertory of noninferential quantitative methods for investigating the characteristics of data and sometimes "improving" them (vis-à-vis the requirements of statistical methods) (Tukey 1977; Velleman and Hoaglin 1981). EDA methods include ways to summarize data (e.g., stem-and-leaf plots), to clarify orderly behavior in the data (e.g., curve smoothing), and to select appropriate transformations needed to improve the fit of data to the assumptions of analytic methods and statistical tests.

Tukey (1977) remarks that "exploratory data analysis is detective in character," while "confirmatory data analysis is judicial or quasi-judicial in character" (p. 3). Just as optimizing multivariate analyses should be done on data other than those on which hypotheses will be formally tested (or other decision made), so exploratory analyses are properly applied to pilot data or data specifically collected for exploratory purposes (Muller, Barton, and Benignus 1984). In field testing, particularly at an early stage of investigations, nearly every study may be more properly considered exploratory than confirmatory, partly because of the limited information at that stage about the characteristics of the variables and partly because of the lack of control inherent in quasi-experimental or observational research. Results of such studies, including statistical tests, can still be reported, but it should be clear in the report that exploratory techniques were used in arriving at the reported results.

Exploratory analyses of the characteristics of data obtained on a battery of tests can provide useful insights into the results of analyses used for the development of a scoring system and reliability evaluation. Another important application is selecting an appropriate nonlinear transformation (e.g., log, square-root) when descriptive analyses suggest that a transformation is needed to improve the fit between the data and the assumptions of analytic methods and hypothesis tests. The two principal types of problems for which nonlinear transformations are useful are (*a*) to permit analysis of a nonlinear relationship using linear regression and (*b*) to improve the fit of the distribution of a variable to the assumptions of homogeneity of variance and symmetry of within-cell distributions that underlie analysis of variance.

Nonlinear relationships. If the shape of a bivariate relationship is linear, the strength of the relationship between the two variables will be accurately represented in linear methods such as correlation or regression analysis on the raw data. Unfortunately, there are many cases in which the relationship between two variables is systematic but not linear (e.g., an exponential growth curve). In this case, a regression equation obtained on raw data will underestimate the strength of the relationship. If the bivariate plot of the data has been examined, the investigator knows that the data do not meet the assumption of linearity and can take appropriate steps to improve the quantitative representation of the actual relationship between the variables. One alternative is to apply a nonlinear transformation to one or both variables to linearize their relationship (Tukey 1977, chap. 6), thus permitting use of linear-regression analysis; another is to attempt to fit a nonlinear function to the data (Gallant 1975). The first is most likely to be successful if the bivariate relationship is monotonic and regular. Given the advances in computing, the second may be the best route when the appropriate transformation is not apparent or when a transformation will not suffice (as in periodic data).

An example of a frequently used nonlinear transformation is tests on quadratic and higher-order trends in regression analysis (e.g., Smith, Langolf, and Goldberg 1983). Smith and colleagues tested the value of both linear and quadratic forms of various independent variables as predictors in a linear regression on the score on a digit-span task in two data sets. In both data sets, they found that for some variables the quadratic form accounted for more variance than did the untransformed (linear) form.

Valciukas et al. (Central nervous system dysfunction, 1978) provided an example of the use of a regular nonlinear function: they fitted a power function to the age-related decline in Embedded Figures performance. In monotonic nonlinear functions (such as the power function), the *nonlinear* function on *raw* data is mathematically equivalent to a *linear* function on *transformed* data. For example, if the log transformation is applied to the power function developed by Valciukas et al. (ibid.), the result is a linear-regression model in which the predictor (obtained) and predicted (corrected) scores are both logs of the raw measures, and the exponent in the power function becomes the slope in the linear regression. Both forms of the function account for the same amount of variance and thus are equivalent for predictive purposes, but the log transformation can be analyzed using a linear-regression program, while the power form of the same relationship requires a nonlinear modeling program.

Homogeneity of variance. When the frequency distribution of a variable systematically deviates from that assumed in a statistical test, a nonlinear transformation may be called for. Two particularly important assumptions are (*a*) that the variance and mean of observations in each group in a study are independent across groups and (*b*) that variances across levels of the independent variable(s) are equivalent; these are assumed in both analysis of variance and regression analysis. For example, the mean and variance of a distribution of measures are typically correlated in reaction times (RTs) and in test scores obtained by summing dichotomous scores (right/wrong) over a set of items. Which process accounts for the correlation in RTs is not always clear. Subjects may become slower and more variable simultaneously; alternatively, subjects who are more variable may simply have a mean RT inflated by outliers. In test scores, variance over subjects is reduced as the mean score of the group approaches the lowest or highest score possible; these are boundaries that limit the amount of variation possible. When exposure to a neurotoxicant either increases variability (in RTs) or produces test performance near the lowest score, the resulting systematic difference in within-group variance between the exposed and control groups results in a biased F-test.

One way to treat this problem (of heterogeneity of variance) is to apply a variance-stabilizing transformation to the data (Natrella 1966; Smith 1976). For example, Eckerman et al. (1984) investigated the effects of alcohol on RTs in a counterbalanced repeated-measures design (N = 17). The data were first cleaned by dropping error trials and "far out" trials within subject (using Tukey's [1977] "schematic summary" methods). Then RTs were transformed to the inverse square root, and finally subject means were calculated. This transformation was selected after investigating the regression of log variances on log means in several RT tasks and subject samples (Smith 1976). Subject means based on the transformed data were normally distributed within cells, while means on the raw data were not.

Eckerman et al. (1984) found that they were more likely to detect an effect in the transformed than in the raw RTs, apparently because the transformation reduced the inflated error variability in the slower group and thus reduced the mean squared error overall. For example, the effect of alcohol on simple RT was significant in the transformed data ($p < 0.037$) but just short of significance in the raw data ($p < 0.051$).

A transformation can be found to accomplish just about any desired "improvement" in one's data. Budescu and Wallsten (1979) urge that a transformation be chosen and used responsibly and offer guidelines for this process (see also Smith 1976). Finally, the effect of a transformation should be evaluated before it is used, since it sometimes differs from what was intended. For instance, too "strong" an inverse transformation can reverse the direction of a correlation between mean and variance from positive to negative instead of achieving the zero correlation that was the aim of the transformation.

Controlling for Confounded Effects

A major problem in field testing for neurotoxic effects is controlling for confounded variables in the selection and assignment of subjects to groups. The most damaging consequence of nonrandom assignment to groups is that uncontrolled factors confounded with level of exposure (e.g., motivation to cooperate in the study, intelligence, age, level of education) pose a serious threat to the external validity of the study (e.g., Repko, Morgan, and Nicholson 1975).

The basic principles used to control confounding variables in experimental research also can be used in neurotoxicity assessment; these include, for example, blocking on confounding factors in selection of the subject sample, use of corrected scores or norms (e.g., age-corrected scores), and use of covariates in the statistical analysis (Winer 1971; Cook and Campbell 1979). The objective in each case is to reduce unwanted variance in the *dependent* measure (to reduce error variance) while leaving variation attributable to the independent variable unaffected. It is counterproductive to use statistical methods (e.g., covariance analysis or partial correlation) to remove the effect of a confounded variable when it is correlated with both the independent and the dependent variables (Cook and Campbell 1979). This is because statistically removing a component of variance shared with the independent variable reduces the size of the very component of variance that is being evaluated by the statistical test.

Field testing for psychological effects of neurotoxicants has special problems in the use of covariates because extent of exposure is often correlated with the covariates needed to remove confounded sources of variance in the dependent variable(s). Even when the relationship between exposure criteria and behavioral tests is studied using a correlational design, exposure is still conceptually the independent measure, and the assumptions of covariance analysis apply, particularly that the covariate or partialed variable is not correlated with the independent variable. For example, Tuttle, Wood, and Grether (1977) obtained partial correlations between exposure measures and psychological test scores, controlling for the effect of age in both measures. In this case, age was directly related to amount of exposure and inversely related to raw scores on behavioral tests. The partial-correlation analysis removed the component of exposure correlated with age, thus probably resulting in underestimates of the correlations between exposure and behavioral measures.

A more appropriate way to remove the effect of age is to partial it from the dependent variable only. For instance, Baker et al. (1983) developed a prediction equation for each of the tests in a battery based on the regression of demographic characteristics on behavioral test performance in an unexposed group. The deviation from predicted performance in an exposed group (Baker et al., Occupational lead, 1985) was obtained by computing a *percent-predicted score* (the ratio of observed to predicted score × 100), and this score was then used to study the effects of lead.

To summarize, controlling for confounding factors in field testing calls for a careful analysis of the hypothesized relationships among independent, dependent, and confounding variables *prior to* designing the study, since some confounded variance cannot be removed using statistical methods but must be controlled by using appropriate sampling procedures or by correcting scores on the basis of norms.

Conclusions

Field study of behavioral toxicology is still at an early stage of development. Knowledge of the behavioral effects of toxic substances in humans is generally based on small samples of both persons and tests. Systematic studies of the reliability and construct validity of tests in the exposed population have not been done. Norms for performance on these tests in the unexposed population have been obtained on similarly small samples of subjects, frequently with a relatively narrow range of demographic characteristics.

The general inattention to methodological consistency makes it difficult to integrate the research to date into a clear picture of what is known and not known about the effects of toxic substances on human behavior. In view of the variation in methods of subject selection, measurement, and statistical analysis, the completion of a series of studies of a particular toxic substance does not assure that there has been a concurrent accumulation of reliable knowledge about the effects of that substance. Apparent replications or failures to replicate a significant relationship must be evaluated carefully, since different studies may have measured different things in different populations.

As detailed in the first part of this chapter and in chapter 15, a substantial amount of groundwork has already been done in test development, development of test-administration technology, and both field and laboratory studies of these tests under limited conditions. What is needed next is systematic evaluation of the testing methods now available, with particular attention to *reliability,* to *norms* in subgroups of the normal human population, and to *construct validity.* We hope the material covered in this chapter will serve as a useful tool in this process, both by providing a summary of test development to date and by providing access to the methods and literature relevant to psychometric problems in field testing.

Acknowledgments

Preparation of this manuscript was supported by cooperative agreement CR-808834 from the Neurotoxicology Division, Health Effects Research Laboratory, U.S. Environmental Protection Agency.

References

Allen, G. L., and Morgan, B. B., Jr. 1985. Assessment of learning abilities using complex experimental learning tasks. *Neurobehav. Toxicol. Teratol.* 7:355–58.

Alluisi, E. A. 1975. Optimum uses of psychobiological, sensorimotor, and performance measurement strategies. *Hum. Factors* 17:309–20.

Alluisi, E. A.; Beisel, W. R.; Bartelloni, P. J.; and Coates, G. D. 1973. Behavioral effects of tularemia and sandfly fever in man. *J. Infect. Dis.* 128:710–17.

American Psychological Association, American Educational Research Association, and National Council on Measurement in Education. 1974. *Standards for educational and psychological tests.* Washington, D.C.: American Psychological Association.

Anders, T.; Fozard, J.; and Lillyquist, T. 1972. Effects of age upon retrieval from short-term memory. *Dev. Psychol.* 6:214–17.

Anderson, J. R. 1978. Arguments concerning representations for mental imagery. *Psychol. Rev.* 85:249–77.

Anger, W. K. 1984. Neurobehavioral testing of chemicals: Impact on recommended standards. *Neurobehav. Toxicol. Teratol.* 6:147–53.

Anger, W. K., and Johnson, B. L. 1985. Chemicals affecting behavior. In *Neurotoxicity of industrial and commercial chemicals,* edited by J. L. O'Donoghue. Boca Raton, Fla: CRC Press.

Arezzo, J. C., and Schaumburg, H. H. 1980. The use of the Optacon® as a screening device. *J. Occup. Med.* 22:461–64.

Arlien-Søborg, P.; Bruhn, P.; Gyldensted, C.; and Melgaard, B. 1979. Chronic painters' syndrome: Chronic toxic encephalopathy in house painters. *Acta Neurol. Scand.* 60:149–56.

Baker, E. L.; Feldman, R. G.; White, R. F.; Harley, J. P.; Dinse, G. E.; and Berkey, C. S. 1983. Monitoring neurotoxins in industry: Development of a neurobehavioral test battery. *J. Occup. Med.* 25:125–30.

Baker, E. L.; Feldman, R. G.; White, R. F.; Harley, J. P.; Niles, C. A.; Dinse, G. E.; and Berkey, C. S. 1984. Occupational lead neurotoxicity: A behavioural and electrophysiologic evaluation: I. Study design and year one results. *Br. J. Ind. Med.* 41:352–61.

Baker, E. L.; Letz, R.; Fidler, S.; Shalat, S.; Plantamura, D.; and Lyndon, M. 1985. Computer-based neurobehavioral testing for occupational and environmental epidemiology. *Neurobehav. Toxicol. Teratol.* 7:369–78.

Baker, E. L.; White, R. F.; Pothier, L. J.; Berkey, C. S.; Dinse, G. E.; Travers, P. H.; Harley, J. P.; and Feldman, R. G. 1985. Occupational lead neurotoxicity: Improvement in behavioural effects after reduction of exposure. *Br. J. Ind. Med.* 42:507–16.

Bornschein, R.; Pearson, D.; and Reiter, L. W. 1980. Behavioral effects of moderate lead exposure in children and animal models: Part 1, clinical studies. *CRC Crit. Rev. Toxicol.* 8:43–99.

Branconnier, R. J. 1985. Dementia in human populations exposed to neurotoxic agents: A portable microcomputerized dementia screening battery. *Neurobehav. Toxicol. Teratol.* 7:379–86.

Branconnier, R. J.; DeVitt, D. R.; Cole, J. O.; and Spera, K. F. 1982. Amitriptyline selectively disrupts verbal recall from secondary memory of the normal aged. *Neurobiol. Aging* 3:55–59.

Brennan, R. L. 1983. *Elements of generalizability theory.* Iowa City: American College Testing Program.

Brown, G. G., and Nixon, R. K. 1979. Exposure to polybrominated biphenyls: Some effects on personality and cognitive functioning. *JAMA* 242:523–27.

Brown, G. G.; Preisman, R. C.; Anderson, M. D.; Nixon, R. K.; Isbister, J. L.; and Price, H. A. 1981. Memory performance of chemical workers exposed to polybrominated biphenyls. *Science* 212:1413–15.

Budescu, D. V., and Wallsten, T. S. 1979. A note on monotonic transformations in the context of functional measurement and analysis of variance. *Bull. Psychon. Soc.* 14:307–10.

Campbell, D. T., and Fiske, D. W. 1959. Convergent and discriminant validation by the multitrait-multimethod matrix. *Psychol. Bull.* 56:81–105.

Carroll, J. B. 1978. How shall we study individual differences in cognitive abilities?—Methodological and theoretical perspectives. *Intelligence* 2:87–115.

———. 1980. *Individual difference relations in psychometric and experimental cognitive tasks.* L. L. Thurstone Psychometric Laboratory Report No. 163. NTIS No. AD-A086 057. Chapel Hill: University of North Carolina.

Cochran, W. G. 1970. Some effects of errors of measurement on multiple correlations. *Am. Stat. Assoc. J.* 65:22–34.

———. 1983. *Planning and analysis of observational studies.* New York: John Wiley & Sons.

Cook, T. D., and Campbell, D. T. 1979. *Quasi-experimentation: Design and analysis issues for field settings.* Boston: Houghton-Mifflin Co.

Cooper, L. A., and Regan, D. T. 1982. Attention, perception, and intelligence. In *The handbook of human intelligence,* edited by R. J. Sternberg, 123–69. Cambridge: Cambridge University Press.

Cronbach, L. J.; Gleser, G. C.; Nanda, H.; and Rajaratnam, N. 1972. *The dependability of behavioral measurements: Theory of generalizability for scores and profiles.* New York: Wiley.

Cronbach, L. J.; Rajaratnam, N.; and Gleser, B. 1963. Theory of generalizability: A liberaliza-
tion of reliability theory. *Br. J. Stat. Psychol.* 16:137–63.

Crook, T.; Ferris, S.; and McCarthy, M. 1979. The misplaced-objects task: A brief test for
memory dysfunction in the aged. *J. Am. Geriatr. Soc.* 27:284–87.

Crook, T.; Ferris, S.; McCarthy, M.; and Rae, D. 1980. Utility of digit recall tasks for assessing
memory in the aged. *J. Consult Clin. Psychol.* 48:228–33.

Davis, K. L.; Mohs, R. C.; Tinklenberg, J. R.; Pfefferbaum, A.; Hollister, L. E.; and Kopell,
B. S. 1978. Physostigmine: Improvement of long-term memory processes in normal
humans. *Science.* 201:272–74.

Davis, L. J., Jr., and Swenson, W. M. 1970. Factor analysis of the Wechsler Memory Scale. *J.
Consult. Clin. Psychol.* 35:430.

Eckerman, D. A.; Carroll, J. B.; Foree, D.; Gullion, C. M.; Lansman, M.; Long, E. R.; Waller,
M. B.; and Wallsten, T. S. 1985. An approach to brief field testing for neurotoxicity.
Neurobehav. Toxicol. Teratol. 7:387–94.

Eckerman, D. A., Elliott, S. L.; Long, E. R.; Robinson, G. S.; Gullion, C. M.; and Otto, D. A.
1984. Sensitivity of a field testing battery for evaluating neurobehavioral toxicity: Effects
of ethanol and carbon monoxide. Paper presented at the Society of Toxicology meeting,
Atlanta, Ga., March 1984. Abstract published in *Toxicologist* 4:24.

Erickson, R. C., and Scott, M. L. 1977. Clinical memory testing: A review. *Psychol. Bull.*
84:1130–49.

Feldman, R. G.; Ricks, N. L.; and Baker, E. L. 1980. Neuropsychological effects of industrial
toxins: A review. *Am. J. Ind. Med.* 1:211–27.

Ferris, S. H.; Crook, T.; Clark, E.; McCarthy, M.; and Rae, D. 1980. Facial recognition memory
deficits in normal aging and senile dementia. *J. Gerontol.* 35:707–14.

Foree, D.; Eckerman, D. A.; and Elliott, S. L. 1984. M.T.S.: An adaptable microcomputer-
based testing system. *Behav. Res. Meth. Instr. Comput.* 16:223–29.

Fyans, L. J., Jr. 1983. Multilevel analysis and cross-level inference of validity using generalizability theory. In *Generalizability theory: Inferences and practical applications,* edited by
L. J. Fyans, Jr., 49–66. San Francisco: Jossey-Bass.

Gallant, A. R. 1975. Nonlinear regression. *Am. Statistician* 29:73–81.

Gamberale, F.; Annwall, G.; and Olson, B. A. 1976. Exposure to trichloroethylene. III.
Psychological functions. *Scand. J. Work Environ. Health* 4:220–24.

Golden, C. J.; Hammeke, T. A.; and Purisch, A. D. 1978. Diagnostic validity of a standardized neuropsychological battery derived from Luria's neuropsychological tests. *J. Consult. Clin. Psychol.* 46:1258–65.

Grandjean, P.; Arnvig, E.; and Beckmann, J. 1978. Psychological dysfunctions in lead-exposed workers: Relation to biological parameters of exposure. *Scand. J. Work Environ.
Health* 4:295–303.

Hane, M.; Axelson, O.; Blume, J.; Hogstedt, C.; Sundell, L.; and Ydreborg, B. 1977. Psychological function changes among house painters. *Scand. J. Work Environ. Health* 3:91–99.

Hänninen, H. 1971. Psychological picture of manifest and latent carbon disulfide poisoning.
Br. J. Ind. Med. 28:374–81.

———. 1979. Psychological test methods: Sensitivity to long term chemical exposure at
work. *Neurobehav. Toxicol. Teratol.* 1:157–61.

Hänninen, H.; Eskelinen, L.; Husman, K.; and Nurminen, M. 1976. Behavioral effects of
long-term exposure to a mixture of organic solvents. *Scand. J. Work Environ. Health* 4:240–
55.

Hänninen, H.; Hernberg, S.; Mantere, P.; Vesanto, R.; and Jalkanen, M. 1978. Psychological
performance of subjects with low exposure to lead. *J. Occup. Med.* 20:683–89.

Hänninen, H., and Lindström, K. 1979. *Behavioral test battery for toxicopsychological studies used
at the Institute of Occupational Health in Helsinki.* 2d ed., rev. Helsinki: Institute of
Occupational Health.

Hänninen, H.; Nurminen, M.; Tolonen, M.; and Martelin, T. 1978. Psychological tests as indicators of excessive exposure to carbon disulfide. *Scand. J. Psychol.* 19:163–74.

Harbeson, M. M.; Bittner, A. C., Jr.; Kennedy, R. S.; Carter, R. C.; and Krause, M. 1983. Performance evaluation tests for environmental research (PETER): Bibliography. *Percept. Mot. Skills* 57:283–93.

Humphreys, L. G. 1967. Critique of Cattell's "Theory of fluid and crystallized intelligence: A critical experiment." *J. Ed. Psychol.* 58:129–36.

Irons, R. C., and Rose, P. V. 1985. Naval biodynamics laboratory human performance computerized testing. *Neurobehav. Toxicol. Teratol.* 7:395–98.

Joe, G. N., and Woodward, J. A. 1976. Some developments in multivariate generalizability. *Psychometrika* 41:205–17.

Johnson, B. L., and Anger, W. K. 1983. Behavioral toxicology. In *Environmental and occupational medicine*, edited by W. N. Rom, 329–50. Boston: Little, Brown & Company.

Johnson, B. L.; Cohen, H. H.; Struble, R.; Setzer, J. V.; Anger, W. K.; Gutnik, B. D.; McDonough, T.; and Hauser, P. 1974. Field evaluation of carbon monoxide exposed toll collectors. In *Behavioral toxicology: Early detection of occupational hazards*, edited by C. Xintaras, B. L. Johnson, and I. de Groot, 306–28. DHEW (NIOSH) Publication No. 74-126. Washington, D.C.: Government Printing Office.

Kane, M., and Brennan, R. L. 1980. Agreement coefficients as indices of dependability for domain referenced tests. *Appl. Psychol. Meas.* 4:105–26.

Kear-Colwell, J. J. 1973. The structure of the Wechsler Memory Scale and its relationship to "brain damage." *Br. J. Soc. Clin. Psychol.* 12:384–92.

Kintsch, W. 1977. *Memory and cognition.* New York: John Wiley & Sons.

Kirk, R. E. 1968. *Experimental design: Procedures for the behavioral sciences.* Belmont, Calif.: Brooks/Cole.

Knave, B.; Olson, B. A.; Elofson, S.; Gamberale, F.; Isaksson, A.; Mindus, P.; Persson, H. E.; Struwe, G.; Wennberg, A.; and Westerholm, P. 1978. A cross-sectional epidemiologic investigation of occupationally exposed industrial workers with special references to the nervous system. *Scand. J. Work Environ. Health* 4:19–45.

Langolf, G. D.; Chaffin, D. B.; Henderson, R.; and Whittle, H. P. 1978. Evaluation of workers exposed to elemental mercury using quantitative tests of tremor and neuromuscular functions. *Am. Indus. Hyg. Assoc. J.* 39:976–84.

Lawrence, S. W., Jr. 1962. The effects of anxiety, achievement motivation and task importance upon performance on an intelligence test. *J. Ed. Psychol.* 53:120–26.

Lezak, M. D. 1983. *Neuropsychological assessment.* 2d ed., rev. New York: Oxford University Press.

Lindström, K. 1980. Changes in psychological performances of solvent-poisoned and solvent-exposed workers. *Am. J. Ind. Med.* 1:69–84.

Lindström, K.; Härkönen, H.; and Hernberg, S. 1976. Disturbances in psychological functions of workers occupationally exposed to styrene. *Scand. J. Work Environ. Health* 3:129–39.

Lord, F. M., and Novick, M. R. 1968. *Statistical theories of mental test scores.* Reading, Mass.: Addison-Wesley.

Luria, A. R. 1973. *The working brain.* New York: Basic Books.

MacLeod, C. M.; Dekaban, A. S.; and Hunt, E. 1982. Memory impairment in epileptic patients: Selective effects of phenobarbital concentration. *Science* 202:1102–4.

Maurissen J. 1985. Psychophysical testing in human populations exposed to neurotoxicants. *Neurobehav. Toxicol. Teratol.* 7:309–18.

Mohs, R. C., and Davis, K. L. 1980. Choline chloride effects on memory: Correlation with the effects of physostigmine. *Psychiatry Res.* 2:149–56.

Mohs, R. C.; Tinklenberg, J. R.; Roth, W. T.; and Kopell, B. S. 1980. Sensitivity of some human cognitive functions to effects of methamphetamine and secobarbital. *Drug Alcohol Depend.* 5:145–50.

Morrison, D. F. 1967. *Multivariate statistical methods.* New York: McGraw-Hill.

Mulaik, S. A. 1972. *The foundations of factor analysis.* New York: McGraw-Hill.

Muller, K. E.; Barton, C. N.; and Benignus, V. A. 1984. Recommendations for appropriate statistical practice in toxicologic experiments. *NeuroToxicology* 5(2):113–26.

Natrella, M. G. 1966. The use of transformations. In *Experimental statistics,* 20-1–20-13. U.S. Department of Commerce, National Bureau of Standards Handbook 91. Rev. ed. Washington, D.C.: Government Printing Office.

Nunnally, J. C. 1978. *Psychometric theory.* 2d ed. New York: McGraw-Hill.

Otto, D. A. 1983. The application of event-related slow brain potentials in occupational medicine. In *Neurobehavioral methods in occupational health,* edited by R. Gilioli, 71–78. Oxford: Pergamon Press.

Otto, D. A.; Bauman, S. B.; and Robinson, G. S. 1985. Application of a portable microprocessor-based system for electrophysiological field testing. *Neurobehav. Toxicol. Teratol.* 7:409–14.

Pachella, R. G. 1974. The interpretation of reaction time in information-processing research. In *Human information processing: Tutorials in performance and cognition,* edited by B. H. Kantowitz, 41–82. Hillsdale, N.J.: Erlbaum/Wiley.

Pellegrino, J. W., and Glaser, R. 1979. Cognitive correlates and components in the analysis of individual differences. In *Human intelligence: Perspectives on its theory and measurement,* edited by R. J. Sternberg and D. K. Detterman, 61–88. Norwood, N.J.: Ablex.

Peterson, C. 1985. How much risk is too much? *Washington Post,* 4 February.

Poulton, E. C. 1965. On increasing the sensitivity of measures of performance. *Ergonomics* 8:69–76.

Putz, V. R. 1979. The effects of carbon monoxide on dual-task performance. *Hum. Factors* 21:13–24.

Reitan, R. M., and Davison, L. A. 1974. *Clinical neuropsychology: Current status and applications.* New York: Winston/Wiley.

Repko, J. D.; Corum, C. R.; Jones, P. D.; and Garcia, L. S., Jr. 1978. *The effects of inorganic lead on behavioral and neurologic function.* DHEW (NIOSH) Publication No. 78-128. Washington, D.C.: Government Printing Office.

Repko, J. D.; Morgan, B. B., Jr.; and Nicholson, J. A. 1975. *Behavioral effects of occupational exposure to lead.* DHEW (NIOSH) Publication No. 75-164. Washington, D.C.: Government Printing Office.

Sanes, J. N.; Colburn, T. R.; and Morgan, N. T. 1985. Behavioral motor evaluation for neurotoxicity screening. *Neurobehav. Toxicol. Teratol.* 7:329–37.

Schaumburg, H. H.; Arezzo, J. C.; Markowitz, L.; and Spencer, P. S. 1981. Neurotoxicity assessment. In *Assessment of health effects at chemical disposal sites,* edited by W. W. Lowrance, 82–104. New York: Rockefeller University Press.

Seppäläinen, A. M. 1983. Electrophysiological methods. Paper presented at the World Health Organization and National Institute for Occupational Safety and Health Workshop on the Prevention of Neurotoxic Illness in Working Populations, Cincinnati, Ohio, May 1983.

Seppäläinen, A. M.; Hänninen, H.; Anger, W. K.; Baker, E. L.; Carter, R.; Cherry, N.; Dick, R.; Feldman, R.; Letz, R.; Otto, D.; and Vinson, D. 1983. Report from the work group on recommended test methods. Paper presented at the World Health Organization and National Institute for Occupational Safety and Health Workshop on the Prevention of Neurotoxic Illness in Working Populations, Cincinnati, Ohio, May 1983.

Shavelson, R., and Webb, N. 1981. Generalizability theory: 1973–1980. *Br. J. Math. Stat. Psychol.* 34:133–66.

Sitram, N.; Weingartner, H.; and Gillin, J. C. 1978. Human serial learning: Enhancement with arecholine and choline and impairment with scopolamine. *Science* 201:274–76.

Smith, A. 1975. Neuropsychological testing in neurological disorders. In *Advances in neurology*, edited by W. I. Friedlander, 49–110. vol. 7. New York: Raven Press.

Smith, J. E. K. 1976. Data transformations in analysis of variance. *J. Verb. Learn. Verb. Behav.* 15:339–46.

Smith, P. J. 1979. Short-term memory scanning is related to memory span and mercury exposure. Ph.D. diss., University of Michigan.

———. 1985. Behavioral toxicology: Measures of cognitive functioning. *Neurobehav. Toxicol. Teratol.* 7:345–50.

Smith, P. J., and Langolf, G. D. 1981. The use of Sternberg's memory-canning paradigm in assessing effects of chemical exposure. *Hum. Factors* 23:701–8.

Smith, P. J.; Langolf, G. D.; and Goldberg, J. 1983. Effects of occupational exposure to elementary mercury on short-term memory capacity. *Br. J. Ind. Med.* 40:413–19.

Snow, R. E. 1979. Theory and method for research on aptitude processes. *Human intelligence*, 105–37. *See* Pellegrino and Glaser 1979.

Squire, L. R.; Judd, L. L.; Janowsky, D. S.; and Huey, L. Y. 1980. Effects of lithium carbonate on memory and other cognitive functions. *Am. J. Psychiatry* 37:1042–46.

Stanley, J. C. 1971. Reliability. In *Educational measurement*, edited by R. L. Thorndike, 356–442. Washington, D.C.: American Council on Education.

Sterman, A. B., and Schaumburg, H. H. 1980. The neurological examination. In *Experimental and clinical neurotoxicology*, edited by P. S. Spencer and H. H. Schaumburg, 675–80. Baltimore: Williams & Wilkins.

Sternberg, S. 1966. High speed scanning in human memory. *Science* 153:652–54.

Sutcliffe, J. P. 1980. On the relationship of reliability to statistical power. *Psychol. Bull.* 88:509–15.

Theios, J. 1973. Reaction time measurements in the study of memory processes: Theory and data. *Psychol. Learn. Motiv.* 7:43–85.

———. 1977. Commentary on "Reaction time measurements in the study of memory processes: Theory and data." In *Human memory: Basic processes*, edited by G. Bower, 243–51. New York: Academic Press.

Thorne, D. R.; Genzer, S. G.; Sing, H. C.; and Hegge, F. W. 1985. The Walter Reed performance assessment battery. *Neurobehav. Toxicol. Teratol.* 7:415–18.

Tolonen, M., and Hänninen, H. 1978. Psychological tests specific to individual carbon disulfide exposure. *Scand. J. Psychol.* 19:241–45.

Townsend, J. T. 1974. Issues and models concerning the processing of a finite number of inputs. In *Human information processing: Tutorials in performance and cognition*, edited by B. Kantowitz, 133–86. Hillsdale, N.J.: Erlbaum.

Townsend, J. T., and Ashby, F. G. 1978. Methods of modeling capacity in simple processing systems. In *Cognitive theory*, edited by N. J. Castellan, Jr., and F. Restle, 3:199–239. Hillsdale, N.J.: Erlbaum/Wiley.

Tryon, G. S. 1980. The measurement and treatment of test anxiety. *Rev. Ed. Res.* 50:343–72.

Tukey, J. W. 1977. *Exploratory data analysis.* Reading, Mass.: Addison-Wesley.

Tuttle, T. C.; Wood, G. D.; and Grether, C. B. 1977. *Behavioral and neurological evaluation of workers exposed to carbon disulfide.* DHEW (NIOSH) Publication No. 77-128. Washington, D.C.: Government Printing Office.

Tuttle, T. C.; Wood, G. D.; Johnson, B. L.; and Xintaras, C. 1977. *A behavioral and neurological evalation of dry cleaners exposed to perchloroethylene.* DHEW (NIOSH) Publication No. 77-214. Washington, D.C.: Government Printing Office.

Valciukas, J. A., and Lilis, R. 1980. Psychometric techniques in environmental research. *Environ. Res.* 21:275–97.

Valciukas, J. A.; Lilis, R.; Fischbein, A.; Selikoff, I. J.; Eisinger, J.; and Blumberg, W. E. 1978. Central nervous system dysfunction due to lead exposure. *Science* 201:465–67.

Valciukas, J. A.; Lilis, R.; Wolff, M. S.; and Anderson, H. A. 1978. Comparative neuro-behavioral study of a polybrominated biphenyl-exposed population in Michigan and a nonexposed group in Wisconsin. *Environ. Health Perspect.* 23:199–210.

Valciukas, J. A., and Singer, R. M. 1982. An embedded figures test in environmental and occupational neurotoxicology. *Environ. Res.* 28:183–98.

Van der Kamp, L. J. T. 1976. Generalizability and educational measurement. In *Advances in psychological and educational measurement*, edited by D. N. M. deGruijter and L. J. T. van der Kamp, 173–84. New York: Wiley.

Velleman, P. F., and Hoaglin, D. C. 1981. *Applications, basics, and computing of exploratory data analysis.* Boston: Duxbury Press.

Wang, P.; Kaplan, J.; and Rogers, E. 1975. Memory functioning in hemiplegics: A neuro-psychological analysis of the Wechsler Memory Scale. *Arch. Phys. Med. Rehabil.* 56:517–21.

Webb, N. M.; Shavelson, R. J.; and Maddahian, E. 1983. Multivariate generalizability theory. In *Generalizability theory*, 67–82. *See* Fyans 1983.

Weingartner, H.; Gold, P.; Ballenger, J. C.; Smallberg, S. A.; Summers, R.; Rubinow, D. R.; Post, R. M.; and Goodwin, F. K. 1981. Effects of vasopressin on human memory functions. *Science* 211:601–3.

Weingartner, H.; Grafman, J.; Boutelle, W.; Kaye, W.; and Martin, P. R. 1983. Forms of memory failure. *Science* 221:380–82.

Weiss, B. 1983. Behavioral toxicology and environmental health science: Opportunity and challenge for psychology. *Am. Psychol.* 38:1174–87.

Williamson, A. M.; Teo, R. K. C.; and Sanderson, J. 1982. Occupational mercury exposure and its consequences for behaviour. *Int. Arch. Occup. Environ. Health* 50:273–86.

Winer, B.J. 1971. *Statistical principles in experimental design.* 2d ed. New York: McGraw-Hill.

Xintaras, C., and Burg, J. A. R. 1980. Screening and prevention of human neurotoxic out-breaks: Issues and problems. In *Experimental and clinical neurotoxicology*, 663–74. *See* Sterman and Schaumburg 1980.

Young, F. W. 1986. In *Multidimensional scaling: History theory, and applications*, edited by F. W. Young and R. M. Hamer. Hillsdale, N. J.: Erlbaum.

Workplace Exposures

There are in excess of 850 chemicals found in the workplace for which there is evidence of neurotoxicity at the present time (Anger and Johnson 1985, a review of major secondary reference sources on which this chapter builds). While this number represents only about 1 percent of the total estimated 100,000 chemicals found in the workplace (NIOSH 1983), many are among those to which significant numbers of workers are exposed. As of 1974, the National Occupational Hazard Survey (NOHS) identified 197 chemicals to which over 1 million persons were believed exposed in U.S. workplaces, based on sampling estimates, during all or part of the work day (NIOSH 1977). Of these, 65 (33 percent) are among those listed as neurotoxic in Anger and Johnson (1985), although neurotoxicity is not the primary effect in many cases (e.g., benzene). These chemicals are listed in table 15.1 along with the estimated size of the populations of workers exposed full- or part-time (NIOSH 1977). Some of the 65 are obviously general-usage groups (e.g., solvents), and others are chemicals that are not neurotoxic in the concentrations usually encountered in the workplace (e.g., food additives), but the number of workers exposed to chemicals that are neurotoxic at some level is quite large. While the bulk of these exposures are part-time (of undetermined frequency), the number of workers exposed full-time exceeds 7.7 million.

In view of the large exposure population, which establishes a major potential workplace hazard, this chapter is intended primarily to provide a background on occupational factors related to neurotoxicity of importance to scientists and to suggest steps to undertake when conducting workplace research designed to assess the hazards posed by neurotoxic chemicals. Specific purposes of this chapter are (*a*) to reflect the extent of workplace exposures; (*b*) to identify those behavioral tests most frequently reported as successful in the workplace-testing literature; (*c*) to describe the general methodological approaches used to identify neurotoxicity in workplace settings; (*d*) to relate the major findings reported in the existing workplace literature; (*e*) to describe the steps required to conduct workplace research projects; and (*f*) to outline steps that should be taken at the conclusion of such a study.

Table 15.1 Neurotoxic chemicals with estimated exposure populations over 1 million

Chemical	Population (in millions)	Chemical	Population (in millions)
Acetone (1,000 ppm)[a]	2.8	Ethylene glycol (0.2 ppm ceiling)	2.3
Alcohol	4.3	Food additives	3.7
Aliphatic hydrocarbons	2.9	Formaldehyde (3 ppm)	1.8
Alkanes	2.8	Glycerol	3.3
Alkyl styrene polymers	2.3	Hexane (500 ppm)	2.1
Ammonia (500 ppm)	3.2	Isophorone (25 ppm)	1.5
Amyl acetate, N- (100 ppm)	1.9	Lead (0.05 mg/m^3)	1.4
Aniline (5 ppm)	1.3	Lithium grease	1.6
Antimony sulfide (0.5 mg/m^3)	1.2	Methanol (200 ppm)	2.6
Aromatic hydrocarbons	3.9	Methyl acetate (200 ppm)	1.4
Asphalt	2.2	Nitrous oxide	2.0
Benzene (1 ppm)	1.9	Oil, fuel no. 1	3.7
Butanol	2.2	Oil, lube	2.3
Butyl acetate (150 ppm)	1.9	Petroleum distillates	3.0
Cadmium oxides (0.1 mg/m^3)	1.4	Pine oil	2.6
Carbon disulfide (20 ppm)	1.1	Polymethacrylate resin	2.5
Carbon tetrachloride (10 ppm)	2.0	Products of combustion	2.1
Chlorinated hydrocarbons	1.4	Propanol, 1-	1.3
Chlorobenzene (75 ppm)	1.1	Propylene glycol (200 ppm)	2.6
Chromium oxides	1.5	Shellac	3.0
Cresol (5 ppm)	1.9	Sodium chloride	6.4
Cyclohexanol (50 ppm)	1.3	Solvent	4.1
Cyclohexanone (50 ppm)	1.2	Tetrachloroethylene (100 ppm)	2.0
Degreaser	2.5	Toluene (200 ppm)	4.8
Diacetone alcohol (50 ppm)	1.3	Trichlorobenzene	1.1
Dichlorobenzene, ortho- (50 ppm)	2.0	Trichloroethylene (100 ppm)	3.7
Dichlorodifluoromethane (1,000 ppm)	3.8	Trichlorofluoromethane	2.6
Dichloroethane, 1,2-	1.9	Tricresyl phosphate (0.1 mg/m^3)	2.3
Dichlorotetrafluoroethane	2.5	Tungsten oxides	1.3
Diphenylamine	1.5	Turpentine (100 ppm)	2.0
Dyes	3.3	Vinyl chloride	2.3
Ethanol	8.1	Xylene (100 ppm)	4.3
Ethyl acetate (400 ppm)	2.7		

[a]Federal Permissible Exposure Limits (PELs), or legal maximum average daily concentrations, from 1984 are added where possible; other maxima may also apply and are found in 29 CFR 1910.1000. The level is given in parts of chemical per million parts of air or milligram of chemical per cubic meter of air. Some chemicals also have ceiling concentrations that are not listed; in cases where they are listed, only a maximum ceiling is allowed.

Occupational Exposure to Neurotoxic Chemicals

The exposure maxima found in table 15.1 are listed in terms of inhalation exposures. This should not obscure the fact that environmental exposures may occur through multiple routes, including cutaneous, oral, and inhalation. Inhalation exposures are easily measured in the industrial environment and form the basis for most estimates of chemical exposure in occupational research. The contribution of oral exposures to total industrial exposure is uncertain, but most problems can be avoided through effective hygiene practices. The impact of cutaneous exposures should not be underestimated, although their importance for most substances is unknown, and methods for measuring their impact are not well developed. Lauwerys et al. (1980) concluded that the amount of dimethylformamide (found in polyacrylic fiber production) absorbed through the skin was twice that absorbed through inhalation, assuming that no personal protective devices were used. Tsuruta (1975) estimated that immersion of both hands in methylene chloride (a solvent that penetrates the skin effectively) was equivalent to a one-minute inhalation exposure to 8,540 ppm. Put another way, a one-minute skin exposure could, in select cases, introduce into the body a quantity of chemical equivalent to that produced by an eight-hour inhalation exposure at the maximum allowable U.S. federal occupational exposure standard (Susten 1984).

The neurotoxic chemicals with large exposure populations do not reflect the breadth of exposures in the United States today. In *Patty's Industrial Hygiene and Toxicology,* the most extensive review of the toxicity of industrial chemicals available, 22 major chemical groupings are classified in which 10 or more neurotoxic chemicals are found (Clayton and Clayton 1981–82). These groupings are listed in table 15.2. Even more reflective of the extensive exposure potential is the wide variety of occupations in which neurotoxic chemicals are found. The 850 neurotoxic chemicals mentioned above are readily identified in 38 of the 68 Standard Industrial Classifications (SICs) used in NOHS (NIOSH 1977), including all categories of manufacturing. These are listed in table 15.3, where they are ordered by SIC number. With respect to the primary industrial uses of the many neurotoxic chemicals, the major usage or product categories are solvents, pesticides (especially herbicides and insecticides), fertilizers, chemical synthesis (particularly in products involving petrochemicals, fuels), metal products (all phases), plastics, textiles, pharmaceuticals, photography, glassmaking, and automobile manufacturing (Anger and Johnson 1985). The breadth of occupations underlines the need for a better identification of those products or manufacturing processes where neurotoxic chemicals are involved.

The large number of neurotoxic chemicals has produced some 120 nervous-system-related effects following exposure to industrial chemicals, according to authors' reports. Those behavioral effects that have been reported in the secondary literature for 25 or more chemicals, along with the number of chemicals with which

Table 15.2 Chemical groupings in which 10 or more neurotoxic chemicals are found

Alcohols	Glycol derivatives
Alicyclic hydrocarbons	Halogenated aliphatic hydrocarbons containing Cl, Br, and I
Aliphatic and alicyclic amines	Halogenated cyclic hydrocarbons
Aliphatic carboxylic acids	Ketones
Aliphatic hydrocarbons	Metals
Aliphatic nitro compounds, nitrates, and nitrites	Nitrogen compounds
Aromatic hydrocarbons	Organic phosphates
Cyanides and nitriles	Organic phosphorus esters
Esters of aromatic monocarboxylic acids and monoalcohols	Organic sulfur compounds
Ethers	Phenols and phenolic compounds

Source: Clayton and Clayton 1981–82.

Table 15.3 SIC classifications and industries in which neurotoxic chemicals are found

07	Agricultural services and hunting	34	Fabricated metal products
13	Oil and gas extraction	35	Machinery, except electrical
16	Heavy construction contractors	36	Electrical equipment and supplies
17	Special trade contractors	37	Transportation equipment
19	Ordnance and accessories	38	Instruments and related products
20	Food and kindred products	39	Miscellaneous manufacturing industries
21	Tobacco manufacture	41	Local and interurban passenger transit
22	Textile mill products	42	Trucking and warehousing
23	Apparel and other textile products	44	Water transportation
24	Lumber and wood products	45	Transportation by air
25	Furniture and fixtures	46	Pipeline transportation
26	Paper and allied products	50	Wholesale trade
27	Printing and publishing	54	Food stores
28	Chemicals and allied products	55	Automotive dealers and service stations
29	Petroleum and coal products	58	Eating and drinking places
30	Rubber and plastics products	72	Personal service
31	Leather and leather products	73	Miscellaneous business services
32	Stone, clay and glass products	75	Auto repair, services and garages
33	Primary metal industries	80	Medical and other health services

each has been linked, are listed in table 15.4 (ibid.). "Behavioral changes" or "CNS effects" have been reported for 50 chemicals but were eliminated from consideration because the terms were too vague to be useful. Table 15.4, then, contains the 35 behavioral effects most frequently recognized and reported in the reference literature as occurring following exposure to industrial chemicals.

Functional Tests of Neurotoxicity in Humans

Most of the 35 neurotoxic effects listed in table 15.4 have been identified in humans following chemical exposures, through the use of functional behavioral tests. I describe those behavioral tests next, selecting only from tests found successful in workplace neurotoxicity research.

Within the motor category, tests reflecting incoordination in humans include symmetry drawing (Lindström, Härkönen, and Hernberg 1976) and the Mira test (Hänninen 1971, 1974; Hänninen et al. 1976; Tolonen and Hänninen 1978), which have detected population differences following exposure to styrene, carbon disulfide, and mixed solvents. The Michigan eye-hand coordination test has detected effects in workers following exposures to carbon monoxide (Johnson et al. 1974) and inorganic lead (Repko, Morgan, and Nicholson 1975). Clumsiness has been assessed using toe and finger tapping after mercury (Chaffin and Miller 1974) and mixed solvent exposures (Hänninen et al. 1976), and the Santa Ana dexterity test has been successfully used to identify clumsiness in carbon disulfide–exposed workers (Hänninen 1971, 1974; Tuttle, Wood, and Grether 1976; Tolonen and Hänninen 1978), in workers exposed to solvent mixtures (Hänninen et al. 1976), and in workers using inorganic lead (Milburn, Mitran, and Crockford 1976; Hänninen et al. 1978; Mantere et al. 1979). Simple reaction-time changes have been seen in workers exposed to carbon disulfide (Tuttle, Wood, and Grether 1976), inorganic lead (Milburn, Mitran, and Crockford 1976), jet fuels (Knave et al. 1978), and paint

Table 15.4 Neurobehavioral effects reported following chemical exposures for 25 or more chemicals

Effect	Number of Chemicals	Effect	Number of Chemicals
Motor		*General*	
Activity changes	32	Anorexia	158
Ataxia	89	Autonomic dysfunction	26
Convulsions	183	Cholinesterase inhibition	64
Incoordination/unsteadiness/		CNS depression	131
clumsiness	62	Fatigue	87
Paralysis	75	Narcosis/stupor	125
Pupil size changes	31	Peripheral neuropathy	67
Reflex abnormalities	54		
Tremor/twitching	177	*Affect/Personality*	
Weakness	179	Apathy/languor/lassitude/	
		lethargy/listlessness	30
Sensory			
Auditory disorders	37	Delirium	26
Equilibrium changes	135	Depression	40
Olfaction disorders	37	Excitability	58
Pain disorders	64	Hallucinations	25
Pain, feelings of	47	Irritability	39
Tactile disorders	77	Nervousness/tension	29
Vision disorders	121	Restlessness	31
		Sleep disturbances	119
Cognitive			
Confusion	34		
Memory problems	33		
Speech impairment	28		

solvents (Hänninen et al. 1976; Hänninen et al. 1978; Mantere et al. 1979; Olson et al. 1979). Weakness has been detected in workers exposed to methyl chloride using a dynamometer (Repko et al. 1976). Tests of finger tremor have been developed and used successfully for measurements in persons exposed to mercury (Wood, Weiss, and Weiss 1973) and methyl chloride (Repko et al. 1976), as has a test of arm tremor for mercury exposures (Chaffin and Miller 1974). Other motor functions found in table 15.4 are evaluated in animal research (namely, activity) or in neurological exams, but quantitative behavioral tests for these effects have not been developed in workplace studies published to date.

The functional sensory effects listed in table 15.4 are relatively general in nature, but several tests have been used to differentiate exposed workers from referents. Audiometric and tone decay tests have identified group differences in workers exposed to inorganic lead (Repko et al. 1978), and equilibrium problems have been detected following methyl chloride exposures using rail balancing (Repko et al. 1976). Disorders of olfaction and pain have not been identified in groups exposed to neurotoxic chemicals, but changes in tactile sensitivity have been identified in acrylamide workers using the Optacon® (Arezzo and Schaumburg 1980). Changes in vision have been studied extensively, but few have revealed functional changes following chemical exposure. The Benton visual-retention test has reflected carbon disulfide exposures (Hänninen 1971, 1974), the embedded-figures test has detected effects of polybrominated biphenyl and inorganic lead exposures

(Valciukas et al., Behavioral indicators, 1978; Valciukas et al., Comparative behavioral study, 1978), and the Neisser letter search has identified changes associated with carbon disulfide exposures (Tuttle, Wood, and Grether 1976). The Bourdon-Wiersma has consistently identified exposure-related changes in visual perception as seen in workers exposed to carbon disulfide (Hänninen 1971, 1974; Tolonen and Hänninen 1978), styrene (Lindström, Härkönen, and Hernberg 1976), and jet fuels (Knave et al. 1978).

Cognitive tests used to identify confusion and speech impairment have not been reported in the workplace literature, but such changes may best be determined through conversation with test subjects by a trained observer. The Wechsler Memory Scale has identified memory deficits, in comparison with controls, in workers exposed to solvents in auto painting (Hänninen et al. 1976), in storage-battery workers exposed to inorganic lead (Hänninen et al. 1978), and in farmers exposed to polybrominated biphenyls (Brown and Nixon 1979).

Changes in general functions in table 15.4 have not been individually studied using behavioral tests in humans, but neurophysiological tests have been used to identify peripheral neuropathy, and, of course, cholinesterase inhibition is a measure of reduced cholinesterase detectable in the blood. Evaluations of changes in affect or personality have been attempted in a number of studies. The Multiple Affect Adjective Checklist identified changes in lead-exposed smelter workers (Johnson et al. 1980), as has the Manifest Anxiety Scale in organophosphate-exposed workers (Levin 1974). Personality tests that have been reported as successful are the Minnesota Multiphasic Personality Inventory following polybrominated biphenyl exposures (Brown and Nixon 1979) and the Rorschach inkblot test following exposures to carbon disulfide (Hänninen 1971, 1974; Tolonen and Hänninen 1978), styrene (Lindström, Härkönen, and Hernberg 1976), and solvents in auto painting (Hänninen et al. 1976).

The tests listed above are those that have been reported successful in workplace evaluations and under field conditions. While the tests listed under all functional categories above may not be the best tests available for those functions, they have been found useful in distinguishing between persons who were exposed to chemicals from those who were not.

General Approaches to Workplace Testing

Three interrelated approaches have been taken to workplace testing for neurobehavioral effects; each has considerable merit. Historically the first and most consistent approach to workplace testing is best represented by the work of the Finnish Institute of Occupational Health (FIOH). Investigators at FIOH developed a test battery that is well adapted to studying the main problems found in Finland, particularly exposure to a limited number of solvents. Their tests, which have gone through a series of refinements over the years, include the Benton visual-retention test, Bourdon-Wiersma, symmetry drawing, the Mira test, reaction time, Santa Ana, and elements of the Wechsler Adult Intelligence Scale and the Wechsler Memory Scale (Hänninen and Lindström 1979). The battery is now used routinely in neurotoxicity evaluations of worker groups in Finland.

The second approach to workplace testing has its origins in the wide variety of neurobehavioral problems and neurotoxic chemicals found in the United States.

Because of this diversity, standardized batteries of tests for identifying and characterizing neurotoxicity following exposures of occupational origin in humans were not developed in the United States. Indeed, investigators in the field typically adopt a unique battery of tests for each particular situation, and one may not use the same test in the same fashion as another. The tests used in particular studies have been selected based on two factors: (1) the type of symptoms reported by the exposed group to be tested and (2) the established neurotoxic effects of the chemical under study and/or related chemicals. This approach has characterized National Institute for Occupational Safety and Health (NIOSH) research in the past (Anger 1985). While there is considerable overlap in the tests that have been used in the United States, this is due more to the lack of proven, valid, and reliable tests available to the researchers for workplace testing than to any attempt to develop a consistent approach or battery of tests to assess the various problems. However, the recognition in the United States that there is a need to screen diverse populations for unknown effects has brought about a change in philosophy in some laboratories, and test batteries are now in the validation stages in the United States (e.g., Rush et al. 1983; Foree, Eckerman, and Elliott 1984; and Baker et al. 1985).

The third approach represents a melding of the first two and was well articulated in the World Health Organization meeting held in Cincinnati in May 1983 (WHO n.d.). At that meeting, a small group of established researchers in neurotoxicology assembled to recommend a battery of tests that could be used as a basic screen to identify a broad range of neurotoxic effects, particularly in developing countries. This group suggested a core test battery that would be used in virtually all settings. Tests were selected into the core set if they had been used successfully in workplace studies (i.e., if they had identified group differences) and if they could be transported easily to other cultures and undeveloped settings. In addition, a series of other tests was identified as supplemental to the core battery, their use being dependent on the chemical involved, the type of personnel available to conduct the tests, and the setting in which the tests were to be administered. The core set of tests was intended to generate more uniform, more consistent data from a broad variety of worker types, occupations, and neurotoxic exposure conditions, while the supplemental tests were intended to provide more in-depth information based on the known effects of the chemical under study and symptoms reported by the exposed workers.

As indicated above, several investigators in the United States are in the process of developing or validating test batteries. Two rationales can be formulated for selecting tests into a broad-based battery of the sort needed to assess the variety of chemicals found in a country as diverse as the United States. The most comprehensive rationale would attempt to assess all major functional nervous-system effects in order to identify all potential problems that might be produced by chemical exposures. This would require a taxonomy of nervous-system effects. Such taxonomies have been developed by Carroll (1980) for cognitive functions and Fleischman (1954) for motor functions. However, there is no widely accepted taxonomy that attempts to specify all nervous-system functions.

A second rationale would be to select tests on the basis of neurotoxic effects typically found following occupational or environmental exposures. The effects found in table 15.4 form a basis for such a battery of tests, though one far less thorough than the former rationale would produce. This rationale for developing a battery of tests is likely to be an evolutionary one. As certain effects replaced others as the most frequently reported problems, the make-up of the battery would be altered. Undoubtedly, this would be a healthy process, since changes in technology and test development would provide further reasons for evolution. However, as implied by the strategy used in the United States in the past, the chemical(s) under study should also be carefully considered when preparing a workplace or community neurotoxicity evaluation. The investigator should include a set of tests that will identify known symptoms of the chemicals under study, as well as a battery of general tests for those effects that are not (yet) known. Clearly, this is an important area for future development.

Results of Workplace Research on Industrial Chemicals

Neurobehavioral research conducted at the workplace to identify effects of chronic chemical exposures, using the approaches listed above, has produced a relatively small body of information. By and large, the chemicals studied are among those that are well established as producing neurotoxicity. The findings have been critically reviewed recently (Anger and Johnson 1985) and thus are only summarized below, with emphasis on those neurotoxic effects seen at the lowest exposure levels evaluated at the workplace.

Solvents have been investigated rather extensively owing to their pervasive use and established effects on the nervous system. Carbon disulfide (CS_2) is perhaps the most thoroughly studied, particularly in Europe, where it figured prominently in the industrial revolution. High concentrations have produced broad changes in psychomotor performance, intelligence, and personality. Workers exposed to slightly less than 20 ppm demonstrate significant cognitive losses (intelligence, memory, vigilance), as well as psychomotor changes and reductions in nerve-conduction velocity (Hänninen 1971; Seppäläinen and Tolonen 1974). In the 1–10 ppm range, the easily measurable cognitive effects disappear, and the reductions in nerve conduction velocity are smaller but still statistically significant (Johnson et al. 1983). Worker populations in the United States exposed at approximately these concentrations also report a greater degree of symptoms historically related to CS_2 exposure (blurred vision, memory problems, tremor, and dizziness) than do unexposed comparison subjects (Putz-Anderson et al. 1983).

Methyl chloride has been studied in workers exposed to 35 ppm in the manufacturing of foam products (Repko et al. 1976). Reaction time and signal detection in a light-display monitoring task were slower in the exposed workers, as was performance on a dual task. Increased tremor was seen in exposed subjects, but a neurological exam was generally negative, reflecting a lack of clinical abnormality. Coordination was reduced, although exposed subjects displayed greater strength. Styrene, used extensively in the production of plastics, has also received attention. It is narcotic at high concentrations (Sittig 1979) and has produced impairments in perceptual speed and accuracy, memory, and cognitive performance (Gutewort et al. 1978) at above 100–170 ppm. Headaches, fatigue, and concentration difficulty are reported when styrene concentrations are in the 50–100 ppm range (Zielhuis 1962). Psychomotor decrements are found in workers exposed to 50–75 ppm, and EEG abnormalities have been seen in significant proportions of workers exposed to concentrations above 30 ppm styrene (Lindström, Härkönen, and Hernberg 1976; Härkönen 1977; Härkönen et al. 1978).

The evidence on trichloroethylene, a solvent used primarily in vapor-degreasing operations, reflects few neurobehavioral effects at low concentrations. Workers believed to have been heavily exposed to trichloroethylene in the past demonstrated significantly worse performance than a comparison group on tests of visual perception, dexterity, and the Mira test of psychomotor ability (Lindström 1973). The lack of information on the groups' exposure history and the lack of effects in a small group of offset press workers exposed to 50 ppm trichloroethylene (Triebig et al. 1977) make it difficult to draw conclusions about the level at which effects of chronic trichloroethylene exposure begin to affect the nervous system.

Workplace research in the United States has particularly concentrated on two metals that were also two of the earliest known neurotoxic chemicals, inorganic lead and mercury, but European research has provided some of the most critical data. Storage-battery and smelter workers exposed to lead have been studied most extensively. Owing to the difficulty of relating airborne lead exposures to body burden levels, most research involving this metal has related effects to measures of lead in the blood at the time of testing. At 50–70 µg lead per dl of blood, changes are reported in cognitive function, including spatial relations, symbol manipulation, visual perception, memory, and verbal/visuospatial abstraction (Grandjean, Arnvig, and Beckmann 1978; Valciukas et al., Behavioral indicators, 1978; Valciukas et al., Central nervous system dysfunction, 1978). Reductions are also seen in conduction velocity of the ulnar and median nerves (Seppäläinen et al. 1975) at 50–70 µg/dl. Effects are less marked in workers with blood lead concentrations between 30 and 60 µg/dl. Spatial organization and eye-hand coordination were reduced in workers with blood lead concentrations in this range as compared with controls (Mantere et al. 1979).

Because of the long biological half-life of mercury following exposure, behavioral data collected in the occupational setting, generally in the chloralkali industry, are related to either blood or urine mercury concentrations, rather than airborne exposure levels, at the time of testing. At above 500 µg mercury per liter of urine, tremor is the predominant effect (Langolf et al. 1978; Langolf, Whittle, and Henderson 1979). Tremor may also be seen at mercury concentrations as low as 250 µg/l (Langolf et al. 1978; Langolf et al. 1981) using surface EMG or linear accelerometers but not by visual inspection of the outstretched arm. Other changes have also been seen, but at higher mercury levels. At 400–450 µg/l (urine), reductions in nerve conduction velocity have been reported. There are indications of changes in memory at and below 400 µg/l (Langolf et al. 1981) and in concept formation in workers with peak concentrations above 300 µg/l (Hänninen 1982). Reduced performance on the Michigan eye-hand coordination test has been seen in workers with urinary mercury concentrations of about 375 µg/l. Urinary mercury concentrations below 250 µg/l, but with periodic excursions above 500 µg/l, produced changes in the stretch reflex and finger tapping in workers (Langolf et al. 1978).

Finally, workplace evaluations of persons exposed to carbon monoxide (Johnson et al. 1974), formaldehyde (Wayne, Bryan, and Ziedman 1977), perchloroethylene (Tuttle et al. 1977), and polybrominated biphenyls (Valciukas et al., Comparative neurobehavioral study, 1978; Brown and Nixon 1979) have been conducted, but those studies do not contain a sufficient body of information to draw general conclusions regarding the relation between exposure or body burden levels and behavioral effects. The paucity of research in the area of workplace neurotoxicity evaluations reflects the logistical difficulties of conducting such studies. The steps in conducting this type of research project, and the problems, are outlined below.

Steps in Conducting Workplace Research

There have been only about 50 workplace studies devoted to neurobehavioral evaluations of chemical effects (Hänninen 1983). One reason is that a workplace or field study might best be described as a logistical and experimental nightmare. Based on the experience of NIOSH personnel, and particularly my own, the following identifies important steps to be followed in conducting a workplace research project and significant pitfalls to be avoided. Of course, this section also reflects the experience of an agency that has a legal mandate to conduct such research, and private or academic groups might well not receive the same treatment as has NIOSH.

Invariably, the amount of available information regarding the projected research problem is extremely limited. Identification of a suitable work group is a difficult first step. The investigator must consider company willingness to allow worker participation, as well as the representativeness of the selected worker sample to the overall workforce. This is further complicated by the likelihood that workplace conditions may differ considerably in different locales within a country, certainly in one as diverse as the United States. Information from the NIOSH National Occupational Environmental Survey (the successor to the National Occupational Hazard Survey) will soon be available to describe the distribution of companies and exposures across the United States based on statistical projections.

Prior to initiating testing, the subject companies and prospective test subjects must be sought out and convinced of the value of the study in order to ensure an acceptable degree of participation. The methods used in such efforts need to be documented and eventually should become a part of the published report in order to provide information on the subject participation rate in different groups or companies. Essential to convincing companies or workers to participate in the study is the perception that a professional, competent operation is being undertaken and that some potential benefit can come from the study. An honest, open approach to discussions with all groups is probably the most successful and proper posture to take in these efforts. A slide presentation or actual demonstration of the tests by the investigators can be quite compelling and serves as an important aid in test description, one that anchors the presentation and tends to dispel fears of persons that are unfamiliar with such tests.

Questions of concern to employers generally relate to intentional cheating by workers and the value of each of the tests—irrelevant tests are seen as an opportunity for problems to surface, or as a fishing expedition by the investigators. I should note that most companies have been responsive to my attempts to convince them of the benefit of such a study to their workers and their company. Workers, too, are generally concerned about their working conditions and the chemicals with which they work. Most cooperate enthusiastically as long as they are convinced that their data will be kept confidential. Healthy, unexposed workers serving as a reference group for evaluating effects of interest are usually necessary and also tend to be cooperative, since a research project brings them attention and a break from the routine—both of which are enticements to any potential subject. Needless to say, management and worker attitudes can either enhance or reduce cooperation considerably.

Study design is usually limited by the nature of the workplace study (Melius and Schulte 1981), but a statistician should be involved for design and power calculations to determine a suitable N needed to identify an effect at various alpha levels. Any cross-sectional workplace study deals with the survivors—those who are still healthy or sufficiently unimpaired to continue working. Attempts should be made to determine patterns of sickness in the test population and their predecessors. The level of chemical exposures prior to testing is necessary information, as is some biological indicator of subject body burden. Industrial hygienists and biochemists are invaluable here. Unfortunately, determination of both exposure and body burden often is not possible, but documented evidence of one or the other is essential. Where an estimate is necessary, subject grouping can only be made on a crude basis, since fine distinctions would be specious and misleading (and an accurate historical reconstruction of a lifetime of exposures is rare at best). This may lead to misclassification of the exposure, a bias that plagues such studies. The need to distinguish between acute and chronic effects must be considered in scheduling testing in order to avoid confounding the two. Generally, there will be two or at most three groups, and between-groups comparison is essential when chronic effects are the focus of the study. Statistical analyses generally have to contend with the problems of multiple measures and the need to control for age and educational variables.

Testing conditions are typically determined by the industry involved and past experience with the selected tests. Compromises always have to be made in obtaining a test setting. NIOSH has generally used company clinics, laboratories, motel rooms, conference centers, or union halls. Perhaps more important than the appearance of the test site is the demeanor of the investigators. A competent, professional attitude and a familiarity with the tests is essential, particularly in the early stages, when the first persons tested are relaying impressions to their coworkers. This may affect cooperation of later workers, as well as test performance. Test answers cannot be transparent, since the extensive social network in any company will soon spread such information despite requests by the investigators not to do so. We have also experienced the deliberate spread of misinformation about the tests as a practical joke on the untested workers.

A number of important considerations fall in the category of necessary ancillary matters. The test subjects, including the comparison group, must give genuinely informed consent. Subjects should be told the purposes and benefits of the study, be informed of any unpleasant tests with which they will be confronted (and any alternative tests that they would be allowed to substitute for them), and be told who is responsible for the study and how to contact them should questions arise. Perhaps most important is explaining clearly to the subjects that they may withdraw from the testing at any time if they find it unsatisfactory in any way, and without prejudice to them. This is helpful in convincing them to undertake the tests, but it is also necessary because most subjects will not read the consent form thoroughly. Moral, ethical, and right-to-know issues that transcend the study itself are obviously involved. For such issues, the institutional Human Subjects Review Board (HSRB) shares some of the responsibility with the investigators and provides a beneficial cross-check.

Records must be kept in a manner that will make them accessible long into the future, for the individuals tested and for potential regulatory purposes. NIOSH has found it helpful to follow the Food and Drug Administration's Good Laboratory Practices (1978) and to keep a thorough log which records and documents day-to-day decisions regarding the study, as well as the unique or unusual events in the study, from its outset.

The manuscript or report written about the study needs to be comprehensive. Few reports in the open literature contain sufficient information to fully characterize and evaluate the results of the respective studies. Necessary information certainly includes (*a*) worker characteristics such as age, sex, race, and education; (*b*) number of years that the worker has been in the current job or profession, along with available information on the pattern of exposures over the years; (*c*) exposure measurements or estimates and the methods used to obtain them; (*d*) time of last exposure to the chemical(s) under study; (*e*) chemicals other than the subject of the study to which the workers were exposed at work and away, over the years (including how recently and to what degree alcohol or drugs that might alter behavior have been used); (*f*) exclusions and their basis (e.g., occurrence of diseases that may mimic the expected chemical effects); (*g*) details on the occupations of subjects in all study groups, including controls; (*h*) percentage of persons approached who agreed to be in the study, by group; (*i*) complete description of (or reference to) all tests and procedures for administering them; (*j*) description of statistical tests used, probabilities obtained, and measures of central tendency and variability for each group on each test; and (*k*) the basis for conclusions drawn. Few published reports of worksite studies contain all this information.

Debriefing and Problem Remediation

Once a workplace study is completed, and the data analyzed, a strategy must be developed for providing clear information about individual test results to all test subjects who request them. Of course, any medical finding with possible health significance should be referred to the subject, with a recommendation that he/she consult a physician. If a personal physician was named by the subject (e.g., on the consent form), he/she too should be notified immediately. In addition, most workers will want to know how they performed individually on the various tests, a very difficult problem with tests that were not designed to be diagnostic and that lack the status and information base of clinical instruments. I feel that some indication of where each individual ranked on each test relative to the entire group should be sufficient. If the worker fell near the bottom of the distribution on each test, then he/she should be advised to consult a physician on those test results, in case there is some medical problem that can be treated. Of course, it is possible that any individual may perform very poorly regardless of his/her environment. Even the normal healthy population, by definition, must have its share of subnormal performers, and the variety of confounding factors (e.g., age, race, education, time of testing, unique distractions, emotional upset) is even more relevant to understanding individual data than to evaluating group performance.

Completion and publication of the report cannot be the conclusion of such a project. Information must reach the companies using the chemicals and the workers exposed to them. Because that population will not have real access to the scientific journals in which the study is likely to be published, a report that is comprehensible to the layman should be provided to each worker and each company involved in the study testing. The local, national, and international unions directly involved should be contacted, along with company management, trade associations, and other companies in the industry under study. Face-to-face meetings with workers and management have the greatest likelihood of providing information and initiating action to ameliorate any identified problems. A brief, written summary is a good second choice when meetings are not possible, but this should, of course, be accompanied by the full report. There are usually industry, trade, and general safety/health magazines that might publish such summaries. In cases where the company studied is a subsidiary or an intermediate in a manufacturing/distribution/sales/use chain, the other members of the chain should be contacted. Regulatory and standard-recommending groups should also receive the reports. If work practices and engineering controls have been identified that can reduce exposures, such recommendations should certainly be mentioned in any report or summary. Finally, where tests used in the study or alternative tests are available to serve as monitoring or screening devices, these can be recommended to the company or representative worker group. In summary, completion of a report is not the end of the road. Occupational health researchers must ensure that measures are taken to disseminate the information gained from research and, where appropriate, to effect changes based on that research.

Summary

This chapter identifies 65 neurotoxic chemicals with exposure populations in excess of 1 million, full- and part-time, and the number of people exposed full-time exceeds 7.7 million. Twenty-two chemical groupings that include 10 or more neurotoxic chemicals are identified, and industries where these chemicals are found are listed by SIC number. The behavioral effects most frequently reported in the secondary literature to occur following exposure to neurotoxic chemicals are also listed under the categories of motor, sensory, cognitive, affect/personality, and general. The tests used in workplace studies to identify those effects are presented, along with a review of the three main approaches to workplace testing—the use of standardized batteries, the adoption of tests based on expected effects of the chemicals under evaluation, and the use of a core set of tests with additions based on the chemical to be studied. The results of workplace studies are presented for those chemicals for which there has been sufficient replication to draw conclusions. These are carbon disulfide, methyl chloride, styrene, trichloroethylene, lead, and mercury. Finally, the steps necessary to undertake a workplace research project, to debrief the worker, and to begin the process of problem remediation are presented.

Acknowledgments

Thanks are due to Wilma Wilson and Pamela Schumacher for typing the various drafts of this paper. Ideas on information to be provided to subjects following study completion reflect comments made at a meeting convened by E. L. Baker at the Harvard School of Public Health in November 1983. Mention of products or company names does not constitute endorsement by the National Institute for Occupational Safety and Health.

References

Anger, W. K. 1985. Neurobehavioral tests used in NIOSH-supported worksite studies, 1973–1983. *Neurobehav. Toxicol. Teratol.* 7:359–68.

Anger, W. K., and Johnson, B. L. 1985. Chemicals affecting behavior. In *Neurotoxicity of industrial and commercial chemicals,* edited by J. L. O'Donoghue, 51–148. Boca Raton, Fla.: CRC Press.

Arezzo, J. C., and Schaumburg, H. H. 1980. The use of the Optacon[R] as a screening device. *J. Occup. Med.* 22:461–64.

Baker, E. L.; Letz, R. E.; Fidler, A. T.; Shalat, S.; Plantamura, D.; and Lyndon, M. 1985. A computer-based neurobehavioral evaluation system for occupational and environmental epidemiology: Methodology and validation studies. *Neurobehav. Toxicol. Teratol.* 7:369–77.

Brown, G. G., and Nixon, R. K. 1979. Exposures to polybrominated biphenyls: Some effects on personality and cognitive functioning. *JAMA* 242:523–27.

Carroll, J. B. 1980. *Individual difference relations in psychometric and experimental and cognitive tasks.* L. L. Thurstone Psychometric Laboratory Report No. 163. Chapel Hill: University of North Carolina.

Chaffin, D. B., and Miller, J. M. 1974. Behavioral and neurological evaluation of workers exposed to inorganic mercury. In *Behavioral toxicology: Early detection of occupational hazards,* edited by C. Xintaras, B. L. Johnson, and I. DeGroot, 214–39. USDHEW (NIOSH) Publication No. 74-126. Cincinnati.

Clayton, G. D., and Clayton, E. F., eds. 1981–82. *Patty's industrial hygiene and toxicology.* Vol. 2, pts. a, b, c. New York: John Wiley & Sons.

Fleischman, E. A. 1954. Dimensional analysis of psychomotor abilities. *J. Exp. Psychol.* 48:437–54.

Food and Drug Administration. 1978. Nonclinical laboratory studies/good laboratory practice regulations. *Federal Register* 43 (247) (22 December).

Foree, D.; Eckerman, D. A.; and Elliott, S. L. 1984. M.T.S.: An adaptable microcomputer-based testing system. *Behav. Res. Meth. Instrum.* 16:223–29.

Grandjean, P.; Arnvig, E.; and Beckmann, J. 1978. Psychological dysfunctions in lead-exposed workers: Relation to biological parameters of exposure. *Scand. J. Work Environ. Health* 4:295–303.

Gutewort, T.; Haublein, H. G.; Seeber, A.; and Zeller, H. J. 1978. Biochemical, neurological, and psychological signs of the effects of styrene on functions of the nervous system and liver. Presented at the XIX International Congress on Occupational Health, Dubrovnik.

Hänninen, H. 1971. Psychological picture of manifest and latent carbon disulfide poisoning. *Br. J. Ind. Med.* 28:374–81.

———. 1974. Behavioral study of the effects of carbon disulfide. In *Behavioral toxicology: Early detection of occupational hazards,* 73–80. *See* Chaffin and Miller 1974.

———. 1982. Behavioral effects of occupational exposure to mercury and lead. *Acta Neurol. Scand.* 66:167–75.

———. 1983. Psychological test batteries: New trends and developments. In *Neurobehavioral methods in occupational health,* edited by R. Gilioli, M. F. Cassitto, and V. Foa, 123–29. New York: Pergamon Press.

Hänninen, H.; Eskelinen, L.; Husman, K.; and Nurminen, M. 1976. Behavioral effects of long-term exposures to a mixture of organic solvents. *Scand. J. Work Environ. Health* 2:240–55.

Hänninen, H.; Hernberg, S.; Mantere, P.; Vesanto, R.; and Jalkanen, M. 1978. Psychological performance of subjects with low exposure to lead. *J. Occup. Med.* 20:683–89.

Hänninen, H., and Lindström, K. 1979. *Behavioral test battery for toxicopsychological studies used at the Institute of Occupational Health in Helsinki.* 2d ed., rev. Helsinki: Institute of Occupational Health.

Härkönen, H. 1977. Relationships of symptoms to occupational styrene exposure and to the findings of electroencephalographic and psychological examinations. *Int. Arch. Occup. Environ. Health* 40:231–39.

Härkönen, H.; Lindström, K.; Seppäläinen, A. M.; Asp, S.; and Hernberg, S. 1978. Exposure-response relationship between styrene exposure and central nervous functions. *Scand. J. Work Environ Health* 4:53–59.

Johnson, B. L., and Anger, W. K. 1983. Behavioral toxicology. In *Environmental and occupational medicine,* edited by W. N. Rom, 329–50. Boston: Little, Brown & Co.

Johnson, B. L.; Boyd, J.; Burg, J. R.; Lee, S. T.; Xintaras, C.; and Albright, B. E. 1983. Effects on the peripheral nervous system of workers' exposure to carbon disulfide. *NeuroToxicology* 4:53–66.

Johnson, B. L.; Burg, J. R.; Xintaras, C.; and Handke, J. L. 1980. A neurobehavioral examination of workers from a primary nonferrous smelter. *NeuroToxicology* 1:561–81.

Johnson, B. L.; Cohen, H. H.; Struble, R.; Setzer, J. V.; Anger, W. K.; Gutnik, B. D.; McDonough, T.; and Hauser, P. 1974. Field evaluation of carbon monoxide exposed toll collectors. In *Behavioral toxicology: Early detection of occupational hazards,* 306–28. *See* Chaffin and Miller 1974.

Knave, B.; Olson, B. A.; Elofsson, S.; Gamberale, F.; Isaksson, A.; Mindus, P.; Persson, H. E.; Struwe, G.; Wennberg, A.; and Westerholm, P. 1978. Long-term exposure to jet fuel: A cross-sectional epidemiologic investigation on occupationally exposed industrial workers with special reference to the nervous system. *Scand. J. Work Environ. Health* 4:19–45.

Knave, B.; Persson, H. E.; Goldberg, J. M.; and Westerholm, P. 1976. Long-term exposure to jet fuel: An investigation on occupationally exposed workers with special reference to the nervous system. *Scand. J. Work Environ. Health* 3:152–64.

Langolf, G. D.; Chaffin, D. B.; Henderson, R.; and Whittle, H. P. 1978. Evaluation of workers exposed to elemental mercury using quantitative tests of tremor and neuromuscular functions. *Am. Indus. Hyg. Assoc. J.* 39:976–84.

Langolf, G. D.; Smith, P. J.; Henderson, R.; and Whittle, H. 1981. Sensitive tests for detection of neurotoxic effects. In *Organ-directed toxicity: Chemical indices and mechanisms,* edited by S. S. Brown and D. S. Davies, 227–33. New York: Pergamon Press.

Langolf, G. D.; Whittle, H. P.; and Henderson, R. 1979. Prospective study of psychomotor function and urinary mercury cell chlor-alkali plant workers. *Arch. Hig. Rada Toksikol.* (Prague) 30 (suppl): 275–88.

Lauwerys, R. R.; Kivits, A.; Lhoir, M.; Rigolet, P.; Houbeau, D.; Bucket, J. P.; and Roeis, H. A. 1980. Biological surveillance of workers exposed to dimethylformamide and the influence of skin protection on its percutaneous absorption. *Int. Arch. Occup. Environ. Health* 45:189–203.

Levin, H. S. 1974. Behavioral effects of occupational exposure to organophosphate pesticides. In *Behavioral toxicology: Early detection of occupational hazards,* 154–64. *See* Chaffin and Miller 1974.

Lindström, K. 1973. Psychological performances of workers exposed to various solvents. *Scand J. Work Environ. Health* 10:151–55.

Lindström, K., Härkönen, H.; and Hernberg, S. 1976. Disturbances in psychological functions of workers occupationally exposed to styrene. *Scand. J. Work Environ. Health* 3:129–39.

Mantere, P.; Hänninen, H.; Hernberg, S.; and Martelin, T. 1979. Exposure-response relationship for neurotoxic lead effects: Psychological performance in a one year follow-up study. *Act. Nerv. Super.* (Prague) 21:292–94.

Melius, J. M., and Schulte, P. A. 1981. Epidemiologic design for field studies: Occupational neurotoxicity. *Scand. J. Work Environ. Health* 7, suppl. 4:34–39.

Milburn, H.; Mitran, E.; and Crockford, G. W. 1976. An investigation of lead workers for subclinical effects of lead using three performance tests. *Ann. Occup. Hyg.* 19:239–49.

National Institute for Occupational Safety and Health (NIOSH). 1977. *National occupational hazard survey, 1972–1974*. USDHEW (NIOSH) Publication No. 73-114. Cincinnati.

———. 1983. *Registry of toxic effects of chemical substances, 1981–2*. USDHHS (NIOSH) Publication No. 83-107. Cincinnati.

Olson, B. A.; Gamberale, F.; Gronquist, B.; and Andersson, K. 1979. Effects of solvents on reaction performance of foundry workers: A longitudinal study. *Arbet och Halsa* (Stockholm) 16:5–16.

Putz-Anderson, V.; Albright, B. E.; Lee, S. T.; Johnson, B. L.; Chrislip, D. W.; Taylor, B. J.; Brightwell, W. S.; Dickerson, N.; Culver, M.; Zentmeyer, D.; and Smith, P. 1983. A behavioral examination of workers exposed to carbon disulfide. *NeuroToxicology* 4:67–78.

Repko, J. D.; Corum, C. R.; Jones, P. D.; and Garcia, L. S., Jr. 1978. *The effects of inorganic lead on behavioral and neurological function*. USDHEW (NIOSH) Publication No. 78-128. Cincinnati.

Repko, J. D.; Jones, P. D.; Garcia, L. S.; Schneider, E. J.; Roseman, E.; and Corum, C. R. 1976. *Behavioral and neurological effects of methyl chloride*. USDHEW (NIOSH) Publication No. 77-125. Cincinnati.

Repko, J. D.; Morgan, B. B., Jr.; and Nicholson, J. A. 1975. *Behavioral effects of occupational exposure to lead*. USDHEW (NIOSH) Publication No. 75-164. Cincinnati.

Rush, A. J.; Weissenburger, J.; Vinson, D. B.; and Giles, D. E. 1983. Neuropsychological dysfunctions in unipolar nonpsychotic major depressions. *J. Affective Disord.* 5:281–87.

Seppäläinen, A. M.; Tola, S.; Hernberg, S.; and Kock, B. 1975. Subclinical neuropathy at "safe" levels of lead exposure. *Arch. Environ. Health* 30:180–83.

Seppäläinen, A. M., and Tolonen, M. 1974. Neurotoxicity of long-term exposure to carbon disulfide in the viscose rayon industry: A neurophysiological study. *Scand. J. Work Environ. Health* 11:145–53.

Sittig, M. 1979. *Hazardous toxic effects of industrial chemicals*. Park Ridge, N.J.: Noyes Data Corp.

Susten, A. L. 1984. Personal communication, 1 February.

Tolonen, M., and Hänninen, H. 1978. Psychological tests specific to individual carbon disulfide exposure. *Scand. J. Psychol.* 19:241–45.

Triebig, G.; Schaller, K. H.; Erzigheit, H.; and Valentik, H. 1977. Biochemische untersuchungen and psychlogische studien an cronisch trichlorathyen-belasteten personen unter berucksichtigung expositionsfrier intervalle [Biochemical and psychological investigations on subjects exposed to trichloroethylene]. *Int. Arch. Occup. Environ. Health* 38:149–62.

Tsuruta, H. 1975. Percutaneous absorption of organic solvents: 1) Comparative study of the in vivo percutaneous absorption of chlorinated solvents in mice. *Indus. Health* 13:227–36.

Tuttle, T. C.; Wood, G. D.; and Grether, C. B. 1976. *Behavioral and neurological evaluation of workers exposed to carbon disulfide*. USDHEW (NIOSH) Publication No. 77-128. Cincinnati.

Tuttle, T. C.; Wood, G. D.; Grether, C. B.; Johnson, B. L.; and Xintaras, C. 1977. *A behavioral and neurological evaluation of dry cleaners exposed to perchloroethylene.* USDHEW (NIOSH) Publication No. 77-214. Cincinnati.

Valciukas, J. A.; Lillis, R.; Eisinger, J.; Blumberg, W. E.; Fischbein, A.; and Selikoff, I. J. 1978. Behavioral indicators of lead neurotoxicity: Results of a clinical field survey. *Int. Arch. Occup. Environ. Health* 41:217–36.

Valciukas, J. A.; Lillis, R.; Fischbein, A.; Selikoff, I. J.; Eisinger, J.; and Blumberg, W. E. 1978. Central nervous system dysfunction due to lead exposure. *Science* 201:465–67.

Valciukas, J. A.; Lillis, R.; Wolff, M. S.; and Anderson, H. A. 1978. Comparative neuro-behavioral study of a polybrominated biphenyl-exposed population in Michigan and a nonexposed group in Wisconsin. *Environ. Health Perspect.* 23:199–210.

Wayne L. G.; Bryan, R. J.; and Ziedman, K. 1977. *Irritant effects of industrial chemicals: Formaldehyde.* Ohio: USDHEW (NIOSH) Publication No. 77-117. Cincinnati.

Wood, R. W.; Weiss, A. B.; and Weiss, B. 1973. Hand tremor induced by industrial exposure to inorganic mercury. *Arch. Environ. Health.* 26:249–52.

World Health Organization (WHO). N.d. Proceedings of Workshop on Prevention of Neurotoxic Illness in Working Populations, Cincinnati, May 1983. Forthcoming.

Zielhuis, R. 1962. Relationships between exposure to solvents and symptoms of intoxication. *Tijdschr. voor Social Geeneskunde* (Amstelveen, Netherlands) 40:225.

Robert B. Dick and
Barry L. Johnson

16

Human Experimental Studies

This chapter describes laboratory research using human subjects to investigate the effects of chemicals on the nervous system as reflected by behavioral indices. There exists an abundance of literature describing laboratory studies of neurotoxic substances. However, the preponderance of this literature describes studies conducted on laboratory animals. The literature on human experimental studies is understandably less plentiful, though it is nonetheless valuable in assessing the neurotoxic properties of chemicals. In the following pages, an overview of human experimental research in neurotoxicology is presented, followed by a review of the findings from published investigations. The chapter concludes with a brief summary of the present state of human laboratory research and some recommendations for future efforts.

The merits of conducting human experimental research on neurotoxic substances are both numerous and obvious, but the principal role played by experimental research is to provide data on the acute effects of neurotoxic chemicals. This role is different from that of epidemiological studies and, in many instances, from that of clinical case reports. In these studies/reports, affected individuals usually have been exposed to chemicals for much longer periods of time, or a significant time period has elapsed since the exposure. Frequently, higher exposure levels are reported than typically found in experimental laboratory studies. For health professionals, information obtained in experimental neurotoxicological research has several important uses. Some of the more important are as follows:

- To identify the presence or absence of acute neurobehavioral effects at low exposure levels that may serve as indicators of subclinical effects.

- To test the adequacy of existing or proposed exposure limits for minimizing acute neurotoxic effects.

- To identify human performance capacities that may be impaired by short-term exposures to toxic chemicals, thereby increasing the risk of unsafe job performance.

- To provide data on the toxicological effects of combined chemical exposures or other workplace conditions (e.g., physical agents, work pace, drugs) that may interact to modify the neurotoxicity of single chemicals.

With the foregoing in mind, and the knowledge that relatively few human experimental studies on neurotoxic chemicals have been undertaken, the question arises, Why have more experimental studies not been performed? There are two principal explanations. First, and the more important of the two, is the ethical issue inherent in conducting *any* form of experimental research on humans. This consideration not only restricts the types of experiments that can be used but limits the nature and range of chemicals to which volunteer subjects can be exposed. Obviously, more elaborate safeguards to such testing must also be in place. Second, the proper conduct of human experimental studies imposes significant facility and staffing requirements which can be complex and costly. Both of these factors are discussed in more detail in the ensuing sections.

Human Exposure Experiments

Human exposure studies to evaluate the toxic effects of chemicals are possibly among the most difficult and expensive controlled laboratory experiments to conduct. Historically, these experiments dealt primarily with such physiological concerns as uptake and excretion using blood, breath, and urine measures, dermal responses, and effects on soft tissues such as eyes, ears, nose, and throat. Subjective feelings, including expressions of depression, excitation, drowsiness, and sleepiness, were also recorded. These could be considered to be measures of central-nervous-system (CNS) response. Although it is difficult to pinpoint an exact date for the introduction of direct, objective neurobehavioral measures, the late 1950s and early 1960s mark the appearance of more published articles using neurobehavioral tests. The measures used were primarily neurological tests such as the Halstead-Reitan, Romberg, heel-to-toe, Crawford Manual Dexterity, and Flanagan coordination tests, and intelligence tests, such as certain mental performance measures from the Wechsler Adult Intelligence Scale. These tests generally measured aspects of coordination, memory, mental control, or organic brain damage. Measurements were somewhat gross, and oftentimes when effects were noted, exposure levels were sufficiently high to produce various physical complaints (Parkhouse et al. 1960; Stewart et al. 1968), which possibly confounded the results. Beginning in the 1970s, neurobehavioral testing was oriented more toward detecting subclinical effects of chemical exposures. More sophisticated tests, designed to detect subtle shifts in behavior such as attention, memory-processing time, motor-response time, perceptual motor coordination, sensorimotor coordination, and other cognitive processes, were utilized. Testing has evolved to include electroencephalograms (EEGs), both visual and auditory evoked potentials (VER and AEP), whole-body sway, vigilance, simple and choice RT, signal detection, performance on dual tasks, time estimation, memory scanning, recognition and recall memory, and so on. With these tests have come increasing use of the computer to present stimuli, record responses, and analyze data.

Their complexity and the relatively limited dose-response range allowable for the exposure conditions of interest make human exposure studies difficult to conduct. Complexity involves several factors, the first of which is the subjects themselves. Medical screening is necessary to eliminate any subjects with either a physical or a mental condition—apart from the exposure conditions of interest—that could affect the performance test measures. Additionally, human beings are complex individuals and bring several attributes into the experiment that can be difficult for an experimenter to control. These are classified as subject variables and include age, sex, class, education, motivational levels, work history, drug usage, and circadian rhythms.

Second, human studies require more experimenter-to-subject interaction than other types of studies, which can be a source of bias. The ethics of human exposure experiments require that subjects be fully informed and have complete confidence in the experiment. Also, for some participants a certain amount of controlled and consistent interaction is probably necessary to reduce the anxiety caused by the test situation. Kiutz et al. (1965) provided a review of interaction effects that lead to data contamination. These include having more than one experimenter, personality of the experimenter (i.e., warm or cold, autocratic or democratic), experimenter experience, sex of the experimenter, and expectancy effects, where the experimenter influences the subject to perform as expected. Interaction effects are also enhanced when subjects are tested in groups in large exposure chambers. Testing subjects in groups of two or more, in groups with mixed sexes, or in pairs or groups where the subjects may be friends introduces factors that could influence the results. Gale (1977) examined some of these factors and showed that most stimulating was being alone in the test situation, followed by the testing of strangers in groups as opposed to friends.

Third, human exposure studies—usually necessitating the collection of biochemical, physiological, and psychological or behavioral measures—require a multidisciplinary team effort. Buck et al. (1977) listed a few of the disciplines involved. These include: psychology, toxicology, medicine, chemistry, physiology, biophysics, biomedical engineering, computer science, and statistics. The involvement of so many disciplines in human exposure studies results in their being rather large, expensive operations requiring considerable coordination and management effort.

Fourth, the dose-response range of the experimental situation is limited by both tolerable concentrations and the duration of exposure. Since humans obviously cannot be exposed to high concentrations of potentially harmful chemical agents, human exposure studies generally operate in the lower range of the dose-response curve. At such low concentrations, behavioral effects are likely to be small and may be overwhelmed by task and procedural problems (Teichner 1975). Duration of chemical exposure is also a limiting factor (Otto 1977) because of economic, social, and ethical considerations. Although a typical test session may run up to eight hours, the actual chemical exposure averages only two to four hours in most studies (ibid.). Many studies have used repeated exposures to increase the duration, but this introduces other problems if the intervening time between exposures is lengthy (several days or weeks).

The basic structure of a human exposure study requires at least the following elements: (1) controlled exposure of the chemical(s) studied; (2) methods for estimating the body burden of chemical(s) in the human organism; (3) appropriate tests and experimental design to reflect the neurobehavioral response of the subjects to the chemical insult; and (4) control groups or control condition(s). The first element refers to the mechanisms for administering and controlling the exposure. Inhalation is the most common method, with subjects exposed in an environmental chamber or an apparatus such as a mask. Ingestion, although less common, has also been used. Dermal absorption, another possible route, has not been used in human exposure studies involving neurobehavioral testing. The second element refers to various biochemical indicators used to evaluate tissue uptake and distribution in the body. It will be discussed only briefly, since the technical issues involved are worthy of a separate chapter. The biochemical measures ordinarily used in human exposure studies are alveolar breath concentrations of expired air, blood concentrations (venous), and urinary excretion values. Blood and breath measures are probably mandatory for any human exposure study. There are instances where one may be superior to the other, as in the work of Stewart and colleagues (Stewart 1974; Stewart et al., Behavioral toxicology, 1974) with trichloroethylene where breath was superior to blood in reflecting the most recent vapor exposure. Both measures taken together, however, seem to give a better picture of chemical body burden levels. Urinary excretion measures have also been used, but to a lesser extent. These measures are more time-consuming, and if 24-hour samples are collected, they require more cooperation on the part of the subject. In addition, urine levels do not correlate well with concentration peaks for some chemicals, especially in acute exposures. There is also the problem that the chemical exposures under study do not necessarily yield excretions but rather metabolites. Metabolic end-product identification is currently lacking for many chemicals.

An important component of human exposure research involves the development of experimental tasks, designs, procedures, and analyses of results—in short, the test protocol. Such discussion would be quite voluminous and beyond the scope of this chapter, although a few relevant points are discussed below. In the design and execution of human studies, special attention should be given to task considerations. Indeed, the task defines the measure of neurotoxic effect. Given the limitations in varying dose levels to obtain effects, the emphasis shifts more to varying the task parameters (difficulty levels, interference, task length, feedback). As Teichner (1975) so aptly stated, "Human toxicology experiments should be interactions between concentrations and task parameters." Furthermore, the choice of parameters, as well as of the task and procedures, implies a selection of processes thought to underlie performance (ibid.). Unfortunately, using task parameters is not always easy, and the behavioral test itself may not relate well to physiological significance. However, the choice of a stable performance measure with good reproducibility is an important criterion for a neurobehavioral task, because it will allow for comparisons between chemicals and provide some standardization when the same tests are used in different laboratories.

The use of control groups is important, and no study should be run without either a separate control group or, in the case of experiments using the same subjects for all expsoure conditions, a control condition. It is recommended that two types of control groups be used in human exposure experiments: blind (or placebo) control groups and a positive control group. The positive control group, or referent control group, as it is sometimes called, refers to a group of subjects receiving a treatment that is used to provide an indication of the sensitivity of the tests used and to serve as a reference on the magnitude of effects. The condition involves exposure to a substance such as ethanol, known to cause effects, on the specified performance measures. Several studies (Klein 1973) have been done to compare the effects of ethanol with those of other CNS depressants. As a corollary to the above, human exposure experiments should be conducted as a minimum in the single-blind condition, or preferably in double-blind conditions.

Findings

Having discussed some of the more important methodological issues attendant to human neurotoxicology studies, it is appropriate to review the findings from the research in this field. The number of such studies is not large, for reasons previously discussed, and it is possible to present findings from several investigations that have enhanced our understanding of chemical agents found at the workplace having acute neurotoxic effects. The studies reported are organized according to classes of chemicals studied and are fairly exhaustive of the total number of human exposure studies completed in the past 20 years that have appeared in the Western literature. An exception is the carbon monoxide (CO) and anesthetics literature, from which only the more definitive studies were selected for inclusion here.

Although it was initially our intent to review and critique the studies based on some standard set of criteria and present them in some sort of tabular format, this task proved difficult because of the lack of uniform reporting in human exposure studies. While some of the studies provided the necessary detail to fit these criteria, many did not, often falling short in adequate descriptions of design and methodology. Table 16.1 lists the criteria that were developed to evaluate the human exposure studies. In the narrative descriptions that follow, these criteria are used to

Table 16.1 Criteria for human exposure studies

Items	Criterion
Subjects	Was the number, age, and sex of subjects described?
	Were the subjects paid or nonpaid volunteers, nonsmokers, homogeneous group, medically screened?
Exposure/route	Type: environmental chamber, air mask, mouthpiece, ingestion
Exposure/measurements	Were the exposure duration and procedures for measuring concentration described, and were they adequate to produce/confirm the desired body burden level?
	Were exposure levels reported in ppm, percent, or mg/M^3?
	Were exposure levels constant or fluctuating?
Experimental design/procedures	Was the type of design described, and was it appropriate?
	Were the experimental procedures and methodology described?
	Were the experimental procedures adequate?
	Was the study conducted single- or double-blind?
Statistical analysis	Was appropriate statistical analysis done?
	Were data and summary statistics reported with probability values?
Biochemical measures	Were adequate biochemical measures (venous blood, alveolar breath) taken to verify body burden levels?
Behavioral measures	Were the behavioral measures adequately described and appropriately used, and were practice and learning effects controlled?
Results	Were the results described supported by the data and analysis?

summarize the studies and to point out their shortcomings. Common deficiencies include too few subjects, poor design, and either inadequate methodology or a poor description of methodology. Based on our laboratory experience with neurobehavioral tests and study designs, a subject group of five or less per cell is considered small, and probably inadequate for most of the measures used. A preferable number would be somewhere between ten and fifteen subjects per exposure condition, but for many of the studies reviewed the number of subjects per condition fell between five and ten. In some cases, small group sizes are possible, providing analysis is done to test for the homogeneity of the error variance. In fairness to some of the foreign studies, the inadequate descriptions of methodology and reporting of results may have been due to faulty translations. Of special importance in describing each study are three factors: the nature of the subjects in the study sample, the behavioral and/or neurological parameters investigated, and the types and extent of the subjects' exposures to the test material.

Organic Solvents

More human laboratory studies have been conducted on organic solvents than on any other chemical class. There are several explanations for this. Organic solvents are used quite extensively in the workplace, which makes them important to study, but as chemicals they are easy to handle, and the volatility of many of them is convenient for inhalation studies. Many organic solvents possess profound toxicity at high concentrations but are generally safe at low concentrations. The known toxicity includes narcotizing effects, and sufficiently long exposure to extremely high concentrations can cause death. Lower exposure levels can result in eye and respiratory irritation and effects on behavior and neurologic processes. These last-named effects have been the subject of investigation in several laboratories, and the important findings are reported in this section.

Chlorinated Hydrocarbons

Methyl chloride. The most widespread use of methyl chloride is as a chemical intermediate, but it is also used as a blowing agent for plastic foams. Industrial exposure occurs when foamed plastic is cut or shaped (Torkelson and Rowe 1981). The neurobehavioral effects were investigated by Putz-Anderson and colleagues (1981). This work was a follow-up to a field investigation that reported that workers chronically exposed to an average of 43 ppm methyl chloride vapor showed increased hand tremor and impaired performance on cognitive time-sharing tasks (Repko et al. 1976). Putz-Anderson and associates were also interested in the possible potentiating effects of diazepam, a prescription drug. Fifty-six participants, whose mean age was 22 years, were divided into six groups, comprising a 3 × 2 factorial design. The first factor (methyl chloride) consisted of three levels of exposure (0, 100, or 200 ppm for three hours), and the second factor (diazepam) consisted of two doses (0 or 10 mg). Blood and breath samples were collected to measure for methyl chloride uptake. Each subject was tested in an environmental room over five continuous hours. The first two hours, used to establish a baseline level of performance, were followed by a three-hour methyl chloride inhalation exposure. The behavioral tests consisted of a visual discrimination, a dual task, and a time discrimination. Diazepam produced a significant 10 percent decrement in task performance, whereas the effect of 200 ppm methyl chloride was marginally significant, reducing task performance by about 5 percent. When methyl chloride and diazepam were combined, the subjects' total performance loss was equal to the sum of the losses resulting from exposure to each chemical alone. There was no performance decrement at 100 ppm methyl chloride.

The findings from the Putz-Anderson et al. study are in general agreement with those from Stewart et al. (Methyl chloride, 1977), who exposed four subjects in several sessions to a 150 ppm level of methyl chloride. Although the small subject size limits the impact of the results, no abnormal effects were found on subjects' EEG, VEP, or behavioral tests, with one exception: a small decrement in subjects' performance on a visual time-discrimination test was found. These two investigations suggest a general lack of behavioral toxicity to acute exposure of methyl chloride at levels of 200 ppm and below.

Methylene chloride. Interest in methylene chloride (dichloromethanol) resulted from two factors: (*a*) its widespread usage (as a degreasing agent, for paint removal, and as an aerosol propellant) and (*b*) the finding that CO is a metabolite of methylene chloride (Stewart et al. 1972). Since CO is known to be a neurotoxicant, the question arose whether methylene chloride possessed similar toxic properties.

An early study by DiVincenzo, Yanno, and Astill (1972) looked at the uptake and elimination of methylene chloride in breath and urine in human subjects exposed by inhalation. A portion of the study examined the effects of these exposures on two simple tests of psychomotor and cognitive performance. Eleven male subjects aged 28–60 were exposed individually in an environmental room to 100 ppm and 200 ppm methylene chloride for two to four hours. Each test lasted about two minutes and involved the placement of colored pegs of various sizes into a pegboard while, at the same time, mentally adding three single-digit numbers presented at five-second intervals. The time to complete this dual psychomotor-cognitive test was the sole performance measure. Performance on the behavioral tasks was reportedly unaffected, but the lack of actual performance data in the report limits the value of this study.

Stewart et al. (1972) conducted the first experimental study to explore the relationship between methylene chloride exposure and elevated carboxyhemoglobin (COHb) levels. Eleven nonsmoking male volunteers aged 23–43 were exposed by inhalation in an environmental room to methylene chloride vapor. Methylene chloride exposures were conducted in four separate experiments. The exposure conditions were 213 ppm for 60 minutes; 986 ppm for two hours; an average exposure of 700 ppm for two hours (514 ppm during the first hour and 862 ppm during the second); and 514 ppm for one hour. In experiments 2 and 3 (three subjects each) the investigators recorded cortical VEP generated in response to a strobe lamp flash after both one and two hours of exposure. Pre-exposure recordings of each subject's VEP were obtained for comparison with those measured under methylene chloride exposure. The results clearly showed that COHb levels were elevated in response to methylene chloride inhalation. For example, after 986 ppm for one hour, the mean COHb was elevated 10 percent over pre-exposure levels. Stewart et al. reported that exposure to methylene chloride vapor in the 500–1000 ppm range resulted in light-headedness in two of the three subjects. There were alterations in certain features of the VEP in all subjects involved in both experiments 2 and 3, although no data were provided to support this contention. Very small sample sizes (N = 3) and sparse description of methodologic details prevent acceptance of any results specific to neurotoxic effects. However, this study remains an important one, since it firmly established that COHb levels were elevated by methylene chloride inhalation.

Winneke and coworkers (1973) reported a series of neurobehavioral investigations on the acute effects of methylene chloride. In one experiment, auditory vigilance and Critical Flicker Frequency (CFF) performance were assessed in 12 female subjects (mean age unstated) exposed for three hours to 300 ppm and 800 ppm methylene chloride. During the exposure, three uninterrupted 45-minute vigilance tests were performed, separated by CFF testing. In a second experiment, 18 female subjects were exposed to 800 ppm methylene chloride for four hours. Auditory vigilance and a battery of psychomotor tests were administered. The psychomotor tests lasted two hours and commenced 100 minutes after initiation of methylene chloride exposure. In both experiments, subjects were tested in a balanced repeated-measures design, with an eight-day interval between sessions. A control condition of 0 ppm was included in each experiment. Results showed that methylene chloride significantly impaired auditory vigilance and CFF performance at both 300 ppm and 800 ppm levels. Furthermore, 800 ppm produced a general impairment of psychomotor performance: motor speed was reduced, RTs were lengthened, and coordination and precision of complex movement patterns were impaired.

Gamberale, Annwall, and Hultengren (1975a) exposed 14 male subjects aged 20–30 to methylene chloride. Study participants were exposed to concentrations of 870 mg/m³ (242 ppm), 1,740 mg/m³ (483 ppm), 2,600 mg/m³ (722 ppm), and 3,470 mg/m³ (964 ppm) for 30 minutes each. The smoking status of the subjects was not reported. The test chemical was administered through a breathing valve and tube connected to a mouthpiece, and the same subjects were tested in a control condition ("0" concentration). Alevolar air was sampled to obtain exposure data on each subject. Though not measured, the maximum COHb concentration was estimated to approach 5 percent. The results showed no significant impairments on visually cued RT, short-term memory (STM), and cognitive function (arithmetic task) for any of these methylene chloride exposure levels when compared with subject performance under control conditions.

Putz, Johnson, and Setzer (1979) also compared the effects of COHb produced by inhalation exposure with those of CO and methylene chloride. Six nonsmoking male and six female subjects aged 18–40 were exposed in a counterbalanced order to methylene chloride, CO, and control air for a four-hour exposure period. The exposure was conducted in an environmental room with the methylene chloride exposure level at 200 ppm. This produced a COHb level of about 5 percent. Performance on a dual task (eye-hand coordination with peripheral brightness monitoring) and an auditory vigilance task were tested continuously during the session at two levels of task difficulty. Both CO and methylene chloride degraded subjects' performance, starting at about two hours' exposure, when COHb levels were approximately 5 percent, and task performances continued to decline thereafter. Significant decrements occurred, however, only under the higher task difficulty condition on each performance measure and near the end of the four-hour exposure period.

The results of these studies show that the acute effects of methylene chloride can be detected in concentrations as low as 200 ppm with exposure durations running for four hours yielding a body burden level of 5 percent COHb. These effects have been demonstrated on several performance measures, including CFF, vigilance, tracking and monitoring, and psychomotor tests (Winneke 1982). Exposures as high as 963 ppm (Gamberale, Annwall, and Hultengren 1975*a*) did not produce any effects, but in this study shorter exposure durations were used, and lack of confirmatory body burden COHb levels leaves some doubt as to whether a 5 percent blood level was reached.

Trichloroethylene. Trichloroethylene (TCE) has been widely used as an industrial solvent, though its use has diminished in recent years owing to pressures from environmental and safety legislation (McNeill 1979). At present, TCE is still used in some degreasing operations, and because of its widespread use at one time, several laboratory experiments were conducted for the purpose of elaborating any acute effects on the nervous system.

One of the earliest studies on the psychophysiological effects of TCE was performed by Stopps and McLaughlin (1967). The sole subject was exposed in an environmental chamber to four separate TCE concentrations (100, 200, 300, and 500 ppm) for 2.75 hours. Two control conditions (0 ppm TCE) bracketed each day's TCE exposure, and behavior performance tests of manual dexterity, card sorting, dial display, and the Necker Cube were used. Below 300 ppm no performance decrements occurred. At 300 ppm (Necker Cube) data showed a decrement, and at 500 ppm Necker Cube and manual dexterity performances showed impairment.

Kylin et al. (1967) reported a lowering of the fusion limit on an optokinetic nystagmus test in 15 subjects exposed to 1,000 ppm TCE for two hours. However, the loss was not as great as that caused by 0.72 gm/kg alcohol ingestion, and the TCE effects were evident only on comparison of exposure and control tests. The design was somewhat novel in that subjects were exposed for two hours and then immediately tested without exposure, and the results were compared against the decline in body burden levels. The study, although interesting, presents graphic results, and only two subjects were used in the alcohol condition. The same two subjects were also used in the chemical exposure condition.

Vernon and Ferguson (1969) evaluated the effects of 0, 100, 300, and 1,000 ppm TCE vapor on measurements of visual-motor performance. Each level was administered for two hours in random order to each of eight male subjects aged 21–30. TCE vapor was inhaled via a breathing tube connected to a gas-mixing chamber, and crystals of unstated content were used to mask the presence of TCE. A battery of six standardized tests was employed to evaluate aspects of sensorimotor performance: CFF, depth perception, form perception, hand steadiness, hand dexterity (Purdue Pegboard), and a "code-substitution" test. During each two-hour session, five tests were given three times to each subject; the Purdue Pegboard test was given prior to and after only the 1,000 ppm exposure. TCE produced performance losses on only three tests at the 1,000 ppm level, namely, depth perception, hand steadiness, and hand dexterity. This study demonstrated that comparatively high levels of TCE were necessary to degrade simple visual-motor capabilities, although dosage levels were not tested between 300 ppm and 1,000 ppm.

Ferguson and Vernon (1970) also studied TCE in combination with three CNS depressants—thorzylamine hydrochloride (Anahist), meprobamate (Equamil), and alcohol—using practically the same design and tests described above. Eight subjects were used in each of the drug-combination conditions, and six in the alcohol combination. Neither 50 mg thorzylamine hydrochloride nor 800 mg meprobamate showed any significance on the behavioral tests, and there was no enhancement when combined with 300 ppm or 1,000 ppm TCE. However, subjects who ingested 35 ml/70 kg (body weight) alcohol and were exposed to TCE evidenced significant deterioration of performance at both the 300 ppm and the 1,000 ppm exposure levels. Hand steadiness was affected most dramatically.

In 1971 Salvini, Binaschi, and Riva (1971*b*) reported effects at 110 ppm. This report sparked considerable controversy, since it suggested that a 100 ppm exposure concentration (then the Threshold Limit Value (TLV) for TCE) could cause neurobehavioral problems. Six male subjects aged 20–22 were exposed to an average TCE vapor concentration of 110 ppm. The subjects were tested on two different days. On one day they were exposed to TCE, and on the other day they were exposed to a "control atmosphere," with a four-day interval between exposures. The exposures were counterbalanced, and each subject was exposed singly in an environmental room. During each exposure session visual perception (perceptive field, span of perception, stimulus organization), STM (Wechsler Memory Scale), RT (compound auditory and visual RT), and manual dexterity (O'Connor test) were evaluated. The results showed a statistically significant decrease in performance on all tests, but no data on the magnitude of reduction were presented. This study was not without its complications and possible shortcomings. The experiment was apparently done nonblind, and the atmospheric sampling methods have been questioned. The atmospheric sampling problems, summarized in Stewart (1974) and Stewart et al. (1974), include both the technique used and the lack of an independent sampling procedure.

Stewart and coworkers (Effects of trichloroethylene, 1973) attempted to replicate the Salvini, Binaschi, and Riva (1971*b*) study. The same behavioral tests and testing regimen were used. Stewart et al. departed from Salvini, Binaschi, and Riva in several ways, which probably strengthened the experiment by allowing the study of successive exposures and the establishment of a dose-response relationship. First, an additional TCE vapor level was included, so subjects were exposed to concentrations of 0, 50, and 100 ppm in a partially counterbalanced design for three days. Second, nine subjects—six males and three females—were used. Third, two additional performance tests were added. The results from Stewart et al. did not confirm any of Salvini and coworkers' findings. No performance decrements relating to either TCE level were found. Although Stewart et al.'s negative outcomes cast doubt on Salvini and coworkers' findings, the study serves more to condemn the experimental procedures and design than to illuminate the effects of TCE. Both studies appear to have major design problems. Too few subjects per cell were tested, so that within-subjects variability was a problem, especially in Stewart et al.'s study. The results also showed that several of the tests evidenced learning effects. This finding, together with the fact that in the latter study the same subjects were tested in groups (of three) at all three concentration levels for three days, suggests some confounding in the data which compromises the final results.

Nakaaki et al. (1973) exposed four male volunteers to both 0 ppm (control) and 100 ppm TCE for six hours for four days in two daily three-hour exposures separated by one hour. Psychophysiological tests used included CFF, simple RT, time estimation, hand steadiness, and cold-sensation thresholds. The tests were apparently administered four times per three-hour exposure period. No significant differences from control values were detected at the 100 ppm level, although there were slight declines in performance.

Winneke (1982) reports on two experiments done at the Medical Institute of Air Hygiene and Silicosis Research, University of Dusseldorf, in the period after the Salvini, Binaschi and Riva (1971*b*) study. In one experiment 18 subjects were exposed to 50 ppm TCE for 3.5 hours, and in the second experiment 12 subjects were exposed, and the TCE effects were compared with those of alcohol at 0.76 ml/kg. Neurobehavioral performance measures used in both studies were CFF, light and tone signal tests (visual and auditory vigilance), psychomotor tests, and AEP. No behavioral deficits were found in the 50 ppm TCE exposure conditions, but ethanol did cause significant effects on the percentage of correct detections on the vigilance task. There was some alteration of the AEP in the TCE exposure conditions.

Gamberale, Annwall, and Olson (1976), in another attempt to resolve the contradiction between the studies by Salvini, Binaschi, and Riva and Stewart et al. exposed 15 subjects to 100 ppm and 200 ppm TCE. The study was similar to the previous ones but used a superior design that negated some of the criticisms of Salvini and coworkers' basic design. The design allowed for the control and analysis of learning effects, and it eliminated the confounding of concentration with day of exposure by dividing the subjects into three groups and partially counterbalancing the order of exposure. The duration of exposure was shortened to minimize effects of motivation and circadian rhythms. Subjects were exposed every other day at the same time to either 0, 100, or 200 ppm and were tested on an addition test, simple RT, short-term memory, and choice RT. Only the addition test, which involved adding briefly presented numbers as fast as possible, showed any significant effect with increasing TCE concentration. The authors concluded that the impairment caused by TCE at these levels was minimal.

An additional report also casts doubt on Salvini, Binaschi, and Riva's findings. Konietzko et al. (1975), in the Federal Republic of Germany, exposed 20 male volunteers with a mean age of 27 for four continuous hours to 95 ppm TCE vapor. The TCE exposure was conducted in an environmental room, on four persons at a time, where tests of hand steadiness, line tracing, aiming, tapping, visual compound RT, and the Viennese determination test were administered. The last-named test required the subject to extinguish a programmed colored light by pressing a buttom of the same color. This series of six tests, which lasted 15 minutes, was given prior to TCE exposure and then was repeated after exposure. The results showed no losses on any psychometric test as a consequence of 95 ppm TCE vapor exposure. Of some concern, however, was the lack of procedural detail in this study.

Nomiyama and Nomiyama (1977), in testing 12 subjects, 3 at each exposure concentration of 0, 27, 81, and 201 ppm, also found no significant effects on tests of CFF and two-point discrimination. Subjects were tested before exposure, four times during exposure, and five times after exposure at hourly intervals. The study was well designed, and the retention, uptake, and excretion procedures and parameters are well described, but the behavioral tests and their analyses are not. In addition, the subject size per exposure condition is small.

Dutch investigators have also studied TCE in single exposures (Ettema, Kleerekoper, and Duba 1975; Ettema et al. 1975), in comparison with alcohol and CO (Ettema et al. 1975), and in combination with alcohol (Windemuller and Ettema 1978). These studies are somewhat unique in that they used behavioral performance tasks as both independent and dependent variables and a physiological measure to evaluate mental load. The physiological measure used was sinus arrhythmia (SA), or irregularity of heart-rate pattern. The authors postulated that mental load would suppress SA and that when it was combined with an exposure to alcohol, further suppression would occur. The behavioral tests were auditory and visual binary choice tasks under both paced (experimenter-controlled) and self-paced (subject-controlled) conditions, the Bourdon-Wiersma test (pattern discrimination and speed), an identification test, a memory test, and dual tasks which were combinations of the binary tests and other tasks. Four ingestion levels of alcohol ranging from 20 ml gin to 120 ml gin were used. Mean blood alcohol levels for each group were roughly 0.06 g/L, 0.10 g/L, 0.25 g/L, and 0.50 g/L. CO exposure levels were 175 ppm for 3.25 hours, and TCE exposures alone were 150 or 300 ppm for 2.5 hours. The alcohol, CO, and TCE studies all had their own control groups and used separate groups of subjects for each exposure (concentration) level. The combination study (TCE + alcohol) used a within-Ss design (the same subjects underwent all exposure conditions) with four exposure conditions: control, alcohol (0.35 gr/kg), alcohol (0.35 gr/kg), and TCE (200 ppm), or TCE at 200 ppm. The studies were well designed, with the final experiments preceded by pilot studies and the use of relatively large numbers of subjects. However, short exposure times and lack of confirming body burden levels, except in the alcohol studies, were significant shortcomings. The results of these studies indicated that TCE at neither 300 ppm nor 150 ppm had any significant effect on the battery of performance tests used, nor did CO at 175 ppm. Only alcohol showed any significant effects on the performance tests, producing a dose-response relationship, with the effective blood alcohol level at about 0.30 g/L. Alcohol and TCE in combination did not affect the performance tests, but significant effects were noted with alcohol and TCE on SA, the postulated indicator of mental capacity or mental state. Although all exposure conditions suppressed SA, the alcohol + TCE combination caused the most suppression. The authors feel that the effects of the various exposure conditions were to lower mental capacity without altering behavioral performance. The hypothesis that SA is a valid indicator of mental state is the most controversial issue in these studies.

The evidence in all the TCE studies indicates that consistent decrements on neurobehavioral tests do not occur below 300 ppm. The Salvini, Binaschi, and Riva (1971b) findings that detected effects at 110 ppm were not replicated by several studies that used presumably superior experimental methods. Of some additional interest in the TCE studies are the effects of alcohol in combination with TCE because of the known instances of degreasers flush observed in TCE-exposed workers. One study (Ferguson and Vernon 1970) showed that performance losses due to TCE exposures in combination with alcohol ingestion were greater than those due to exposures to TCE alone. This effect was noted at 300 ppm, the lowest level tested. Windemuller and Ettema (1978) used a similar combination procedure, but with a 200 ppm TCE exposure level. No effects on the performance tests were noted. The results of these two studies suggest that the combination may not lower the threshold for performance decrement but only enhance performance decrements at higher exposure concentrations.

Tetrachloroethylene (perchloroethylene). Tetrachloroethylene (T_4CE) is a popular industrial solvent used in dry cleaning and degreasing. As the use of TCE has diminished, particularly in dry-cleaning operations, there has been greater use of T_4CE. Stewart and colleagues conducted two investigations to evaluate the acute toxicity of T_4CE (Stewart et al. 1970; Stewart et al., Effects of perchloroethylene, 1977). In the first study, 1 female, aged 30, and 16 male subjects, ranging in age from 24 to 64, were given a series of five seven-hour exposures between 99 ppm and 109 ppm on consecutive days in an environmental room. Each individual experiment involved six to eight subjects, but the selection of subjects for each of the five experiments was not stated, and neither the subjects nor the investigators appeared to be blind to the T_4CE condition. Tests given at various times during the study included recording of subjective responses (odor perception; headache; eye, nose, throat irritation) and a neurological examination that contained a modified Romberg, heel-to-toe, and finger-to-nose tests. After five hours of exposure, the Crawford Manual Dexterity test and the Flannagan coordination, arithmetic, and inspection tests were performed. Also, after six hours of exposure on the fourth and fifth days, visual acuity and depth perception were measured by unstated means. Although not described, the subjects' performances on the psychometric tests were apparently compared with laboratory norms to evaluate the effects of T_4CE. The paper indicated that 25 percent of the subjects reported untoward subjective responses, principally a mild frontal headache, sensory irritation, and light-headedness. The single objective sign observed was an abnormal modified Romberg test occurring in three of the subjects within the first three hours of exposure in at least one of the experiments. This study by Stewart et al. (1970) suggests that 100 ppm T_4CE vapor was a borderline concentration in producing CNS symptoms and signs of toxicity. The study suffers, however, from want of a control condition, lack of a clear presentation of methods, and apparent nonblind exposures.

A subsequent T_4CE experiment by Stewart and coworkers (Effects of perchloroethylene, 1977) was concerned with neurological and behavioral effects of this solvent, alone and in combination with ethanol and diazepam. Six subjects of each sex, aged 19–42, were tested in an environmental room in a partially counterbalanced order for 12 weeks across the following conditions: 0, 25, or 100 ppm T_4CE; 0, 6, or 10 mg/day diazepam; and 0, 0.75, or 1.5 ml 100-proof vodka/kg body weight. Subjects were tested in pairs, and the T_4CE exposure duration was 5.5 hours. All T_4CE vapor exposures were replicated, and all testing was performed in a double-blind mode. A battery of neurological and behavioral tests was administered at the peak blood levels of the drugs: Michigan eye-hand coordination, rotary pursuit, Flannagan coordination, saccade eye velocity, and dual-attention tasks. Each subject was given 2.5 days' training prior to entering the first exposure condition, and in the course of these tests the subjects completed the Lorr-McNair mood evaluation test, and EEGs were recorded. Data analyses revealed a decrement in subject performance on at least one test at the highest dose level of each drug alone, but no interaction with T_4CE could be demonstrated in any test for either combination. Further, there was no consistent effect of T_4CE alone on the EEG or subjective symptoms reported for any subject. These results indicate that under the conditions studied, which simulated worker exposures to T_4CE and the drugs diazepam or alcohol, the subjects demonstrated no decrements in neurological or behavioral performance that could be attributed to the addition of T_4CE exposure to drug consumption. Decrements in performance of the Michigan eye-hand coordination, rotary pursuit, and Flannagan coordination tests due to alcohol consumption reinforce the known hazard of the use of this drug in the workplace, while the decrements in performance associated with diazepam dosing were more subtle, appearing only on the rotary pursuit test. As regards T_4CE exposure, a slight but statistically significant decrement in the performance of the Flannagan coordination test at the highest-level exposure (100 ppm) was noted.

Overall, despite some differences in test results, the two Stewart studies are consistent in indicating that 100 ppm generally produced no adverse effects on the behavioral tests used. The 1977 study was experimentally superior because it contained a control condition, was conducted double-blind, and used two drug conditions that served as positive controls. Whether or not 100 ppm constitutes an upper limit is still in question because experiments using neurobehavioral tests have not been reported with higher exposure concentrations.

1,1,1-Trichloroethane (methyl chloroform). 1,1,1-Trichloroethane is a saturated halogenated hydrocarbon felt to have a low toxicity within the class of chlorinated hydrocarbon solvents. As is the case with T_4CE, the industrial use of 1,1,1-trichloroethane has increased with the reduced utilization of TCE. Some human experimental studies relevant to acute, neurotoxic effects are notable.

Stewart et al. (1969), in a controlled exposure to methyl chloroform, found essentially only marginal neurotoxic effects in subjects exposed for five days at 500 ppm for 6.5–7 hours per day relative to a nonexposure control condition. The effect was manifested in the failure of two out of five subjects tested to perform the modified Romberg test. These same two subjects demonstrated some difficulty on the test before the exposure, but the abnormality was more pronounced during exposure, and it persisted throughout the session. The authors felt that these two subjects may have had an unusual susceptibility to the CNS-depressant effects of methyl chloroform and that the 500 ppm level was an overexposure. However, because the two subjects had performed a normal modified Romberg before the exposure, even with difficulty, other factors, such as test anxiety, may have affected their performance.

In Italy, Salvini, Binaschi, and Riva (1971*a*) employed an experimental design and methods identical to those described for their controversial study on TCE (1971*b*). Six test subjects aged 20–23 were exposed to 450 ppm 1,1,1-trichloroethane vapor for four hours, followed by a two-hour break and then four more hours of exposure. The performance tests consisted of a tachistoscopic test of visual perception, complex (auditory and visual) RT, immediate memory (Wechsler digit span), and manual dexterity (O'Connor test). The investigators reported that 450 ppm exposure produced no statistically significant losses on any performance test, though no data are provided other than analysis of variance tables. It is noteworthy that the authors report decrements of 20 percent on the test of visual perception and 6 percent in immediate memory span, but the results were not statistically significant. This study, though suggestive of an acute effect of 1,1,1-trichloroethane vapor, suffers from use of a small number of subjects.

Gamberale and Hultengren (1973) also evaluated the psychophysiological effects of 1,1,1-trichloroethane in 12 male subjects aged 20–30. The exposure concentrations were 250, 350, 450, and 500 ppm in four contiguous 30-minute periods. The experiment was conducted in a partially counterbalanced order; that is, six subjects received solvent exposures and then seven days later received no solvent. The remaining six subjects were tested in reverse order. The air-gas mixture was supplied via a respiratory valve and low-resistance mouthpiece, and menthol crystals were used to mask the presence of 1,1,1-trichloroethane. In the final 20 minutes of each exposure period, five performance tests were administered. These consisted of manual dexterity (wire spiral), perceptual speed (identical-numbers identification), perceptual speed (spokes), simple RT, and choice RT. Subjective responses were also obtained on six affective scales. The results showed no effect of 1,1,1-trichloroethane on affective states; nor were the subjects able to identify when the solvent was present. However, the performance tests showed clear, significant evidence of solvent-induced impairment. Generally, simple psychomotor tasks (simple RT) were more susceptible to impairment than were those with more cognitive demand. Performance decrements were evident earliest at the 350 ppm exposure and became more severe with increased 1,1,1-trichloroethane concentrations. Acute exposures to 1,1,1-trichloroethane will display effects at the 350 ppm level, even for relatively short (30-minute) exposure periods. Although the other two studies in this group (Stewart et al. 1969; Salvini, Binaschi, and Riva 1971a) did not produce statistically significant decrements at higher exposure levels, there was indication of performance losses on some of the tests used. However, the small number of subjects used in the latter two studies would make it difficult to detect statistically significant changes; hence, one can question their value in defining toxicity thresholds for 1,1,1-trichloroethane.

Aromatic Hydrocarbons

Toluene. Toluene is an alkylbenzene used extensively as a solvent in the chemical, rubber, paint, and drug industries (Sandmeyer 1981). Toluene also is a chemical whose use may be abused (Sharp and Carroll 1978), most notably in "glue sniffing," as it is known to produce hilarity and narcosis in high concentrations. Gamberale and Hultengren (1972) investigated the effects of acute toluene inhalation exposure on psychophysiological functions. Twelve male subjects aged 20–35 were divided at random into two groups of six. Subjects in one group were first exposed to toluene, followed by a control air exposure. The second group was exposed in the reverse order. The toluene exposure consisted of consecutive 20-minute exposure phases of 100, 300, 500, and 700 ppm. All exposures were presented by use of a valve and mouthpiece through which subjects inhaled toluene mixed with air. Menthol crystals placed in the air-delivery system were used to mask the odor of toluene, and samples of subjects' alveolar air were taken throughout the exposure period. Performance tests made in the final 15 minutes of each 20-minute exposure phase measured perceptual speed and visual RT (simple and choice). Results showed that both RT and perceptual speed were impaired by toluene exposure. Simple RT was significantly lengthened when the exposure reached 300 ppm, choice RT was significantly affected at 500 ppm, and perceptual speed was significantly slowed at the 700 ppm toluene level.

Winneke (1982) tested eighteen subjects who were exposed for 3.5 hours in counterbalanced order to either 0 ppm or 100 ppm toluene. CFF was used by the investigators as a measure of CNS activation, and a dual task, consisting in detecting random visual and auditory signals, was used to measure subjects' vigilance throughout the exposure session. At the end of 3.5 hours, a comprehensive battery of psychomotor tests was also administered. No evidence was found of performance losses owing to the 100 ppm toluene exposure.

Suzuki (1973) examined the effects of acute toluene exposure on the autonomic nervous system. The subjects were ten male students aged 18–22, who were divided equally into two groups. One group served as a control, while the other was exposed to 200 ppm toluene for six hours (three hours of exposure, one hour of no exposure, three hours of exposure). Both groups were tested while subjects were at rest over a two-day period, the first day being an acclimation day, the second the exposure day. The subjects were tested for autonomic-nervous-system disturbances during the last hour of each of the two days of testing, and the results for the two days were compared. No significant differences were found on measures of galvanic skin reflex, peripheral vasoconstriction, heart rate, respiration rate, or EEGs. The small sizes of both the control and the experimental groups may not have been sufficient to detect effects because of the wide range of individual differences usually displayed in the measures used.

Stewart et al. (1975) exposed male and female subjects to toluene vapors ranging from 0 ppm to 100 ppm for five (male) and three (female) weeks. Their findings generally support the results of the above-mentioned studies where limited effects were noted below the 300 ppm level. Only females exposed for 7.5 hours showed any performance decrements, and this effect (fewer correct responses) was seen only on one test, a dual task involving visual vigilance and tone detection. Because no performance decrements were noted with male subjects or with female subjects at 3.5 hours of exposure on the alertness test or other cognitive tests, the authors felt that their results were in agreement with the other toluene studies. They concluded that the 100 ppm level may be the upper limit for worker exposure and that the margin of safety for sedentary workers was only two- to threefold.

A recently published study by Anderson et al. (1983) involving a six-hour exposure to toluene did not reveal significant behavioral-test performance effects at the 100 ppm level, although some marginal CNS effects were reported. Sixteen male subjects aged 21–34 were divided into four groups and exposed for six hours to control air and 10 ppm, 40 ppm, and 100 ppm on four consecutive days using a Latin square design. The behavioral test battery included a five-choice serial RT test with an added vigilance component, a rotary-pursuit test, a screw-plate test, Landolt's ring, Bourdon-Wiersma, a multiplication test, a sentence-comprehension test, and a word memory test. The test battery (which included some physiological measurements) took 1.5 hours and was run twice, after 1 hour of exposure and during the fifth and sixth hours of exposure. Although no statistically significant test-performance decrements were detected, subjects did report significantly more frequent incidences of mild headache, dizziness, intoxication, and the feeling that the tests were more difficult at the 100 ppm exposure. This study was well designed and used good experimental procedures with a rigorous statistical analysis. The only noted shortcoming was the use of several paper-and-pencil-type tests, which are used more in field testing, instead of automated tests, which are now generally preferred for laboratory testing.

NIOSH investigators (Dick et al. 1984; Russo et al., personal communication) have recently completed a series of human exposure studies that included toluene, methyl ethyl ketone (see below), and ethanol (at 0.8 ml/kg used as a positive control). One hundred forty-four different subjects were assigned to eight different treatment conditions and exposed in an environmental room to either 0 ppm, 100 ppm toluene, or 50 ppm toluene/100 ppm MEK. Exposure duration was 4 hours, with a 2.5-hour pre-exposure period and a 71-minute post exposure period. Behavioral testing took place in all periods. The studies were done single-blind, with subjects in the control/placebo conditions being given a wiff of 25 ppm toluene for two minutes. Behavioral-performance measures used were a visual-vigilance task (Mackworth Clock), a pattern-recognition task, a choice RT task, and an eyeblink-reflex task. Toluene at 100 ppm produced a small but significant impairment on one measure in the visual-vigilance task by lowering the percentage of correct hits. No decrements owing to toluene were shown on the other tests, but ethanol affected both the visual-vigilance task and the choice RT task. Toluene at 50 ppm in combination with MEK at 100 ppm produced no test decrements.

The toluene-exposure studies are generally consistent in indicating that the 300 ppm level is where significant psychomotor (RT) impairment occurs and that impairment is minimal or nonexistent at 100 ppm. Two studies have detected some apparently isolated effects at the 100 ppm level on vigilance-type tasks, but the lack of consistency of findings at this test level suggests a marginal effect. Stewart et al. (1975) detected effects only in females exposed for 7.5 hours, and the NIOSH investigators found a significant effect on only one of several measures used. In contrast, the Winneke study (1982) and the recent work by Anderson et al. (1983) did not detect an effect at 100 ppm, even though one of the tasks used in these studies contained a vigilance measure. The data are less clear at 200 ppm. Although the Suzuki (1973) study used this concentration, the behavioral-performance measure was not comparable to those in other studies, so evidence of effects at 200 ppm still remains to be adequately evaluated.

Styrene. Styrene is an alkenylbenzene that has been used extensively in the production of plastics. Nasal and eye irritation are present in exposures over 600 ppm, with CNS effects (drowsiness, depression) becoming pronounced at 800 ppm (Sandmeyer 1981).

In one of the first human exposure studies to test for behavioral effects, Stewart et al. (1968) exposed male subjects to several concentrations of styrene (50, 100, 200, and 375 ppm) for different periods of time in a series of single-session experiments. Only at the 375 ppm exposure level for a duration of one hour were behavioral test measures affected. Exposures at 375 ppm beyond one hour were physically not tolerated well by the subjects. Two of five subjects so exposed showed 20–30 percent reductions in the Crawford Manual Dexterity Collar and Pin test scores, and three of the five subjects dropped at least a tenth of a percentile on the Flannagan coordination test. Since the study was devoted primarily to establishing blood, breath, and urinary excretion values, the behavioral tests were only summarized. This brevity, coupled with the small sample size, limits the value of the study.

Gamberale and Hultengren (1974) studied the effects of styrene on psychological functions. Styrene was administered in a manner similar to that described in the toluene study by the same authors (see above), except that it was not possible to disguise the presence of styrene to the subjects. Twelve male subjects aged 21–31 were exposed to 30-minute, stepped concentrations of 50, 150, 250, and 350 ppm over a 120-minute exposure session while perceptual speed, RT, and manual dexterity were measured. Choice RT was slightly (5 percent) yet significantly lengthened only at the 350 ppm exposure level, but no other effects were seen.

Oltramare et al. (1974) exposed six subjects to 50, 100, 200, and 300 ppm styrene for one to three hours in an environmental room. Three psychomotor tests (simple visual RT, compound RT, and RT to multiple stimuli) were administered to three subjects. Owing to the small sample size, only qualitative results were reported. Exposure to 50 ppm produced pre-narcotic symptoms and lengthened simple and compound RT, effects which worsened at higher levels. However, these results are subject to much criticism owing to small sample sizes, wide age range (30–60 years), and the fact that three subjects had prior occupational styrene exposure.

Swedish investigators (Odkvist et al. 1980) examined the effects of styrene on vestibular function. Five males aged 22–34 inhaled 300 ppm of styrene through a breathing valve for one hour while working at an intensity of 50 watts on a bicycle ergometer. Prior to styrene exposure and then immediately after cessation of exposure, electronystagmography, optokinetic testing, and two balance tests were performed by each subject. Results showed no significant effect of styrene on either balance test and no evidence of either spontaneous or fixation nystagmus. The optokinetic test showed mean-eye-speed decreases under styrene exposure, but these did not reach statistical significance. The authors believed that these decreases were indicative of styrene's effects on the cerebellum, which they believed lessened the normal inhibition of the "audiomotor" mechanism controlling eye movement. This argument is weakened, however, by the small sample size and the lack of effect noted on other cerebellar functions (namely, balance tests).

Although the Stewart et al. (1968) and Gamberale and Hultengren (1974) studies show some consistency in terms of effects being noted at the 350–75 ppm level, the styrene studies as a whole are problematic. Exposure duration periods are short, sample sizes are small, and the experimental procedures and data analysis in some of the studies are weak.

Xylene. Xylene is very similar to toluene and occurs in three isomeric forms—are o-, m-, or p-xylene (Sandmeyer 1981). The m-xylene form has been the most extensively studied, although the three forms are assumed to possess similar properties. The xylenes are used as thinners, solvents, paint removers, and chemical intermediates.

Gamberale, Annwall, and Hultengren (1978) studied the effects of xylene singly and in combination with physical exercise. Fifteen male subjects aged 21–33 were divided into three equal groups and run in a 3 × 3 Latin square, repeated measures design. Exposures occurred through a breathing valve and were masked by menthol crystals. Three exposure levels were used: control air (0 ppm), 435 mg/m³ (100 ppm), and 1,300 mg/m³ (300 ppm). Eight of the 15 subjects were additionally run in a second experiment that used a 2 × 2 Latin square, repeated measures design with a control (0 ppm) and the 1,300 mg/m³ (300ppm) exposure level. Both experiments used a 70-minute exposure period, with behavioral testing occurring in the latter 35 minutes, but the second experiment used the first 30 minutes for a physical work condition (bicycle ergometer, 100 watts). Subjective responses (reports of sickness, headaches, and so on) and a mood profile (calm versus hurried, concentrated versus distracted, and so on) were recorded, and the behavioral tests used were CFF, RT, addition, simple RT, short-term memory (STM), and choice RT. No significant impairments were found under the single 100 ppm or the single 300 ppm exposure conditions, but performance on all five tests was impaired when a 300 ppm exposure was paired with physical exercise. Most significantly affected were RT addition, STM, and choice RT.

The effects of xylene on the CNS, singly and in combination with physical exercise and alcohol, were investigated by Savolainen and coworkers in Finland. This exhaustive series of studies basically involved two different types of experimental procedures, and the results are sometimes difficult to interpret because of the numerous publications that evolved from this effort. One procedure involved exposing the same subjects for two weeks under constant and fluctuating concentrations of xylene singly and combined with physical exercise (Savolainen, Riihimäki, and Linnoila 1979; Savolainen et al., Effects of m-xylene exposure, 1980; Riihimäki and Savolainen 1980; Savolainen and Riihimäki 1981a). Subjects were exposed to a constant level of xylene for five successive days, the first four days at 100 ppm and the fifth at 200 ppm. After a two-day weekend break, subjects were exposed for one to three more days to fluctuating concentrations of xylene that ranged from 100 ppm to 400 ppm. Peak concentrations lasted ten minutes, with the rise and fall taking five minutes. Mean concentrations were generally 100 ppm or 200 ppm over the exposure session. Physical exercise, when introduced, was on a bicycle ergometer at a 100-watt load. Exposure durations were either four or six hours per day using this procedure. In the second procedure (Savolainen 1980; Savolainen et al., Effects of xylene and alcohol, 1980b; Savolainen and Riihimäki 1981b; Seppäläinen, Savolainen, and Kovola 1981), subjects were divided into two groups and exposed over a nine-week period to xylene either alone or in combination with ethyl alcohol. Two levels of xylene (150 ppm and 290 ppm) and two levels of ethanol (0.4 g/kg and 0.8 g/kg) were used, and subjects were tested once per week. The nine treatment combinations, which included three control days, were run in reverse order for each group. Duration was usually four hours per session for this procedure. Psychophysiological measurements used in one or both procedures consisted of body sway, choice and simple RT, CFF, finger-tapping speed, extraocular muscle balance, EEG, evoked potentials (visual and somatosensory), electroretinograms, Santa Ana manual dexterity, and a measure of nystagmus.

Inhalation exposures at 100–400 ppm revealed statistically significant increases in average body sway, as well as an increase in and a slowing of both choice and simple RT. The effects were most noted at the 400 ppm level and did not always occur at the lower-concentration levels. In addition, tolerance developed to these effects as they disappeared on days of successive exposure but reappeared following days of nonexposure and under fluctuating concentration conditions. Xylene exposures had little or no effect on nystagmus and other measures such as CFF and extraocular muscle balance. Changes in spontaneous EEG, which consisted of an increased number of slow transients in the occipital region, were detected only in the fluctuating exposure procedure during the ten-minute peak exposure periods. The amplitudes and latencies of VER were unaffected by xylene alone, and only at the 290 ppm level with ethanol ingestion were demonstrable changes noted (Seppäläinen, Savolainen, and Kovala 1981). No effects of xylene, singly or in combination with ethanol, were found on somatosensory evoked potentials and electroretinograms (ibid.). Added physical exercise appeared to enhance losses, since impairments were detected more often on body balance, simple and choice RT, and Santa Ana manual dexterity tests at lower-exposure concentrations.

Combinations of alcohol and xylene produced mixed results. On some performance measures the combination appeared additive, while on others it was not as effective as single doses of alcohol in causing decrements. Alcohol at doses of 0.4 g/kg or 0.8 g/kg caused more impairment on body sway than did a four-hour exposure of xylene at either 140 ppm or 290 ppm. Similar results were true for choice RT and simple RT: xylene and alcohol in combination exerted some impairment, but not as great as that caused by alcohol alone. In one test where alcohol dose dependently caused gaze deviation nystagmus, the combined action of xylene with alcohol seemed to produce antagonistic effects. Since most of the effects noted above were adaptive (i.e., tolerance developed), the authors (Riihimäki and Savolainen 1980) concluded that xylene does cause some effects on the CNS that apparently relate to absolute blood-xylene concentration and the rate of xylene uptake. A rapid rise in concentration levels will apparently overcome the adaptive effects and cause some CNS disturbances.

An investigation of possible interactions between xylene and 1,1,1-trichloroethane was also reported by Savolainen and coworkers (Savolainen et al. 1981; Savolainen, Riihimäki, and Laine 1982). Nine male volunteers were exposed to single atmospheric nonfluctuating concentrations of m-xylene (200 ppm) or 1,1,1-trichloroethane (200 ppm and 400 ppm) plus the combination 200 ppm xylene + 400 ppm 1,1,1-trichloroethane for four hours per day at six-day intervals. Psychophysiological tests consisted of body sway, RT, finger tapping, gaze nystagmus, and CFF. Although results did not reveal any marked impairments of those behavioral functions measured for either xylene, 1,1,1-trichloroethane, or a combination of the two, the authors devote considerable discussion to the opposite tendencies caused by high and low concentrations of xylene and 1,1,1-trichloroethane. The lower-level exposures of each solvent (200 ppm) tended to improve test performances, while the higher 1,1,1-trichloroethane concentrations alone or in combination with xylene impaired performance. The results were only suggestive, since statistically significant differences from control scores were not present, but they do agree with other studies that have found biphasic changes using ethyl alcohol and anesthetic gases (Savolainen, Riihimäki, and Laine 1982).

This series of studies on exposures to xylene tends to show that the effective level for consistent decrements in neurobehavioral performance occurs near a 400 ppm exposure concentration. When decrements were noted at lower concentrations, they were not consistent and seemed to be related to periods when the uptake of the chemical was most rapid (concentration increase or physical exercise).

Ketones

Ketones are compounds that contain a carbonyl group (C = 0) attached to two carbon atoms. They are used commonly as solvents and share many of the same properties of the other organic solvents described, including dizziness, drowsiness, and CNS depression. They also cause irritation of the eyes and respiratory passages and are sometimes referred to as irritants. Not many studies involving human exposures have been conducted, although their widespread usage seems to warrant it.

Acetone. Two Japanese studies have evaluated the effects of acetone on human performance tasks. In the first study, Nakaaki (1974) simultaneously exposed four sedentary subjects, two males (ages 46 and 31) and two females (28 and 23), to acetone vapor concentrations ranging from 170 ppm to 690 ppm. All exposures occurred in an environmental room. A two-hour exposure occurred in the morning, followed by a two-hour rest period (0 acetone) and then another two-hour afternoon exposure, for a total exposure of four hours. This pattern continued for four days and was repeated three times, for a total of twelve exposure sessions. Time-estimation performance was tested during each exposure period at 0, 30, 60, 90, and 120 minutes; the task consisted in estimating 5-, 10-, and 30-second intervals. No details were provided on subject training or task presentation. A control condition (0 acetone) was employed, but its length was not stated. There was slight eye and throat irritation at concentrations below 200–300 ppm and severe irritation above this range. The investigator reported that acetone exposure, particularly at 450 ppm or greater, produced "a tendency of elongation of time estimation in men and women." Because of the small sample size (four subjects), limited data reporting, fluctuating exposure concentrations, and brief descriptions of the experimental procedures, test methods, and subject training, it is difficult to draw conclusions from this study.

A more robust investigation on acetone was conducted by Matsushita et al. (1979). Groups of six male subjects, with an average age of 22 years, were exposed to acetone in an environmental room at vapor concentrations of 0, 250 (twice), or 500 ppm. The exposure regimen consisted of two three-hour daily exposure periods (three hours in the morning, one hour's rest, three hours in the afternoon) for six consecutive days, followed by four days of recovery. All subjects were sedentary, except one 250 ppm group, which underwent moderate exercise during acetone exposure. Subjective symptoms were recorded at 0, 10, 30, and 90 minutes in each acetone exposure period, and simple visual RT was measured before acetone exposure and after two hours in each exposure period. The results showed eye and throat irritation at 250 ppm, which was pronounced at 500 ppm. Simple RT values significantly increased in a dose-response relationship as a function of acetone exposure. The major increase in RT occurred between the control condition and days 2, 3, and 4 of the 500 ppm exposure. On all three days the RTs increased by about 10 percent. At 250 ppm, irrespective of exercise, the RT increased by about 5 percent.

Methyl ethyl ketone. Nakaaki (1974), using the same procedures described above for acetone, exposed the same four subjects to concentrations of methyl ethyl ketone (MEK) from 90 ppm to 270 ppm. Time estimation was the performance measure used, and males gave judgments indicating underestimates for both the long and short performance times, whereas females showed only slight under-estimation during short performance times. As with the acetone study, conclusions from this report are difficult because only four subjects were used and the results are not directionally consistent with the acetone exposure. There are also sex differences in the MEK results.

Dick et al. (1984) and Russo et al. (personal communication), in an experiment described above (see the section on toluene), exposed 16 subjects to 200 ppm MEK and 20 subjects to 100 ppm MEK and 50 ppm toluene simultaneously. Twenty-two subjects served as a control group. No significant differences were noted on perfor-mance measures of choice RT, visual-vigilance, pattern recognition, or eyeblink in any of the exposure conditions, although there was some indication of a marginal effect with the MEK exposure (200 ppm) on the eyeblink test.

It is difficult to make comparisons across the studies evaluating organic sol-vents because of the variety of experimental procedures used, as well as the differ-ent chemicals involved. However, a review of all the studies suggests some com-monalities. For several of the organic solvents (toluene, xylene, TCE, methylene chloride) the range of consistent performance decrements on neurobehavioral tests appears to occur between 200 ppm and 400 ppm. Winneke (1982) has also present-ed this argument in a recent paper comparing the effects of methylene chloride, toluene, and TCE, although being somewhat more restrictive in the concentration range (200–300 ppm). Consistent performance decrements below 200 ppm gener-ally are not present, and when they do occur, they primarily show up on vigilance-type tasks. These tasks may be more affected by the specified chemicals or subject to still unknown influences of the experimental procedures employed.

Metals

Lead. There appears in the literature but one recent report bearing on human laboratory exposure to a metal. Verberk (1976) presented the neurological findings from a group of ten subjects who ingested inorganic lead for 49 days. All study participants were males aged 20–30. A control group of nine persons was also included in the study. The lead-treated group ingested 30 micrograms Pb per kilogram of body weight (the frequency of Pb ingestion was unstated), yielding a blood lead level of 200–400 parts per billion (i.e., 20–40 micrograms per 100 ml blood) from day 14 and thereafter. The nerve-conduction velocity of the left ulnar nerve, both for the fast- and slow-conducting fibers, was determined for each study participant once every two weeks. The results showed no significant differences between groups for either measure of motor-nerve-conduction velocity at the end of the study. While this finding differs from the reports of reduced nerve-conduc-tion velocities in workers chronically exposed to inorganic Pb, this disparity may be attributable to any of several possibilities, including uncontrolled factors (e.g., laboratory temperature, which can affect nerve-conduction velocity), lower Pb levels in the lab study, or lack of sufficient time for Pb administration. It can be stated, however, that under the conditions of this study, the neurological effects of subchronic exposure to Pb may differ from the effects of chronic exposure.

Organophosphates

Several organophosphorous (OP) compounds have severe neurotoxic effects through stimulation of the central and autonomic nervous systems. Acute exposure experiments with OP compounds and testing for neurotoxic effects are not common, which is not surprising considering their toxic potential. Their potential for human exposure comes through their use as pesticides in agricultural settings.

Mevinphos. Verberk and Salle (1977) investigated the acute neurotoxicity of mevinphos in eight male volunteers who were compared with a control group of equal number. The test group received mevinphos dissolved in corn oil, 25 µg/kg, by ingestion of a gelatin capsule. After a two-week pre-exposure phase to determine baseline values, the test phase of this experiment began, lasting 28 days, followed by a two-week recovery phase. Each study participant was examined twice weekly for red-blood-cell cholinesterase and once weekly for neurological function. Tests of the latter consisted of: (*a*) Achilles tendon reflex (force and duration), (*b*) ulnar motor-nerve-conduction velocity of fast fibers and slow fibers, and (*c*) neuromuscular transmission. The results showed that the mevinphos group had a mean cholinesterase depression of 19 percent at the end of the 28-day exposure. Verberk and Salle also found a significant 7 percent decrease in slow-fiber motor-nerve-conduction velocity and a 38 percent increase in the force of the Achilles tendon reflex. Other test measures did not differ between the two groups. These findings of acute effects are in general agreement with those from studies on pesticide workers.

Parathion. The effects of small doses of ethyl and methyl parathion on the CNS were investigated in two male volunteers (aged 62 and 53) by Rodnitzky, Levin, and Morgan (1978). Each subject completed four five-day periods of parathion ingestion separated by one to eight weeks in the following order: 2 mg methyl parathion; 4 mg methyl parathion; 1 mg ethyl parathion; and 2 mg ethyl parathion. Plasma and red-blood-cell (RBC) cholinesterase levels were measured before and after each ingestion period. Each subject was tested on four occasions—(1) ingestion baseline, (2) at the end of the peak methyl parathion ingestion period, (3) at the end of the peak ethyl parathion ingestion period, and (4) one month after the last ingestion. Each subject's performance was assessed on tests of memory, visual retention, complex RT, language, vigilance, and proprioception. In addition, anxiety and depression were measured by use of the Taylor Manifest Anxiety and Beck Depression scales, respectively. The results showed that serum and RBC cholinesterase levels were not depressed by any parathion administration; nor were there performance decrements or psychological manifestations when compared with the pre-ingestion baselines. In fact, tendencies for improved psychomotor and cognitive performance were noted in both subjects. Rodnitzky, Levin, and Morgan (1978) suggested that these changes could indicate a facilitating property of low doses of OP compounds. Such an interpretation must be viewed with caution, since the improved performance could simply represent learning effects by the subjects. The study is also limited by use of only two subjects and the absence of a control (placebo) condition.

Two studies do not provide a sufficient data base for gauging the neurotoxicity of a class of chemical compounds that has such widespread usage and potential for worker exposure. The outlook for more laboratory studies using OP compounds is probably limited. As the aforementioned studies indicate, apparently several days of successive exposure are required in order to influence the body burden indicator with the low dosage level involved, and the safety aspects of OP compounds would certainly be of concern to most investigators.

Noxious Gases

Carbon monoxide. More human experimental studies have been reported on CO than on any other chemical. Perhaps the principal reason stems from the fact that CO is a ubiquitous contaminant. It is found at workplace settings wherever carbonaceous material is burned, as well as in the ambient air of cities due to automobile emissions. Further, since the neurotoxic—indeed, lethal—properties of CO at high exposure concentrations are well known, it has been of interest to investigate the effects at low exposure levels. The result has been an outpouring of investigations conducted under laboratory conditions. In fact, a recent review of the behavioral effects of CO lists 150 references (Laties and Merigan 1979). Unfortunately, as we point out in this review, the CO behavioral literature abounds in disparate results, conflicting findings, and failures to replicate study results. These conflicting outcomes can be attributed to a multitude of factors: different experimental designs, uncontrolled factors, a lack of standardized behavioral tests, and errors in generating and monitoring experimental atmospheres. Nevertheless, there does seem to be one common feature in those studies: low-level CO exposure impairs elements of human performance. This feature involves an interaction between the type of behavioral test administered and the functional status of the subject. Therefore, this section is organized to point out the effects of CO on various task parameters, an organization made possible because many studies have been designed to investigate the effects of CO on task parameters. Specifically, CO is most likely to impair performance if the task presented is sufficiently difficult and the subject's performance capacity has been diminished through experimental means. This thesis is based in part on the investigation reported by Wright and Shephard (1978), who found subjects' errors on an auditory-duration discrimination task increased by task difficulty, test environment, and the subjects' arousal level. Representative studies are described below.

Most investigations have reported that CO at low concentrations exerts little effect on routine measurements of vision, although there are exceptions. McFarland (1970) exposed four male subjects aged 16–25 to measured amounts of CO metered into a close-fitting oronasal mask. The usual duration of testing was three to four hours, although CO exposure persisted for only 10–15 minutes, which achieved COHb levels of up to 20 percent. Visual-threshold determinations were made at 10-minute intervals throughout the experiments. The visual threshold determination required the dark-adapted subject to distinguish the presence of an 0.1-second light flash presented against a dim background while sitting in a darkened room. The results showed a progressive degradation in visual threshold, starting at a COHb level of 5 percent. This experiment had a number of unique features. The subjects were well-practiced—that is, learning effects were minimal—and the performance task was a relatively difficult threshold determination. Furthermore, continued presentation of the performance task over an extended period—three to four hours—had a fatiguing effect that even moderate amounts of CO could enhance.

A study by Salvatore (1974) bears similarity to the McFarland experiment. Six subjects, each of whom served as his or her own control, were exposed by mask to CO for 20 minutes in order to produce COHb levels of 4–8 percent. They were then evaluated on tests that measured their time to detect static and dynamic visual targets after practice on the previous day. In the static phase the subject, adapted for one minute to an illumination of 17 foot-lamberts, detected low-contrast targets when the ambient illumination dropped to 0.02 foot-lambert. In the dynamic phase the illumination was constant at 6 foot-lamberts, and the subjects detected the targets moving into the visual field. There was a significant decrement in target-detection time due to CO for the dynamic task, but not for the less demanding static test.

McFarland (1973), Wright, Randell, and Shephard (1973), and Rummo and Sarlanis (1974) reported results of experiments on the effects of CO on automobile-driving performance, but with different outcomes. In a double-blind experiment, Wright, Randell, and Shephard administered CO by adding 80 ml to a rebreathing bag, which in turn was used for breath analysis for CO content. A control condition consisted in adding no CO to the air bag. Following a training period of unstated duration, 50 subjects of each sex were tested on a driving simulator for 30–40 minutes. Results showed that an elevation of 3.4 percent COHb produced a small but significant decrement in "careful driving" skills, although individual performance tests were not significantly impaired, unless all data were grouped together. Wright, Randell, and Shephard included smokers in their study, so the results must be viewed as being confounded somewhat by possible differences in subjects' reactions to CO due to acclimatization. McFarland (1973) also tested driving performance under the influence of CO. Twenty-seven subjects were tested under laboratory conditions at COHb levels of 6 percent, 11 percent, and 17 percent by breathing from a bag containing room air or 700 ppm CO. When the desired COHb level was achieved, subjects were tested on visual RT, peripheral vision, depth perception, dark adaptation, and glare recovery over an unstated period of time. No significant impairment of performance was found at any of the three COHb levels. It is possible that failure to conduct the study in double-blind fashion, the small number of subjects, and the lack of control of task difficulty could have led to McFarland's obtaining different results from those reported by Wright, Randell, and Shephard (1973). Rummo and Sarlanis (1974) tested seven subjects aged 19–27 for auditory and visual vigilance performance using an automobile simulator. CO was administered from a tank containing 800 ppm and connected to a scuba-type mouthpiece. The CO exposure, as well as a sham air exposure, lasted for 20 minutes. Subjects were then tested continuously for two hours on a simulator. Subjects' detection of randomly appearing dashboard lights, as well as RT and steering-wheel (psychomotor) performance, were recorded. The study was apparently single-blind. Results showed COHb levels of 6–8 percent produced significantly slower RTs and fewer steering-wheel corrections.

Dual-task performance and task difficulty levels have been investigated with some consistent results. Putz and associates examined the effects of CO on compensatory psychomotor tracking and vigilance tasks presented concurrently. In the first experiment (Putz 1979), 30 subjects were exposed to 5, 36, and 74 ppm CO for four hours, producing COHb levels of 1 percent, 3 percent and 5 percent, respectively, at the end of the exposure. The 5 ppm "exposure" represented the laboratory ambient air level. The compensatory tracking task required keeping a spot on an oscilloscope centered in a target ring positioned on the oscilloscope's face. This was effected by the subject's adjusting a hand control to cancel out random (to the subject) vertical oscillations of the dot controlled by a computer. The subjects worked on this tracking task for 30 minutes hourly over the full four hours of CO exposure. The subject concurrently reported the presence of a light placed in the subject's peripheral visual field. Both the tracking task and the vigilance task involved two distinct levels of difficulty. The results showed that a COHb level of 5 percent was sufficient to degrade tracking performance by about 10 percent when the tracking task was set at its higher level of difficulty.

In a separate experiment, Putz, Johnson, and Setzer (1979) utilized the same methods and tests to compare the effects of CO and methylene chloride. (The findings relevant to methylene chloride were described previously.) The results were also the same. CO impaired subjects' performance on the dual task and an auditory vigilance test when COHb levels reached 5 percent and when the performance tasks were demanding. The main differences between the two experiments conducted by Putz and by Putz, Johnson, and Setzer were the experimental design and the addition of an auditory vigilance task. In the first study, testing across groups was performed without replication of subjects; that is, a particular subject was tested only under one treatment condition. In the second experiment, each subject was tested across all three conditions (CO, methylene chloride, control). The results bearing on CO decrements were the same from both studies, lending support to the generalizability of the finding.

Mihevic, Gliner, and Horvath (1983) have also studied dual-task performance with CO exposure and reported similar findings, but they believe that the effect has some task specificity to a secondary task rather than the primary motor performance task. Sixteen subjects (eight male, eight female) with an average age of 25 years were exposed to room air and 100 ppm CO in two different 2.5-hour sessions. Subjects were tested during the last 60 minutes of exposure, with this period divided into three 20-minute intervals. The mean venous COHb levels per interval were 1.86 percent, 4.33 percent, and 5.67 percent. Performance tests consisted of a reciprocal tapping test with two levels of difficulty as the primary task and a digit manipulation test with two levels of difficulty as the secondary task. Results indicated that tapping performance was not affected by CO exposures, indicating that CO had little effect on motor performance either alone or combined with the digit manipulation test. However, tapping performance and digit manipulation when performed together were affected by CO exposures at a COHb level of 5 percent. The effect was present through a significant increase in response time on the digit manipulation task at its most difficult level.

The effects of CO on vigilance have also been investigated. As expressed by Laties and Merigan (1979), "On this type of task the subject is asked to detect and report small environmental changes ('signals') occurring at infrequent intervals and therefore requiring continuous attention. These signals may or may not be embedded among closely similar stimuli that are not signals." As previously described, the studies of Putz and coworkers also included an auditory vigilance task. The auditory vigilance task was conducted for 30 minutes out of each hour of the four-hour CO exposure period. Subjects listened by earphone to a train of pulses of white noise. At random intervals with a probability of 0.20 a slightly less intense or more intense pulse was presented. The less intense pulse, called the signal, was to be reported by the subject. Results showed that a COHb level of 5 percent significantly impaired vigilance, both in terms of fewer correct responses and in terms of response time to those signals correctly identified.

In contrast to the findings of Putz, Johnson, and Setzer (1979), two other investigations specific to the effects of CO on vigilance were negative in outcome. Benignus et al. (1977) exposed male subjects aged 18–34 to 0, 100, or 200 ppm CO in a controlled-environment room during a numeric-monitoring task shown previously to be sensitive to low-frequency noise and psychoactive drugs. The performance task consisted in viewing a pseudorandom series of digits and pressing a hand-held button whenever three consecutive even or odd digits appeared. Subjects performed this task, in the double-blind experiment, for 16.7 minutes repeated over a 3.3-hour period with 3.3-minute rest periods between tests. Each subject was tested in one group comprised of 17 (0 ppm), 16 (100 ppm), or 19 (200 ppm) subjects. In order to reduce the effects of intersubject differences, each subject's performance was gauged against a pre-exposure baseline performance. The group mean COHb levels attained were 0.01 percent (0 ppm), 4.61 percent (100 ppm), and 12.62 percent (200 ppm), but there was no impairment on task performance at any CO exposure level. The results from this well-designed study clearly demonstrate the lack of effect of acute, low-level CO exposure on a monitoring task. It is possible that the task employed was too simple and that subjects' reserve performance capacity may not have been taxed.

Davies et al. (1981) also found no effect of acute CO exposures on what they termed vigilance performance. In their study, six different groups (ranging from six to nine persons per group) of nonsmoking male subjects were studied separately for 18 consecutive days, each in a controlled human exposure chamber. Each group was subjected to a five-day control period within the closed chamber followed by an eight-day period of continuous CO exposure for eight hours each day. The CO exposure levels were 0, 15, or 50 ppm. A post-exposure period of five days followed. During the course of each CO exposure, always at the same time of day, a one-hour auditory vigilance task was performed. The auditory vigilance task consisted in listening through earphones to regularly repeated fixed-frequency tones. The subject pressed a hand-held buttom switch when the 440 ms pulses decreased by 80 ms. Subjects had had one practice session prior to CO exposures. The results showed that COHb levels reached 7 percent at the 50 ppm exposure and 2.4 percent at the 15 ppm level. Subjects' vigilance performance, assessed in terms of successful hits and misses of target signals, was unaffected by any CO exposures.

In addition to the studies previously described, one last area of CO research merits mentioning. Several investigators have examined the effect of low-level, acute CO exposure on subjects' performance of time-discrimination tasks. The origin of this interest resides in the report by Beard and Wertheim (1967), who exposed singly 18 young (sex and age range unstated) subjects to 0, 50, 100, 175, and 250 ppm in different sessions. Each exposure session lasted four hours and was conducted in a single-blind manner using CO introduced into a small audiometric booth. An auditory time-discrimination task required the subject to estimate, responding by pressing a lever, whether the second of two tones of fixed frequency (1,000 Hz) was longer, shorter, or equal in duration to the first. There were 600 total trials per session. Beard and Wertheim reported that subjects' performance, measured by the percentage of correct responses, was significantly degraded at 50 ppm after 90 minutes of exposure. Further, increased CO levels resulted in an impressive, essentially linear, dose-response decrement in performance.

The Beard and Wertheim report produced intense interest owing to its implications for the setting of environmental limits for CO. This led to attempts by other investigators to reproduce the findings. All have been unsuccessful, though great efforts have been exerted in the interests of closely comparable test conditions and methods. The attempts by Stewart et al. (Effect of carbon monoxide, 1973), Wright and Shephard (1978), and especially Otto, Benignus, and Prah (1979) are particularly noteworthy. In none of these investigations were CO exposures found to impair auditory time discrimination. Stewart et al. used CO levels ranging up to 500 ppm for 75 minutes, achieving COHb levels near 20 percent, and Otto, Benignus, and Prah exposed subjects to 150 ppm CO for 2.3 hours. The exposure levels from both studies therefore included a portion of the CO range used by Beard and Wertheim, but the results were clearly at variance with Beard and Wertheim's. A number of explanations for this disparity have been suggested, but it seems sufficient to say that the Beard and Wertheim results at best possess no applicability beyond the situation imposed by their test conditions.

Anesthetics

Anesthetics occur either as gases or liquids and produce severe CNS depression. Inadvertent, uncontrolled use may result in death. The chemicals reported on in this section are used primarily as anesthetics. Some chemicals, such as TCE, are used both as industrial solvents and as anesthetics and have been covered in previous sections. Human exposure can arise from medical workers' being exposed during surgical procedures or by patients' undergoing dental work or surgical procedures. Studies at subanesthetic or subhypnotic concentrations are numerous, so only a selected sample are reported here, since more comprehensive reviews are available (Porter 1972; Smith and Shirley 1978). Studies involving trace concentrations (less than 1,500 ppm nitrous oxide (N_2O) or 150 ppm halothane) are limited, so the review in this area is more exhaustive.

Subanesthetic Studies

Subanesthetic studies generally involve exposure to high concentrations for relatively short durations during which the subject remains conscious and usually does not experience amnesia. Such studies have been used to study mental performance, memory processing, undersea-diving performance, and aftereffects of anesthetic administration. An early series of experiments (Parkhouse et al. 1960; Henrie, Parkhouse, and Bickford 1961) used a neurobehavioral test battery to study the effects of N_2O. Parkhouse et al. (1960) exposed 24 subjects (medical personnel), divided into three groups, to N_2O mixtures of 20 percent (200,000 ppm), 30 percent (300,000 ppm), and 40 percent (400,000 ppm) and to compressed air (0 ppm) using a partially repeated exposures design. The purpose of the experiment was to determine how intact mental performance was at various levels of N_2O analgesia, so a pain test was included. The mental-performance tests consisted in date and time reporting, alphabet repetition, counting backwards, meaningful story recitation, paired designs, and nonsense syllables. The last three tests were under an immediate-recall condition during exposure and a delayed-recall condition 30 minutes after exposure. Analgesic effects began to occur at the 20 percent level, and significant deterioration of mental performance was most evident between the 30 percent and 40 percent N_2O levels on the paired-design and nonsense-syllable tests. The differences between the delayed- and immediate-recall conditions were most prevalent at the 40 percent level, and this level produced the most physical symptoms (nausea, irritability, and so on) in some subjects, which may have contributed as much to the subjects' performance as did the depressant effects of N_2O.

Henrie, Parkhouse, and Bickford (1961) essentially repeated this experiment without the pain condition and using only the 30 percent N_2O exposure level. One of the purposes was to compare behavior alterations as measured by electroencephalography and psychological tests. Eighteen subjects were used, and significant behavioral test impairment was noted, but the EEG tracings revealed no consistent changes due to the exposure to N_2O. The EEG results were somewhat surprising, because at this exposure level most subjects reported marked CNS symptoms, such as drowsiness, blurred vision, impaired memory, and so on. The authors concluded that the psychological tests provided a more sensitive measure of N_2O effects than the EEG.

Biersner (1972) exposed 21 military divers to N_2O in an experiment to test the effects of inert gas narcosis. To simulate the anesthetic properties of air at a depth of 210 feet, a gas mixture consisting of 30 percent (300,000 ppm) N_2O, 20 percent (200,000 ppm) oxygen, and 50 percent (500,000 ppm) nitrogen was used. Subjects were exposed for ten minutes to either the gas mixture or control air in a counterbalanced order through a conventional face mask and then took tests of visual function (acuity, accommodation, steropsis, nystagmus), memory (Wechsler Memory Scale), gross motor skill (Bennett Dexterity Test), and fine motor control (Purdue Pegboard). Results demonstrated that visual function, fine and gross motor performance, and intact long-term memory (LTM) were unaffected after N_2O exposure, while learning and STM were significantly impaired. The STM finding was somewhat controversial, and a follow-up study comparing the 1972 study data with a hyperbaric nitrogen group (Biersner et al. 1977) offered some clarification of the results. As measured by a digit-span test, STM and attention were unaffected, but the poorer recall of the simple and paired-associate items under the N_2O condition indicated that LTM was affected.

In a series of experiments designed specifically to evaluate the narcotic effects of N_2O on memory and auditory perception Fowler et al. (1980) reported impairment of LTM but not of STM. This was indicated by examination of the serial position curves on a recall test (15-item word lists) designed to test both STM and LTM. The greatest effects on recall were at the beginning and middle of the curve (word positions 1–8) and not in the recency (word positions 9–15) portion. The effect occurred with a 30-minute exposure to 35 percent (350,000 ppm) N_2O. Like other experimenters, the authors felt that their results indicated that the effect was not on retrieval of information but possible interference with rehearsal strategies in STM.

Effects on memory have also been evaluated using other anesthetics. Adam (1973) revealed in a series of studies using several chemicals that subanesthetic concentrations affected the long-term registration of material presented verbally (verbal memory) more than stimuli presented acoustically or visually. STM functions were left relatively intact. Tests included word lists, digit spans, cards with figures, and so on. Both recognition and recall memory were tested for these different forms of presentation on both conscious and unconscious subjects. The anesthetics tested and the inspired exposure concentrations when memory effects were noted in fully conscious subjects were as follows: enflurane, 0.35 percent or 3,500 ppm; penthrane, 0.67 percent or 6,700 ppm; cyclopropane, 1.91 percent or 19,100 ppm; ether, 1.04 percent or 10,400 ppm; and forane, 0.076 percent or 760 ppm to 0.32 percent or 3,200 ppm. Exposure durations varied between 30 minutes and 120 minutes depending on the time needed to achieve stable end tidal concentrations. Only a small number of subjects were used in these experiments, which were not designed specifically to determine dose-effect levels, although control conditions were used.

The time course for effects of anesthetics using neurobehavioral tests has also been reported in the literature. Such studies are important in determining the time for release of patients and their activity restrictions after outpatient surgery. Korttila et al. (1977) compared anesthetic mixtures (halothane or enflurane with N_2O) with control air and tested subjects for up to seven hours after administration with a variety of psychomotor tasks. Thirty-four subjects were randomly assigned to the three separate conditions (halothane-N_2O, enflurane-N_2O, control air), and the gas mixture ratios for halothane and enflurane were 2 to 1 O_2 and 4 to 1 N_2O. The peak concentrations of halothane and enflurane were 1.5 percent (15,000 ppm) and 3.0 percent (30,000 ppm), respectively, during an exposure of approximately five minutes. Duration of analgesia was measured as the time during which the subject did not react to abdominal pinching. The experiment was conducted double-blind, and the psychomotor tasks were the Bourdon-Wiersma test, Santa-Ana Dexterity, tapping speed, choice RT, and simulated automobile driving. Driving simulation was tested two, four, five, and seven hours after anesthesia, while the other tests were performed one and five hours after anesthesia. Results showed that psychomotor performance was significantly impaired for the halothane and enflurane groups as compared with the control groups, but the difference between the two anesthetics was marginal. Performance on the Santa Ana, choice RT, and simulated-driving tests remained significantly impaired for five hours after anesthetic administration.

Korttila et al. (1981) tested the time course of an anesthetic agent (N_2O) on still other measures of behavioral performance. Two experiments were run and 30 subjects were tested both during exposure to 30 percent (300,000 ppm) N_2O or control air and after exposure at 2-, 12-, 22-, and 32-minute intervals. Performance tests used included target tapping, free recall (words), math problems, and CFF. The peak effects of N_2O inhalation occurred as soon as 2 minutes after the 30 percent end tidal concentration was achieved. Compared with baseline or control conditions, N_2O exposure impaired tapping rate, number of words recalled, and arithmetic performance, but it improved CFF discrimination. Total recovery took about 22 minutes, and there was no evidence of tolerance development to the mental and psychomotor effects after a repeated administration of the chemical.

Trace Anesthetic Studies

Trace anesthetic studies have received their inpetus because of concern for adequate protection of health personnel working in operating theaters during surgical or dental procedures from waste anesthetic gases. One study (Bruce and Bach 1976) was apparently instrumental in the recommendation of permissible concentration levels of 25 ppm for N_2O and 2 ppm for halogenated anesthetics in the environment of medical workers (Smith and Shirley 1978). Bruce and Bach (1976) exposed male subjects aged 20–30 to N_2O alone (50 and 500 ppm) or combined with halothane by way of a face mask. The combination exposures were 500 ppm and 10 ppm; 50 ppm and 1.0 ppm; and 25 ppm and 0.5 ppm N_2O and halothane, respectively. In all there were five sets of exposures. Twenty subjects were used for each exposure condition, and each participant was tested twice, in pure air or pure air plus anesthetic gas, for periods of four hours. During the course of exposure a test battery was given consisting of tests of vigilance, STM, cognition, manual dexterity, dual task, and visual acuity. Findings showed that those exposure conditions containing N_2O at 50 ppm or higher produced significant losses on an audiovisual RT task that required detection of abnormal electrocardiograms. The addition of halothane exacerbated the performance impairment, affecting tests of memory, visual acuity, and vigilance. However, as reported below, verification of these results has not been forthcoming, even when other investigators used comparable tests and procedures.

Cook et al. (Behavioral effects, 1978; Subanesthetic concentrations, 1978), using both trace and subanesthetic levels, were not able to verify the Bruce and Bach findings in a series of experiments that included 10-, 30-, 120-, and 150-minute exposures to halothane (0.002 percent or 20 ppm to 4 percent or 400 ppm), N_2O (1 percent or 1,000 ppm to 30 percent or 300,000 ppm), enflurane (0.2 percent or 2,000 ppm to 0.53 percent or 5,300 ppm), and N_2O combined with halothane (0.05 percent or 500 ppm to 0.002 percent or 20 ppm). Results indicated that behavioral performance was significantly affected only with 30-minute exposures to N_2O, halothane, and enflurane at the 20 percent (200,000 ppm), 0.2 percent (2,000 ppm), and 0.42 percent (4,200 ppm) levels, respectively. Nitrous oxide (500 ppm) and halothane (20 ppm) in combination for a 150-minute exposure did not signficantly impair behavioral performance. Thirty-nine participants inhaled the gases through a mouthpiece, and the experiments were repeated-measures designs wherein all exposures were both preceded and followed by control-air measurements. The behavioral tests used were audiovisual choice RT, digit span, and the Purdue Pegborad assembly test. The levels of impairment were above trace concentrations yet below amnesic levels, as verified by word pairs and picture-recall tests.

British researchers (Smith and Shirely 1977; Allison, Shirley, and Smith 1979) reported on experiments using similar tests and procedures that also failed to reproduce Bruce and Bach's (1976) findings. In a first experiment, one female and nine male anesthetists and anesthetic technicians were exposed in a counterbalanced order to either control air or 100–150 ppm halothane on two separate occasions. Subjects inhaled the gas through a venti-mask, and the exposure duration was 3–4 hours. In a second experiment 15 male psychology students were exposed (via mask) on two separate sessions to either control air or a mixture of 500 N_2O and 15 ppm halothane for 3.5 hours. Gas odors were masked by spraying the nasal mucosa with lignocaine. Performance tests used were an audiovisual RT test (experiments 1 and 2), Wechsler Memory Scale (experiment 2), and pattern recall (experiment 2). In both studies results indicated no decrements in performance at any of the exposure levels used. One criticism of this study (Smith and Shirley 1977) was that subjects were allowed to drink a cup of coffee during the exposure period in experiment 2. Allison, Shirley, and Smith repeated this experiment including some higher exposure levels and not permitting subjects to ingest caffeine during the N_2O exposure. No effects were noted on the audiovisual RT test with exposures for 1.5 hours at the levels tested below 8 percent N_2O (80,000 ppm). Effects were evident at the next highest level, using 12 percent (120,000 ppm), so the threshold of N_2O effect was felt to be 8–12 percent.

Frankhuizen et al. (1978) in another verification attempt found no adverse effects of N_2O (1,600 ppm) and halothane (16 ppm) versus control air exposures for 2 hours in a climatic chamber. Twenty-four male subjects were used in a two-session, counterbalanced, double-blind procedure. The tests used were an audiovisual RT test, word-number recall, and anagram problem solving. Unlike the other studies mentioned above, this study used a double-blind procedure. The most recent verification effort (Venables et al. 1983) tested for effects at the 50 ppm exposure level of N_2O, which was the lowest level at which Bruce and Bach (1976) detected neurobehavioral impairments. Twenty-four subjects were exposed in an environmental chamber to either 50 ppm N_2O or a placebo for 4 hours in a counterbalanced design. Four performance tasks (an audiovisual task, a simple RT, a four-choice RT, and a pursuit-tracking task [Stressalyzer]) were tested in the last 40 minutes of exposure. No significant effects were evident at the 50 ppm exposure level.

The studies included in this section demonstrate the applicability of neurobehavioral testing in classifying the effects of anesthetic gases. The nature of the study designs and the results makes it difficult to define effective dose levels for significant neurobehavioral effects to occur for acute exposure to anesthetic gases for several reasons: (1) a wide range of concentrations has been used, and the concentration measurement units reported are not consistent; (2) duration of exposure is obviously critical in measuring the effects of the chemicals, and these may vary from study to study; (3) many of the experiments cited were designed for purposes other than dose-effect measurements; and (4) many of the studies reported used available medical personnel instead of naive subjects. It appears, however, that some conclusions can be extracted. Anesthetic exposures at subanesthetic concentrations affect memory processes probably by interfering with the learning of new material rather than by causing forgetting of older, previously learned material. More specific conclusions, such as interfering with rehearsal strategies, transfer from STM to LTM, and so on, are supportable but only when encrusted in a particular memory theory. In addition, the low levels of trace concentrations of N_2O and halothane reported by Bruce and Bach (1976) where test performance decrements were significant have not been replicated, and in fact the minimum levels of effect appear to be several times higher.

Miscellaneous Chemicals

Three additional chemicals that have been used in human exposure studies are summarized below. These chemicals are basically industrial preparations and do not fit into the classification scheme used in this chapter. They are included primarily for informational purposes and as examples of study design.

White spirit. White spirit, which is also called Stoddard solvent, contains paraffins, naphthenes, alkylbenzenes, and a trace of benzene (Sandmeyer 1981). Its pharmacological and toxicological effects are similar to those of gasoline. It is used as a dry-cleaning agent and a paint solvent and especially as a substitute for turpentine (Browning 1965). Gamberale, Annwall, and Hultengren (1975b) investigated the acute effects of white spirit on the CNS by studying its consequences in 14 males aged 18–34 in two experiments. In the first of two experiments all 14 subjects, in partially counterbalanced order with a control condition, were exposed to 625, 1,250, 1,875, and 2,500 mg/m³ white spirit in inspiratory air (via breathing valve) in four continuous 30-minute periods. In the second experiment, eight of these subjects were exposed to 4,000 mg/m³ white spirit in inspiratory air for 50 minutes. Using the 1984 TLV tables published by the American Conference of Governmental Industrial Hygienists, the conversion for Stoddard solvent to ppm is 525 mg/m³ = 100 ppm. The 4,000 mg/m³ dose would be roughly equivalent to 760 ppm, although these investigators probably used a European preparation for Stoddard solvent, which may be different from those used in the United States. Tests of perceptual speed, simple visual RT, STM, manual dexterity, and numerical ability (addition of digits) were administered in the final 20 minutes of each 30-minute exposure period in both experiments. Some CNS symptoms (dizziness, unsteadiness, and so on) were reported by subjects, but no effects of white spirit exposure occurred in experiment 1 on any performance measure. In experiment 2, however, with the 4,000 mg/m³ exposure, simple RT and STM were significantly impaired.

Freon-113. Stopps and McLaughlin (1967) exposed two male subjects (ages unstated) to Freon-113 (1,1,2-trichloro-1,2,2-trifluroethane). The exposure regimen started at 1,500 ppm and proceeded by 1,000 ppm steps to 4,500 ppm. Overall, the Freon-113 exposure lasted 2.75 hours, and air controls alternated with each Freon-113 session. Subjects were tested on manual dexterity, the Necker Cube test, card sorting, and vigilance (coding task). Performance deteriorated progressively, with increased Freon-113 concentration, starting at 2,500 ppm on all tasks.

Propylene glycol dinitrate. Stewart and coworkers (1974c) investigated the acute effects of propylene glycol dinitrate (PGD). PGD is a constituent of OTTO Fuel II, which is a torpedo propellant. Twenty subjects aged 22–51 were exposed in a controlled-environment room to PGD vapor concentrations of 0, 0.03, 0.1, 0.2, 0.35, 0.5, and 1.5 ppm with exposure durations of 8 hours (0–0.35 ppm), 7.3 hours (0.5 ppm), and 3.2 hours (1.5 ppm). Tests/measurements administered included a checklist of subjective symptoms; a modified Romberg test; time estimation; the Flannagan arithmetic, coordination, and inspection tests; spontaneous EEG, and VEP. Exposure to 0.2 ppm or greater produced headache and disruption of the VER in the majority of the subjects. Marked impairment in balance occurred after exposure to 0.5 ppm for 6.5 hours, while 40 minutes at 1.5 ppm added eye irritation to the list of symptoms. The psychomotor-test results were unremarkable at all PGD exposure concentrations.

It is difficult to form any definitive conclusions based on one human exposure study carried out on each of these mixtures. The exposure levels that caused the first indication of neurobehavioral impairment on the performance tests for Stoddard solvent and Freon-113 are quite high in comparison with those for the organic solvents, but these are mixtures and not chemical compounds. Of some interest are the subjects' reports of CNS symptoms of light-headedness, unsteadiness, and dizziness at the lower exposure levels for white spirit. On the other hand, PGD appears to be very potent, demonstrating neurobehavioral effects at the lowest concentrations of any chemical reported in this chapter from an acute exposure.

Comment

The preceding sections of this chapter describe the findings from many studies. Few of these findings, if any, can be readily extrapolated to disease conditions. However, many findings do reflect the three principal benefits of human experimental neurobehavioral studies: (1) the establishment of the nature and extent of short-term neurotoxic effects produced by acute exposure to single chemicals; (2) relationships between combination chemical exposures; and (3) the accrual of information that could contribute to safe exposure levels. We believe comments on the outcome of each of these three are in order.

Information about the acute neurobehavioral effects of chemicals has been obtained for many occupationally relevant compounds. However, a perusal of the literature reveals few studies that could be termed complete. Our knowledge of a chemical's acute effects still relies heavily on the synthesis of results across studies. An example is TCE. Several reports are available, each one characteristic to some extent of the experiments' differences in methods and procedures. Assessing the effects of TCE, therefore, requires comparing results across studies before ascribing any neurobehavioral effects. While this cross-laboratory approach is often valuable in showing that a particular chemical evidences effects under several different experimental approaches, it can be confusing when the results are contradictory. An alternative approach might be to conduct within the same laboratory a series of experiments exploring a broader range of chemical exposures and neurobehavioral consequences. An example of this approach is the series of studies on xylene conducted at the Finnish Institute of Occupational Health.

The second area in which experimental studies can make valuable contributions is that of combination exposures. The number of studies has been disappointingly small, as has the number of chemicals studied. Five areas of interest can be briefly identified: (1) the combination of various chemical agents to investigate whether the effects are additive, antagonistic, or potentiating; (2) the combination of chemical exposures with ethanol ingestion; (3) the combination of chemical exposures with drug ingestion; (4) the combination of exposures with physical agents such as noise, heat, and so on; and (5) the combination of chemical exposures with stress. The above interest areas are more representative of actual exposure situations, such as would occur in a workplace environment, than they are of the exposure to a single chemical under controlled laboratory conditions.

Finally, the portent of human neurobehavioral studies for safety is still unclear. Neurobehavioral findings have not become a requirement for the establishment of safe exposure limits by standards-setting or standards-recommending bodies. This is not surprising, since there have been no studies conclusively demonstrating that acute chemical intoxication leads to increased workplace accidents. Definitive information is needed, because it appears from available data that the neurobehavioral effects found after chemical exposures in the human laboratory situation are not generally marked by overt changes in behavior.

Recommendations for Research

A number of recommendations can be put forth for future research. These recommendations are briefly mentioned below and pertain to either the type of investigation that needs to be undertaken or areas where the research methodology can be strengthened.

First, the number of chemicals studied and the inclusion of chemical exposure combinations in the research design should be expanded. The conduct of such studies will, by design, also contain exposures to single chemicals, but the use of combination exposure conditions is more representative of a typical exposure situation. Combination conditions need not be limited to other chemicals but could also include noise, stress, and so on. We also recommend that such investigations routinely include ethanol or a similar reference substance for comparative purposes, as has been stressed previously (Horvath and Frantik 1973).

Improved research designs and protocols are also needed. Too many studies have been conducted in which group size was too small, learning effects were not controlled, or non-blind testing conditions were used. Many studies could have been improved by the use of pilot studies to identify design faults prior to undertaking the main effort. Despite the increased sophistication of testing methods and data analysis during the past three decades, opportunities for major improvement still exist.

Experimental investigations into the effects of chemicals on a variety of task parameters are sorely needed. Little attention has been paid to fine neuromotor control, to the broad range of sensory abilities, or to many areas of complex cognitive functions. The possibility that exposed individuals will take unnecessary risks needs attention. Tests of personality and affect are not routinely used in exposure studies, yet there is some indication that high concentrations of many toxic chemicals can produce profound changes in personality and behavior.

Another area of need relates to the development of valid testing methods for use in laboratories that can also be applied to field test situations. The benefits of portability and standardization are obvious. Test methods must be developed and validated in the laboratory and standardized for purposes of interlaboratory comparisons. Expanded use of interlaboratory comparisons of methods and chemicals studied would reap additional rewards. Exchange across national laboratories is presently lacking, and it appears that the number of laboratories conducting human exposure studies is not increasing. With scarce resources, there is also a need to maximize resource use by the adoption of proper research designs. In addition, we must develop strategies to assign priorities to chemicals for study and to foster coordination in laboratories conducting such research to maximize the yield. The literature review above testifies to the need for improvements and coordination in this area of research, owing particularly to the unique contribution that it makes to our knowledge of chemical effects.

Dedication

The authors dedicate this chapter to the memory of a colleague, Dr. Warren Teichner, a scholar who provided inspiration to many who followed.

Acknowledgments

The following individuals contributed significantly to the outcome of the study: Nadine Dickerson, who typed the revisions; and W. Kent Anger, Ph.D., and Alex Cohen, Ph.D., who reviewed the chapter.

References

Adam, N. 1973. Effects of general anesthesia on memory functions in man. *J. Comp. Physiol. Psychol.* 83(2):294–305.

Allison, R. H.; Shirley, A. W.; and Smith, G. 1979. Threshold concentration of nitrous oxide affecting psychomotor performance. *Br. J. Anaesth.* 51:177–79.

American Conference of Governmental Industrial Hygienists (ACGIH). 1984. *Threshold limit values for chemical substances and physical agents in the work environment and biological exposure indices with intended changes for 1984–85.* Cincinnati.

Anderson, I.; Lundqvist, G. R.; Mølhave, L. O.; Pedersen, F.; Proctor, D. F.; Vaeth, M.; and Wyon, D. P. 1983. Human response to controlled levels of toluene in six-hour exposures. *Scand. J. Work Environ. Health* 9:405–18.

Beard, R. R., and Wertheim, G. A. 1967. Behavioral impairment associated with small doses of carbon monoxide. *Amer. J. Pub. Health* 57:2012–22.

Benignus, V. A.; Otto, D. A.; Prah, J. D.; and Benignus, G. 1977. Lack of effects of carbon monoxide on human vigilance. *Percept. Mot. Skills* 45:1007–14.

Biersner, R. J. 1972. Selective performance effects of nitrous oxide. *Hum. Factors* 14(2):187–94.

Biersner, R. J.; Hall, D. A.; Neuman, T. S.; and Linaweaver, P. G. 1977. Learning rate equivalency of two narcotic gases. *J. Appl. Psychol.* 62(6):747–50.

Browning, E. 1965. *Toxicology and metabolism of industrial solvents*, 156–58. New York: Elsevier.

Bruce, D. L., and Bach, M. J. 1976. *Effects of trace concentrations of anesthetic gases on behavioral performance of operating room personnel.* DHEW-NIOSH Technical Report No. 76-169. Cincinnati.

Buck, W. B.; Hopper, D. L.; Cunningham, W. L.; and Karas, G. G. 1977. Current experimental considerations and future perspectives in behavioral toxicology. In *Behavioral toxicology: An emerging discipline*, edited by H. Zenick and L. W. Reiter, chap. 2, pp. 1–10. EPA Technical Report No. 600/9-77-042. Washington, D.C.

Cook, T. L.; Smith, M.; Starkweather, J. A.; Winter, P. M.; and Eger, E. I., II. 1978. Behavioral effects of trace and subanesthetic halothane and nitrous oxide in man. *Anesthesiology* 49:419–24.

Cook, T. L.; Smith, M.; Winter, P. M.; Starkweather, J. A.; and Eger, E. I., II. 1978. Effect of subanesthetic concentrations of enflurane and halothane on human behavior. *Anesth. Analg.* 57:434–40.

Davies, D. M.; Jolly, E. J.; Pethybridge, R. J.; and Colquhoun, W. P. 1981. The effects of continuous exposure to carbon monoxide on auditory vigilance in man. *Int. Arch. Occup. Environ. Health* 48:25–34.

Dick, R. B.; Setzer, J. V.; Wait, R.; Hayden, M. B.; Taylor, B. J.; Tolos, B.; and Putz-Anderson, V. 1984. Effects of acute exposure of toluene and methyl ethyl ketone on psychomotor performance. *Int. Arch. Occup. Environ. Health* 54:91–109.

DiVincenzo, G. D.; Yanno, F. J.; and Astill, B. D. 1972. Human and canine exposures to methylene chloride vapor. *Am. Indus. Hyg. Assoc. J.* 33(3):125–35.

Ettema, J.; Kleerekoper, L.; and Duba, W. C. 1975. Study of mental stresses during short-term inhalation of trichloroethylene. *Staub* 35(11):409–10.

Ettema, J. H.; Zielhuis, R. L.; Burer, E.; Meier, H. A.; Kleerekoper, L.; and de Graaf, M. A. 1975. Effects of alcohol, carbon monoxide and trichloroethylene exposure on mental capacity. *Int. Arch. Occup. Environ. Health* 35:117–32.

Ferguson, R. K., and Vernon, R. J. 1970. Trichloroethylene in combination with CNS drugs. *Arch. Environ. Health* 20(4):462–67.

Fowler, B.; White, P. L.; Wright, G. R.; and Ackles, K. N. 1980. Narcotic effects of nitrous oxide and compressed air on memory and auditory perception. *Undersea Biomed. Res.* 7(1):35–46.

Frankhuizen, J. L.; Vlek, C. A. J.; Burm, A. G. L.; and Rejger, V. 1978. Failure to replicate negative effects of trace anaesthetics on mental performance. *Br. J. Anaesth.* 50:229–34.

Gale, A. 1977. Some EEG correlates of sustained attention. In *Human factors III,* edited by R. R. Mackie, 263–83. New York: Plenum Press.

Gamberale, F.; Annwall, G.; and Hultengren, M. 1975a. Exposure to methylene chloride II. Psychological functions. *Scand. J. Work Environ. Health* 1:95–103.

———. 1975b. Exposure to white spirit II. Psychological functions. *Scand. J. Work Environ. Health* 1:31–39.

———. 1978. Exposure to xylene and ethylbenzene III. Effects on central nervous functions. *Scand. J. Work Environ. Health* 4:204–11.

Gamberale, F.; Annwall, G.; and Olson, B. A. 1976. Exposure to trichloroethylene. III. Psychological functions. *Scand. J. Work Environ. Health* 4:220–24.

Gamberale, F., and Hultengren, M. 1972. Toluene exposure II. Psychophysiological functions. *Work Environ. Health* 9:131–39.

———. 1973. Methylchloroform exposure II. Psychophysiological functions. *Work Environ. Health* 10:82–92.

———. 1974. Exposure to styrene II. Psychological functions. *Work Environ. Health* 11:86–91.

Henrie, J. R.; Parkhouse, J.; and Bickford, R. 1961. Alteration of human consciousness by nitrous oxide as assessed by electroencephalography and psychological tests. *Anesthesiology* 22:242–59.

Horvath, M., and Frantik, E. 1973. Quantitative interpretation of experimental toxicological data: The use of reference substances. In *Adverse effects of environmental chemicals and psychotropic drugs,* edited by M. Horvath, 1:11–21. 2 vols. Amsterdam: Elsevier.

Kiutz, B. L.; Delprato, D. J.; Mettel, D. R.; Persons, C. E.; and Schappe, R. H. 1965. The experimenter effect. *Psychol. Bull.* 63:223–32.

Klein, K. 1973. Alcohol as reference substance for the quantitative prediction of maximum allowable drug concentrations in relation to traffic safety. In *Adverse effects of environmental chemicals and psychotropic drugs,* 1:41–52. See Horvath and Frantik 1973.

Konietzko, H.; Elster, J.; Benesath, A.; Drysch, K.; and Weichardt, H. 1975. Psychomotor reactions under standardized trichloroethylene load. *Arch. Toxicol.* 33(2):129–39.

Korttila, K.; Ghoneim, M. M.; Jacobs, L.; Mewaldt, S. P.; and Peterson, R. C. 1981. Time course of mental and psychomotor effects of 30 per cent nitrous oxide during inhalation and recovery. *Anesthesiology* 54:220–26.

Korttila, K.; Tammisto, T.; Ertama, P.; Pfaffli, P.; Blomgren, E.; and Hakkinen, S. 1977. Recovery, psychomotor skills and simulated driving after brief inhalational anesthesia with halothane or enflurane combined with nitrous oxide and oxygen. *Anesthesiology* 46:20–27.

Kylin, B.; Axell, K.; Samuel, H. E.; and Lindborg, A. 1967. Effect of inhaled trichloroethylene on the CNS. *Arch. Environ. Health* 15(1):48–52.

Laties, V. G., and Merigan, W. H. 1979. Behavioral effects of carbon monoxide on animals and man. *Annu. Rev. Pharmacol. Toxicol.* 19:357–92.

McFarland, R. A. 1970. The effects of exposure to small quantities of carbon monoxide on vision. *Ann. N.Y. Acad. Sci.* 174:301–12.

———. 1973. Low level exposure to carbon monoxide and driving performance. *Arch. Environ. Health* 27:355–59.

McNeill, W. C. 1979. Trichloroethylene. In *Kirk-Othmer encyclopedia of chemical technology.* edited by M. Grayson, 5:745–53. 3d. ed. New York: John Wiley.

Matsushita, T.; Goshima, E.; Miyakaki, H.; Maeda, K.; Takeuchi, Y.; and Inoue, T. 1979. Experimental studies for determining the MAC value of acetone. 2. Biological reactions in the "six-day exposure" to acetone. *Sangyo Iqaku* 11(10):507–15.

Mihevic, P. M.; Gliner, J. A.; and Horvath, S. M. 1983. Carbon monoxide exposure and information processing during perceptual-motor performance. *Int. Arch. Occup. Environ. Health* 51:355–63.

Nakaaki, K. 1974. Experimental study on the effect of organic solvent vapors on human subjects. *Rodo Kagaku* 50(2):89–96.

Nakaaki, K.; Onishi, N.; Iida, H.; Kimotsuki, K.; Fukabori, S.; and Morikiyo, Y. 1973. An experimental study on the effect of exposure to trichloroethylene vapor in man. *J. Science Labour* 49(8):449–63.

Nomiyama, K., and Nomiyama, H. 1977. Dose-response relationship for trichloroethylene in man. *Int. Arch. Occup. Environ. Health* 39(4):237–48.

Odkvist, L. M.; Astrand, I.; Larsby, B.; and Kall, C. 1980. Does styrene disturb the balance apparatus in man? *Arbete och Halsa* 2:4–19.

Oltramare, M.; Desbaumes, E.; Imhoff, C.; and Michiels, W. 1974. *Toxicology of styrene monomer: Experimental and clinical research in man*, 84–100. Geneva: Medicine & Hygiene.

Otto, D. A. 1977. Neurobehavioral toxicology: Problems and methods in human research. In *Behavioral toxicology: An emerging discipline*, chap. 10, pp. 1–31. *See* Buck et al. 1977.

Otto, D. A.; Benignus, V. A.; and Prah, J. D. 1979. Carbon monoxide and human time discrimination: Failure to replicate Beard-Wertheim experiments. *Aviat. Space Environ. Med.* 50:40–43.

Parkhouse, J.; Henrie, J. R.; Duncan, G. M.; and Rome, H. P. 1960. Nitrous oxide analgesia in relation to mental performance. *J. Pharmacol. Exp. Ther.* 128:44–54.

Porter, A. L. 1972. Analytical review of the effects of non-hydrogen bonding anesthetics on memory processing. *Behav. Biol.* 7:291–309.

Putz, V. R. 1979. The effects of carbon monoxide on dual-task performance. *Hum. Factors* 21:13–24.

Putz, V. R.; Johnson, B. L.; and Setzer, J. V. 1979. A comparative study of the effects of carbon monoxide and methylene chloride on human performance. *J. Environ. Pathol. Toxicol.* 2:97–112.

Putz-Anderson, V.; Setzer, J. V.; Croxton, J. S.; and Phipps, F. C. 1981. Methyl chloride and diazepam effects on performance. *Scand. J. Work Environ. Health* 7:8–13.

Repko, J. D.; Jones, P. D.; Garcia, L. S.; Schneider, E. J.; Roseman, E.; and Corum, C. R. 1976. *Behavioral and neurological effects of methyl chloride*. DHEW-NIOSH Publication No. 77-125. Cincinnati.

Riihimaki, V., and Savolainen, K. 1980. Human exposure to m-xylene. Kinetics and acute effects on the CNS. *Ann. Occup. Hyg.* 23:(4)411–22.

Rodnitzky, R. L.; Levin, H. S.; and Morgan, D. P. 1978. Effects of ingested parathion on neurobehavioral functions. *Clin. Toxicol.* 13(3):347–59.

Rummo, N., and Sarlanis, K. 1974. The effect of carbon monoxide on several measures of vigilance in a simulated driving task. *J. Safety Res.* 6:126–30.

Salvatore, S. 1974. Performance decrement caused by mild carbon monoxide levels on two visual functions. *J. Safety Res.* 6:131–34.

Salvini, M.; Binaschi, S.; and Riva, M. 1971*a*. Evaluation of the psychophysiological functions in humans exposed to threshold limit value of 1,1,1-trichloroethane. *Br. J. Ind. Med.* 28:286–92.

———. 1971*b*. Evaluation of the psychophysiological functions in humans exposed to trichloroethylene. *Br. J. Ind. Med.* 28:293–95.

Sandmeyer, E. 1981. Aromatic hydrocarbons. In *Patty's industrial hygiene and toxicology*, edited by G. D. Clayton and E. F. Clayton. 2B:3253–3431. New York: Wiley.

Savolainen, K. 1980. Combined effects of alcohol on the central nervous system. *Acta Pharmacol. Toxicol. (Copenh)* 46:366–72.

Savolainen, K., and Riihimäki, V. 1981*a*. An early sign of xylene effect on human equilibrium. *Acta Pharmacol. Toxicol. (Copenh)* 48:279–83.

———.1981*b*. Xylene and alcohol involvement on the human equilibrium system. *Acta Pharmacol. Toxicol. (Copenh)* 49:447–51.

Savolainen, K.; Riihimäki, V.; and Laine, A. 1982. Biphasic effects of inhaled solvents on human equilibrium. *Acta Pharmacol. Toxicol. (Copenh)* 51:237–42.

Savolainen, K.; Riihimäki, V.; Laine, A.; and Kekoni, J. 1981. Short-term exposure of human subjects to m-xylene and 1,1,1-trichloroethane. *Int. Arch. Occup. Environ. Health* 49:89–98.

Savolainen, K.; Riihimäki, V.; and Linnoila, M. 1979. Effects of short-term xylene exposure on psychological functions in man. *Int. Arch. Occup. Environ. Health* 44(4):201–11.

Savolainen, K.; Riihimäki, V.; Seppäläinen, A. M.; and Linnoila, M. 1980. Effects of short-term m-xylene exposure and physical exercise on the CNS. *Int. Arch. Occup. Environ. Health* 45:105–21.

Savolainen, K.; Riihimäki, V.; Vaheri, E.; and Linnoila, M. 1980. Effects of xylene and alcohol on vestibular and visual functions in man. *Scand. J. Work Environ. Health* 6:94–103.

Seppäläinen, A. M.; Savolainen, K.; and Kovala, T. 1981. Changes induced by xylene and alcohol in human evoked potentials. *Electroencephalogr. Clin. Nuerophysiol.* 51:148–55.

Sharp, C. W., and Carroll, L. T. 1978. *Voluntary inhalation of industrial solvents.* Rockville, Md.: National Institute on Drug Abuse.

Smith, G., and Shirley, W. 1977. Failure to demonstrate effect of trace concentrations of nitrous oxide and halothane on psychomotor performance. *Br. J. Anaesth.* 49:65–70.

———. 1978. A review of the effects of trace concentrations of anesthetics on performance. *Br. J. Anaesth.* 50:701–12.

Stewart, R. D. 1974. Solvent seminar keynote address. In *Behavioral toxicology,* edited by C. Xintaras, B. Johnson, and I. de Groot, 35–41. DHEW-NIOSH Technical Report No. 74-126. Cincinnati.

Stewart, R. D.; Baretta, E. D.; Dodd, H. C.; and Torkelson, T. R. 1970. Experimental human exposure to tetrachloroethylene. *Arch. Environ. Health* 20:224–29.

Stewart, R. D.; Dodd, H. C.; Baretta, E. D.; and Schaffer, A. W. 1968. Human exposure to styrene vapor. *Arch. Environ. Health* 16(5):656–62.

Stewart, R. D.; Fisher, T. N.; Hosko, M. J.; Peterson, J. E.; Baretta, E. D.; and Dodd, H. C. 1972. Experimental human exposure to methylene chloride. *Arch. Environ. Health* 25:342–48.

Stewart, R. D.; Gay, H. H.; Schaffer, A. W.; Erley, D. S.; and Rowe, V. K. 1969. Experimental human exposure to methyl chloroform vapor. *Arch. Environ. Health* 19(4):467–72.

Stewart, R. D.; Hake, C. L.; Forster, H. V.; Lebrun, A. J.; Peterson, J. E.; and Wu, A. 1975. *Toluene: Development of a biological standard for the industrial worker by breath analysis.* DHEW-NIOSH Contract Report No. 99-72-84. Cincinnati.

Stewart, R. D., Hake, C. L.; Lebrun, A. J.; Kalbfleisch, J. H.; Newton, P. E.; Peterson, J. E.; Cohen, H. H.; Struble, R.; and Busch, K. A. 1973. *Effects of trichloroethylene on behavioral performance capabilities.* DHEW-NIOSH Contract Report No. HSM-99-72-84. Cincinnati.

Stewart, R. D.; Hake, C. L.; Peterson, J. E.; Forster, H. V.; Newton, P. E.; Soto, R. J.; and Lebrun, A. J. 1974. In *Behavioral toxicology,* 81–92. See Stewart 1974.

Stewart, R. D.; Hake, C. L.; Wu, A.; Graff, S. A.; Forster, H. V.; Keeler, W. H.; Lebrun, A. J.; Newton, P. E.; and Soto, R. J. 1977. *Methyl chloride: Development of a biological standard for the industrial worker by breath analysis.* DHEW-NIOSH Report No. 77-1. Cincinnati.

Stewart, R. D.; Hake, C. L.; Wu, A.; Kalbfleisch, J. H.; Newton, P. E.; Marlow, S. K.; and Vucicevic-Salama, M. 1977. *Effects of perchloroethylene/drug interaction on behavioral and neurological function.* DHEW-NIOSH Technical Report No. 77-191. Cincinnati.

Stewart, R. D.; Newton, P. E.; Hosko, M. J.; and Peterson, J. E. 1973. Effect of carbon monoxide on time perception. *Arch. Environ. Health* 27:155–60.

Stewart, R. D.; Peterson, J. E.; Newton, P. E.; Hake, C. L.; Hosko, M. J.; Lebrun, A. J.; and Lawton, G. M. 1974. Experimental human exposure to propylene glycol dinitrate. *Toxicol. Appl. Pharmacol.* 30(3):377–95.

Stopps, G. J., and McLaughlin, M. 1967. Psychophysiological testing of human Ss exposed to solvent vapors. *Am. Indus. Hyg. Assoc. J.* 28:43–50.

Suzuki, H. 1973. Autonomic nervous responses to experimental toluene exposure in humans. *Sangyo Igaku* 15(4):379–84.

Teichner, W. 1975. Carbon monoxide and human performance: A methodological exploration. In *Behavioral toxicology,* edited by B. Weiss and V. Laties, 77–103. New York: Plenum Press.

Torkelson, T. R.; and Rowe, V. K. 1981. Halogenated aliphatic hydrocarbons containing chlorine, bromine and iodine. In *Patty's industrial hygiene and toxicology,* 2B:3433–3601. *See* Sandmeyer 1981.

Venables, H.; Cherry, N.; Waldron, H. A.; Buck, L.; Edling, C.; and Wilson, H. K. 1983. Effects of trace levels of nitrous oxide on psychomotor performance. *Scand. J. Work Environ. Health* 9:391–96.

Verberk, M. M. 1976. Motor nerve conduction velocity in volunteers ingesting inorganic lead for 49 days. *Int. Arch. Occup. Environ. Health* 38:141–43.

Verberk, M. M., and Salle, H. J. 1977. Effects on nervous function in volunteers ingesting mevinphos for one month. *Toxicol. Appl. Pharmacol.* 42:351–58.

Vernon, R. J., and Ferguson, R. K. 1969. Effects of trichloroethylene on visual-motor performance. *Arch. Environ. Health* 18:894–900.

Windemuller, F. B., and Ettema, J. 1978. Effects of combined exposure to trichloroethylene and alcohol on mental performance. *Int. Arch. Occup. Environ. Health* 41:77–85.

Winneke, G. 1982. The behavioral effects of exposure to some organic solvents: Psychophysiological aspects. In *Occupational neurology.,* edited by J. Juntunen. *Acta Neurol. Scand.* 69, suppl. 92:117–29.

Winneke, G.; Kastka, J.; and Fodor, G. G. 1973. Disturbances of vigilance and visual-motor performance resulting from air pollutants and drugs. In *Adverse effects of environmental chemicals and psychotropic drugs,* 193–201. *See* Horvath and Frantik 1973.

Wright, G. R.; Randell, P.; and Shephard, R. J. 1973. Carbon monoxide and driving skills. *Arch. Environ. Health* 27:349–54.

Wright, G. R.; and Shephard, R. J. 1978. Carbon monoxide exposure and auditory duration discrimination. *Arch. Environ. Health* 32:226–35.

V

Regulatory and Statistical Considerations

William F. Sette and
Tina E. Levine

17

Behavior as a Regulatory Endpoint

Regulatory agencies concerned with toxic chemicals may be influenced by prevailing public opinion, industrial pressures, congressional demands, as well as the results of research. To date, behavioral effects have not been considered particularly important either within the toxicology community or within most regulatory agencies. However, behavior has played, and will continue to play, a role in environmental regulation.

Research scientists are often unaware of the considerations (both scientific and other) that contribute to regulatory decisions. This impedes their ability to directly communicate the utility of their experimental results to regulatory decision makers and to design experiments maximally useful in making public-health decisions. This chapter describes some of the considerations involved in regulatory decision making and focuses on the aspects of behavior that are most relevant to these decisions. This chapter also explains how behavioral testing is being integrated into the evaluation of chemicals subject to regulation by the Environmental Protection Agency (EPA) under the Toxic Substances Control Act (TSCA).

Are Behavioral Effects Indicative of Toxicity?

Criticism has been directed both at behavior as an endpoint and at the field of behavioral toxicology: behavioral effects have been criticized as being merely pharmacological rather than toxic effects, and behavioral toxicology has been criticized as too young a scientific discipline to be methodologically prepared for the development of standardized testing procedures. The traditional domain of toxicology is pathology, structural damage to target tissue. Functional changes, of which behavioral changes represent one type, have been considered only cursorily. For example, the guidelines for acute and subchronic toxicity testing issued by the EPA refer only in passing to "behavioral observation" (e.g., USEPA 1983). The primary foci of these guidelines are death and morphological changes on target organs, predominantly the liver and kidney. Thus, in the same tradition, neurotoxicity is considered to be limited to those effects that are expressed as neuropathological changes, while the acute effects of solvents on behavior, for example, are considered to be pharmacological and outside the proper scope of toxicology.

From a semantic point of view, it is simple to assert that what distinguishes pharmacological from toxicological effects is intent, that is, whether such effects were intended or inadvertent. It is hard to imagine such intent for most chemical products other than drugs or pesticides. Thus, any behavioral effect of an industrial chemical may be considered to be a toxic effect. What is more important, acute behavioral effects have indeed served as the basis for recommending exposure controls to chemicals. Anger (1984) has reviewed the standards recommended by the American Council of Government Industrial Hygienists (ACGIH) and noted that for roughly one-fourth of these chemicals, effects on the nervous system or behavior served as a basis for recommending an acceptable exposure level. Narcosis or other behavioral effects were cited as explicit bases for 20 of those recommendations and were undoubtedly important for many others. On 27 June 1974 the Occupational Safety and Health Administration (OSHA), without evaluation, adopted virtually all of the ACGIH recommendations from 1968 as their permissible exposure limits (29CFR 1910.1000 and 39CFR 23502). Thus, behavioral effects have served as the basis for regulation of many industrial chemicals.

While undoubtedly a young technology, behavioral toxicology shares its youth with much of regulatory science. Agencies have focused on the impact of chemical exposures on human health only recently and are now seeking to protect the public from the consequences of such exposure. Since the thalidomide tragedy in 1961, teratology testing of chemicals has become widespread. Genetic toxicology was recognized as a discipline around 1969 with the formation of the Environmental Mutagen Society. The linking of environmental mutagens with mammalian carcinogens was largely developed from 1969 to 1971. The Fifth Rochester Conference on Environmental Toxicity in 1972 was devoted to behavioral toxicology (Weiss and Laties 1975). Thus, the relatively young regulatory sciences developed fairly concurrently out of the older basic disciplines of experimental psychology and psychopharmacology, molecular genetics and developmental biology.

In criticism of the youthful technology of behavioral toxicology, a major comment often voiced by the toxicology community has been that it lacks validity. *Validity* is a term that is widely used and often misused. Anastasi (1976) noted that "the validity of a test concerns what the test measures and how well it does so." Often in regulatory agencies tests are described as being "validated" or undergoing "validation." This usually means that several laboratories are using the same test to see whether they get the same results, or that many chemicals with known effects are being tested with the procedure under study to see whether the test gives the expected result. The ability of a procedure to produce consistent results either within or across laboratories is termed *reliability*. The ability of a test to predict or reflect what may happen to exposed humans is termed *predictive validity*. Predictive validity and reliability are test characteristics of great importance to the regulator.

A survey of known neurotoxicants clearly indicates that similar neurological (i.e., behavioral) signs are produced in humans and experimental animals. For example, in Spencer and Schaumburg's *Experimental and Clinical Neurotoxicology* there are detailed descriptions of neurotoxic effects for more than 21 agents. For those agents with documented human disease (approximately 16), the effects produced in animals are similar to those seen in humans. Thus, behavioral testing has clear predictive validity. Unfortunately, most neurotoxicants have been discovered in humans on the basis of neurobehavioral signs. Animal models have been developed later. In addition, the reliability of behavioral techniques has been amply demonstrated during the more than 25 years of experience in the field of psychopharmacology, where chemicals have been studied over a broad range of laboratories as well as repeatedly within a single laboratory.

A Brief Overview of Environmental Laws

The regulation and testing of chemicals in the United States to prevent adverse health effects is mandated by a number of different laws that govern specific uses of chemicals or the site of exposure. Under these laws, agencies differ in their ability to require premarketing approval, toxicity testing, and regulation of exposure. Four agencies—the Consumer Product Safety Commision (CPSC), EPA, the Food and Drug Administration (FDA), and OSHA—have authority to restrict exposure or use of chemicals and to require data reporting. Two of these, EPA and FDA, can require testing by manufacturers. Only EPA and FDA have authority for the premarketing approval of drugs and food, and pesticides, respectively (Fisher 1980).

Table 17.1 lists some of the legal language included in several prominent environmental acts. As can be seen, definitions of health concerns to be regulated are worded very generally. Concerns and priority are usually focused on serious irreversible effects. Acute effects, including behavioral effects, are of lower priority and often are discounted or ignored.

Risk assessment involves the qualitative and quantitative characterization of the adverse health effects of chemicals. Several of the laws require the balancing of

Table 17.1 Illustrative definitions of hazards of concern and legal language for regulating exposure

Act	Agency	Degree of Protection	Hazards of Concern
Occupational Safety and Health Act (OSHA)	OSHA	"Adequately assures to the extent feasible that no employee will suffer"	"Material impairment of health or functional capacity" (sec. 6.*b*.5)
Clean Air Act (CAA)	EPA	"An ample margin of safety"	"An increase in serious irreversible, or incapacitating reversible illness" (sec. 112.*a*.1)
Federal Insecticide, Fungicide, and Rodenticide Act (FIFRA)	EPA	"Unreasonable risk to man or the environment taking into account the economic, social and environmental costs and benefits"	"Unreasonable adverse effects"
Toxic Substances Control Act (TSCA)	EPA	"To protect adequately against such risk using the least burdensome requirement" (sec. 6.*a*)	"An unreasonable risk of injury to health or the environment" (sec. 6.*a*)
Consumer Product Safety Act (CPSC)	CPSC	"Standard shall be reasonably necessary to prevent or reduce an unreasonable risk of injury" (15 USC, sec. 2056)	"Unreasonable risk of injury . . . in commerce . . . a risk of death, personal injury or serious or frequent injury" (15 USC, sec. 2051)

Source: NAS 1983.

risks with other factors to support actions (Ricci and Molton 1981; NAS 1983). The process of evaluating alternative regulatory options and selecting among them is called *risk management* (ibid.). In FIFRA, for example, "unreasonable adverse effects" are defined as "unreasonable risk to man or the environment taking into account the economic, social and environmental costs and benefits." This definition, as well as others cited in table 17.1, does not clearly distinguish between risk assessment and risk management. Recently, an NAS committee advocated that regulatory agencies distinguish more clearly between risk assessment and risk management processes in the hope that the description of health hazards would not be obscured by the necessary trade-offs involved in risk management decisions (ibid.).

The Toxic Substances Control Act (TSCA) and Risk Assessment

TSCA gives EPA authority to require the testing of chemicals in commerce and control exposure to them. According to section 4 of TSCA, three legal findings must be made before testing of an existing chemical can be required: (1) that exposure to the chemical may present an unreasonable risk of injury or that the chemical is or will be produced in substantial quantities, and exposure may be substantial or significant; (2) that the current data are inadequate to reasonably determine or predict the health effects of the chemical; and (3) that testing is necessary to develop such data (see fig. 17.1). Pending development of data under section 5.*e*, similar findings are required to control exposure to new chemicals. Under section 6, action may be taken to control exposures to existing chemicals if their risks are judged to be unreasonable. Therefore, EPA must decide (1) which data are adequate to determine whether or not a chemical is toxic and (2) if a chemical is determined to be toxic, the relationship between exposure and the frequency or extent of toxic effects. These data will then permit the estimation of the extent of the risk posed to humans by the chemical under a particular set of exposure conditions—that is, a risk assessment. A complete risk assessment involves four steps: (1) the qualitative assessment of the hazard, (2) a description of dose-effect relationships, (3) an analysis of actual human exposures, and (4) the characterization of the risk to humans.

In evaluating whether a behavioral effect may present an unreasonable risk to human health, several parameters of the behavioral effect are of interest. The *severity* of behavioral effects may range from the subtle acute impairment of vigilance performance by low-level, short-term exposures to carbon monoxide (Laties and Merigan 1979) to severe mental retardation following lead encephalopathy (Byers and Lord 1943). The nonfatal chronic (47 years) motor spasticity produced by acute triorthocresyl phosphate exposure (Morgan and Penovich 1978) illustrates the fact that the *duration* of effect may far exceed the duration of exposure. The onset of effects may occur within seconds after initiation of exposure, or it may be delayed by weeks or months. The *reversibility* of behavioral effects may be a function of the nature of the effect, the anatomic site, or the rate of excretion of the agent. In addition, it has long been known that the reserve capacity within the nervous system for many functions can lead to behavioral recovery even after massive physical damage (Lashley 1929).

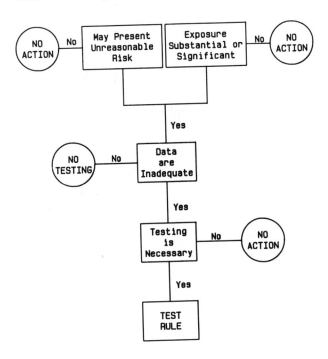

Fig. 17.1 The decision making involved in promulgating a test rule under TSCA. The exposure case is considered only if production is substantial.

An additional complication in the evaluation of behavioral effects is the development of tolerance. A reduction in response to a chemical following repeated exposure, it may develop to only some of the effects and at different rates, and it may be a function of the method used to measure the effects (Bignami et al. 1975; Jaffe 1975; NAS 1975). These adaptations to chronic dosing may have long-term consequences that emerge only after long-term treatment or after cessation of exposure. For example, haloperidol, a butyrophenone used as a tranquilizer, often produces acute dyskinesias which disappear as treatment is continued. Years later, either during or shortly after treatment, more persistent and sometimes permanent dyskinesias, aptly called tardive or late dyskinesias, may emerge. Thus, acute tolerance to an effect does not mean that adaptation does not have a long-term cost.

Finally, while acute, subtle effects can be less serious than chronic, profound effects, they can often have significant toxicological consequences. The acute and graded effects of ethanol on driving illustrate this point. In order to assess these parameters, we must evaluate the indirect evidence that stems from physical-chemical data and the known toxicity of structural analogues and the direct evidence on the chemical under consideration.

Indirect Evidence

Physical-chemical data may suggest certain pharmacokinetic properties, such as routes of absorption, distribution, metabolism, and excretion. Zbinden (1973) lists 14 physical-chemical variables that are important. The property most specifically relevant to neurotoxicity is lipid solubility, as estimated by the octanol/water partition coefficient. This property provides an estimate of how readily a chemical may penetrate cell membranes in general and the blood-brain barrier in particular.

Nonpolar compounds and those that do not bind to plasma proteins also cross the blood-brain barrier more easily (Klaasen 1975). Chemicals with these properties, then, are more likely to be neurotoxic, because they have access to the target tissue.

Knowledge of a chemical's structure and the known properties of other members of the same chemical class may also suggest an increased chance of certain health effects. For example, structural similarity to known neurotransmitters may suggest behavioral effects.

Direct Evidence

Direct evidence includes both human and animal data. Human data may come from clinical case reports, epidemiological studies, or controlled laboratory experiments. They provide direct evidence of human poisoning and the best evidence of health effects. In general, clinical case reports are limited both by the poorly quantified nature of the signs and symptoms reported and by the nature of the exposure data. By definition, case reports constitute too small a sample size for statistical analysis and estimation of population incidence. Epidemiological studies employ statistically adequate population samples and may employ tests that provide well-quantified measures of toxicity, although like case studies, surveys of population incidences of poorly quantified signs and symptoms, which are most common, often provide only qualitative estimates of the exposure conditions. Controlled laboratory studies use precisely quantified exposures, small but statistically adequate group sizes, and the best available quantitative test methods; however, ethical considerations and limited resources place moral and practical limits on such studies (see chapters 15 and 16).

Acute and subchronic toxicity studies in animals can also provide evidence of potential human toxicity. Neurological signs such as paralysis and convulsions are among the behavioral effects reported in toxicity studies. Behavior is the most general level of analysis and reflects the total integrated activity of all the biological systems, both neural and nonneural, of the organism. Thus, behavioral changes may indicate neurotoxicity or may be secondary to other systemic toxicity. Traditional toxicology has paid lip service to the utility of behavior as a general indicator of health status by including behavioral observations as a standard component of general toxicity testing. However, behavioral changes that may be attributed to a direct impact on the nervous system are the major concern within EPA's Office of Toxic Substances.

Estimating "safe" exposure levels in humans involves both qualitative and quantitative comparison of available data derived from the scientific literature, as well as specific, usually animal, testing. Animal tests generally provide the quantitative data on the relation between exposure and effects. Ideally, a complete dose-effect curve should be described, from an exposure level that produces a small (or no) effect to an exposure level that produces marked effects.

Given the exposure levels that define apparent thresholds for effects in animals, one can estimate "safe" exposure levels in humans by the application of appropriate safety factors. This approach can be succinctly described as follows: "safe" exposure level = threshold exposure level/margin of safety. Kushner, Wands, and Fong (1983) have recently reviewed the margins of safety used for different types of data. While not formally the policy of any agency, they are illustrative of the types of factors considered in risk-management decisions. These may be summarized as follows:

1. If human data are available, then a margin of safety of 10 is used to allow for variation in population sensitivity.
2. If chronic animal data are used, then a margin of safety of 100 is used to allow for species extrapolation (10) and variation in population sensitivity (10).
3. If subchronic rather than chronic animal data are used, then an additional margin of safety of 10 may be applied.
4. If a lowest-effect level rather than a no-effect level is used, then an additional safety factor may be applied.
5. For very serious effects, an additional factor may be added.

Estimates based on simple application of these safety factors should be modified by any knowledge of the factors extrapolated.

The final product of any technical risk assessment should be a series of conclusions and scientific judgments rather than a single "acceptable" exposure level presumed to represent all of the scientific judgments involved in its derivation.

Neurotoxicity Guidelines

Under section 4 of TSCA, if evaluation of the data on an existing chemical indicates that the statutory findings can be made, a rule requiring industry to develop the needed test data may be promulgated. However, such a rule must include "standards for the development of test data," that is, test guidelines. The primary question of the Office of Toxic Substances needed to answer in order to develop these guidelines was, What kinds of test data will allow us to determine the risks posed by a given chemical? A number of expert panels have considered this question with regard to behavioral toxicity.

In 1973, in anticipation of TSCA, EPA joined forces with the National Academy of Sciences-National Research Council to sponsor the first such panel (NAS 1975). The panel considered the use of behavioral data both as a general indicator of toxicity to any organ system and as a specific indicator of CNS function. They recommended that behavioral observations be an important component of all toxicity studies and that more comprehensive behavioral testing be performed if preliminary screening indicated effects but the socioeconomic benefits of the chemical warranted continued interest in its development.

The behavioral observations recommended for acute-toxicity studies included activity changes; objective signs, such as tremors, convulsions, ptosis, salivation, lacrimation, defecation, and abnormal posture; reflex changes; and body-weight changes. These measures were derived from procedures used in the pharmaceutical industry to screen for central-nervous-system (CNS) activity.

The panel recommended that if CNS effects were revealed by the preliminary screen, it should be determined whether CNS activity was present over a wide dose range by using spontaneous motor activity. The results of such testing would also guide dose selection for specific procedures. The specific procedures recommended comprised the categories of sensory processes, motor processes, and complex functions (i.e., learning). In addition, measures of tolerance and dependence and measures of behavior following prenatal exposures were recommended (ibid.).

In 1976, CPSC requested that the NAS review and amplify its earlier publication *Principles and Procedures for Evaluating the Toxicity of Household Substances* (NAS 1977). The behavioral toxicity panel for this review recommended two general screening tests: operant behavior and circadian cycle of activity. They also suggested many of the same procedures for assessment of specific functions discussed above, namely, measurement of sensory function, ataxia, tremors, and reflexes (ibid.).

Most recently, another panel of the NAS/NRC has been evaluating compounds that have been tested for neurotoxicity (NAS 1982). While they have developed criteria to assess the adequacy of such testing, they have reiterated their previous recommendation that both conditioned and unconditioned behaviors be studied and that spontaneous motor activity and schedule-controlled behavior are good measures of unconditioned and conditioned behavior, respectively (NAS 1984).

The Office of Toxic Substances has used these recommendations to develop an approach to testing industrial chemicals. The behavioral tests for which we have developed guidelines are (1) a functional observational battery, (2) motor activity, and (3) operant behavior.

The Functional Observational Battery

The range of complexity of techniques for neurotoxicity assessment is matched only by the range of complexity of functions governed by the nervous system. The functional observational battery is designed to apply a low level of technical complexity to a range of behaviors indicative of neurological function. Such a battery should "screen" chemical agents that are suspect neurotoxicants but for which there is little information on potential sites of action. The battery may identify neurotoxic end points and thus suggest more complex, focused evaluation upon which risk assessments may be based. It should aid in evaluating the significance of morphological changes. Absence of both functional and morphological changes provides some assurance that an unstudied agent does not have a high potential for causing neurotoxic damage.

Ideally, a neurotoxicity screening battery should be capable of detecting deficits in the major functions governed by the nervous system: sensation, movement, cognition, emotion, and life maintenance. In addition, it should be simple, rapid, and inexpensive to conduct so that a large number of chemicals may be evaluated. In reality, techniques for properly detecting sensory and cognitive deficits are complex, expensive, and narrow in scope. The reflex techniques for assessing vision and hearing that are included in the battery will detect only almost total blindness or deafness. Thus, research to develop simpler and less expensive procedures for these endpoints would be very useful. One promising technique in this area is the use of stimuli modifying the startle reflex as a rapid test of sensory thresholds (Ison and Hoffman 1983). When available data on structurally related chemicals indicate that an agent may cause specific deficits in these areas, more complex testing may be justified. In the meantime, screening for most chemicals will be limited to detection of the gross deficits induced by very high doses.

Observations of animals are called for in certain sections of the Test Guidelines for Acute and Subchronic Health Effects. Among the signs of toxicity to be observed daily are behavioral signs; yet, no suggestions for what behaviors to observe or how to score the data are provided. The functional observational battery provides this guidance. It is recommended that this type of behavioral testing be combined routinely with the testing for other health effects.

Motor Activity

The functional state of the nervous system is often reflected in an animal's motor activity. Overall activity may reflect the influence of a host of nonneurally mediated effects, but activity is critical to the animal's survival (Reiter 1978). Measurement of motor activity is relatively rapid and simple; no training is necessary, and there are many commercially available devices that yield reliable measurements and continuous quantitative data (Kinnard and Watzman 1966; Robbins 1977; Reiter and Mac-Phail 1979). Motor activity has been studied extensively in both behavioral pharmacology and behavioral toxicology, and these studies have indicated that it is sensitive to the effects of a wide variety of agents (e.g., Dews 1953; Fibiger and Campbell 1971; Vasko, Lutz, and Domino 1974; Silverman and Williams 1975; Waldeck 1975).

Operant Behavior

Schedule-controlled operant behavior has been used widely in both behavioral pharmacology (Thompson and Schuster 1968; Harvey 1971; McMillan and Leander 1976) and, more recently, behavioral toxicology (Weiss and Laties 1975; Geller, Stebbins, and Wayner 1979). It is used by all of the federal laboratories concerned with behavioral effects of chemicals and drugs (EPA, NIEHS, NIOSH, and FDA), and its use has been endorsed by three committees of the NAS (for EPA, 1975; for CPSC, 1977; and for the National Toxicology Program [NTP], 1982).

There are many reasons why schedule-controlled operant behavior is both heuristically and empirically valuable:

1. Operant behavior, as behavior modified by its consequences, is a broad biological phenomenon critical for the adaptation and long-term survival of individuals and their species.

2. Tests of schedule-controlled behavior allow the reliable and quantitative examination of the effects of substances on behavior (Dews 1972; Thompson and Boren 1977).

3. The extensive literature on operant behavior provides a conceptual framework for analysis of behavior effects (Thompson and Boren 1977).

4. Simpler procedures, such as unconditioned reflexes or motor activity, measure different aspects of behavior.

5. Operant conditioning allows the experimenter to tailor the behavior to the needs of the experiment (e.g., to examine the effects of a substance on a variety of response rates [Laties 1978; Dews and Wenger 1979]).

6. Tests of schedule-controlled behavior have been used to evaluate the effects of a variety of chemicals: metals (Evans, Laties, and Weiss 1975); solvents (Colotla et al. 1979; Glowa 1981; Wood, Rees, and Laties 1983); anoxic agents (Laties and

Merigan 1979); and pesticides (Dietz and McMillan 1979a, 1979b; Reiter et al. 1981).

The extent of the need for testing of industrial chemicals has recently been emphasized by a group that assessed the toxicity-testing needs for substances to which there is known or anticipated human exposure (NAS 1984). They identified a select universe of chemicals consisting of a wide variety of those used in commerce, food additives, cosmetic ingredients, and pesticides and inert ingredients. A set of reference protocol guidelines was established against which to determine the adequacy of existing neurobehavioral toxicity evaluation. These guidelines included neuropathologic evaluation and functional evaluation of both unconditioned and conditioned behavior. Neurobehavioral toxicity evaluation was the area of greatest testing need in two categories: pesticides and inert ingredients in pesticide formulations, and cosmetic ingredients. For food additives and for three separate categories of chemicals in commerce, neurobehavioral toxicity evaluation ranked in the top five areas of greatest testing need.

Much concern has been expressed that the adoption of strictly prescribed test procedures might not protect the public health and might retard the growth of an interesting toxicological literature (e.g., Weiss and Laties 1979). From our perspective, it is striking how few chemicals have been subjected to *any* systematic behavioral study. The adoption of general procedural guidelines to allow more chemicals to be tested in a similar fashion can only enhance the potential of behavioral toxicology to aid in public-health decision making.

Application of Test Guidelines to Research Needs

Two applications of these guidelines would be of greatest help to toxicologists in evaluating new and existing industrial chemicals. First, screening information on parent compounds of different chemical classes would aid in identifying classes of chemicals with the potential to produce adverse behavioral effects and would alert toxicologists to look very closely at any new chemical belonging to one of the potentially toxic classes. Second, more information on the effect of subchronic or chronic exposure to chemicals known to have no or only transient acute effects is needed. Studies in these areas would have much more utility to the regulatory scientist than the development of increasingly "sensitive" behavioral endpoints to study popular, well-characterized behavioral toxicants.

The functional-observational-battery and motor-activity guidelines can also be used to study behavioral teratogens. However, the area of behavioral teratology offers interpretive challenges to the regulatory scientist. For the regulator, there are two situations in which special risk analyses must be done for the developing organism because analyses based on the adult will not be valid. The first concerns those agents that exert long-term behavioral effects following prenatal or neonatal exposure owing to an irreversible toxic effect of the agent on the developing nervous system. These effects may be qualitatively different from the behavioral effects of such agents in the adult. The second concerns agents that are concentrated by the fetus such that exposure is much higher than would be predicted on the basis of adult data (see also chapter 7).

In order to determine whether either of these situations exists for a chemical of concern, additional data should be collected in the course of behavioral teratology testing. First, an internal dose should be determined for both the adult (for example, the dam) and the offspring. If the doses are comparable, a more careful behavioral analysis of the dam should reveal whether she shows behavioral toxicity at dose levels affecting the fetus. Often, a detailed behavioral study done in the offspring is compared to cursory observation of the mother. If the doses are not comparable—for instance, if the fetus concentrates the toxin as happens with methylmercury—then comparison of behavioral toxicity should be made between adults and fetuses with comparable *internal* doses. Kinetic determinations are also important in the neonatal period to determine whether developmental delays reflect residual exposure to the agent in the neonatal period. These data, in combination with the data on chemical classes discussed earlier, would help us to predict which new chemical agents should be subjected to behavioral teratology testing in addition to adult testing.

It is often stated in behavioral teratology papers and proposals that the developing nervous system is particularly vulnerable to toxic insult. We must take greater care to determine when this is indeed the case and distinguish this situation from those where neonatal exposure leads to behavioral toxicity qualitatively and quantitatively similar to that of the adult.

Summary

Behavioral effects are important in evaluating toxicity. Behavior has been the basis of many exposure standards; the validity of behavioral testing has long been established; and a series of government committees have endorsed and defined uses of behavioral testing.

We have described the basic steps involved in regulatory decision making and the aspects of behavior most relevant to these decisions. We have also described how behavioral data are evaluated and the types of behavioral test guidelines developed to support the recommendation of behavioral testing. Finally, we have suggested areas of research that we feel would be most helpful in providing scientific support for regulatory decisions.

Acknowledgments

The authors wish to acknowledge the unique perspective of Dr. Ronald Wood, whose suggestions contributed materially to this chapter. We also wish to thank Dr. Victor Laties for his helpful comments on the manuscript and Bobbe Ward for her assistance in preparing the manuscript. This chapter represents the opinions of the authors. No official support or endorsement by the U.S. Environmental Protection Agency of the opinions expressed is intended or should be inferred.

References

Anastasi, A. 1976. *Psychological testing*. 4th ed. New York: Macmillan.
Anger, W. K. 1984. Neurobehavioral testing of chemicals: Impact on recommended standards. *Neurobehav. Toxicol. Teratol.* 6:147–53.
Bignami, G.; Roxic, N.; Michalek, M.; Milsevic, M.; and Gatti, G. L. 1975. Behavioral toxicity of anticholinesterase agents. In *Behavioral toxicology*, 155–215. *See* Weiss and Laties 1975.

Byers, R. K., and Lord, E. E. 1943. Late effects of lead poisoning on mental development. *Am. J. Dis. Child* 66:471–94.

Colotla, V. A.; Bautista, M.; Lorenzana-Jimenez, M.; and Rodriguez, R. 1979. Effects of solvents on schedule-controlled behavior. In *Test methods for definition of effects of toxic substances on behavior and neuromotor function*, 113–18. *See* Geller, Stebbins, and Wayner 1979.

Dews, P. B. 1953. The measurement of the influence of drugs on voluntary activity in mice. *Brit. J. Pharmacol. Chemother.* 8:46–48.

———. 1972. Assessing the effects of drugs. In *Methods in psychobiology,* edited by R. D. Myers, 2:83–124. New York: Academic Press.

Dews, P. B., and Wenger, G. R. 1979. Testing for behavioral effects of agents. In *Test methods for definition of effects of toxic substances on behavior and neuromotor function*, 119–27. *See* Geller, Stebbins, and Wayner 1979.

Dietz, D. D., and McMillan, D. E. 1979a. Comparative effects of Mirex and Kepone on schedule-controlled behavior in the rat: I. Multiple fixed-ratio 12 fixed-interval 2-min schedule. *Neurotoxicology* 1:369–85.

———. 1979b. Comparative effects of Mirex and Kepone on schedule-controlled behavior in the rat: II. Space-responding, fixed-ratio, and unsignalled avoidance schedules. *Neurotoxicology* 1:387–402.

Evans, H. E.; Laties, V. G.; and Weiss, B. 1975. Behavioral effects of mercury and methyl mercury. *Fed. Proc. Am. Soc. Exp. Biol.* 34:1858–67.

Fibiger, H. C., and Campbell, B. A. 1971. The effect of parachlorophenylalanine on spontaneous locomotor activity in the rat. *Neuropharmacology* 10:25–32.

Fisher, F. 1980. Neurotoxicology and government regulation of chemicals in the United States. In *Experimental and clinical neurotoxicology*, 874–82. *See* Spencer and Schaumburg 1980.

Geller, I.; Stebbins, W. C.; and Wayner, M. J. 1979. *Test methods for definition of effects of toxic substances on behavior and neuromotor function. Neurobehav. Toxicol.* 1, suppl. 1.

Glowa, J. R. 1981. Some effects of sub-acute exposure to toluene on schedule-controlled behavior. *Neurobehav. Toxicol. Teratol.* 3:463–65.

Harvey, J. A., ed. 1971. *Behavioral analysis of drug action: Research and commentary.* Glenview, Ill.: Scott, Foresman.

Ison, J. R., and Hoffman, H. S. 1983. Reflex modification in the domain of startle: II. The anomalous history of a robust and ubiquitous phenomenon. *Psychol. Bull.* 94:3–17.

Jaffe, J. 1975. Drug addiction and drug abuse. In *The pharmacological basis of therapeutics,* edited by L. Goodman and A. Gilman, 284–324. 5th ed. New York: Macmillan.

Kinnard, E. J., and Watzman, N. 1966. Techniques utilized in the evaluation of psychotropic drugs on animal activity. *J. Pharmacol. Sci.* 55:995–1012.

Klaasen, C. D. 1975. Absorption, distribution and excretion of toxicants. In *Toxicology: The basic science of poisons,* edited by L. J. Caserett and J. Doull, 26–44. New York: Macmillan.

Kushner, L. M.; Wands, R. C.; and Fong, V. 1983. *The potential use of the ADI in superfund implementation.* Unpublished report, MTR-83W16. McLean, Va.: MITRE Corporation. EPA Contract No. 68-02-3660.

Lashley, K. S. 1929. *Brain mechanisms and intelligence.* Chicago: University of Chicago Press.

Laties, V. G. 1978. How operant conditioning can contribute to behavioral toxicology. *Environ. Health Perspect.* 26:29–35.

Laties, V. G., and Merigan, W. H. 1979. Behavioral effects of carbon monoxide on animals and man. *Annu. Rev. Pharmacol. Toxicol.* 19:357–92.

McMillan, D. E., and Leander, J. D. 1976. Effects of drugs on schedule-controlled behavior. In *Behavioral pharmacology,* edited by S. D. Glick and J. Goldfarb, 85–139. St. Louis: C. V. Mosby.

Morgan, J. P., and Penovich, P. 1978. Jamaica ginger paralysis. *Arch. Neurol.* 35:350.

National Academy of Sciences (NAS). 1975. *Principles for evaluating chemicals in the environment.* Washington, D.C.

NAS. 1977. *Principles and procedures for evaluating the toxicity of household substances.* Washington, D.C.

———. 1983. *Risk assessment in the federal government: Managing the process.* Washington, D.C.

———. 1984. *Toxicity testing: Strategies to determine needs and priorities.* Washington, D.C.

Occupational Safety and Health Administration (OSHA). 1974. *Subpart Z—toxic and hazardous substances.* CFR 1910.1000.

Reiter, L. W. 1978. Use of activity measures in behavioral toxicology. *Environ. Health Perspect.* 26:9–20.

Reiter, L. W., and MacPhail, R. C. 1979. Motor activity: A survey of methods with potential use in toxicity testing. *Neurobehav. Toxicol.* 1, suppl. 1:53–66.

Reiter, L. W.; MacPhail, R. C.; Ruppert, P. H.; and Eckerman, D. A. 1981. Animal models of toxicity: Some comparative data on the sensitivity of behavioral tests. In *Proceedings of the eleventh conference on environmental toxicology,* 11–23. AFAMRL-TR-80-125. Springfield, Va.: National Technical Information Services.

Ricci, P. F., and Molton, L. S. 1981. Risk and benefit in environmental law. *Science* 214:1096–1100.

Robbins, T. W. 1977. A critique of the methods available for the measurement of spontaneous motor activity. In *Handbook of psychopharmacology,* edited by L. L. Iversen, S. D. Iversen, and S. H. Snyder, 7:37–82. New York: Plenum Press.

Silverman, A. P., and Williams, H. 1975. Behaviour of rats exposed to trichloroethylene vapour. *Br. J. Ind. Med.* 32:308–15.

Spencer, P. S., and Schaumburg, H. H., eds. 1980. *Experimental and clinical neurotoxicology.* Baltimore: Williams & Wilkins.

Thompson, T., and Boren, J. J. 1977. Operant behavioral pharmacology. In *Handbook of operant behavior,* edited by W. K. Honig and J. E. R. Staddon, 540–69. Englewood Cliffs, N.J.: Prentice-Hall.

Thompson, T., and Schuster, C. R. 1968. *Behavioral pharmacology.* Englewood Cliffs, N.J.: Prentice-Hall.

U.S. Congress. 1976. *Toxic substances control act.* 94th Cong. Public Law 94-469.

U.S. Environmental Protection Agency (USEPA). 1983. *Health effects test guidelines.* EPA 560/6-83-001. PB 83-257691. Springfield, Va.: National Technical Information Services.

Vasko, M. R.; Lutz, M. P., and Domino, E. F. 1974. Structure-activity relations of some idolealkylamines in comparison to phenethylamines on motor activity and acquisition of avoidance behavior. *Psychopharmacology* 36:49–58.

Waldeck, B. 1975. On the interaction between caffeine and barbiturates with respect to locomotor activity and brain catecholamines. *Acta Pharmacol. Toxicol.* 36:172–80.

Weiss, B., and Laties, V. G., eds. 1975. *Behavioral toxicology.* New York: Plenum Press.

Weiss, B., and Laties, V. G. 1979. Assays for behavioral toxicology: A strategy for the Environmental Protection Agency. In *Test methods for definition of effects of toxic substances on behavior and neuromotor function,* 213–15. *See* Geller, Stebbins, and Wayner 1979.

Wood, R. W.; Rees, D. C.; and Laties, V. G. 1983. Behavioral effects of toluene are modulated by stimulus control. *Toxicol. Appl. Pharmacol.* 68:462–72.

Zbinden, G. 1973. *Progress in toxicology: Special topics,* 12:8–18. New York: Springer-Verlag.

18

Design and Analytical Methods

Behavioral toxicology places stringent requirements on design and analysis because the costs to society of research decisions are high. Thus, the highest standards of validity and reliability must be met if the effects of most interest, those near the threshold, are to be detected. Since behavioral effects are typically small, subtle responses, the appropriate application of experimental design and statistical analysis is of paramount importance to this field. Behavioral toxicology has been recognized as a distinct field for approximately two decades. Therefore, it is not surprising that most research is compound-oriented. This has often been at the expense of the development and application of sound study design and analysis strategies. It is hoped that this work will serve as a resource survey of available methods.

Gad (1982) discussed five types of data: observational scores, response rates, error rates, times to endpoints, and teratology/reproduction data. Based on a review of procedures used in existing articles and the scale of measurement involved, Gad suggested analysis methods for each type of data. Weil (1982) and Gad and Weil (1982) reiterated this position. The latter article gave detailed accounts of many specific data analysis methods for toxicology data, including recommendations for the widespread use of *nonparametric* statistics. The concern for matching data type to analysis method is commendable, and related papers appeared in supplement 5 (1982) of the *Archives of Toxicology*.

Mitchell and Tilson (1982) discussed problems and research needs in behavioral toxicology. They included some treatment of certain statistical problems. They described the present widespread practice of conducting many statistical tests on data from a single, small set of subjects. Both Type I error rate (false positive decisions) and Type II error rate (false negative decisions) are thereby usually inflated. They suggested looking for internal consistency and avoiding taking any single results too seriously. Similar advice was provided by Gad and Weil (1982) in their distinction between statistical and biological significance.

The need to control error rates dominates design and analysis recommendations made here. The goal is to provide techniques in which statistical and biological significance coincide. Such thinking motivated earlier articles on the topic. Muller, Otto, and Benignus (1983) focused on the issues in the context of psychophysiological research. The present common practice of conducting many tests may lead to nonreplicable findings. Muller, Barton, and Benignus (1984) provided recommendations for statistical practice sufficient to solve the problems. Their suggestions are described in detail below.

Valciukas and Lilis (1980) discussed psychometric techniques in environmental research. They focused on studies of human exposures in the work environment rather than in the laboratory. Such work involves epidemiological concerns for sample formation, control variables, and the difficulty of causal inference in observational studies. It entails problems different from those encountered in experimental laboratory research.

Basic Concepts

Some Useful Statistical Ideas

All variables can be considered to be nominal, ordinal, interval, or ratio scales of measurement, a classification generally credited to Stevens (1951). A nominal (or *categorical*) scale has values that indicate only group membership, such as species, with possible values dog, cat, and rat. Ordinal-scale numeric values indicate ranking of the objects, such as symphony number. An interval scale has numeric values that in addition allow meaningful comparison among and between differences (intervals), for example, degrees Celsius. A ratio scale has numeric values for which ratios of values are meaningful and can be thought of as an interval scale with a true zero. This allows comparison of ratios of values. A good example is degrees Kelvin. More generally, each scale has the properties of all scales listed before it.

Variables also can be classified according to their role in a data analysis. The outcome measure is often called the *response* variable. In turn, the treatment or potentially correlated variable is often called the *predictor* variable. Important special cases are *dependent* and *independent* variables, respectively. The latter two terms are often reserved for situations in which random assignment to treatment has occurred. A variable that is important but not of central interest is often called a *control* or *nuisance* variable. More specialized terms are *covariate* and *confounder*, whose distinction depends on the analysis and field of study.

In some analyses it is important to classify predictor and control variables as either *fixed* or *random*. Such variables are said to be random if the values are sampled from an infinite population of values and then assigned to subjects (observational units). Predictor or control variables whose values are assigned by nature (that is, they come with the subject) or chosen by the scientist are fixed. The distinction implies different analyses in many cases and also affects the generality of conclusions that may be properly drawn.

Certain simple ideas about sets and their properties are useful in discussing study design and analysis. For the purposes of this paper, a *set* may be taken to be any collection of elements of interest, which are members of the set. One set is a *subset* of another if every member of the first is a member of the second. A *population* is any set of interest. Usually the term describes some set of humans or animals of sufficient scope and/or importance to demand attention. A *sample* is any subset of a population, whether or not the selection rule is well founded. A *parameter* is any property of a population, and a *statistic* is any property of a sample.

The two activities of statistics are parameter estimation and hypothesis testing. Both are based on probability theory, which is a collection of methods for evaluat-

Table 18.1 Decision outcomes in hypothesis testing

True State of Nature	Decision	
	H_0: No Difference	H_A: Difference
H_0: No difference	Correct negative $(1 - \alpha)$	False positive (α), Type I error
H_A: Difference	False negative (β), Type II error	Correct positive $(1 - \beta)$

ing the likelihood of occurrence of events (statistics), given assumptions about a population and rules for sampling. Estimation (of a parameter) provides a value, the *estimator,* which is a statistic (a property of a sample) thought to be a good estimate of a parameter (a property of a population). Goodness of estimation can be defined in many ways depending on the nature of the parameter. Estimators that satisfy particular criteria are described as, for example, least squares or maximum likelihood.

Hypothesis testing consists in estimating the likelihood of a statement about a parameter's being true. The statement is often called H_0, the null hypothesis, since it often corresponds to some parameter's, such as a difference in means, being zero. The competing hypothesis is specified to be mutually exclusive (and usually exhaustive) and is H_A, the alternative hypothesis. In testing a hypothesis, one evaluates a significance level (p value), which is an estimate of a probability. The p value is a statistic itself, therefore, and may be a good or a bad estimator.

If a decision is made as to whether the hypothesis is true, based on the p value, then one of four outcomes must occur (see table 18.1). In behavioral toxicology a null hypothesis usually corresponds to a compound's not being a toxicant, and the alternative hypothesis corresponds to a compound's being a toxicant. In this context, a Type I error is deciding that a compound is toxic when it is not. The probability of such a false positive decision is usually called α. A false negative, a Type II error, arises if a compound that is toxic is declared nontoxic. It is customary to call the probability of a Type II error β. In turn, the probability of a correct decision is either $1 - \alpha$ or $1 - \beta$, depending on the true state of nature. The probability of a correct decision, $1 - \beta$, is often referred to as the power of a test. It is simply the chance of declaring a difference when in fact a true difference exists, such as declaring a compound nontoxic when it is toxic. This interpretation of hypothesis testing stems from a classical frequentist interpretation of probability and decision making. Alternate models of hypothesis testing are preferred by some statisticians, the most popular being a Bayesian approach (see Bickel and Doksum 1977, sec. 2.4, for an introduction to the Bayesian approach).

The above discussion of decision making must be extended in order to accurately describe the practice of using multiple tests in behavioral toxicology. Type I and Type II error rates must be discussed in two important situations: (1) many tests on a single set of data and (2) a number of independent sets of data all of which address the same compound's toxicity. The former situation arises naturally in behavioral toxicology in situations in which many dependent variables are measured on the same set of subjects. If a separate analysis is done for each, as is usually the case, then each gives rise to a hypothesis test of toxicity. Furthermore, an analysis of a particular variable may involve more than one test of toxicity, or methods of exploratory data analysis may lead to many tests. Elementary probability theory can describe the possible consequences of such repeated testing (see Hoel, Port, and Stone 1971). If the probability of a Type I error for a single test is α, then the Bonferroni inequality states that for any k tests the probability of one or more Type I errors for the set of tests is $p \leq k\alpha$. This can be a very conservative bound if the tests overlap a great deal. If, however, the tests are statistically independent, then $p = 1 - (1 - \alpha)^k$. The Bonferroni inequality is quite accurate for independent or nearly independent tests and small α and/or small k. This problem is widely recognized as the reason to conduct a single analysis of variance rather than a collection of many t-tests (Kirk 1968).

The Bonferroni inequality suggests a simple strategy for controlling error rate for any set of hypotheses. If one conducts each test at the α/k level, with k being the number of tests, then one can be assured that the overall error rate is at most the level sought, α. Abt (1981) discussed this application of the Bonferroni inequality in hypothesis testing. Unfortunately, application of the Bonferroni inequality by itself may lead to research with little sensitivity to true differences as a result of Type II error–rate inflation. The goal of the design solutions to be discussed below, therefore, is to provide both α control and β control simultaneously.

Applications of combining significance tests from independent sets of data occur naturally in review articles and in the formulation of regulatory standards. Littell and Folks (1971) reviewed combining significance tests. An important example is a technique known in epidemiology as *stratified analysis*. Assume, for example, that one tests a hypothesis separately in the male population and the female population. Such methods are usually preferable only when a single overall analysis is not available. Rosenthal (1978, 1979, 1980, 1982) provided introductions to many issues in combining tests and meta-analysis. In meta-analysis one usually attempts to estimate the strength of an effect, as well as the presence or absence of an effect. This goes beyond the goal of simply combining p values in order to provide a single decision (see also Rosenthal and Rubin 1979; Cooper and Rosenthal 1980; Hsu 1980; Hedges 1982; and Kraemer and Andrews 1982).

Research Questions in Behavioral Toxicology

Three research questions may be posed in behavioral toxicology. The most basic is whether or not a particular compound is toxic. Only after clearly establishing that an effect exists at some level is it sensible to consider the question of the dose-effect curve, although this argument admittedly assumes a monotone increasing dose-response function and a single response. One should not confuse results from two different responses, since they need not be affected similarly by the same compound. Only after establishing a dose-effect relationship is it sensible to attack the question of mechanism. Behavioral toxicologists should not lose sight of the ordering of these three goals and their relationship to a particular study goal.

Types of Research

Research strategies may be conveniently divided into experimental, quasi-experimental, and observational. The most common type in behavioral toxicology is the true *experiment*, a term reserved for a study in which subjects have been randomly assigned to treatments. The importance of the random-assignment assumption cannot be overemphasized, because it eliminates the need to consider most nuisance variables and permits causal inference. Without random assignment, it is less certain that all nuisance variables have been either eliminated from consideration or properly controlled.

The second type of research, quasi-experimental, has come to be associated with the names Campbell and Stanley (1963). A quasi experiment is characterized by some strategy of assignment of subjects to treatments other than true random assignment. An example of such a design would be a case in which one of two factories received equipment to clean the air and the other did not, the workers at both factories being measured both before and after the introduction of the equipment. Such research constitutes both toxicology and epidemiology.

The third type of research is the observational study (or survey). Most commonly, this type of research is retrospective, looking backward in time. It may also be prospective, collecting data in a planned fashion starting at a fixed point in time. Behavioral toxicology observational studies have been conducted in neighborhoods where contamination from toxic waste was suspected.

All types of studies can be conducted either in a field or a laboratory setting. The classification of a particular study depends not on where data are collected but on how. The most important characteristic is the method of assignment of subjects to treatments. Most commonly, field studies are surveys, and laboratory studies are experiments. The least defensible results are therefore collected in conditions that make them seem most important to someone outside the field. Some relevant references are Kleinbaum, Kupper, and Morgenstern (1982), an excellent survey of methods in epidemiology; Anastasi (1968), a review of tests and measurements at an applied level; and Lord and Novick (1968), a theoretical description of testing.

Design Methods

In order to evaluate design methods, study purposes and design pitfalls are reviewed below. Then five solution strategies are described that can help produce a correct decision about a potential toxicant. The five strategies are (1) top-down planning, (2) designing efficient experiments, (3) balancing α and β in choosing hypotheses, (4) selecting hypotheses for confirmatory analysis, and (5) using appropriate statistical-analysis methods.

Study Purpose

The purpose for any part of a study may be classified as (1) methods development, (2) confirmatory analysis, or (3) exploratory analysis. A study entirely committed to testing and evaluating methodology is commonly known as a pilot study. Since during a pilot study methods may be changed in an attempt to improve them for subsequent work, it usually cannot be published. A pilot study is required if a data-collection protocol has not been used previously. Attempting to avoid conducting a pilot study simply leads to the planned experiment's first few subjects' becoming pilot subjects.

A confirmatory analysis is one designed to confirm or deny a hypothesis. All hypothesis tests must have been specified exactly, and α fixed a priori. This implies restrictions on the scientist: (1) none of the data can be known to the scientist before the tests are fixed, (2) a fixed design and analysis must be used, and (3) no transformation of any variable or additional tests are allowed.

Violation of any of the criteria for a confirmatory analysis requires that the analysis be considered exploratory (Mulaik 1972; Muller, Otto, and Benignus 1983). Since an analysis is considered to be exploratory if any part of it is exploratory, all reasonable analyses in an exploratory analysis should be encouraged; this is sometimes called data snooping. The distinction between exploratory and confirmatory research is the approach to data analysis and thus may be applied when appropriate to the entire set of analyses for a single study.

Methods development, confirmatory analysis, and exploratory analysis are all valid study purposes. All three can be mixed in any single study, although they are usually spread among a series of studies. The design and analysis methods discussed here are intended to help allocate efforts toward these purposes among and within studies and to promote accurate reporting of what has actually occurred.

Design Pitfalls

Three specific problems tend to inflate Type I error rate: (1) the existence of many dependent variables, (2) the existence of many tests on a variable, and (3) data snooping. The first problem tends to arise because it is less expensive to perform multiple tests on one subject than to perform each test on a separate subject. Depending upon the analysis, many tests may be conducted for a single variable and yield the same problem. Data snooping tends to inflate Type I error rate in a less obvious way. First, exploratory analysis usually includes many different tests of the same hypothesis. Second, exploratory analysis tends to capitalize on chance by searching for the maximum difference. Any time a choice is made based upon the smallest p value by (1) comparing different transformations of the independent or dependent variables, (2) comparing subsets of many dependent variables, or (3) selecting a subset of many independent variables, then exploratory analysis has occurred. The inflation of α increases as the amount of exploratory analysis increases.

A second set of design problems leads to inflated β, Type II error rate, which results in a lack of power. The best-known reasons for a lack of power are too small a sample size and inadequate control of error in the laboratory. Interest in small effects, choosing the wrong dependent measure, and choosing a low-power testing method can also inflate Type II error rate. Finally, a conscientious scientist's controlling α through the use of a Bonferroni correction while testing many hypotheses may also inflate β. The solution strategies discussed below all help resolve the antagonism between Type I and Type II error control.

Top-Down Planning

Top-down planning has received great attention in the fields of computer-programming (Yourdon 1979; Yourdon and Constantine 1979; Williams 1981) and research-data management (Muller, Christiansen, and Smith 1981). Top-down planning will be applied first to planning a single study and later to planning a series of studies. The top-down-planning process comprises five steps: (1) specify the experimental questions of interest; (2) specify testable hypotheses implied by the questions; (3) specify target analyses, based on the hypotheses, in sufficient detail to determine the computations giving significance levels and estimates of effect size; (4) determine which data are needed to compute the target analyses; and (5) specify the data-collection protocol for generating the raw data. The reversal from the usual planning approach helps avoid discovering that only bad data-analysis alternatives exist at the completion of a study.

Appropriate Design

Six different design approaches are compared here (see table 18.2), with the goal of providing maximum information at minimum cost prior to specifying confirmatory data-analysis hypotheses. Two approaches to avoid are the one-shot confirmatory study and the standard study (or boiler-plate) study. The recommended approaches are all sequences of studies: (1) exploratory then confirmatory, (2) sequential split sample, (3) simultaneous split sample, and (4) leapfrog series. All four recommended approaches allow accurate estimates of p values and provide excellent sensitivity by separating confirmatory and exploratory analyses. The choice of design controls the amount and type of information that can be gathered for a fixed amount of effort and laboratory planning.

An example of a one-shot confirmatory study would be the investigation of a compound not studied previously using a response variable that has not been tested. Although the amount of time to completion is short, the likelihood of guessing properly as to paradigm and choice of response variables is very low, and choice of sample size is necessarily strictly a guess.

Standard studies are a common part of toxicity screening, and standardized batteries of response measures have been developed for physiological responses such as carcinogenicity. Whether a battery of behavioral toxicity tests should or can be created continues to be debated. From a design perspective, such a study has many of the same disadvantages as a one-shot confirmatory study, because its inflexibility disallows the refinement of protocol and analysis that is the nature of science. Despite that, the pressure to screen the large number of new compounds produced every year will probably force the creation of a screening battery.

The simplest and most common sequential study design involves a pilot study followed by a confirmatory study. This sequence allows modification and refinement of methods in the pilot, followed by planned analyses conducted on the confirmatory study data. With a slight amount of additional work, the two study sequences can be improved substantially, since in a pilot study enough subjects usually are tested to allow simple exploratory analysis. Two large benefits accrue. First, different dependent variables can be examined for sensitivity, but only large effects should be used to modify the planning of the confirmatory study. Second, estimates of variability and treatment differences can be obtained from the pilot study and used to estimate the sample size needed to achieve the power sought. In univariate analysis, power methods are almost always available for almost any kind of response variable. For regression and analysis of variance, important references include Cohen (1977), Koele (1982), O'Brien (1982), and Muller and Peterson (1983, 1984). Cohen's book is highly recommended as easily accessible to the practicing scientist. Pilot-study data should also be used to examine whether the assumptions of the planned data analysis are met by the data. An important example is the evaluation of whether the variables are normally distributed, an important assumption in many analyses.

The second multiple-study approach consists of an exploratory study preceding a confirmatory study. A sample of data is collected under a fixed protocol and analyzed in a thoroughly exploratory fashion. Such results, of course, are not

Table 18.2 Study performance ratings

Study Sequence	Refine Methods	Select Variables and Hypotheses	Select Analysis Techniques	Detect Small Differences	Determine Sample Size	Minimize Time Required	Gain Information
			Characteristics				
One-shot confirmatory	--	--	--	-	--	+	-
Standard	++	-		-	.	++	-
Pilot then confirmatory	+	++	+	++	++	-	+
Exploratory then confirmatory	--	+	+	+	+	+	
Sequential split sample	--	+	+	+	--		
Simultaneous split sample	--	++	++	++	++	--	
Leapfrog series	++	++	++	++	++		++

Source: Muller, Barton, and Benignus 1984. Reprinted by permission of the publisher.

Note: -- represents the worst ratings, and ++ the best. Only ordinal information is included. A specific application may radically alter the assessments of the designs.

published. Method changes can be made for the subsequent study. Furthermore, sample-size calculations can be performed, and choices of dependent variables, independent variables, transformations of variables, and analysis method can be completed before the second study is begun.

A third recommended strategy is a sequential-split-sample design. A sequential split sample proceeds in a manner similar to the exploratory-confirmatory sequence, with the important difference that in a sequential-split-sample design both samples' data must be collected under exactly the same protocol. Hence, data collection for the second sample can proceed while exploratory data analysis is being conducted on the first sample's data, thus saving a great deal of time. The disadvantages are that methods cannot be changed as a function of knowledge gained in the exploratory study, and sample-size calculations are difficult to complete in time to be useful. People involved in doing the exploratory data analysis must remain completely blind to the data from the second sample. Any subsequent change in the analysis of the second sample, as well as any analysis involving data from both samples, is necessarily exploratory.

A recommended split-sample technique that has long been used in psychometric testing (Mosier 1951) is cross validation. It usually involves two samples of equal size. First, a sample of data is collected. Subjects are then randomly assigned to one of two samples, one used for exploratory analysis and the other reserved for confirmatory analysis. Usually the majority of subjects are included in the confirmatory sample in order to ensure at least as much power for confirmatory analysis. The fraction allocated to exploratory analysis can be as little as one-tenth. Factors in the decision include the total sample size, the number of variables, the purpose of the study, the types of analyses, and how much exploratory analysis is planned. Advantages over a sequential split sample include greater control over nuisance variables such as method drift, subjection-population drift, and seasonal effects. As with the sequential split sample, the main disadvantage is the inability to modify experimental methods after the exploratory analysis. Furthermore, sample-size calculations cannot be done to modify the confirmatory sample size to be collected.

The most important and useful method to be discussed is a leapfrog series (Muller, Otto, and Benignus 1983), an approach that attempts to formalize the natural iterative refinement of knowledge inherent in the scientific approach. The key feature is the inclusion of both exploratory and confirmatory work in the same study, with all confirmatory analyses fixed a priori and only confirmatory analyses published. A leapfrog series capitalizes on the fact that a laboratory usually conducts a series of studies on a compound.

A typical leapfrog sequence begins with a pilot study to collect enough data to allow some exploratory analysis of the pilot data (see fig. 18.1). Based on the pilot results, a small amount of confirmatory analysis is planned for the subsequent study, which is conducted and appropriately reported. Efficiency gains are realized from using the same data set for any exploratory analysis of interest and from collecting any measures of potential interest as long as they do not interfere with the planned confirmatory variables. The exploratory variables and results are not reported unless they are *all* negative, but are used to determine the design and analysis plan for the next study. As for the first study, many exploratory analyses are planned and conducted but not reported, a few confirmatory hypotheses are

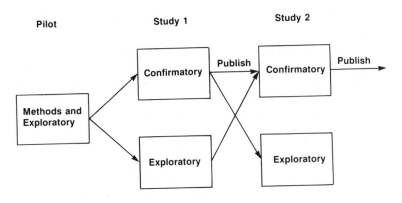

Fig. 18.1 The typical leapfrog study sequence

planned and conducted, and results of the preceding study are used for power analysis. The sequence can be continued, iteratively refining knowledge in leapfrog fashion through a series of studies.

One must take care that no data from a study are used to choose any aspect of a test if that test is to be considered to be confirmatory. This places a burden on the scientist to ensure the validity of reports. Of course, any confirmatory analysis can be followed by as many unreported exploratory analyses as are interesting. Exploratory data analysis can be published if two conditions are met: first, the results from a study must be all nonsignificant; second, sufficient power analysis must be done on the data to indicate that nontrivial interesting differences would have been detected with high probability. Taken together, these two conditions ensure that Type I errors are impossible and Type II errors are improbable.

The most important feature of the leapfrog strategy is that it allows controlling Type I error rates while still providing high power. Furthermore, the natural process of refining methods and hypotheses between studies is exploited with little additional work. Table 18.2 compares these characteristics of the leapfrog and the other five study types described.

Balancing α and β

Three methods exist to minimize Type I error rate. They include (1) using the appropriate aggregate analysis method, (2) using the Bonferroni correction (if an appropriate aggregate method is not available), and (3) reducing the number of tests (in the absence of a Bonferroni correction). An important example of an aggregate method rather than a collection of simpler methods is an analysis of variance in lieu of a collection of t-tests. Simplifying a design by removing factors and eliminating dependent variables reduces the number of tests. This must be done a priori to a confirmatory analysis, based on an earlier study.

Five basic single study methods are available for decreasing Type II error rate (increasing power) without increasing α: (1) observing a larger sample, (2) limiting error variance, (3) limiting interest to large effects, (4) reducing the number of tests in the presence of a Bonferroni correction, and (5) selecting a set of nonoverlapping dependent variables. Considering larger treatment effects is relevant to the discussion of research questions (i.e., Is there an effect? versus What is the dose-effect curve? versus What is the mechanism?). If the goal is simply to detect toxicity, then the use of fewer larger doses will almost always be strongly preferred because it should provide more power. Of course, if the dose-response function is not monotone, then this conclusion may not hold. Reducing the number of tests in the presence of a Bonferroni correction can dramatically increase power. Often this will simply mean designating analysis of one or more dependent variables exploratory rather than confirmatory, thereby dividing α by a smaller number. The price is that the exploratory analysis should not be published.

Selecting Hypotheses for Confirmatory Analyses

Selecting hypotheses for confirmatory analysis of a single study in order to balance Type I and Type II error rates can be very frustrating. Removing some hypotheses from confirmatory status increases the power for those remaining but reduces the power to zero for those excluded, since the exploratory results will not be published. With a Bonferroni correction, of course, Type I error rate can always be controlled, although including more tests almost always reduces power.

Multiple-analysis design involving more than one study resolves this dilemma. The most likely candidate tests yield confirmatory tests immediately, and interesting but less likely candidate tests are included in confirmatory analysis of the next study if exploratory analysis of them indicates that they should be. Great power is achieved for the most likely candidates, and responsive tests are not likely to be missed.

Five criteria should be used in selecting hypotheses for confirmatory analysis: (1) the smallness of the exploratory-analysis p value, which is implicitly a power calculation; (2) the scientific importance of an effect of the size observed; (3) the scientific interpretability of the exploratory result; (4) the scientific importance of the dependent variable involved; and (5) the uniqueness of the dependent variable relative to other candidate dependent variables. Choosing a set of confirmatory hypotheses from the results of exploratory analysis based on these criteria is much easier than selecting confirmatory hypotheses for a one-shot study. Usually, if any of the criteria are met singly by a hypothesis, it probably deserves testing at least in an unreported exploratory analysis in the next study. Typically, most variables and tests in an exploratory step will meet none of the inclusion criteria. If prior scientific preference demands that one or two variables be included in subsequent analyses, then lack of exploratory-analysis support for them may relegate them to unreported exploratory status in the subsequent study.

Analysis Methods

The final design-solution strategy is to use appropriate statistical analysis methods. No fixed rules for data analysis can be given, since it is how, rather than which, methods are applied that determines the utility of the analysis. The three most important characteristics in specifying a data-analysis method are (1) the purpose of the analysis, (2) the measurement scale of the variables involved, and (3) the distributional properties of the variables. Analysis methods are sketched separately below for categorical, ordinal, interval non-Gaussian, interval Gaussian nonlinear, interval Gaussian linear, and certain other models, and some specific comments on particular paradigms and problems are made.

Categorical Data

The analysis of purely categorical variables has seen great progress in the last two decades and can be roughly divided into small- and large-sample results. For small-sample situations many exact tests have been described for specific cases. Alternately, general approaches to hypothesis testing with categorical variables have also been described. Perhaps the most natural approach is to cast the question of relationship between a categorical response and a set of categorical predictors in such a way as to use asymptotic theory concerning general linear models (Grizzle, Starmer, and Koch 1969). (For detailed reviews of this and alternate approaches see Seigel 1956; Bradley 1968; Cox 1970; Hollander and Wolfe 1973; Kritzer 1979; and Forthofer and Lehnen 1981.) Both approaches can treat extremely general cases with a single approach. Computer programs to do the calculations conveniently are becoming widely available.

Typical behavioral toxicology laboratory research often involves samples large enough for these techniques to be appropriate. The methods are now widely used in epidemiology and survey research fields. An important analogy should be drawn to the analysis of variance: doing a large collection of chi-square tests rather than a single overall categorical data analysis is as inappropriate as doing a large collection of t-tests rather than an analysis of variance.

Ordinal Data

The term *nonparametric statistics* has come to be associated with the collection of techniques treating either categorical or ordinal scale measurements. Nonparametric tests and associated estimation theory are available for a large number of special cases of interest to behavioral toxicologists (see Seigel 1956; Bradley 1968; Hajek 1969; Cox 1970; Puri and Sen 1971; Hollander and Wolfe 1973; Bock 1975; and Lehmann 1975). The methods are mostly univariate tests, requiring the use of the Bonferroni correction if more than one dependent variable is to be analyzed. A general hypothesis-testing approach in the sense of the general linear model does exist (see Puri and Sen 1971).

Interval Non-Gaussian Data

Interval-scale data with non-Gaussian error distributions are typically treated either with nonparametric statistics or with special-purpose models assuming a particular alternate distribution function. Since the latter covers a vast range of techniques, each for a specific situation, they cannot be discussed here. Using ordinal-theory methods with non-Gaussian interval variables is often preferred. Proponents of distribution-free statistics argue that the efficiency gain of normal-theory statistics is often small. With properly done analyses, of course, the only difference can be in the power of the test. Typically, if the assumptions are not met, Type I error rate is inflated.

Many data-collection protocols lead to truly non-Gaussian data. Some situations arise in which the data appear nonnormal but are inherently normal. Important examples of the latter are data that have data-entry errors leading to *outliers* and data that when transformed by some simple, monotone transformation are normal. In many cases, simple transformations, such as the reciprocal transformation or the logarithmic transformation, lead to new metrics that are just as meaningful as the original scale. Ratio-scale data, such as toxicant concentrations, often require logarithmic transformation. If errors are proportional to the size of measurements, the transformed variable has an additive Gaussian error distribution. It would be foolish not to use the additional power of normal-theory-test statistics in this situation.

A strategy for interval-scale non-Gaussian data is to assure oneself that the process is inherently non-Gaussian first. Extreme values must be evaluated as possible data-entry or method errors, and values that are clearly impossible should be eliminated from analysis. Next consider possible transformations. If this process fails to produce Gaussian additive errors, then ordinal-theory statistics are the best alternative, unless specific methods exist. Randomization tests are becoming more attractive as computing power increases (see Bradley 1968). Note that choosing transformations is an exploratory analysis usually performed with pilot data and cannot be included as part of a study reported as confirmatory.

Interval Gaussian Data with Nonlinear Models

Until now no distinction has been made between linear and nonlinear models. The latter, more accurately described as nonlinearizable, occur naturally in considering the pharmacokinetics of toxicants and potential toxicants. This field has a rich literature (see Notari 1975; Finney 1978; and O'Flaherty 1981). Convenient and easily accessible software is now available for analyzing such inherently non-linearizable models (Gallant 1975b). Most of the techniques are univariate, although some techniques are available for certain multivariate situations (i.e., Gallant 1975a). Unfortunately, no general multivariate hypothesis-testing techniques have been validated.

Interval Gaussian Data for Linear Models

Interval-scale data with normally distributed errors are common in behavioral toxicology, although some data demand transformation to meet the normality assumption. Some version of the multivariate general linear model should be applied if a linear model is appropriate. The most underutilized method is multivariate analysis of variance (MANOVA). Excellent software and a number of texts are available (Rao 1973; Finn 1974; Harris 1975; Timm 1975). The advantage of MANOVA is its ability to control Type I error rate without the need of a Bonferroni correction. In many applications MANOVA can provide more power than a collection of Bonferroni corrected univariate tests.

Two specific situations are so common as to demand separate comment. When a number of variables have been collected, each in different metrics, then the experimenter faces a decision as to whether to use MANOVA or a collection of Bonferroni corrected ANOVAs. If the number of such dependent variables is small (less than 5 and perhaps less than 10) and the variables do not overlap much, then the Bonferroni corrected univariate approach is likely to be preferred. With this approach, the hypotheses being tested are often the ones of most interest to the experimenter. Furthermore, high power can still be available. As the number of dependent variables gets larger and the amount of variable overlap increases, the multivariate approach becomes more attractive, because it is likely to have more power. Note that adding redundant variables tends to dilute any significant effect and lower the power.

The second important situation involves repeated measurements on subjects. Assume that d dependent variables have been measured at t times, a situation so common that it may be the norm. Two defensible approaches, as well as two less acceptable ones, may be suggested. The completely wrong approach is to analyze each response at each time separately, giving $d \cdot t$ analyses, at a nominal significance level. A valid approach, but typically of low power, is to analyze each of the $d \cdot t$ responses separately using a Bonferroni correction. The two preferred approaches are a univariate mixed-model approach to repeated measures and a multivariate approach to repeated measures. With the univariate approach, d separate ANOVAs would be conducted, each at the α/d level. The univariate approach to repeated measures assumes that the variance of the response at each time is the same (within an analysis). Furthermore, it is assumed that the correlation between any distinct pair of responses (any pair of repeated measures) is a constant. Many, if not most, behavioral measures do not meet this assumption.

When the univariate ANOVA assumption of homogeneity just described is violated, then p values are typically inflated; that is, the α level is not accurately controlled. This weakness of the univariate approach is well documented (see Keselman and Rogan 1980; and Keselman et al. 1980). Two solutions are available. First, various conservative approaches for correcting the p values are available. Huynh and Feldt (1970, 1980) and Huynh (1978) reviewed earlier corrections and proposed new ones. The earlier work, known as the Geisser-Greenhouse correction, leads to approximate tests that may be equivocal in some situations. Nevertheless, the Geisser-Greenhouse or Huynh-Feldt correction should almost always be used in univariate-repeated-measures analysis of behavioral data.

A multivariate approach will often be preferred. For each of the d dependent variables a separate MANOVA (with t responses) is conducted at the α/d significance level. This approach may require collected data on more subjects than the univariate approach requires, but does not need the restrictive homogeneity assumption; hence it is much more likely to have validity for any application, and exact tests are always available. Convenient, easy-to-use multivariate software is already available or will soon be available in all three statistical packages (BMDP, SPSS, and SAS). A single fully multivariate analysis with $d \cdot t$ responses can also be used, although the d separate MANOVAs are usually preferable in terms of interpretability and power.

Recent work has explored the concept of multivariate mixed-model approaches to such data, which demands that the homogeneity of the variance-covariance assumption be met separately by each dependent variable (see Reinsel 1982 and Thomas 1983). Since homogeneity assumption often is not met in behavioral toxicology and the robustness of such approaches has not been thoroughly studied, they will not be considered further.

Mixed models, whether univariate or multivariate, have important limitations. In the context of repeated-measures design the validity of the homogeneity assumption is questionable. Furthermore, no generally preferred strategies exist for estimation and hypothesis testing for general mixed-models design. In fact, estimation and hypothesis testing in mixed models remains a very active area of statistical research. If the models are accurate (for example, if genetic applications often demand them), then they should be used.

Other Models

Specific methodologies that are potentially applicable in behavioral toxicology have been developed for a number of situations. All are associated with dichotomous outcomes, some involving continuous information. These include logistic-regression techniques (Kleinbaum and Kupper 1978), survival analysis (Gross and Clark 1975), proportional-hazard models (Cox 1972), and stochastic-process models (Karlin 1969). Each has an entire literature devoted to it. In some cases fully developed machinery may be readily available for new situations. For example, survival analysis may properly model time to complete a maze, with censoring occurring by limiting all animals to three minutes, for example.

Computing and Research-Data Management

The Importance of Research-Data Management

Toxicology testing outcomes have enormous social and financial effects and often result in the banning of suspect substances or the setting of regulatory standards. The costs associated with toxicity decisions, the standard of evidence needed to support regulatory decisions, and the high potential for lawsuits challenging data analysis all militate toward maintaining the highest possible standards of scientific research. Just as the above reasons motivate the need to control Type I and Type II error rate, they also motivate the need for competent management of all research data.

Whether data are collected by hand, by computer, or by some combination, standards must be the same. An important automatic consequence of application of research-data management principles is the greatly increased defensibility of one's conclusions and data in the face of adversary attack. The goal—based upon the question, What if we had all of our data subpoenaed tomorrow?—is to achieve the subpoena standard.

Research-data management is a field nearly as youthful as behavioral toxicology, its growth having coincided with the growth of the use of computers. Research-data management, as distinguished from business-data management, only became a recognized field when large numbers of scientists could finally afford access to computing. Since then the access has outgrown the techniques used to manage it.

Methods for Research-Data Management

Muller, Christiansen, and Smith (1981) provided an overview of research-data-management methods. Benignus and Muller (1982) gave an overview of computer requirements for EEG data acquisition and analysis that also applies to many other physiological recording situations.

Muller, Christiansen, and Smith (1981) considered four topics in managing data sets, programs, and printouts and made the following recommendations: (1) consistent rules for naming programs and data sets should be used; (2) appropriate techniques for storing and archiving the programs and data sets must be used; (3)

printouts must be managed appropriately; and (4) proper documentation must be included as part of the process.

One of the most important ideas in their data-management approach is using simple naming conventions. Naming conventions should be applied to everything, including disks, tapes, source files, raw-data files, job names, and folders. The important feature is not the particular naming conventions chosen but rather that naming conventions should always be used to create self-documenting data analysis.

They next discussed archiving source programs and data sets. Every program that produced an output that was kept or used for a paper, as well as any data set that met the same standard, was to be archived. On larger computers archiving today usually involves storing the files and programs on computer tapes, which provide inexpensive, long-term storage. The files stored must also be named using naming conventions. These comments also apply to programs used to run laboratory microcomputers helping in data collection. An important rule is to never modify a program that (1) produced output that was kept or (2) collected data that was kept.

Printout management is based on the very simple rule that any printout that is kept must be associated with the exact program that created the printout. This completes the documentation that occurs automatically: each published number can, with some effort, be traced back to the raw-data point. Without such documentation, defending oneself on a witness stand or in the face of a subpoena can be quite difficult. For example, when (not if) errors are discovered in the course of data analysis, it is easy to return to the point before which no errors occurred and rerun all subsequent jobs.

Eventually any laboratory following these recommendations will produce mounds of computer printout, and the best solution is to have all of the computer printout microfilmed. Microfilm records, with even an inexpensive microfilm reader, are more conveniently accessible than printouts. Finally, photographic film stored in a typical office has an extremely long shelf life.

One goal of the data-management methods just presented is to provide automatic documentation at many points. In addition, certain documentation must be created by actions of the programmer-scientist. At the minimum, a single binder with handwritten notes should exist that allows the user to find all other documentation, printouts, and archived files. Such a master documentation binder typically does not contain the documentation itself but simply defines the location of all documentation and files. Large projects may demand that more detailed records be kept on each run, but a summary for each study is probably sufficient for small laboratory research.

An important payoff of the approach to managing programs and printouts is that producing figures, tables, and numbers for results is greatly simplified. Since printouts should be arranged in a binder in the order in which the jobs were run, producing results for a final report or publication usually consists in simply copying numbers from the appropriate binder.

The above approach focuses on the research rather than on any single program because most programming in a research environment is "one-time" programming. Thus, the emphasis is on the accuracy of the result and not on efficiency, which is conceptually the reverse of the usual approach in business-data processing.

Choosing Software and Hardware

Data collection, analysis, and management have been discussed, but it is the task at hand that dictates the choice of software and hardware. Given the cost and capabilities of existing hardware, many behavioral toxicology laboratories use microcomputers for data collection. Certain data-collection tasks, such as high analogue-to-digital conversion rates associated with EEG or other electrophysiological recording, may even demand the use of minicomputers. It is rarely practical or cost-effective to use large main-frame computers for data collection, since software for data collection usually must operate rapidly in real time, under local control, and interface with laboratory equipment. The control available in prime languages (FORTRAN, PL1, Pascal) is usually needed. Language interpreters should be avoided in preference to compilers because of execution-speed needs.

Although the availability of quality software for data analysis on minicomputers is rapidly improving, it still lags far behind that for large computers. As of this writing, a very small number of quality programs are available for microcomputers. Main-frame computers and associated software have advanced to the point where essentially any analysis that is known can be done with them. If cost accounting (including employee time and software purchase costs) is accurate, they are also less expensive. For these reasons small computers will not be competitive in the area of software availability and affordability for data analysis for a while to come.

If possible, the ideal arrangement is to conduct research-data management and data analysis within the context of one of the large statistical packages on a large computer. A microcomputer can save money as a text-editor work station, uploading programs to a large computer. The three most common statistical packages are BMDP (Dixon 1981), SAS (Ray 1982), and SPSS (Hull and Nie 1981). Using them automatically makes the research-data-management techniques suggested earlier easier to implement. Furthermore, they tend to make it easier to implement the choice of data analysis based on what is proper rather on than what is available.

Small computers can easily transfer data to large computers. The simplest and most efficient means of transfer are magnetic media, including disks and tapes. More attractive in theory, though often much less so in practice, is direct data transfer from computer to computer. In turn, the data analysis and data management can all be conducted on the large computer main frame using one of the statistical packages. This frees the laboratory computer for data collection.

A Strategy for Design and Analysis

Design, analysis, and research-data-management methods form a solid tripod on which to support behavioral toxicologic research. The sequence needed to implement the methods can be sketched as a series of four steps which, in turn, are iteratively refined. First, the research goals are specified in a fuzzy way and then sharpened in the context of the limitations of the situation. Second, specific responses, populations, and manipulations are considered. Third, a rough allocation of research goals to different studies is made. Fourth, the first study is described.

For the first study, hypotheses are specified along with a tentative design and analyses. If the variables have been studied before, or if this is not the first in a series of studies, then power calculations can be done. The same process is then applied to the second study. Looking ahead one study is usually sufficient, although in some cases the following studies are also sketched. Then the entire process is repeated to refine and adjust each step. The planning process should include producing a time schedule of key events along with a data flow sequence. This planning strategy supports implementing the design and analytical methods recommended here.

Acknowledgments

This research was supported by U.S. Environmental Protection Agency contract 68-02-3800.

References

Abt, K. 1981. Problems of repeated significance testing. *Controlled Clin. Trials* 1:377–81.

Anastasi, A. 1968. *Psychological testing*. 3d ed. New York: Macmillan.

Benignus, V. A., and Muller, K. E. 1982. Information flow in the brain: Computer requirements. *Behav. Res. Meth. Instrum.* 14:294–99.

Bickel, P. J., and Doksum, K. A. 1977. *Mathematical statistics: Basic ideas and selected topics*. San Francisco: Holden-Day.

Bock, R. D. 1975. *Multivariate statistics methods in behavioral research*. New York: McGraw-Hill.

Bradley, J. V. 1968. *Distribution-free statistical tests*. Englewood Cliffs, N.J.: Prentice-Hall.

Campbell, D. T., and Stanley, J. C. 1963. *Experimental and quasi-experimental designs for research*. Chicago: Rand McNally.

Cohen, J. 1977. *Statistical power analysis for the behavioral sciences*. Rev ed. New York: Academic Press.

Cooper, H. M., and Rosenthal, R. 1980. Statistical versus traditional procedures for summarizing research findings. *Psychol. Bull.* 87:442–49.

Cox, D. R. 1970. *The analysis of binary data*. New York: Halsted Press.

———. 1972. Regression models and life tables. *J. Royal Stat. Soc.*, Ser. B 34:187–220.

Dixon, W. J., ed. 1981. *BMDP statistical software*. Berkeley: University of California Press.

Finn, J. D. 1974. *A general model for multivariate analysis*. New York: Holt, Rinehart & Winston.

Finney, D. J. 1978. *Statistical method in biological assay*. 3d ed. London: Charles Griffin.

Forthofer, R. N., and Lehnen, R. G. 1981. *Public program analysis: A new categorical data approach*. Belmont, Calif.: Wadsworth.

Gad, S. C. 1982. Statistical analysis of behavioral toxicology data and studies. *Arch. Toxicol.*, suppl. 5:256–66.

Gad, S. C., and Weil, C. S. 1982. Statistics for toxicologists. In *Methods in toxicology*, edited by A. W. Hayes, 273–320. New York: Raven Press.

Gallant, A. R. 1975a. Seemingly unrelated nonlinear regressions. *J. Econometrics* 3:33–50.

———. 1975b. Nonlinear regression. *Am. Statistician* 29:73–81.

Grizzle, J. E.; Starmer, C. F.; and Koch, G. G. 1969. Analysis of categorical data by linear models. *Biometrics* 25:489–504.

Gross, A. J., and Clark, V. A. 1975. *Survival distributions: Reliability applications in the biomedical sciences*: New York: John Wiley.

Hajek, J. 1969. *A course in nonparametric statistics*. San Francisco: Holden-Day.

Harris, R. J. 1975. *A primer of multivariate statistics*. New York: Academic Press.

Hedges, L. V. 1982. Estimation and testing for differences in effect size: A comment on Hsu. *Psychol. Bull.* 91:691–93.

Hoel, P. G.; Port, S. C.; and Stone, C. J. 1971. *Introduction to probability theory.* New York: Houghton Mifflin.

Hollander, M., and Wolfe, D. A. 1973. *Nonparametric statistical methods.* New York: John Wiley & Sons.

Hsu, Louis M. 1980. Tests of differences in p levels as tests of differences in effect sizes. *Psychol. Bull.* 88:705–8.

Hull, C. H., and Nie, N. H. 1981. *SPSS update 7-9.* New York: McGraw-Hill.

Huynh, H. 1978. Some approximate tests for repeated measurement designs. *Psychometrika* 43:161–75.

Huynh, H., and Feldt, L. S. 1970. Conditions under which means square ratios in repeated measures designs have exact F distributions. *J. Am. Stat. Assoc.* 65:1582–85.

———. 1980. Performance in traditional F tests in repeated measures designs under covariance heterogeneity. *Comm. Stat. Thry/Method.* A9:61–74.

Karlin, S. 1969. *A first course in stochastic processes.* New York: Academic Press.

Keselman, H. J., and Rogan J. C. 1980. Repeated measures F and psychophysiological research: Controlling the number of false positives. *Psychophysiology* 17:400–503.

Keselman, H. J.; Rogan, J. C.; Mendoza, J. L.; and Breen, J. L. 1980. Testing the validity conditions of repeated measures F tests. *Psychol. Bull.* 87:479–81.

Kirk, R. E. 1968. *Experimental design for the behavioral sciences.* Belmont, Calif.: Wadsworth.

Kleinbaum, D. G., and Kupper, L. L. 1978. *Applied regression analysis and other multivariate methods.* North Scituate, Mass.: Duxburg Press.

Kleinbaum, D. G.; Kupper, L. L.; and Morgenstern, H. 1982. *Epidemiologic research: Principles and quantitative methods.* London: Lifetime Learning.

Koele, P. 1982. Calculating power in analysis of variance. *Psychol. Bull.* 92:513–16.

Kraemer, H. C., and Andrews, G. 1982. A nonparametric technique for meta-analysis effect size calculations. *Psychol. Bull.* 91:404–12.

Kritzer, H. 1979. Approaches to the analysis of complex contingency tables: A guide for the perplexed. *Sociol. Meth. Res.* 7:305–29.

Lehmann, E. L. 1975. *Nonparametrics.* San Francisco: Holden-Day.

Littell, R. C., and Folks, J. L. 1971. Asymptotic optimality of Fisher's method if combining independent tests. *J. Am. Stat. Assoc,* 66:802–6.

Lord, F. M., and Novick, M. R. 1968. *Statistical theories of mental tests scores.* Reading, Mass.: Addison-Wesley.

Mitchell, C. L., and Tilson, H. A. 1982. Behavioral toxicology in risk assessment: Problems and research needs. *CRC Crit. Rev. Toxicol.* 10(4):265–74.

Mosier, C. I. 1951. Problems and design of cross validation. *Ed. Psychol. Meas.* 11:5–11.

Mulaik, S. A. 1972. *The foundations of factor analysis.* New York: McGraw-Hill.

Muller, K. E.; Barton, C. N.; and Benignus, V. A. 1984. Recommendations for appropriate statistical practice in toxicologic experiments. *NeuroToxicology* 5(2):113–26.

Muller, K. E.; Christiansen, D. H.; and Smith, J. C. 1981 Guidelines for managing datasets, programs and printouts in scientific research. *Comput. Programs Biomed.* 13:281–88.

Muller, K. E.; Otto, D. A.; and Benignus, V. A. 1983. Design and analysis issues and strategies in psychophysiological research. *Psychophysiology* 20:212–18.

Muller, K. E., and Peterson, B. L. 1983. Practical methods for computing power in testing and multivariate general linear hypothesis. *American Statistical Association: Proceedings of the statistical computing section.* Washington, D.C.: American Statistical Association.

———. 1984. Power analysis for multivariate linear models: New results and SAS make it practical. In *SUGI proceedings,* 853–58. Cary, N.C.: SAS Institute.

Notari, R. E. 1975. *Biopharmaceutics and pharmacokinetics.* New York: Dekker.

O'Brien, R. G. 1982. Performing power sensitivity analyses on general linear model hypotheses. In *American Statistical Association,* 114–18. See Muller and Peterson 1983.

O'Flaherty, E. J. 1981. *Toxicants and drugs.* New York: John Wiley & Sons.

Puri, M. L., and Sen, P. K. 1971. *Nonparametric methods in multivariate analysis*. New York: John Wiley & Sons.

Rao, C. R. 1973. *Linear statistical inference and its applications*. 2d ed. New York: John Wiley & Sons.

Ray, A. A., ed. 1982. *SAS user's guide: Basics*. Cary, N. C.: SAS Institute.

Reinsel, G. 1982. Multivariate repeated-measurement or growth curve models with multivariate random effects covariance structure. *J. Am. Stat. Assoc.* 77:190–95.

Rosenthal, R. 1978. Combining results of independent studies. *Psychol. Bull.* 85:185–93.

———. 1979. The "file drawer problem" and tolerance for null results. *Psychol. Bull.* 86:638–41.

———. 1980. On telling tails when combining results of independent studies. *Psychol. Bull.* 88:496–97.

———. 1982. Correction to Rosenthal. *Psychol. Bull.* 91:609–22.

Rosenthal, R., and Rubin, D. B. 1979. Comparing significance levels of independent studies. *Psychol. Bull* 86:1165–68.

Seigel, S. 1956. *Nonparametric statistics for the behavioral sciences*. New York: McGraw-Hill.

Stevens, S. S. 1951. Mathematics measurement and psychophysics. In *Handbook of experimental psychology*, edited by S. S. Stevens. New York: John Wiley & Sons.

Thomas, D. R. 1983. Univariate repeated measures techniques applied to multivariate data. *Psychometrika* 48:451–64.

Timm, N. H. 1975. *Multivariate analysis with applications in education and psychology*. Belmont, Calif.: Wadsworth.

Valciukas, J. A., and Lilis, R. 1980. Psychometric techniques in environmental research. *Environ. Res.* 21(2):275–97.

Weil, C. S. 1982. Statistical analysis and normality of selected hematologic and clinical chemistry measurements used in toxicologic studies. *Arch. Toxicol.* suppl. 5:237–53.

Williams, G. 1981. Is this really necessary? A first look at design techniques. *BYTE* 6 (March):6–10, 200–214.

Yourdon, E., ed. 1979. *Classics in software engineering*. New York: Yourdon Press.

Yourdon, E., and Constantine, L. L. 1979. *Structured design: Fundamentals of a discipline of computer program and systems design*. Englewood Cliffs, N.J.: Prentice-Hall.

Peter B. Dews

19

Some General Problems of Neurobehavioral Toxicology

Behavioral toxicology is the scientific study of nontherapeutic, unintended behavioral effects of agents. This definition reminds us that it is the behavioral changes that are of interest, no matter what the cause. The behavioral changes do not have to be caused by a direct effect of the agent on the central nervous system. For example, a spasm or diarrhea caused by the effects of an agent on the smooth muscle of the gastrointestinal tract may cause important behavioral toxicity—indeed, incapacitation—although the agent is not a neurotoxicant. Behavioral toxicology covers both acute and chronic effects, both reversible and irreversible effects. The effects of ethanol in reasonable doses are completely reversible, but ethanol is an important behavioral toxicant for people on the road or in the workplace.

Commonly, the term *behavioral toxicity* is confined to behavioral effects that are not demonstrably the result of overt pathophysiological changes. The narrower usage provides a convenient descriptor but must not be taken to imply basic differences between agents whose effects can be detected by morphological, physiological, or chemical changes in the subject, notably in the central nervous system, and agents whose direct effects cannot yet be detected by these means. The distinction between behavioral toxicity and neurological toxicity is similar to the distinction between psychiatry and neurology. It is not controversial to call schizophrenia a psychiatric condition and peripheral neuritis a neurological condition, even though, on the one hand, few would want to deny that pathophysiological influences on or in the brain someday will be shown to be causally related to the psychiatric manifestations of schizophrenia and, on the other hand, a trigeminal neuralgia may have more psychiatric than neurological consequences. The distinction between *psycho-* and *neuro-* is a function of our understanding and can change in time. In view of the lack of rigor of the definitions, we may ask whether the distinction is worthwhile. Many have answered no, and terms such as *neuropsychiatric disorders* and *psychoneurotoxicology* are seen. But the distinction does emphasize that behavioral phenomena and neurological phenomena both are legitimate areas of scientific endeavor to explore independently as well in trying to relate the one to the other. One of the attractions of behavioral toxicology is that its study may lead to advances in the understanding of the relation between behavioral activities and neurological phenomena. Such advances are not, however, a requirement for the legitimacy of behavioral toxicology, and the worth of a study in behavioral toxicology should not be judged solely, or even mainly, by what it reveals about neurological phenomena. Do we judge the worth of studies in chemistry by what is revealed about laws of physics? We certainly do not do so as a general rule. A case could be made that neurological effects with no functional, behavioral consequences are of little concern, while significant behavioral deficits without a currently recognizable neurological basis are still significant deficits. A person with a scar in his brain may be judged normal, while, as before, a young schizophrenic is not judged normal. The foregoing does not imply a mysterious, nonmaterial substratum for behavioral phenomena; it simply asserts that the types of behavioral phenomena that we study should not be constrained by the limitations of present methods of neurobiology.

Explicit concern with behavioral toxicology is of relatively recent origin, within the last 25 years, although specific instances of behavioral toxicity, such as Maria Theresa's interest in the mad miners of mercury, have been known for centuries. Behavioral toxicology has commanded interest for its potential regulatory implications: Can behavioral methods yield results to help guide regulatory decisions? Are there agents that cause "only" behavioral effects, so far as present methods can detect, over a range of concentrations? Are behavioral effects of some agents detectable at lower exposures than other effects, so that behavioral results are important in determining acceptable exposures? What are the "no behavioral effect levels" of agents? That such questions should arise is understandable. Most of the work on behavioral toxicology has been supported either by agencies of government—the Environmental Protection Agency, the National Institute of Environmental Health Sciences, the National Institute of Occupational Safety and Health—with direct or indirect responsibilities for specification of acceptable public exposures, or by companies concerned with the impact of their products on their workers and the public. It should be noted, however, that the legitimacy of behavioral toxicology as a science does not depend on its usefulness to regulators, although the financial support for the subject may be strongly influenced by such considerations. The use of toxicants has been invaluable in the analysis of physiological phenomena. There is no apparent reason why toxicants should not be similarly valuable in the analysis of behavioral phenomena, so there is scientific justification for the study of behavioral toxicity. It must be admitted that contributions of behavioral toxicology to the analysis of behavioral phenomena have been disappointingly small so far. The potential of behavioral toxicology may have been ineffectively exploited for science because of a preoccupation with detecting minimal effects, arising from the similar preoccupation of the sponsors. Big effects lend themselves much more readily to analysis and the furthering of scientific understanding.

There are three main classes of problems for toxicology: (1) identification of polluting agents that even in trace amounts or with transient contact can cause harm; (2) identification of even slight degrees of harm from agents to which the public is exposed continuously; and (3) identification of peculiarly hazardous materials in the work environment. Before I address these main classes, however, more general comments are necessary.

In what follows, a number of strictures on current practice in toxicology are made. It is to be emphasized that the shortcomings are characteristic of toxicology as a whole and are by no means peculiar to behavioral toxicology.

What Behavioral Effects Constitute Behavioral Toxicity?

Behavioral toxicologists are regularly asked how they recognize a demonstrated behavioral effect of an agent in a laboratory animal as behavioral toxicity rather than as a benign drug effect of potential therapeutic usefulness. Behavioral toxicologists have generally taken the view that any behavioral effect of a nontherapeutic agent seen at levels as low as human exposure may approach should be considered a toxic effect until it is demonstrated not to be so. Such an approach avoids the problem of identifying the effects themselves as toxic or therapeutic and is surely reasonable. The demonstration that nontherapeutic behavioral effects are benign must be made in the human population, either by overwhelming experience or by controlled trials. That the behavioral effects of caffeine as consumed are not toxic may be said to have been demonstrated by overwhelming experience. That other agents, including medicaments, with unsought behavioral side effects are not behaviorally toxic has rarely been demonstrated; many need to be examined in controlled trials. Behavioral toxicities include detriment to work performance or automobile driving and like activities or increase in the likelihood of criminality or suicide or a decrease in the quality of life. Despite the multiplicity of possible behavioral effects, most fit into one of these few categories. The last category is unfortunately vague, but an example illustrates. If a worker exposed to an agent throughout the work day is able to complete his work without impairment but is regularly incapacitated by, for example, "lethargy" in the evening and impotence later as a demonstrated consequence of the exposure, then those effects would surely be recognized as toxic. Instances of impairment of quality of life may be easy to recognize in the particular, though a general definition may be difficult, in part because different people have very different normal life styles.

The whole field of behavioral toxicity of medicaments, while recognized, is grossly underinvestigated. We know little about the contribution of medicinal agents to industrial and traffic accidents and to impaired work performance. For instance, does hypoglycemia in diabetics or anti-hypertension or "anti-anxiety" medication tend to lower safety and performance? The quantitative contributions of medicinal agents and alcohol to lowering safety and performance need continuing study. In recent years, temporary roadblocks have been established, and every driver on the highway has been screened for gross inebriation. The tactic seems to have been socially acceptable. It may be that the public would tolerate a breath test on every driver in such a situation. It is not likely that the public would presently tolerate the taking of a blood sample from every driver. Would drivers be willing to moisten a piece of filter paper with their saliva? Will unannounced checks in the workplace of urine and saliva become socially acceptable? Routine methods may be developed to estimate body burdens of a wide variety of agents from a minute sample of saliva or urine. Such efforts would hasten our understanding of the hazards of agents. Do the risks justify invasion of personal privacy and great expense? Abridgement of personal liberty for the common good is becoming increasingly accepted. It will be interesting to see whether the present fear of AIDS leads to public insistence that diagnosis no longer be permitted to be a private matter between patient and physician. We have come a long way since our great-grandfathers were outraged at the suggestion that they disclose their income to the government for purposes of taxation. It is difficult even to guess at risks without pilot data, but it is unlikely that money would be spent better in pilot studies in many areas of behavioral toxicity than in trying to eliminate the last microgram of dioxin or the last microcurie of added ionizing radiation in the environment. Information on humans is needed to validate assessments on laboratory animals.

Good Laboratory Practices Regulations and Protection of the Public

Everybody recognizes that members of the population may come in contact with an enormous number of potentially toxic agents. If we are to identify the serious hazards, we need quick and cheap ways of screening vast numbers of components. Yet the regulatory emphasis in recent years has been on the development of more and more highly formalized and stipulated methods of testing. Implementation of Good Laboratory Practices (GLP) regulations consumes scarce manpower that could otherwise be devoted to good applied science. The introduction of GLP was prompted by revelations that fraudulent information had been submitted to the Food and Drug Administration. It is not obvious that GLP regulations will help appreciably in the detection of fraudulent submissions without on-site audits, which detect fraud without GLP regulations. GLP regulations need to be justified by showing that the public is better protected from toxic hazards, with due regard to cost in money and resources, than if they had not been promulgated. The opposite may be the case. The regulations emphasize process, rote, and redundancy so that agents are examined less intelligently, more expensively, and perhaps more slowly so that more remain unexamined.

There have been no documented incidents of serious toxicity that could have been avoided only by full-scale GLP assessment of toxicity. Even though ethylene glycol is several times more toxic to people than to mice, observations on only a few mice would have sufficed to indicate that ethylene glycol was too toxic to be used as a solvent for sulfanilamide in an elixir for children. The problem in the case of Minamoto disease was in showing that methylmercury was formed in the sea, not in demonstrating the toxicity of methylmercury, and the poisoning of people with mercury-treated grain was not attributable to inadequately conducted studies on the toxicity of mercury compounds.

Among the large number of agents whose toxicity is known, very few are harmful in trace amounts or with transient exposure. What we need is warning of unexpectedly very high toxicity of an agent proposed for distribution or use in manufacture, toxicity higher than expected by orders of magnitude rather than by 50 percent or 100 percent. If the toxicity is lethality, then if we choose the right species, very few laboratory animals will signal that toxicity, or if we have chosen an animal species grossly different to man with respect to the agent, no number of animals nor carefully documented testing will provide a warning. The law of diminishing returns operates, with a steep decline in returns for increasing numbers of animals.

It has been suggested that if the toxicity is less conspicious than acute lethality, then behavioral assessments may be useful in detecting in a nonspecific way even selective toxicants. The argument is that impairment of any system is likely to manifest itself in changes in the integrated functioning of the whole subject, that is, as changes in behavior. The argument is plausible, but convincing evidence has not been marshaled to validate the approach. Such an enterprise would appear to deserve high priority in the development of risk science. People tend to be so preoccupied in trying to consolidate behavioral and neurological toxicities that the potential of behavioral toxicity as an early warning of toxicity of many kinds has not been adequately pursued. It may be that information already exists to validate or refute the value of the approach. Failure to gain weight is a well-recognized example of a nonspecific detectable effect of even a selective toxicant. Maybe assessment of behavioral toxicity could give information earlier and therefore more cheaply. Rapid and cheap screening methods should be developed, and their predictive ability assessed. Until the tests have been validated and shown to detect agents with unexpectedly high behavioral toxicity or to be useful, efficient indicators of nonspecific toxicants, they should not be prescribed or required by regulations.

Classes of Toxicity

Trace Pollutants

It is reasonable to expect that the distribution of toxicities in populations of new agents in the future will be similar to the distribution in populations of agents that have been studied already. If so, only very rarely will new agents pose a hazard if people are exposed only transiently or to only trace amounts. That is why the tests must be rapid enough to assess great numbers of agents.

With respect to behavioral toxicity, the question arises, Are there trace pollutants with peculiarly behavioral effects? In the workplace at least one agent, lysergic acid diethylamide (LSD), has been found to have profound behavioral effects at levels that are orders of magnitude lower than the levels for other toxic effects. No environmental pollutants seem to have been shown to have such selective behavioral effects, but in view of LSD, it would be rash to assume that they do not exist. It would be easy to build an apparatus that would assess effects of agents on schedule-controlled responding of mice that was entirely automatic. Very short time samples of behavioral assessment, of, say, 10 minutes, would serve to indicate catastrophic behavioral toxicity, so a single apparatus could assess nearly 144 mice each day. No human intervention in training of the mice is needed, so the only demands on personnel are to administer agents. Repeated, progressively increasing doses of an agent could be given to the same mouse on succeeding days until the behavioral performance was severely impaired. Thus, a rough approximation to a dose-effect curve and its slope could be obtained, and the rate of elimination, for agents that persist in pharmacologically active form for more than 24 hours, estimated by time to restoration of normal performance. A low ED.20 (the level reducing performance by 20 percent) would be an indication for further scrutiny. The mouse test could be supplemented by a primate test. A well-trained macaque could be given a single dose of, say, the mouse ED.20. A much larger than expected effect would be an indication for further studies. The use of a primate permits the detection of agents peculiarly toxic to primates. Similar objective behavioral assessments should be made repeatedly on at least some of the subjects in subacute and chronic toxicity studies.

Some features of the examples of procedures just given are rejected out of hand by conventional toxicologists; for example, the notion of giving a whole series of agents, one after the other, to the same monkey is abhorrent to many. It is not likely, however, that such a procedure will lead to many false negatives because of the multiple agents, although the frequency of false positives could be unacceptably high. Only experience will tell. Certainly, the administration of multiple drugs to the same subject not only is acceptable in behavioral pharmacology but is the preferred approach; and in real life everybody is exposed to many agents. Only objective information will serve to guide us to useful and efficient procedures. The point to be emphasized is that if we are going to make an even cursory examination of the very many agents that may merit attention, we cannot afford to reject on doctrinaire grounds any means of increasing speed and efficiency.

The foregoing remarks are intended as no more than an indication as to how one might start searching for efficient and reliable screens. A mandated general requirement for particular screening is not justified at present and would freeze development. In view of the billions of dollars being devoted to other branches of applied toxicology, however, some of which might be saved by judicious use of behavioral tests, abundant support for research and pilot experiments on the value of behavioral screening methods is imperative.

Chronic Consumption

When large populations are to be exposed to appreciable quantities of an agent, such as a new food additive, then just a quick screen to rule out high toxicity is clearly inadequate. The agent must not cause significant harm to the great majority of people with nonabusive usage. If an agent is new, then evidence on its safety can be obtained only in laboratory animals. Then in traditional toxicology comes the agonizing question, How to extrapolate from the results in laboratory animals to expectations for man?

An extrapolation in the sense of a leap in the dark is never scientifically acceptable and should not be used as a basis for regulation. But knowledge about matters that cannot be measured directly need not involve extrapolation. Our knowledge as to where the moon is to be found at any particular time was based on evidence strong enough to be recognized as factual even before direct confirmation, to a high degree of accuracy, by sending things and people there. For strong inferences, we usually need to know about mechanism, although we can sometimes make good inferences on the basis of context. If we know quantitatively the operating characteristics of a test in laboratory animals over a large variety of agents and we can measure the selective amount of harm and lack of harm in appropriately exposed humans, then we may be able to make quantitative inferences from results of the test to hazards in man. Unfortunately, these minimal requirements for sound inferences are lacking for most tests in toxicology, as, for example, in bioassays for almost all carcinogens.

In general, agents producing behavioral effects have more uniform effects across species than agents producing other types of effects. Many of the differences that do exist depend on pharmacokinetic differences rather than on differences in the nature of the behavioral effects themselves. Thus, inferences can be made with rather more confidence in behavioral toxicology than in most other areas of toxicology. Unfortunately, we do not know whether the uniformity extends to those exceptional agents that produce behavioral toxicity at levels far lower than other toxicities, the very agents of greatest concern.

Workplace Exposures

In the workplace a larger variety of agents are encountered, and a larger proportion of them are new agents, than in the general environment. Not infrequently, higher levels of exposure also occur in the workplace. Hence, protection of workers is a particularly important aspect of toxicology. Maximum automation, maximum separation of worker from agent, and good working practices are clearly the first line of protection. As for dietary and environmental exposures, it is not established at present what behavioral toxicology has to contribute to identifying unanticipated hazards from new agents in industrial production or to helping to establish acceptable exposures to agents, although a large role seems likely. Here again, research is necessary. For volatile agents, it would be interesting to expose working laboratory animals to the actual environment of the workplace. Perhaps someday potentially harmful work stations will have squirrel monkeys working under mult FRFI, just as coal miners used to have a canary in a cage to warn of hazard.

More Problems

"No-Effect" Levels

It is not surprising that regulators, lawyers, legislators, and the public want toxicologists to tell them what are "safe" levels (as opposed to "hazardous" levels) of exposure to agents. What is surprising is the insouciance with which toxicologists have accepted the responsibility of establishing safe levels, that is, of proving that there are no effects at or below particular levels. Everyone accepts that it is formally impossible to prove the null hypothesis, but people say that for practical purposes there are levels that one can be "virtually certain" have no effects. But, it is for practical reasons that the concept of an identifiable "no-effect" level is unacceptable.

The difficulty is not the lack of existence of "no-effect" levels. There may be a few lawyers, an occasional statistician, and a few scientists-turned-politicians who believe that there are effects with no threshold, that is, that smaller and smaller exposures to an agent cause smaller and smaller effects without limit, but never *no* effect with non-zero exposure. Essentially no pharmacologist accepts as a viable concept the notion of no minimum threshold for a real effect. Their practical experience demonstrates that there are doses of agents that are too small to affect experimental animals. Nevertheless, pharmacologists gave up the concept of a minimum effective dose (MED) 60 years ago, following Trevan (1927), because MEDs could not be determined satisfactorily. The minimum effective dose below which there is no effect is the lower asymptote of the dose-effect curve. The slope of the sigmoid dose-effect curve becomes less and less as the asymptote of the "no-effect" level is approached. The lower the slope, the greater is the effect of errors, random or nonrandom, in the measurement of effect on the estimates of dose. For example, the death or survival of a single mouse can cause a large change in the estimate of the LD.001. At levels where the effect has become so low as to be virtually "no-effect," the precision with which the level can be measured is also so low that the estimate is useless for practical, as well as theoretical, purposes.

The falling precision of estimates of doses for particular levels of effect can be illustrated by consideration of the integrated normal curve as a reasonable approximation to most dose-effect curves. The curve has its greatest slope at an effect level equal to half of maximum effect. If we take this slope to be 1, then the slope at ED.10 is 0.44; at ED.01, 0.066; and at ED.001, 0.008. Thus at around ED.001 we need 125 mice to give the information that 1 mouse gave at around ED.50. As the slope becomes lower, the change in x (our estimate of the level needed for effect y) for a given change in y (the level of effect that we are measuring, with error) becomes greater; that is, the precision of our estimate falls. Another example can be derived from binomial sampling errors. If we choose a dose that causes a true mortality of 0.001 (1 in 1,000) and give it to groups of 300 mice, then in about 3 groups out of 4 none of the mice will die. Thus, in real life, we cannot reliably detect an LD.001 even with such large groups, and if we cannot detect the effect, we cannot measure the dose necessary to cause it or not to cause it. The "no-effect" level is indeterminate.

It is interesting to speculate on why an unsound concept such as (largest) no-effect level (as well as maximum tolerated dose) should have persisted in regulatory toxicology. It is probably attributable to the major roles played by pathologists and lawyers in regulatory toxicology. Morbid histology is not inherently quantitative in the manner of physiology and pharmacology, and lawyers strive for dichotomies such as guilty/not guilty and safe/unsafe. Quantitative risk assessments do not come naturally to either group.

Statistics in Behavioral Toxicology

In toxicology in general, the estimates of the extremely low levels that purport to cause no more than an acceptable level of hazard—for example, 1 in 1 million or 1 in 10 million cancers from lifetime exposure—are arrived at by calculation, not by determination. The calculations may conceal unreasonable extrapolations. For example, an experiment was conducted on over 24,000 mice to determine the ED.01 for carcinogenesis by 2-acetylaminofluorene (2-AAF) (Cairns 1980). Eight dose levels from 0 to 150 ppm were studied. From the results, the level that would cause bladder cancer in only 1 in 1 million mice was arrived at as follows (Gaylor 1979). In the mice receiving no 2-AAF, the incidence of bladder cancer was 1.0 percent. In mice that had had 30 ppm 2-AAF in the diet for 2 years the incidence was 1.2 percent. From these figures, 30 ppm was said to cause an 0.2 percent increase in cancer. The level, y, of 2-AAF to cause an increase in cancers of 1 in 1 million, $10(E - 6)$, was calculated from the proportionality relation: $y/[30 \times 10(E - 6)] = 10(E - 6)/[2 \times 10(E - 3)]$, whence $y = 15 \times 10(E - 9)$ (Linear Extrapolation; Gaylor [1979] gives 10 ppb).* Note that a "signal" (0.2 percent) that was only one-fifth of the "noise" (1.0 percent in the controls) was extrapolated to 3 orders of magnitude below the putatively measured effect. How can a biologist take such a blind leap seriously? In the data themselves the very existence of any effect not only at the 30 ppm dose level but also at the next two higher levels is unconvincing (for raw data see Farmer, Kodell, and Greenman 1980). Effects at 75 ppm are convincing. If the results in mice only after 24 months' feeding are used (mice were killed at other time intervals), linear extrapolation from effects at 30 ppm gives an estimate of the level for 1 in 1 million of 18 ppb. If, however, we take 60 ppm as the lowest dose with any effect for linear extrapolation, the estimate of the level for 1 in 1 million

---

*$10(E - a)$ signifies 10 with the exponent $-a$.

becomes 11 ppb. Thus, assuming that the lowest measurable effect is seen at a dose level two times higher leads to lower estimate of the level for 1 in 1 million. Such inconsistencies are well known. The example was chosen from a carcinogenesis assay, because that is the field in which extrapolations have been most rampant.

Bioassays for measuring toxic effects, as opposed to just detecting them in a search, should have the following characteristics:

1. They should seek the best estimates of doses for measurable effects and of the slope of the dose-effect curve—not "conservative" estimates but the best estimates.

2. The error of the estimates should be determined from replications. Even if the entire assay is conducted by the same people in the same laboratory, it should be designed in the form of replications. The reason for replications is that there are errors in bioassay additional to sampling errors (Dews and Berkson 1954). There are errors in dosing, measuring, and recording; differences arising from position in the room (Lagakos and Mosteller 1981); and a host of other errors not included in conventional formulae for estimates of errors of sampling from a hypothetical population of subjects. Only replications can give an indication of the size of these errors. If the experiment is conducted as a single whole, then errors are assumed to be just subject sampling errors and so are underestimated.

3. The report of a bioassay should be an account of measured effects at stated exposures. In most ordinary assays, effects of less than 10 percent of full range cannot be measured, and often effects of less than 20 percent cannot be measured reliably.

We have been told repeatedly that the setting of acceptable levels of exposure for human populations involves social, economic, and political considerations, with the estimates of hazard from clinical or field studies or studies on experimental animals providing only a starting point. The assertion is correct. Unfortunately, most promulgators promptly forget the premise and arrive at recommendations of levels for human exposure that appear to be obtained from results in humans or experimental animals by science and statistics but, in fact, are obtained by invalidated extrapolation. Real estimates and not hypothetical, extrapolated derivatives of them should be used in the explicit social, economic, and political discussions that decide the upper limits of permissible human exposure. It is possible that in the future there will be good epidemiological information on enough agents that also have been assayed in the laboratory to permit us to infer expected effects in humans at much lower levels of hazard than we can at present.

Turning now to particular concerns of behavioral toxicity, the following procedure for design and handling of the results of assays is suggested (Dews 1982; Glowa et al. 1983; Glowa and Dews 1983; Dews 1986): From the log dose-effect curve, estimate the dose for the lowest reliably measurable effect, say, the dose for a 0.1 reduction in performance. Estimate the precision from the variance between the replications. Then with conventional normal distribution statistics calculate the level of exposure that would be expected to cause a 0.1 decrement in, say, no more than 1 individual in 100. That is as far as one can go. Note that two parameters are chosen: a level of decrement and a probability of its occurring. Use of two parameters is somewhat reminiscent of the choices of α and β in significance testing. The above procedure has the following advantages over conventional risk assessments by extrapolation.

1. The effect level, for example, reduction by 0.10 of control, is chosen to be on a part of the curve that is directly, or almost directly, determinable. Extrapolation, therefore, is not required for the estimate.

2. The data from all the usable points on the concentration-effect curve contribute to the estimates, avoiding the inefficiency of using only a single point, as, for example, in linear extrapolation. Usable points are points for doses not less than those causing no clearly measurable effect or higher than those causing 100 percent of the measured effect, for example, abolition of the behavioral performance.

3. Selecting the 0.10 point rather than the more familiar 0.50 point allows the slope of the function to enter substantially into the estimation. Other things being similar, the lower the slope, the lower the concentration that may cause toxicity in an occasional subject.

4. By using the normal distribution as the basis for estimation, we replace the unknown function relating dose to effect at low dose levels by the well-known Gaussian function. The several independent observations that go into each estimated 0.10 point help bring the distribution of the estimates toward the normal. Further, the probability estimates from the t-distribution are not sensitive to reasonable departures from normality of the data values. Finally, if the same distribution is used consistently, information will accumulate to assess the performance of the procedure from its actuarial characteristics in an accumulating number of assays. When extrapolations are made to the lower regions of dose-effect curves, each extrapolation is made ad hoc, so there is no way, even in principle, of examining the performance of the procedure.

5. Since the individual estimates of 0.10 points are from independent experiments, the variance reflects the true experimental error of replications, not a value derived from formulae for asymptotic sampling variance. The latter values seriously underestimate the real errors of the estimates.

6. The logarithmic transform of the concentration is standard pharmacological practice and should become so in toxicology. It is based on log normality rather than normality of the distribution of sensitivity to therapeutic or toxic effects of an agent (Gaddum 1945). The transform also prevents estimates of 0.10 points from being negative; a negative concentration is meaningless.

7. The principles of risk estimation can be applied equally to quantitative dose-effect curves or to quantal dose-effect curves based on frequency of all-or-more phenomena, such as occurrences of cancer.

8. The better the assay and the fewer the experimental errors, the smaller will be the variance and therefore the higher will be the concentration at which one has confidence that less than 1 in 100 will be significantly affected. Companies testing potential products will, therefore, be rewarded for good work by justifying a higher permissible level of an agent for any specified risk estimate. Extrapolation procedures are generally insensitive to quality of work, and poor work, which increases variance, has unpredictable effects on estimates and on occasion may grossly understate hazard.

The procedure appears to have the disadvantage of not providing estimates of levels for acceptable risk. It is contended that other procedures do not yield acceptable estimates. My approach has two components not characteristic of conventional risk assessments. First, the dose level estimated is the dose level for a measurable risk. Second, lower risks are estimated from variances based on replications, preferably as independent as possible. Whether the procedures will lead to estimates of risk that more nearly agree with what is found in the field is not known. Little systematic information on the performance of any predictors of toxicity for populations is available. Much of the discussion of risk assessment has been in the context of carcinogenesis, where acceptable risks are too low for it to be possible to measure the accuracy of performance of the estimates. If inhaled gasoline is estimated to cause 43 cancers per year in the United States, we can never hope to measure how good that estimate is, even within orders of magnitude. Many behavioral toxicities, however, are rapidly reversible with no aftermath, and they occur more frequently than do geneses of cancers. While episodes are to be avoided, less conservatism is demanded than for carcinogens, so the incidence of behavioral toxicities may be sufficiently high for it to be possible, in principle, to make quantitative comparisons between effects of load of agents in humans and the dose-effect curves of the same agents in a variety of laboratory animals. Thus, it is possible that behavioral toxicology, apart from its intrinsic merits, will be able to make a contribution to toxicology as a whole on how assays in laboratory animals may be used in quantitative risk assessments for people.

References

Cairns, T. 1980. The ED.01 study: Introduction, objectives and experimental design. *J. Environ. Pathol. Toxicol.* 3:1–7.

Dews, P. B. 1982. Epistemology of screening for behavioral toxicity. In *Nervous system toxicology*, edited by C. L. Mitchell, 229–36. New York: Raven Press.

———. 1986. On the assessment of risk. In *Developmental behavioral pharmacology*, edited by N. Krasnegor, T. Thompson, and D. Gray. Hillside, N.J.: Lawrence Erlbaum Associates. In press.

Dews, P. B., and Berkson, J. 1954. On the error of bio-assay with quantal response. In *Statistics and mathematics in biology*, edited by O. Kempthorne, T. Bancroft, J. W. Gowen, and J. L. Lush, 361–70. Ames: Iowa State College Press.

Farmer, J. H.; Kodell, R. L.; and Greenman, D. L. 1980. Dose and time response models for the incidence of bladder and liver neoplasms in mice fed 2-acetylaminofluorene continuously. *J. Environ. Pathol. Toxicol.* 3:55–68.

Gaddum, J. H. 1954. Lognormal distributions. *Nature* 156:463–66.

Gaylor, D. W. 1979. The ED.01 study: Summary and conclusions. *J. Environ. Pathol. Toxicol.* 3:179–83.

Glowa, J. R.; DeWeese, J.; Natale, M. E.; Holland, J. J.; and Dews, P. B. 1983. Behavioral toxicology of volatile organic solvents. I. Methods: Acute effects. *J. Am. Coll. Toxicol.* 2:175–85.

Glowa, J. R., and Dews, P. B. 1983. Behavioral toxicology of organic solvents. II. Comparison of results on toluene by flow-through and closed chamber procedures. *J. Am. Coll. Toxicol.* 2:319–23.

Lagokos, S., and Mosteller, F. 1981. A case study of statistics in the regulatory process: The FD&C red No. 40 experiments. JNCI 66:197–212.

Trevan, J. W. 1927. The error of determination of toxicity. *Proc. Roy. Soc. B.* 101:483.

Contributors

W. Kent Anger, Division of Biomedical and Behavioral Science, National Institute for Occupational Safety and Health, Cincinnati, Ohio.

Zoltan Annau, Neurotoxicology Program, Department of Environmental Health Sciences, The Johns Hopkins University, Baltimore, Md.

Diane L. DeHaven, Nova Pharmaceutical Corporation, Baltimore, Md.

Peter B. Dews, Laboratory of Psychobiology, Department of Psychiatry, Harvard University Medical School, Boston, Mass.

Robert B. Dick, Division of Biomedical and Behavioral Science, National Institute for Occupational Safety and Health, Cincinnati, Ohio.

Robert S. Dyer, Neurophysiology Branch, Neurotoxicology Division, U. S. Environmental Protection Agency, Research Triangle Park, N.C.

Christine U. Eccles, Department of Pharmacology and Toxicology, University of Maryland School of Pharmacy, Baltimore, Md.

David A. Eckerman, Department of Psychology, University of North Carolina, Chapel Hill, N.C.

Laurence D. Fechter, Neurotoxicology Program, Department of Environmental Health Sciences, The Johns Hopkins University, Baltimore, Md.

Christina M. Gullion, Department of Psychology, University of North Carolina, Chapel Hill, N.C.

Barry L. Johnson, Division of Biomedical and Behavioral Science, National Institute for Occupational Safety and Health, Cincinnati, Ohio.

Victor G. Laties, Environmental Health Sciences Center, Division of Toxicology, Department of Radiation Biology and Biophysics, University of Rochester School of Medicine and Dentistry, Rochester, N.Y.

Tina E. Levine, U.S. Environmental Protection Agency, Washington, D.C.

Richard B. Mailman, Departments of Psychiatry and Pharmacology and Toxicology, Biological Sciences Research Center, University of North Carolina School of Medicine, Chapel Hill, N.C.

Diane B. Miller, U.S. Environmental Protection Agency, Research Triangle Park, N.C.

Keith E. Muller, Department of Biostatistics, University of North Carolina, Chapel Hill, N.C.

Herbert L. Needleman, Department of Psychiatry, University of Pittsburgh, Pittsburgh, Pa.

Stata Norton, Department of Pharmacology, Toxicology, and Therapeutics, University of Kansas Medical Center, College of Health Sciences and Hospital, Kansas City, Kans.

David S. Olton, Department of Psychology, The Johns Hopkins University, Baltimore, Md.

435

Lee S. Rafales, Division of Toxicology and Bioenvironmental Sciences, Department of Environmental Health, University of Cincinnati College of Medicine, Cincinnati, Ohio.

Patricia H. Ruppert (deceased), formerly of the Neurotoxicology Division, U.S. Environmental Protection Agency, Research Triangle Park, N.C.

William F. Sette, Office of Toxic Substances, U.S. Environmental Protection Agency, Washington, D.C.

Hugh A. Tilson, Laboratory of Behavioral and Neurological Toxicology, National Institute of Environmental Health Services, Research Triangle Park, N.C.

Thomas J. Walsh, Laboratory of Behavioral and Neurological Toxicology, National Institute of Environmental Health Sciences, Research Triangle Park, N.C.

Bernard Weiss, Division of Toxicology, Department of Radiation Biology and Biophysics, University of Rochester School of Medicine and Dentistry, Rochester, N.Y.

Gary L. Wenk, Department of Psychology, The Johns Hopkins University, Baltimore, Md.

Ronald W. Wood, Environmental Health Sciences Center, Division of Toxicology, Department of Radiation Biology and Biophysics, University of Rochester School of Medicine and Dentistry, Rochester, N.Y.

John S. Young, Neurotoxicology Program, Department of Environmental Health Sciences, The Johns Hopkins University, Baltimore, Md.

Index

Acetone, 368
2-Acetylaminofluorene (2-AAF), 431
Acetylcholine. *See* Cholinergic systems
Acrylamide
    amphetamine challenge, 63–64
    balance, 46
    locomotory effects, 58–59, 63–64, 254
    neurotransmitters, 63–64, 228, 253–54
    somatosensory effects, 4–8, 335
    workplace, 335
Adjunctive drinking, 18–19
AF64A, 222–23
Aggression, 28
Aging, 15–16, 119–20, 124–25, 206–7, 308
Alcohol. *See* Ethanol
Aluminum, 101–2
Amphetamine, 29–30, 45, 84–86, 201, 249–50
    challenge, 59, 63–64, 104, 157, 223–24, 248–
        55, 257–60
Amygdala, 28
Analgesia, 32–33, 260–61, 375–76
Anesthesia and anesthetics, 197, 375–79
Animal models
    caveats, 8, 15, 24
    of memory and learning, 97, 118, 124
    for regulatory purposes, 396, 431–34
    in teratology, 155–56, 171
Apomorphine, 29, 165, 253–54, 255, 257, 259
Area postrema, 104
Asthma, 11–14
Athletic activity. *See* Locomotor activity
Atropine, 261
Avoidance tasks, 109–10, 156–57, 160, 162, 165,
    226
Axonopathies, 5
5-Azacytidine, 154, 159

Balance, 46–47, 335

Behavior
    sexual, 25, 27, 173–74, 176–77
    social, 47–48, 173–74
Benzene, 250–51
Blood-brain barrier, 155, 395–96

Cadmium, 177–78, 225
Caffeine, 378–79
Carbon disulfide
    amphetamine challenge, 252–53
    field testing, 291, 293, 294, 305
    neurotransmitters, 229, 252–53
    schedule-controlled behavior, 79–80
    visual/motor impairment, 293, 312, 334, 335–
        36, 338
    workplace, 291, 293, 294, 334, 335–36, 338
Carbon monoxide
    avoidance, 109–10
    coordination, 296–97, 334, 355, 372–73
    evoked potentials, 160, 165, 200, 354–55
    and methylene chloride, 354–55
    motor activity, 160
    prenatal exposure, 109–10, 160, 165,
        200
    time-discrimination, 374–75
    vigilance, 355, 373–74, 394
    vision, 371–72
    workplace, 296–97, 334, 339, 371
Carcinogenesis, 8, 431–32
Caudate nucleus, 60, 62
Cerebellum
    ataxia, 44
    irradiation, 175, 180
    methylmercury, 180
    motor dysfunction, 159, 175, 180
    neurotransmitters, 164, 247
    synapses, 155
Chloramphenicol, 109–10

Chlordecone (Kepone®), 4, 225–26, 254–56
Chlordiazepoxide, 252, 254, 260–61
Chlordimeform, 200, 225
Chlorinated hydrocarbons, 248
Chlorpromazine, 252
Cholinergic systems
  insecticides, 226, 260–62
  lead, 259
  learning, 101
  lesions, 222–23
  pharmacologic agents, 247–48
Circadian rhythm, 29, 45
Clonidine, 30, 165, 254
Cognitive functions. *See also* Learning; Memory
  evoked potentials, 207–8
  impairment, 94, 96, 282–84
  testing, 290–301, 307–11, 336
Colchisine, 269
Computers in testing, 298, 301
Conditioning. *See also* Schedule-controlled
    behavior
  classical, 100–107, 118
  operant, 9–10, 106–13
Convulsions, 165–66
Corpus callosum, 207
Cortex, frontal, 28

DDT, 248, 256
Degenerative neurological syndromes, 16
Demyelination, 269
Depression, 310
Development of nervous system, 153–55. *See
    also* Teratology
Dexamethasone, 130–31
Diazepam, 36, 252, 353–54, 360–61
Diencephalon, 165
Diethyldithiocarbamate (DDC), 29, 30
Dihydroxyphenylacetic acid (DOPAC), 62
Dihydroxytryptamine (DHT), 221–23
Diisopropulflorophosphate (DFP), 260–62
Dimethylformamide, 333
Diphrenorphine, 126
Dipropylacetic acid, 201
Dopaminergic systems
  kinetics, 165, 259
  lesions, 164, 221–22, 272
  motor activity, 62, 164
  neurotransmitters, 219
  pharmacologic agents, 247
  receptors, 30, 219
  startle reflex, 29–30
  toxicants
    acrylamide, 228, 253
    cadmium, 225
    carbon disulfide, 252–53
    chlordecone, 254–55
    lead, 223–24, 256–60
    manganese, 224–25, 272

  methylmercury, 165, 226–27
  tins, 181

Enflurane, 377–78
Estrous cycle, 29, 56–57
Ethanol
  activity, 160, 161
  balance, 46
  comparison with other toxins, 351, 359–61,
    364, 366–67, 382
  driving, 395, 426
  evoked potentials, 206
  hippocampal damage, 161
  nutrition, 161, 162
  prenatal exposure, 155, 159–60, 161, 162
  reaction time, 322
  schedule-controlled behavior, 86, 160
  stress, 162
Ethylene glycol, 427
Evoked potentials, 193–213
  cognition-related, 207–8
  flash, 195–203, 354–55
  hippocampal, 204–7
  intrahemispheric, 207
  measurement, 194–97, 202–3, 290
  toxologic alterations, 197–201, 354–55
Eyeblink, 100–103

Feeding, 18–19, 105
Fetal alcohol syndrome, 155, 159–60, 161, 162–64
Field testing, 288–330. *See also* Risk assessment;
    Toxicologic testing; Workplace exposures
  method design, 94–97, 305–13, 323–24
  reliability, 317–20
  scoring, 313–17
  sensitivity, 308–13
  statistical issues, 314–23
  test batteries, 289, 292, 295, 299–300, 302–4,
    306
Finnish Institute of Occupational Health
    (FIOH), 292–93, 336
Food coloring, 12–14
Formaldehyde, 339
Fostering, 161–63
Freon, 380

Geotaxis, 49

Habituation, 97–100, 201, 202
Halothane, 377–79
Halperidol, 29–30, 246, 395
Hearing impairment, 34, 203, 296, 335. *See also*
    Startle response
Hemispheres, of brain, 207
2,5-Hexanedione, 47
Hexobarbitol, 248
High-performance liquid chromatography, 215

Index

Hippocampus
  aging, 206–7
  development, 172, 175
  evoked potentials, 204–7
  exploratory behavior, 45
  irradiation, 175
  lead, 177, 178–79, 182
  learning, 102–3, 159, 161, 175
  lesions, 273
  memory, 118, 128, 273
  motor activity, 60, 175
  startle reflex, 28
  tins, 182, 228, 273
Human experimentation, 348–87
  chemicals
    acetone, 368
    anesthetics, 375–79
    carbon monoxide, 354–55, 371–75
    diazepam, 353–54, 361
    ethanol (as control), 351, 359–61, 364, 366–
      67, 382
    freon, 380
    lead, 369
    methyl chloride, 353–54
    methyl chloroform, 361–62
    methylene chloride, 354–56
    methyl ethyl ketone, 368–69
    mevinphos, 370
    nitrous oxide, 375–77
    parathion, 370
    perchloroethylene, 360–61
    propylene glycol dinitrate, 380–81
    styrene, 364–65
    toluene, 362–64
    trichloroethylene, 351, 356–60, 381
    white spirit, 379–80
    xylene, 365–67
  ethics, 349
  experimental design, 299–301, 349–52, 381–82
6-Hydroxydopamine, 164, 221–23
Hyperactivity, 12–14, 45, 46, 161, 175, 177–78,
      181–82, 257. See also Locomotor activity
Hypothermia, 199, 262

Ibotenic acid, 108
Imipramine, 246
Inhalation route, 33, 160, 332
Intelligence testing and IQ, 282–84, 293, 307–8
Irradiation. See Radiation
Irritation, respiratory, 33

Jet fuel, 294, 336

Kainic acid, 200
Kepone®. See Chlordecone

Lactation, 161–63, 179
Lateral geniculate, 196

Lead
  activity patterns, 46, 59, 62, 178–79
  developmental stage sensitivity, 8–10, 178–
    79, 257, 260
  epidemiology, 281, 282–86
  evoked potentials, 199, 200
  field testing, 282–85, 294, 296, 297, 323, 334–
    35, 339
  hearing, 296, 335
  human experimentation, 369
  individual variation, 121
  intelligence, 282–83, 308, 394
  learning, 101, 182
  memory, 121, 130–32, 336
  neurotransmitters, 62, 223–24, 249, 258–59
  organic, 178–79, 260–61
  personality, 336
  pharmacologic challenge, 59, 249, 256–60
  prenatal exposure, 285–86
  reaction time, 296
  schedule-controlled behavior, 71–72, 101
  sensory impairment, 296, 335
  undernutrition, 257–59
  visuomotor impairment, 334
  workplace, 296, 323, 334–36, 339
Learning, 94–149. See also Conditioning; Memo-
    ry; Schedule-controlled behavior
  measurement, 96–113
  relationship to memory, 96, 107–8, 129
  of skills, 117–18
Lesions, 268–75. See also specific chemicals and
    brain structures
  correlation with functional damage, 164, 272,
    274–75
  prenatal, 154–55, 164
Locomotor activity, 54–69
  measurement, 44–46, 54–56, 64, 399
  non-neuronal components, 56–58
  risk assessment, 397, 399
  sensitivity to toxins, 56, 58–59, 64–65
  toxologic alterations, 19, 59–65, 157, 160, 164,
    165, 177–78
Lordosis, 27
Lysergic acid diethylamide (LSD), 428

Manganese, 224–25, 272
Maze-learning, 121–31, 164, 176, 180, 182, 273
Memory, 94–149. See also Learning
  development of, 113–18
  long-term, 116, 125
  mazes, 121–30
  measurement in animals, 118–33
  measurement in humans, 96, 113–18, 300,
    310, 336
  retrieval, 109, 113–14
  short-term, 118–21, 273, 376–77
  for skills, 117–18
  and stress, 94–95

Mercury vapor
  memory, 113, 115, 294, 298
  motor impairment, 334–35, 339
  schedule-controlled behavior, 77–79
  workplace, 113, 115, 297, 339
Methazoxymethanol (MAM), 165–66, 175
Methimazole, 48
Methylatropine, 261
Methyl chloride, 335, 338, 353–54
Methyl chloroform, 361–62
Methylene chloride, 333, 354–56
Methyl ethyl ketone, 364, 368–69
Methylmercury
  activity, 157, 226
  avoidance tasks, 156–57, 162, 165, 226
  cerebellum, 180
  evoked potentials, 165, 200
  learning, 180
  neurotransmitters, 164–65, 226–27
  pharmacological challenge, 157, 251–52
  postnatal exposure, 179–80, 227
  prenatal exposure, 154, 155, 156–58, 160, 162,
    164–65, 179–80, 226–27, 251, 401
  regulation, 427
  schedule-controlled behavior, 72–76, 157–58
  toxicokinetics, 11, 155
Methylphenidate, 257
2-Methyl-pyridine, 199
α-Methyltyrosine, 200, 256, 261
Mevinphos, 370
Microwaves. *See* Radiation
Minimal brain dysfunction, 257
Monamine systems
  insecticides, 225
  locomotion, 61, 62
  neurotransmitters, 220
Monomethyl tin, 182–83
Monosodium glutamate (MSG), 250
Morphine, 84
Motor impairment. *See also* Locomotor activity;
    Visuomotor impairment
  measurement, 101
MPTP, 16
Myelination, 172

Naloxone, 124–26, 260–61
Neomycin, 36
Neurotransmitters, 214–43. *See also neurochemi-
    cal systems:* Cholinergic; Dopaminergic;
    Monamine; Noradrenergic; Opiate;
    Serotonergic
  in vitro measurement, 214–18
  in vivo measurement, 62–64, 218–21, 246–52
  kinetics, 216–18, 248
  receptors, 217–20, 245–46
  toxologic alterations, 29, 221–30
Nitrous oxide, 375–79

Noradrenergic systems
  methylmercury, 165
  pharmacologic agents, 247
  startle reflex, 30
Nucleus accumbens, 60
Nucleus reticularis, 28
Nursing, 49
Nutrition
  and evoked potentials, 206
  influence on behavior, 57, 249, 257–59
  standards, 9
  toxicologic alterations, 57, 161
Nystagmus, 33–34

Open-field tests, 44–45, 49, 250
Opiate systems
  memory, 124–26
Organic solvents, 4, 117, 334, 353, 369
Organophosphates, 117, 226, 336, 369–71
Oxidants and ozone, 11, 19, 72–73

Pain, 32–33
Paints, 293–94, 334–35, 336
Parathion, 370
Parkinsonism, 16, 224, 272
PBB. *See* Polybromated biphenyls
Pentylenetetrazol, 200, 201
Perchloroethylene, 294, 339, 360–61, 367
Perfusion, of brain, 218, 220
Perseveration, 45
Pharmacologic challenge, 244–67
  by amphetamine, 59, 63–64, 104, 223–24,
    248–55, 257–60
  by apomorphine, 181
  and development, 249–51
  kinetics, 248–49, 251–52, 259
  by phenobarbitol, 248–49, 257
  toxologic tool, 246, 248, 250–51, 262–63
Phencyclidine (PCP), 98, 100, 273–74
Phenobarbitol, 172
  challenge, 248–49, 257
Phenylephrine, 30
Phenytoin, 46
Physostigmine, 201
Pilocarpine, 262
Pimozide, 30
Pizotifen, 256
Polybromated biphenyls (PBBs)
  memory, 94–95, 310, 336
  pharmacologic challenge, 248–49
  stress, 94–95, 310
  visual impairment, 335
  workplace, 297, 310, 339
Polychlorinated biphenyls (PCBs), 229
Postnatal exposure, 170–89. *See also* Teratology
  cadmium, 177–78
  hormones, 175–77

Index

lead, 178–79
methylmercury, 179–80, 227
radiation, 174–75, 180
tins, 180
Prenatal exposure, 153–69. *See also* Teratology
  carbon monoxide, 109–10, 160, 165, 200
  continuous, 158–61
  ethanol, 155, 159–60, 161, 162
  goitrogens, 48
  lead, 285–86
  methylmercury, 154, 155, 156–58, 160, 162, 164–65, 179–80, 226–27, 251, 401
Propylene glycol dinitrate, 380–81
Pyrethrums, 225

Radiation
  microwave, 70–71
  pharmacological challenge, 252
  X-ray, 46, 154, 164, 174–75
Reaction time, 115
Reactivity, generalized, 27–28, 201. *See also* Hyperactivity
Reflexes, 23–42
  lordosis, 25, 27
  measurement, 26–27, 31–34, 36
  modulation, 25–26, 34–37
  neonatal, 48–49
  Preyer's, 34
  startle, 25, 28–30, 35–37, 98–100, 398
  suspension, 48
  toxologic impairment, 23–24, 48
Regulation of toxins, 391–403. *See also* Risk assessment
  behavior as endpoint, 1–2, 391–93, 401, 425
  chronic exposure, 429
  effect levels, 431–34
  EPA requirements, 86, 394, 397
  Good Laboratory Practices, 427
  laws, 393–94
  pharmaceuticals, 426
  schedule-controlled behavior in, 87–90, 399–400
  teratology, 400–401
  trace pollutants, 428–29
  workplace, 342–43, 430
Reserpine, 26, 29
Risk assessment, 391–403. *See also* Field testing; Toxicologic testing
  chemical interactions, 16–18, 354, 359–61, 367, 381–82, 428–29
  dose-response functions, 2, 11, 69, 156–58, 166, 312, 431–34
  indirect evidence, 395–96
  individual variability, 11–14, 312
  multiple exposures, 16, 430
  for regulatory purposes, 1–2, 4, 10–11, 19, 87–90, 391–93, 401, 425

safety factors, 2–3, 396–97
test batteries, 3, 89, 410
thresholds, 357–60, 369, 375, 396, 430–31
of trace pollutants, 428–29
Rotating rod test, 46

Schedule-controlled behavior, 69–93. *See also* Conditioning; Learning
  fixed-interval, 9–10, 71–73
  fixed-number, 72–76, 82, 112
  fixed-ratio, 70–71, 84
  multiple, 76–80, 82–84, 157–58
  sensitivity, 74–76, 79–80, 84–86
  specificity, 79, 82–83
  toxicologic testing, 86–91, 399–400, 428
Scopalamine, 101, 126
Sensitization, 97–98
Sensory impairment. *See also specific modalities*
  measurement, 35, 46, 98, 398
Septal nucleus
  medial, 126–27
  septal rage syndrome, 28
Serotonergic systems
  cadmium, 225
  lesions, 222
  methylmercury, 165, 226–27
  pharmacologic agents, 247
  startle reflex, 26, 30
  tremor, 256
Sexual behavior, 25, 27, 173–74, 176–77
Social behavior, 47–48, 173–74
Sodium pentobarbital, 201
Sodium valproate, 201
Somatosensory impairment, 5–7, 203, 290, 335
Spiroperidol, 254
Startle response, 25, 28–30, 35–37, 98–100, 398
Statistical issues, 404–23
  analysis of variance, 315–17, 416–17
  computer analysis, 418–20
  confirmatory analysis, 414
  confounding, 280, 322–23
  data types, 313, 315, 321–23, 415–18
  dependent and independent variables, 313–14, 410
  design principles, 280–81, 409–13, 420–21
  errors and reliability, 317–20, 392, 406–7, 409
    Type I, 407, 413, 416
    Type II, 413–14
  exploratory analysis, 320–22, 410–12
  for regulatory purposes, 431–34
  significance levels, 284–85
Stress, 94–95, 162
Striatum, 224
Strychnine, 201
Styrene, 335, 336, 338–39, 364–65
Substantia nigra, 272
Suckling, 173

Sulfolane, 200
Sulfur dioxide, 12
Superior colliculus, 197

Tardive dyskinesia, 395
Taste aversion, 102, 104–6
TCE. *See* Trichloroethylene
Telencephalon, 164
Temperature, body, 262
    behavioral regulation, 70–71, 84–86
    hypothermia, 199
    sensitivity, 202, 290
Teratology, 153–69, 170–89. *See also* Postnatal exposure; Prenatal exposure; Toxicologic testing
    developmental basis, 153–55, 163–64, 170–72
    dose-response functions, 156–58, 161, 166, 177
    epidemiology, 285–86
    fostering, 161–63
    neurochemistry, 164–66
    nutrition, 161, 162
    observational studies, 43–44, 48–49, 160, 165, 173
    pharmacokinetics, 155, 158, 249–51
    prolonged exposure, 158–61, 178
    reflex studies, 31
    regulatory aspects, 400–401
    routes of administration, 159–60
    test batteries, 31–32
TET. *See* Triethyl tin
Tetrachloroethylene. *See* Perchloroethylene
Thallium, 46
Thermoregulation. *See* Temperature, body
Thiamine deficiency, 132–33
Thyroid hormones, 175–76
Tin. *See* Monomethyl tin; Triethyl tin; Trimethyl tin
Tolerance, 244–45, 260–62, 366, 395
Toluene, 82–83, 111–12, 229, 362–64
Toxicologic testing, 404–23. *See also* Risk assessment; Teratology
    animal models, 8
    baseline determination, 8, 250, 308
    dose-response functions, 2, 11, 69, 156–58, 166, 312, 350
    experimental design, 279–81
    field (*see* Field testing)
    kinetics and metabolism of toxins, 11, 155
    neurochemistry, 229–30
    observational methods, 43–44, 47, 49–50, 64–65, 397–99
    pharmacologic challenge, 246, 248, 250–51, 262–63
    regulatory aspects, 1–2, 10–11, 86–90
    reversability, 8, 11, 29, 95
    schedule-controlled behavior, 87–90, 399–400
    screening, 28, 55–56, 58–59, 80, 88–89, 270–71, 397–98, 427–28
    sensitivity, 58–59, 64, 74–76, 79–80, 84–86, 269–71, 308–13
    single-subject, 14–15, 74
    specificity, 59–61, 79, 82–83, 271
    statistical aspects (*see* Statistical issues)
    test batteries, 31, 289–300, 306–8, 336–38
    time-series, 4–7, 10, 274, 312–13
    workplace (*see* Workplace exposures)
Tremor, 226, 256
Trichloroethane. *See* Methyl chloroform
Trichloroethylene (TCE), 294, 339, 351, 356–60, 381
Triethyl lead. *See* Lead, organic
Triethyl tin
    activity, 180–82
    cerebellum, 180
    demyelination, 269
    evoked potentials, 198–99
    learning, 129
    neonatal exposure, 129, 180–82
    neurotransmitters, 181
    startle reflex, 28, 36–37
Trihexyphenidyl, 256
Trimethyl tin
    activity patterns, 45, 130, 182
    evoked potentials, 199–200, 201, 206
    hippocampus, 45, 182, 201, 206, 228, 272–73
    learning, 182–83
    maze tests, 45, 129–30, 182, 273
    neonatal exposure, 129, 182
    neurotransmitters, 227–28
    visual impairment, 200, 201
Triorthocresyl phosphate, 394

Undernourishment. *See* Nutrition

Vestibular system, 33–34, 365. *See also* Balance
Vibration. *See* Somatosensory impairment
Visual cortex evoked potentials, 195–98
Visual impairment
    by acrylamide, 8
    by lead, 296
    measurement, 8, 195, 197–203, 335–36
    by organotins, 198, 200
    progression, 8, 11
Visuomotor impairment, 8, 11, 293–94, 356–58, 360, 362
    measurement, 47, 334–35
Voltammetry, in vivo, 220–24

Weight loss, 159–60, 162, 177
White spirit, 379–80
Workplace exposures, 331–47. *See also* Field testing; Risk assessment; Toxicologic testing
    chemicals
        acrylamide, 335
        carbon disulfide, 291, 293, 294, 334, 335–36, 338

Index

carbon monoxide, 296–97, 334, 339
dimethylformamide, 333
jet fuel, 294, 336
lead, 296, 323, 334–36, 339
mercury vapor, 113, 115, 297, 339
methyl chloride, 335, 338
methylene chloride, 333
organophosphates, 336
paints, 293–94, 334–35, 336

polybromated biphenyls, 297, 310, 339
solvents, 336
styrene, 335, 336, 338–39
trichloroethylene, 294, 339
relative importance, 332–34
study design, 340–43
testing, 334–38
X-rays. *See* Radiation
Xylene, 365–67